Medical-Surgical Nursing

made Incredibly Easy!®

3rd edition

Wolters Kluwer | Lippincott Williams & Wilkins
Health

Philadelphia · Baltimore · New York · London
Buenos Aires · Hong Kong · Sydney · Tokyo

Staff

Publisher
J. Christopher Burghardt

Clinical Director
Joan M. Robinson, RN, MSN

Clinical Project Manager
Lorraine M. Hallowell, RN, BSN, RVS

Clinical Editor
Marian Pottage, RN, MS

Product Director
David Moreau

Product Manager
Diane Labus

Editors
Margaret Eckman, Karen Comerford

Editorial Assistants
Karen J. Kirk, Jeri O'Shea, Linda K. Ruhf

Art Director
Elaine Kasmer

Design Assistant
Kate Zulak

Illustrator
Bot Roda

Project Manager, Electronic Products
John Macalino

Vendor Manager
Beth Martz

Manufacturing Manager
Beth J. Welsh

Production Services
SPi Global

Printed in China

MSNIE3010711-030314

Library of Congress Cataloging-in-Publication Data
Medical-surgical nursing made incredibly easy!. —
3rd ed.
    p. ; cm.
    Includes bibliographical references and index.
    ISBN-13: 978-1-60913-648-2 (alk. paper)
    ISBN-10: 1-60913-648-9 (alk. paper)
    1. Surgical nursing—Handbooks, manuals, etc.
2. Nursing—Handbooks, manuals, etc.
I. Lippincott Williams & Wilkins.
    [DNLM: 1. Nursing Care—methods—Handbooks.
2. Perioperative Nursing—methods—Handbooks.
WY 49]
    RT51.M436 2012
    617'.0231—dc22   2011007519

CCS0114

Contents

Contributors and consultants

Natalie Burkhalter, RN, MSN, ACNP, FNP, CNS, CCRN
Associate Professor
Texas A&M International University
Laredo, Tex.

Kimberly Clevenger, RN, MSN, EdDc
Associate Professor of Nursing
Morehead State University
Morehead, Ky.

Shelba Durston, RN, MSN, CCRN
Professor of Nursing
San Joaquin Delta College
Stockton, Calif.

Ginger E. Fidel, RN, MSN, CNL
Instructor
Medical College of Georgia
Athens, Ga.

Stephen Gilliam, RN, PhD, FNP-BC
Assistant Professor
Medical College of Georgia, School of
  Nursing
Athens, Ga.

Eileen Danaher Hacker, PhD, AOCN, APN
Clinical Associate Professor
University of Illinois at Chicago
Chicago, Ill.

Juanita Hickman, RN, PhD
Assistant Dean
Cochran School of Nursing
Yonkers, N.Y.

Julia Isen, RN, MS, FNP-C
Assistant Clinical Professor
University of California, San Francisco,
  School of Community Health Nursing
Nurse Practitioner
University of California, San Francisco,
  Primary Care, Women's Health
  Center
San Francisco, Calif.

Lynn D. Kennedy, RN, MN, CCRN
Assistant Professor of Nursing
Francis Marion University
Florence, S.C.

Wanda Lamont
Director, Learning Resource
Cochran School of Nursing
Yonkers, N.Y.

Mary Jane Nottoli, RN, MSN, CNS
Adjunct Faculty
Cuyahoga Community College, Eastern
  Campus
Cleveland, Ohio.

Donna Scemons, PhD, FNP-BC, CNS
President
Healthcare Systems, Inc.
Castaic, Calif.

Marilyn J. Schuler, RN, MSN, CNE
Nursing Instructor II
Mercy Hospital School of Nursing
Pittsburgh, Pa.

Kendra S. Seiler, RN, MSN
Associate Professor
Rio Hondo College
Whittier, Calif.

Beth H. Snitzer, RN, MSN, GCNS-BC, CS
Clinical Nurse Specialist
Bon Secours St. Francis Medical
  Center
Midlothian, Va.

Foreword

This is a transformative time in information management and technology! Multitudes of resources are available—online, digital books and, of course, the printed text. The sheer volume of resources can be overwhelming at times. The concept of information overload dates back as early as 3rd or 4th century BCE and the Roman philosopher Seneca wrote that the "abundance of books is a distraction." So, with as many references available to today's students and nurses, why choose another medical-surgical text? The third edition of *Medical-Surgical Nursing Made Incredibly Easy!* is a must-have for students, working nurses, and nurses returning to practice. Medical-surgical nursing is a complex and varied field with many subspecialties practiced in an ever-expanding variety of settings. Our place is no longer just at the bedside. Whatever your practice setting, this unique reference has it all in one convenient volume, complete with common disorders, their etiology, pathophysiology, clinical manifestations, and updated diagnostics and treatments.

Content begins with the essentials of medical-surgical nursing and the nursing process, then covers basic concepts of care, including fluids and electrolytes, acid-base balance, pain management, and perioperative nursing. Thirteen chapters follow, covering common disorders organized by body systems. Additional chapters include cancer care, obesity, gerontology care, and end-of-life care. New to the third edition is complete coverage of blood transfusion reactions, including transfusion-related acute lung injury.

All content is presented in an easy-to-read format with bullet points highlighting important data. The disorders chapters begin with a review of anatomy and physiology, history taking, and physical assessment; followed by diagnostic testing, including patient preparation, monitoring, and teaching points; and lastly current NANDA nursing diagnoses. Common disorders include etiology, pathophysiology, clinical manifestations, diagnostics, treatments, and nursing interventions that include evidence-based practice recommendations.

Graphic icons quickly identify special features to enhance and reinforce the reader's understanding of content:

A closer look provides illustrations and charts depicting anatomy, physiology, and complex pathways.

Education edge offers practical patient teaching tips.

What do I do? identifies steps to take in emergency situations.

Weighing the evidence includes updated evidence-based practice pointers to support nursing actions.

Memory jogger relies on helpful mnemonics to jar the memory and reinforce important concepts.

Quick quiz tests the reader's understanding of material covered in the chapter.

Additional features include cartoon drawings to highlight important points and the use of full color throughout the text. Included with the text are online ancillary materials geared toward the student nurse, including:
• 1,000 NCLEX-style questions in the latest format
• NCLEX tutorials
• Clinical simulation case studies
• Test-taking strategies and study techniques.

Relevant content and exciting features presented in an extremely readable and enjoyable format add up to a must-have book for nurses, students, and faculty alike. Students will enjoy the friendly style of writing and can use the text as an adjunct to classroom materials. Faculty may recommend it as a study aid to help clarify difficult concepts or as NCLEX preparation. Practicing nurses can keep it at their fingertips for a review when caring for a patient with an unfamiliar diagnosis or use it as a refresher. Regardless of your practice setting or background, *Medical-Surgical Nursing Made Incredibly Easy!*, Third Edition, will prove to be a useful and fun way to learn or refresh your knowledge and understanding of medical-surgical nursing, the practice field we all love.

Jane F. Marek, MSN, RN
Clinical Specialist and Adult Nurse Practitioner
Instructor of Nursing
Frances Payne Bolton School of Nursing
Case Western Reserve University
Cleveland, Ohio

1

Medical-surgical nursing practice

Just the facts

In this chapter, you'll learn:

♦ roles and functions of a medical-surgical nurse

♦ definitions for the terms *health* and *illness*

♦ the importance of health promotion in patient care.

A look at medical-surgical nursing

Medical-surgical nursing focuses on adult patients with acute or chronic illness and their responses to actual or potential alterations in health. Medical-surgical nursing is one of many specialties in nursing, yet its scope is much broader than such specialties as cardiovascular or orthopedic nursing.

Thanks to the Academy

The Academy of Medical-Surgical Nurses was created in 1991 and now has more than 50 chapters across the United States. Medical-surgical nurses assume diverse roles and responsibilities. They may work in any health care setting, but most are employed by acute care facilities.

What you need to know

Because they care for a wide range of patients in terms of age and illness, medical-surgical nurses need a broad knowledge of the biological, psychological, and social sciences. In addition, because the typical medical-surgical patient is older than age 65, a strong background in gerontology is required.

> The typical med-surg patient is over age 65, so I need a strong background in gerontology.

Roles and functions

Recent changes in health care reflect changes in the populations requiring nursing care and a philosophical shift toward health promotion rather than treatment of illness. The role of the medical-surgical nurse has broadened in response to these changes. Medical-surgical nurses are caregivers, as always, but now they're also educators, advocates, coordinators, change agents, discharge planners, and researchers.

Caregiver

Nurses have always been caregivers, but the activities this role encompasses changed dramatically in the 20th century. Increased education of nurses, expanded nursing research, and the consequent recognition that nurses are autonomous and informed professionals have caused a shift from a dependent role to one of independence and collaboration. (See *Critical thinking: An essential skill.*)

A model of independence

Medical-surgical nurses conduct independent assessments and plan patient care based on their knowledge and skills. They also collaborate with other members of the health care team to implement and evaluate that care.

I'm so proud of my new work... I call her "The Critical Thinker."

Critical thinking: An essential skill

In the complex, rapidly changing health care environment, critical thinking is a skill necessary for providing safe, effective nursing care. Critical thinking takes basic problem solving one step further by considering all related factors, including the patient's unique needs as well as any of the nurse's thoughts and beliefs that may influence her decision-making ability. Critical-thinking skills enable the nurse to take a step outside of the situation and look at the whole picture more objectively.

Truth seekers

Critical thinkers don't rely on tradition to provide all the answers. Instead, they have the desire to seek truth and actively pursue answers to questions to obtain this complete picture. They're also open-minded and creative, and can draw from past clinical experience to come up with all possible alternatives and then zero in on the best solution for the patient.

Practice for your practice

Books, articles, and online courses are available to hone nurses' critical-thinking skills. When nurses engage in critical thinking, their patients have the best chances for success!

Educator

With greater emphasis on health promotion and illness prevention, the nurse's role as educator has become increasingly important. The nurse assesses learning needs, plans and implements teaching strategies to meet those needs, and evaluates the effectiveness of the teaching. To be an effective educator, the nurse must be skilled at interpersonal communication and familiar with principles of adult learning. The nurse must also consider the educational, cultural, and socioeconomic background of the patient when planning and providing patient teaching.

Before you go

Patient teaching is also a major part of discharge planning. Education of patients, family members, and caregivers has greater importance because patients are discharged sooner, and often sicker, than before. Along with teaching come responsibilities for making referrals, identifying community and personal resources, and arranging for necessary equipment and supplies for home care.

Advocate

The nurse's first responsibility as an advocate is to ensure the health, welfare, and safety of the patient. Being an advocate also means that the nurse makes every attempt to respect the patient's decisions and to communicate those wishes to the other members of the health care team. The nurse must accept a patient's decision, even if it differs from the decision the nurse would make.

Coordinator

All nurses practice leadership and manage time, people, resources, and the environment in which they provide care. They carry out these tasks by directing, delegating, and coordinating activities. (See *How to delegate safely*, page 4.)

Call a huddle

All health care team members, including the nurse, provide patient care. Although the doctor is usually considered the head of the team, the nurse plays an important role in coordinating the efforts of all team members to meet the patient's goals, and she may conduct team conferences to facilitate communication among team members.

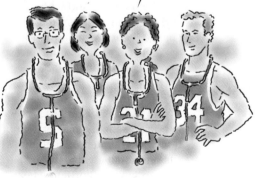

The nurse plays an important role in coordinating the efforts of all health care team members.

How to delegate safely

Nurses must have a clear understanding of their responsibilities to ensure that delegating is done safely and successfully. Nurses must remember that although responsibility for a task has been delegated, accountability hasn't. When a nurse delegates a task, she should make sure that the person assigned the task understands what's expected of her. The delegating nurse should also receive regular updates from that person, ask specific questions, and evaluate the outcome.

Five "rights"

The National Council of State Boards of Nursing identifies five "rights" of delegation that must be satisfied by the delegating nurse:

Right task — The task being assigned or transferred must be within the scope of abilities and practice of the individual receiving the responsibility.

Right circumstance — The individual variables involved (patient condition, environment, caregiver training) must be appropriate for delegation.

Right person — The individual receiving the responsibility must have the legal authority to perform the task. Institutional policies regarding delegation must be consistent with the law.

Right direction and communication — Instructions and expectations must be clear, specific, and understood.

Right supervision and follow-up — The delegating nurse must supervise, guide, and evaluate the performance of individuals to whom she delegates. In addition to ensuring that a particular task has been successfully carried out, the delegating nurse must also provide additional training and feedback to coworkers who function under her direction.

Change agent

As a change agent, the nurse works with the patient to address his health concerns, and with staff members to address organizational and community concerns. This role demands a knowledge of change theory, which provides a framework for understanding the dynamics of change, human responses to change, and strategies for effecting change.

Doing what's right

In the community, nurses serve as role models and assist consumers in bringing about changes to improve the environment, work conditions, or other factors that affect health. Nurses also work together to bring about change through legislation by helping to shape and support laws that promote health and safety, such as those that mandate the use of car safety seats and motorcycle helmets.

Discharge planner

As a discharge planner, the nurse assesses the patient's needs for discharge starting at the time of admission. This includes the patient's support systems and living situation. The nurse also links the patient with available community resources.

Researcher

The primary tasks of nursing research are to promote growth in the science of nursing and to develop a scientific basis for nursing practice. Every nurse should be involved in nursing research and apply research findings to her nursing practice.

The evidence is in

Nurses provide the best possible patient care when they base their practices on scientific evidence. In evidence-based practice, nursing practice is based on the conscientious and consistent use of scientific research to make informed decisions. Nurses can obtain the latest scientific information from several sources, including electronic and print media. But, to use that information appropriately, they must evaluate the evidence. Nurses should evaluate scientific research, especially research studies, for strength and quality to determine the best scientific information to use in their practice. A strong scientific study has conclusions that are valid—that is, truthful or correct. A quality study is well designed and implemented, with data that is well collected and evaluated. (See *Types and strength of evidence*.)

Weighing the evidence

1.5 lbs

Types and strength of evidence

To determine the strength of the evidence used to support a particular theory or intervention, first identify the type of evidence presented. Then rank the type of evidence according to its relative strength, going from weak to strong, as shown below:

Synthesis of multiple randomized controlled clinical trials
Single randomized controlled clinical trial
Cohort studies and case-control studies   *Strength of evidence increases*
Qualitative and descriptive studies
Consensus expert opinion

The health-illness continuum

We may talk about health all the time, but defining the word isn't easy!

How people view themselves — as individuals and as part of the environment — affects the way health is defined. Many people view health as a continuum, with wellness — the highest level of function — at one end and illness and death at the other. All people are somewhere on this continuum and, as their health status changes, their location on the continuum also changes.

Health defined

Although health is a commonly used term, definitions abound. No single definition is universally accepted. A common one describes health as a disease-free state, but this presents an either-or situation: A person is either healthy or ill.

WHO says...

The World Health Organization (WHO) calls health "a state of complete physical, mental, and social well-being and not merely the absence of disease or infirmity." This definition doesn't allow for degrees of health or illness. It also fails to reflect the concept of health as dynamic and constantly changing.

It's about culture

Sociologists view health as a condition that allows for the pursuit and enjoyment of desired cultural values. These include the ability to carry out activities of daily living, such as working and performing household chores.

It's about levels

Many people view health as a level of wellness. According to this definition, a person is striving to attain his full potential. This allows for a more holistic and subjective view of health.

Factors affecting health

One of the nurse's primary functions is to assist patients in reaching an optimal level of wellness. When assessing patients, the nurse must be aware of factors that affect their health status and plan to tailor interventions accordingly. Such factors include:
• genetics (biological and genetic makeup that causes illness and chronic conditions)

- cognitive abilities (which affect a person's view of health and ability to seek out resources)
- demographic factors, such as age and sex (certain diseases are more prevalent in a certain age-group or sex)
- geographic locale (which predisposes a person to certain conditions)
- culture (which determines a person's perception of health, the motivation to seek care, and the types of health practices performed)
- lifestyle and environment (such as diet, level of activity, and exposure to toxins)
- health beliefs and practices (which can affect health positively or negatively)
- previous health experiences (which influence reactions to illness and the decision to seek care)
- spirituality (which affects a person's view of illness and health care)
- support systems (which affect the degree to which a person adapts and copes with a situation).

Illness defined

Nurses must understand the concept of illness, particularly how illness may affect the patient. Illness may be defined as a sickness or deviation from a healthy state. It's considered a broader concept than disease. Disease commonly refers to a specific biological or psychological problem that's supported by clinical manifestations and results in a body system or organ malfunction. It may result from external factors such as infectious agents or from internal factors such as atherosclerosis. Illness, on the other hand, occurs when a person is no longer in a state of perceived "normal" health. A person may have a disease, but not be ill all the time because he has adapted to the disease.

Yes, you say you're ill. But tell me, what does this all mean to you?

What does it mean to you?

Illness also encompasses how the patient interprets the disease's source and importance, how the disease affects his behavior and relationships with others, and how he tries to remedy the problem. Another significant component is the meaning that a person attaches to the experience of being ill.

Types of illness

Illness may be acute or chronic. Acute illness usually refers to a disease or condition that has a relatively abrupt onset, high intensity, and short duration. If no complications occur, most acute illnesses end in a full recovery and the person returns to the previous or a similar level of functioning.

Regain and maintain

Chronic illness refers to a condition that typically has a slower onset, less intensity, and a longer duration than acute illness. Chronic illnesses typically include periods of exacerbation, (when symptoms increase) and remission (when symptoms are well controlled or absent). The goal is to help the patient regain and maintain the highest possible level of health, although some patients fail to return to their previous level of functioning.

Effects of illness

When a person experiences an illness, one or more changes occur that signal its presence. These may include:
- changes in body appearance or function
- unusual body emissions
- sensory changes
- uncomfortable physical manifestations
- changes in emotional status
- changes in relationships.

  Most people experience a mild form of some of these changes in their daily lives. However, when the changes are severe enough to interfere with usual daily activities, the person is usually considered ill.

Perception and reaction

People's reactions to feeling ill vary. Some people seek action immediately and others take no action. Some may exaggerate their symptoms and others may deny that their symptoms exist. A patient's perception and reaction to illness is unique and is usually based on his culture, knowledge, view of health, and previous experiences with illness and the health care system.

Effects of illness on the family

The presence of illness in a family can have a dramatic effect on the functioning of the family as a unit. The type of effect depends on the following factors:
- which family member is ill
- the seriousness and duration of the illness

What makes you think I'm in denial? I know I've lost a little weight...and maybe some skin...but really, I feel perfectly fine.

• the family's social and cultural customs (each member's role in the family and the tasks specific to that role).

Which member?

The types of role change that occur also vary, depending on the family member affected. For example, if the affected member is the primary breadwinner, other members may need to seek employment to supplement the family income. As the primary breadwinner assumes a dependent role, the rest of the family must adjust to new roles. If the affected family member is a working single parent, serious economic and child care problems may result. That person must depend on support systems for help or face additional stress.

Health promotion

Research shows that poor health practices contribute to a wide range of illnesses, a shortened life span, and increased health care costs. Good health practices can have the opposite effect: fewer illnesses, a longer life span, and lower health care costs.

Better late than never

Good health practices can benefit most people no matter when they're started. Of course, the earlier in life good practices are started, the fewer poor habits have to be overcome. Even so, later is better than never. For example, stopping cigarette smoking has immediate and long-term benefits. Immediately, the patient will experience improved circulation, pulse rate, and blood pressure. After 10 years without smoking, he'll cut his risk of dying from lung cancer in half.

Better late than never when it comes to certain health practices. For example, smoking cessation has immediate benefits.

What is health promotion?

Quite simply, health promotion is teaching good health practices and finding ways to help people correct their poor health practices.

But what specifically should you teach? The project *Healthy People 2020* sets forth comprehensive health goals for the nation with the aim of reducing mortality and morbidity in all ages. These objectives make a useful teaching plan. (See Healthy People 2020: *Goals and objectives*, page 10.)

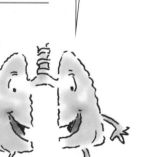

Healthy People 2020: Goals and objectives

Each decade, the U.S. Department of Health and Human Services identifies a set of health improvement objectives for the nation to achieve over the next decade. The overarching goals of the current initiative, *Healthy People 2020*, include:
• Eliminate preventable disease, disability, injury, and premature death
• Achieve health equity, eliminate disparities, and improve the health of all groups
• Create social and physical environments that promote good health for all.
• Promote healthy development and healthy behaviors across every stage of life.
Specific, measurable objectives in a wide range of areas support these goals. These include objectives for nutrition, fitness, and access to care as well as disease-specific objectives, such as objectives for human immunodeficiency virus, diabetes, and cancer.

Healthy People is managed by the Office of Disease Prevention and Health Promotion, U.S. Department of Health and Human Services. http://www.healthypeople.gov/

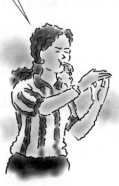

Time out on smoking and other unhealthy habits!

Adult health care

Adults between ages 25 and 64 may fall victim to several health problems, including heart disease and cancer. Although some of these problems stem from genetic predisposition, many are linked to unhealthy habits, such as overeating, smoking, lack of exercise, and alcohol and drug abuse. Your teaching can help an adult recognize and correct these habits to ensure a longer, healthier life.

Geriatric health care

Today, people live longer than ever before. In the past century, life expectancy in the United States has increased from 47 years to about 78 years. Fortunately, most elderly people maintain their independence, with few needing to be institutionalized.

Cope and avoid

Even so, most elderly people suffer from at least one chronic health problem. With the nurse's help, they can cope with existing health problems and learn to avoid new ones. Doing so will improve their quality of life and allow them to continue contributing to society.

State of mind

Emphasize that aging is a state of mind as well as of body. Urge the elderly patient to continue as many activities as possible, depending on his mobility. Also, help him explore new interests or hobbies. Recommend that he attend a hospital- or community-sponsored seminar on retirement. Such seminars usually cover topics like budgeting and health and fitness.

> Aging is a state of mind and body.

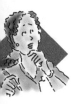

Quick quiz

1. Which trait isn't a characteristic of a critical thinker?
   A. Relying on tradition
   B. Creativity
   C. Open-mindedness
   D. Desire for truth

   Answer: A. Critical thinkers don't rely on tradition but rather actively pursue answers to questions and consider all alternatives in making a decision. This requires creativity, a desire for truth, and being open-minded.

2. A nurse who is preparing to delegate:
   A. can delegate a task to whomever she chooses.
   B. can delegate whichever task she chooses.
   C. has no responsibility for follow-up.
   D. makes sure the person to whom she delegates has the legal authority to perform the task.

   Answer: D. To delegate safely, nurses must observe several "rights": the right task, right circumstance, right person, right direction and communication, and right supervision and follow-up.

3. Which action is an example of health promotion?
   A. Administering antibiotics to a patient
   B. Splinting a patient's fractured bone
   C. Assisting a patient in smoking cessation
   D. Inserting an I.V. catheter

Answer: C. Health promotion involves teaching good health practices as well as helping people correct their poor health practices. Helping a patient to stop smoking helps him to correct a poor health practice.

4. The effect of illness on a family unit depends on several factors, including:
   A. when the illness occurs.
   B. which family member is affected.
   C. whether the illness is due to poor health habits.
   D. at what point the patient sought care.

Answer: B. The effect of illness on a family unit depends on which family member is affected, the seriousness and duration of the illness, and the family's social and cultural customs.

Scoring

☆☆☆ If you answered all four questions correctly, super! You surge ahead of the pack in med-surg!

☆☆ If you answered three questions correctly, great! You sure have been practicing your nursing practice!

☆ If you answered fewer than three questions correctly, don't despair! Reviewing the chapter will promote a healthy understanding!

2

Nursing process

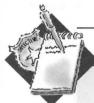

Just the facts

In this chapter, you'll learn:

♦ five key steps of the nursing process

♦ tools for effectively communicating with your patient while taking a health history

♦ components of a health history

♦ the proper techniques for performing inspection, palpation, percussion, and auscultation.

A look at the nursing process

One of the most significant advances in nursing has been the development and acceptance of the nursing process. This problem-solving approach to nursing care offers a structure for applying your knowledge and skills in an organized, goal-oriented manner. Closely related to the scientific method, it serves as the cornerstone of clinical nursing by providing a systematic method for determining the patient's health problems, devising a care plan to address those problems, implementing the plan, and evaluating the plan's effectiveness.

> Staying goal-oriented is the cornerstone of clinical nursing. The nursing process helps achieve that focus.

Five alive

The five phases of the nursing process are dynamic and flexible. Because they're interrelated, they often overlap. Together, they resemble the steps that many other professions rely on to identify and correct problems. They include:

☝ assessment

✌ nursing diagnosis

🤟 planning

EVALUATION

IMPLEMENTATION

PLANNING

NURSING DIAGNOSIS

ASSESSMENT

implementation

evaluation.

Process pluses

When used effectively, the nursing process offers several important advantages:
• The patient's specific health problems, not the disease, become the focus of health care. This emphasis promotes the patient's participation and encourages his independence and compliance — factors important to a positive outcome.
• Identifying a patient's health problems improves communication by providing nurses who care for the patient with a common list of recognized problems.
• The nursing process provides a consistent and orderly professional structure. It promotes accountability for nursing activities based on evaluation and, in so doing, leads to quality improvement.

> Dynamic and flexible, that's me — and the nursing process!

Assessment

Assessment involves data collection used to identify a patient's actual and potential health needs. According to American Nurses Association guidelines, data should accurately reflect the patient's life experiences and his patterns of living. To accomplish this, you must assume an objective and nonjudgmental approach when gathering data. You can obtain data through a health history, a physical assessment, and a review of pertinent laboratory and medical information.

Health history

A health history is used to gather subjective data about the patient and explore past and present problems. First, ask the patient about his general physical and emotional health; then ask him about specific body systems and structures. Information may come from the patient himself, from the patient's significant other or caregiver, or from other health care professionals.

The accuracy and completeness of your patient's answers largely depend on your skill as an interviewer. Before you start asking questions, review the communication guidelines in the following sections.

Effective techniques

To obtain the most benefit from a health history interview, try to ensure that the patient feels comfortable and respected and understands that he can trust you. Use effective interview techniques to help the patient identify resources and improve problem-solving abilities. Remember, however, that successful techniques in one situation may not be effective in another. Your attitude and the patient's interpretation of your questions can vary. In general, you should:
- allow the patient time to think and reflect
- encourage the patient to talk
- encourage the patient to describe a particular experience
- indicate that you have listened to the patient such as through paraphrasing the patient's response.

Know right from wrong

Although there are many right ways to communicate with a patient, there are also some wrong ways that can hamper your interview. (See *Interview techniques to avoid*.)

Conducting the interview

Physical surroundings, psychological atmosphere, interview structure, and questioning style can all affect the interview flow and outcome; so can your ability to adopt a communication style to fit each patient's needs and situation. Close the door to help prevent interruptions and try to arrange yourself so you're facing the patient, slightly offset from him, to create a friendly feeling. Sit down, if possible, to communicate your willingness to spend time listening to him.

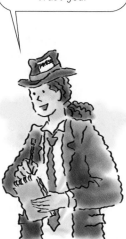

Use effective interview techniques to encourage your patient to talk about his problems and experiences and to show that he can trust you.

Interview techniques to avoid

Some interview techniques create communication problems between nurse and patient. Techniques to avoid include:
- asking "why" or "how" questions
- asking probing or persistent questions
- using inappropriate or confusing language
- giving advice
- giving false reassurance
- changing the subject or interrupting.

Also avoid using clichés or stereotypical responses, giving excessive approval or agreement, jumping to conclusions, and using defensive responses.

Start at the very beginning

Begin by introducing yourself. Establish an assessment time frame and ask if the patient has questions about the assessment procedure. Spend a few minutes chatting informally before beginning the interview.

A note on notes

You'll need to take some notes so that you can accurately remember what the patient tells you, but make sure your note taking doesn't interfere with your communication. If you need to document your findings during the interview using a handheld device or computer terminal, make sure your back isn't toward the patient. Making eye contact and nodding to indicate understanding are cues that will assure the patient that you are listening to him.

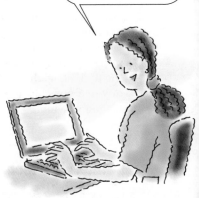

If you need to document your findings during the interview on a computer terminal, make sure your back isn't toward the patient.

Short and sweet

A patient who's ill, experiencing pain, or sedated may have difficulty completing the health history. In such instances, obtain only the information pertaining to the immediate problem. To avoid tiring a seriously ill patient, obtain the history in several sessions or ask a close relative or friend to supply essential information.

Two types

Typically, the health history includes two types of questions: open-ended, which permit more subtle and flexible responses, and closed-ended, which require only a yes-or-no response. Open-ended questions usually result in the most useful information and give patients the feeling that they're actively participating in and have some control over the interview. Closed-ended questions help eliminate rambling conversations. They're also useful when the interview requires brevity — for example, when a patient reports extreme pain or digresses frequently.

Logical and patient

Whatever question type you use, move logically from one history section to the next. Also allow the patient to concentrate and give complete information on a subject before moving on.

Obtaining health history data

The health history has five major sections: biographic data, health and illness patterns, health promotion and protection patterns, role and relationship patterns, and a summary of health history data.

Biographic data

Begin obtaining the patient's health history by reviewing personal information. This data section identifies the patient and provides important demographic information, such as the patient's address, telephone number, age, sex, birth date, Social Security number, place of birth, race, nationality, marital status, occupation, education, religion, cultural background, and emergency contact person.

Health and illness patterns

This information includes the patient's chief complaint; current, past, and family health history; status of physiologic systems; and developmental considerations.

Mind his P's and Q's

Determine why the patient is seeking health care by asking, "What brings you here today?" If the patient has specific symptoms, record that information in the patient's own words. Ask the patient with a specific symptom or health concern to describe the problem in detail, including the suspected cause. To ensure that you don't omit pertinent data, use the PQRST mnemonic device, which provides a systematic approach to obtaining information. (See *PQRST: What's the story?*, page 18.)

For a patient who seeks a health maintenance assessment, health counseling, or health education, expect to take few notes.

Think back

Next, record childhood and other illnesses, injuries, previous hospitalizations, surgical procedures, immunizations, allergies, and medications taken regularly.

Tell me about your mother

Information about the patient's relatives can also unmask potential health problems. Some diseases, such as cardiovascular disease, alcoholism, depression, and cancer, may be genetically linked. Others, such as hemophilia, cystic fibrosis, sickle cell anemia, and Tay-Sachs disease, are genetically transmitted.

Genogram and grampa, too

Determine the general health status of the patient's immediate family members, including maternal and paternal grandparents, parents, siblings, aunts, uncles, and children. If any are deceased, record the year and cause of death. Use a genogram to organize family history data.

Ask the patient with a specific concern to describe the problem in detail. Be sure to record the information using his own words.

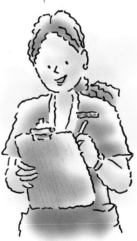

PQRST: What's the story?

Use the PQRST mnemonic device to fully explore your patient's chief complaint. When you ask the questions below, you'll encourage him to describe his symptom in greater detail.

    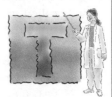

Provocative or palliative
Ask the patient:
• What provokes or relieves the symptom?
• Do stress, anger, certain physical positions, or other things trigger the symptom?
• What makes the symptom worsen or subside?

Quality or quantity
Ask the patient:
• What does the symptom feel like, look like, or sound like?
• Are you having the symptom right now? If so, is it more or less severe than usual?
• To what degree does the symptom affect your normal activities?

Region or radiation
Ask the patient:
• Where in the body does the symptom occur?
• Does the symptom appear in other regions? If so, where?

Severity
Ask the patient:
• How severe is the symptom? How would you rate it on a scale of 1 to 10, with 10 being the most severe?
• Does the symptom seem to be diminishing, intensifying, or staying about the same?

Timing
Ask the patient:
• When did the symptom begin?
• Was the onset sudden or gradual?
• How often does the symptom occur?
• How long does the symptom last?

Information about the patient's past and current physiologic status (also called *review of systems*) is another health history component. Starting from the head and systematically proceeding to the toes, ask the patient about any past or present symptoms of disease in each body system. A careful assessment helps identify potential or undetected physiologic disorders.

Health promotion and protection patterns

What a patient does or doesn't do to stay healthy is affected by such factors as health beliefs, personal habits, sleep and waking patterns, exercise and activity, recreation, nutrition, stress and coping, socio-economic status, environmental health patterns, and occupational health patterns. To help assess health promotion and protection patterns, ask the patient to describe a typical day and inquire about which behaviors the patient believes are healthful.

Role and relationship patterns

A patient's role and relationship patterns reflect his psychosocial (psychological, emotional, social, spiritual, and sexual) health. To assess role and relationship patterns, investigate the patient's self-concept, cultural influences, religious influences, family role and relationship patterns, sexuality and reproductive patterns, social support patterns, and other psychosocial considerations. Each of these patterns can influence the patient's health.

Summary of health history data

Conclude the health history by summarizing all findings. For the well patient, list the patient's health promotion strengths and resources along with defined health education needs. If the interview points out a significant health problem, tell the patient what it is and begin to address the problem. This may involve referral to a doctor or other practitioner, education, or plans for further investigation.

Physical assessment

Perform hand hygiene in front of the patient before begining the physical assessment. Use drapes so only the area being examined is exposed. Develop a pattern for your assessments, starting with the same body system and proceeding in the same sequence. Organize your steps to minimize the number of times the patient needs to change position. By using a systematic approach, you'll be less likely to forget an area.

Count 'em—four

No matter where you start your physical assessment, you'll use four techniques:

- inspection
- palpation
- percussion
- auscultation.

Use these techniques in sequence except when you perform an abdominal assessment. Because palpation and percussion can alter bowel sounds, the sequence for assessing the abdomen is inspection, auscultation, percussion, and palpation. Let's look at each step in the sequence.

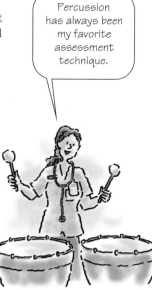

Percussion has always been my favorite assessment technique.

Inspection

Inspect the patient using vision, smell, and hearing to observe normal conditions and deviations. Performed correctly, inspection can reveal more than other techniques.

Inspection begins when you first meet the patient and continues throughout the health history and physical examination. As you assess each body system, observe for color, size, location, movement, texture, symmetry, odor, and sounds.

Palpation

Palpation requires you to touch the patient with different parts of your hands, using varying degrees of pressure. To do this, you need short fingernails and warm hands. Always palpate tender areas last. Tell your patient the purpose of your touch and what you're feeling with your hands.

Palpate to evaluate

As you palpate each body system, evaluate the following features:
- texture — rough or smooth?
- temperature — warm, hot, or cold?
- moisture — dry, wet, or moist?
- motion — still or vibrating?
- consistency of structures — solid or fluid-filled?

Percussion

Percussion involves tapping your fingers or hands quickly and sharply against parts of the patient's body, usually the chest or abdomen. The technique helps you locate organ borders, identify organ shape and position, and determine if an organ is solid or filled with fluid or gas. (See *Percussion types.*)

Do you hear what I hear?

Percussion requires a skilled touch and an ear trained to detect slight variations in sound. Organs and tissues, depending on their density, produce sounds of varying loudness, pitch, and duration. For instance, air-filled cavities, such as the lungs, produce markedly different sounds than do the liver and other dense tissues. (See *Sounds and their sources,* page 22.)

As you percuss, move gradually from areas of resonance to those of dullness and then compare sounds. Also, compare sounds on one side of the body with those on the other side.

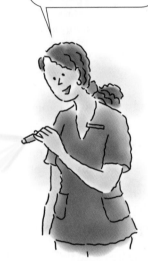

Inspection begins when you first meet the patient. Performed correctly, it can reveal more than the other techniques in your physical assessment.

Percussion types

You can perform percussion using the direct or indirect method. Direct percussion reveals tenderness. Indirect percussion elicits sounds that give clues to the makeup of the underlying tissue.

Direct percussion
Using one or two fingers, tap directly on the body part. Ask the patient to tell you which areas are painful and watch his face for signs of discomfort. This technique is commonly used to assess an adult patient's sinuses for tenderness.

Indirect percussion
Press the distal part of the middle finger of your non-dominant hand firmly on the body part. Keep the rest of your hand off the body surface. Flex the wrist of your dominant hand. Using the middle finger of your dominant hand, tap quickly and directly over the point where your other middle finger touches the patient's skin. Listen to the sounds produced.

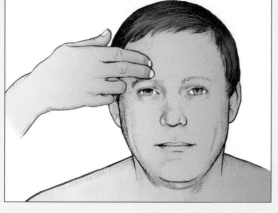

Auscultation

Auscultation, usually the last assessment step, involves listening for various breath, heart, and bowel sounds with a stethoscope. To prevent the spread of infection among patients, clean the heads and end pieces of the stethoscope with alcohol or a disinfectant after every use.

Diagnostic test findings

Diagnostic test findings complete the objective database. Together with the nursing history and physical examination, they form a significant profile of the patient's condition.

Sounds and their sources

As you practice percussion, you'll recognize different sounds. Each sound is related to the structure underneath. This chart offers a quick guide to percussion sounds and their sources.

Sound	Quality of sound	Where it's heard	Source
Tympany	Drumlike	Over enclosed air	Air in bowel
Resonance	Hollow	Over areas of part air and part solid	Normal lung
Hyperresonance	Booming	Over air	Lung with emphysema
Dullness	Thudlike	Over solid tissue	Liver, spleen, heart
Flatness	Flat	Over dense tissue	Muscle, bone

Analyzing the data

The final aspect of assessment involves analyzing the data you've compiled. In your analysis, include the following steps:
• Group significant data into logical clusters. You'll base your nursing diagnosis not on a single sign or symptom but on a cluster of assessment findings. By analyzing the clustered data and identifying patterns of illness-related behavior, you can begin to perceive the patient's problem or risk of developing other problems.
• Identify data gaps. Signs, symptoms, and isolated incidents that don't fit into consistent patterns can provide the missing facts you need to determine the overall pattern of your patient's problem.
• Identify conflicting or inconsistent data. Clarify information that conflicts with other assessment findings, and determine what's causing the inconsistency. For example, a patient with diabetes who says that she complies with her prescribed diet and insulin administration schedule, but whose serum glucose is greatly elevated, may need to have her treatment regimen reviewed or revised.
• Determine the patient's perception of normal health. A patient may find it harder to comply with the treatment regimen when his idea of "normal" doesn't agree with yours.
• Determine how the patient handles his health problem. For instance, is the patient coping with his health problem

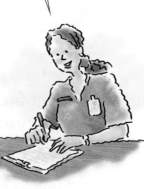

Cluster all the data you've gathered to identify patterns of illness-related behaviors and your patient's perception of health. Use this information, along with your knowledge of the patient's coping skills, to formulate nursing diagnoses.

successfully, or does he need help? Does he deny that he has a problem, or does he admit it but lack solutions to the problem?
- Form an opinion about the patient's health status. Base your opinion on actual, potential, or possible concerns reflected by the patient's responses to his condition and use this to formulate your nursing diagnosis.

Nursing diagnosis

In 1990, NANDA International (NANDA-I) defined the nursing diagnosis as "a clinical judgment about individual, family, or community responses to actual or potential health problems or life processes. Nursing diagnoses provide the basis for the selection of nursing interventions to achieve outcomes for which the nurse is accountable."

Identify, diagnose, and validate

In forming a nursing diagnosis, you'll identify the patient's problem, write a diagnostic statement, and validate the diagnosis. You'll establish several nursing diagnoses for each patient. Arrange the diagnoses according to priority so that you address the patient's most crucial problems first.

Identifying the problem

The first step in developing a nursing diagnosis is to identify the problem. To do this, you must assess the patient and obtain clinical information. Then organize the data obtained during the assessment and determine how the patient's basic needs can be met. The problem identified can be either actual or potential. The diagnosis must be one that can be resolved by a nurse working within her scope of practice.

The NANDA-I taxonomy helps nurses form clear and accurate nursing diagnoses for their patients.

Writing the diagnostic statement

The diagnostic statement consists of a nursing diagnosis and the etiology (cause) related to it. For example, a diagnostic statement for a patient who's too weak to bathe himself properly might be *Bathing or hygiene self-care deficit related to weakness*. A diagnostic statement related to an actual problem might be *Impaired gas exchange related to pulmonary edema*. A statement related to a potential problem might be *Risk for injury related to unsteady gait*.

Stress present, balance absent

The etiology is a stressor or something that brings about a response, effect, or change. A stressor results from the presence of a stress agent or the absence of an equilibrium factor. Causative agents may include birth defects, inherited factors, diseases, injuries, signs or symptoms, psychosocial factors, iatrogenic factors, developmental phases, lifestyle, or situational or environmental factors.

Validating each diagnosis

Next, validate the diagnosis. Review clustered data. Are they consistent? Does the patient verify the diagnosis? If not, you may need to relook at the data and modify the diagnosis.

Prioritizing the diagnoses

After you've established several nursing diagnoses, categorize them in order of priority. Obviously, life-threatening problems must be addressed first, followed by health-threatening concerns. Also, consider how the patient perceives his health problem; his priority problem may differ from yours.

Maslow's hierarchy

One system of categorizing diagnoses uses Maslow's hierarchy of needs, which classifies human needs based on the idea that lower-level, physiologic needs must be met before higher-level, abstract needs. For example, if a patient has shortness of breath, he probably isn't interested in discussing his relationships. (See *Maslow's hierarchy of needs*.)

Planning

After you establish the nursing diagnoses, you'll develop a written care plan. A written care plan serves as a communication tool among health care team members that helps ensure continuity of care. The plan consists of two parts: patient outcomes, or expected outcomes, which describe behaviors or results to be achieved within a specified time; and the nursing interventions needed to achieve those outcomes.

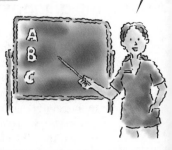

Prioritize your patient's needs, addressing life-threatening problems first, followed by health-threatening concerns.

Maslow's hierarchy of needs

To formulate nursing diagnoses, you must know your patient's needs and values. Of course, physiologic needs — represented by the base of the pyramid in the diagram below — must be met first.

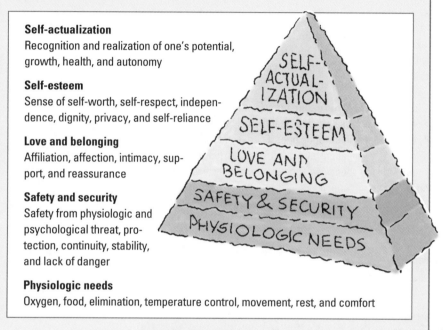

Self-actualization
Recognition and realization of one's potential, growth, health, and autonomy

Self-esteem
Sense of self-worth, self-respect, independence, dignity, privacy, and self-reliance

Love and belonging
Affiliation, affection, intimacy, support, and reassurance

Safety and security
Safety from physiologic and psychological threat, protection, continuity, stability, and lack of danger

Physiologic needs
Oxygen, food, elimination, temperature control, movement, rest, and comfort

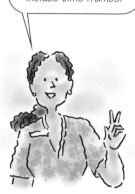

Be sure to include two parts in your written care plan: patient outcomes and the nursing interventions needed to achieve them. Equally important, state both parts of the care plan in measurable, observable terms and include time frames.

Measure and observe

Be sure to state both parts of the care plan in measurable, observable terms and dates. The statement, "The patient will perceive himself with greater self-worth," is too vague, lacks a time frame, and offers no means to observe the patient's self-perception. A patient outcome such as, "The patient will describe himself in a positive way within 1 week," provides an observable means to evaluate the patient's behavior and a time frame for the behavioral change. (See *Ensuring a successful care plan*, page 26.)

Intervention options

Before you implement a care plan, review your intervention options and then weigh their potential to succeed. Determine if you can obtain the necessary equipment and resources. If not, take steps to get what you need or change the intervention accordingly. Observe the patient's willingness to participate in the various interventions and be prepared to postpone or modify interventions if necessary.

Ensuring a successful care plan

Your care plan must rest on a solid foundation of carefully chosen nursing diagnoses. It also must fit your patient's needs, age, developmental level, culture, strengths and weaknesses, and willingness and ability to take part in his care. Your plan should help the patient attain the highest functional level possible while posing minimal risk and not creating new problems. If complete recovery isn't possible, your plan should help the patient cope physically and emotionally with his impaired or declining health.

Using the following guidelines will help ensure that your care plan is effective.

Be realistic
Avoid setting a goal that's too difficult for the patient to achieve. The patient may become discouraged, depressed, and apathetic if he can't achieve expected outcomes.

Tailor your approach
Individualize your outcome statements and nursing interventions. Keep in mind that each patient is unique; no two patient problems are exactly alike.

Avoid vague terms
Use precise, quantitative terms rather than vague ones. For example, if your patient is restless, describe his specific behavior, such as "constantly tossing and turning in bed" rather than "patient restless." To indicate that the patient's vital signs are stable, document specific measurements, such as "heart rate 100 beats/minute" rather than "heart rate stable."

Implementation

The implementation phase is when you put your care plan into action. Implementation encompasses all nursing interventions directed at solving the patient's problems and meeting health care needs. While you coordinate implementation, you also seek help from the patient, the patient's family, and other caregivers.

Monitor and gauge

After implementing the care plan, continue to monitor the patient to gauge the effectiveness of interventions and adjust them as the patient's condition changes. Documentation of outcomes achieved should be reflected in the care plan. Expect to review, revise, and update the entire care plan regularly, according to facility policy. Keep in mind that the care plan is usually a permanent part of the patient's medical record.

Evaluation

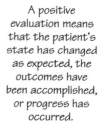

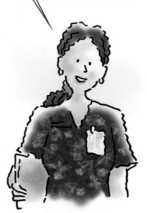

A positive evaluation means that the patient's state has changed as expected, the outcomes have been accomplished, or progress has occurred.

After enough time has elapsed for the care plan to effect desired changes, you're ready for evaluation, the final step in the nursing process. During evaluation, you must decide if the interventions carried out have enabled the patient to achieve the desired outcomes.

Start with the finish

Begin by reviewing the patient outcomes stated for each nursing diagnosis. Then observe your patient's behavioral changes and judge how well they meet the outcomes related to them. Does the patient's behavior match the outcome or fall short of it?

Consider the evaluation to be positive if the patient's behavior has changed as expected, if the outcomes have been accomplished, or if progress has occurred. Failure to meet these criteria constitutes a negative evaluation and requires new interventions.

Process success

The evaluation phase also allows you to judge the effectiveness of the nursing process as a whole. If the process has been applied successfully, the patient's health status will improve. Either his health problems will have been solved or progress will have been made toward achieving their resolution. He'll also be able to perform self-care measures with a sense of independence and confidence, and you'll feel assured that you've fulfilled your professional responsibility.

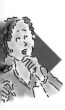

Quick quiz

1. When obtaining a health history from a patient, ask first about:
    A. biographic data.
    B. his chief complaint.
    C. health insurance coverage.
    D. family history.

Answer: A. Take care of the biographic data first; otherwise, you might get involved in the patient history and forget to ask basic questions.

2. The first technique in your physical assessment sequence is:
   A. palpation.
   B. auscultation.
   C. inspection.
   D. percussion.

Answer: C. The assessment of each body system begins with inspection. It's the most commonly used technique, and it can reveal more than any other technique.

3. When palpating the abdomen, begin by palpating:
   A. lightly.
   B. firmly.
   C. deeply.
   D. the most tender area.

Answer: A. Light palpation is always done first to detect surface characteristics. Tender areas should always be palpated last.

4. Expected outcomes are defined as:
   A. goals the patient should reach as a result of planned nursing interventions.
   B. what the patient and his family ask you to accomplish.
   C. goals a little higher than what the patient can realistically reach to help motivate him.
   D. goals set by the medical team for each patient.

Answer: A. Expected outcomes are realistic, measurable goals and their target dates.

Scoring

✰✰✰ If you answered all four questions correctly, bravo! You're a process pro.

✰✰ If you answered three questions correctly, way to go! You've got the nursing process pretty down pat.

✰ If you answered fewer than three questions correctly, chin up! Process this chapter one more time and try again.

3

Fluids and electrolytes

Just the facts

In this chapter, you'll learn:

♦ the way in which fluids and electrolytes are distributed throughout the body

♦ the meanings of certain fluid- and electrolyte-related terms

♦ types of I.V. fluids and how they're used

♦ complications associated with I.V. therapy

♦ nursing considerations for patients receiving I.V. therapy.

A look at fluids

Where would we be without body fluids? Nowhere. Fluids are vital to all forms of life. They help maintain body temperature and cell shape, and they help transport nutrients, gases, and wastes. Let's take a close look at fluids and the way the body balances them.

Making gains = losses

The skin, the lungs, the kidneys — just about all major organs — work together to maintain a proper balance of fluid. To maintain proper balance, the amount of fluid gained throughout the day must equal the amount lost. Some of those losses can be measured (sensible losses); others can't (insensible losses).

> Together with the body's other major organs, we help orchestrate fluid balance.

Fluid compartments

This illustration shows the primary fluid compartments in the body: intracellular and extracellular. The extracellular compartment is further divided into interstitial and intravascular fluids. Capillary walls and cell membranes separate intracellular fluids from extracellular fluids.

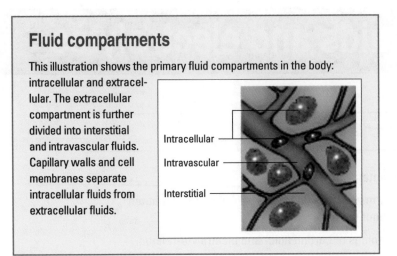

Intracellular

Intravascular

Interstitial

Following the fluid

The body holds fluid in two basic areas, or compartments — inside the cells and outside the cells. Fluid found inside the cells is called *intracellular fluid* (ICF); fluid found outside them, *extracellular fluid* (ECF). Capillary walls and cell membranes separate the intracellular and extracellular compartments. (See *Fluid compartments.*) To maintain proper fluid balance, the distribution of fluid between the two compartments must remain relatively constant.

ECF can be broken down further into interstitial fluid, which surrounds the cells, and intravascular fluid, or plasma, which is the liquid portion of blood. In an adult, interstitial fluid accounts for about 75% of the ECF. Plasma accounts for the remaining 25%.

A look at electrolytes

Electrolytes work with fluids to maintain health and well-being. They're found in various concentrations, depending on whether they're inside or outside the cells. (See *Understanding electrolytes.*) Electrolytes are crucial for nearly all cellular reactions and functions. Let's take a look at what electrolytes are, how they function, and what upsets their balance.

Memory jogger

To help you remember which fluid belongs to which compartment, keep in mind that **INTER** means between (as in **inter**val—between two events) and **INTRA** means within or inside (as in **intra**venous—inside a vein).

Understanding electrolytes

Electrolytes help regulate water distribution, govern acid-base balance, and transmit nerve impulses. They also contribute to energy generation and blood clotting. This table summarizes what the body's major electrolytes do. Check the illustration to see how electrolytes are distributed in and around the cell.

Potassium (K)
- Main intracellular fluid (ICF) cation
- Regulates cell excitability
- Permeates cell membranes, thereby affecting the cell's electrical status
- Helps to control ICF osmolality and, consequently, ICF osmotic pressure

Magnesium (Mg)
- A leading ICF cation
- Contributes to many enzymatic and metabolic processes, particularly protein synthesis
- Modifies nerve impulse transmission and skeletal muscle response (Unbalanced Mg concentrations dramatically affect neuromuscular processes.)

Phosphorus (P)
- Main ICF anion
- Promotes energy storage and carbohydrate, protein, and fat metabolism
- Acts as a hydrogen buffer

Sodium (Na)
- Main extracellular fluid (ECF) cation
- Helps govern normal ECF osmolality (A shift in Na concentrations triggers a fluid volume change to restore normal solute and water ratios.)
- Helps maintain acid-base balance
- Activates nerve and muscle cells
- Influences water distribution (with chloride)

Chloride (Cl)
- Main ECF anion
- Helps maintain normal ECF osmolality

- Affects body pH
- Plays a vital role in maintaining acid-base balance; combines with hydrogen ions to produce hydrochloric acid

Calcium (Ca)
- A major cation in teeth and bones; found in fairly equal concentrations in ICF and ECF
- Also found in cell membranes, where it helps cells adhere to one another and maintain their shape
- Acts as an enzyme activator within cells (Muscles must have Ca to contract.)
- Aids coagulation
- Affects cell membrane permeability and firing level

Bicarbonate (HCO₃⁻)
- Present in ECF
- Primary funcion is regulating acid-base balance

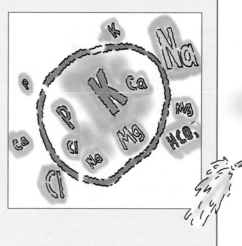

Electrolytes influence water distribution to the cells.

Anions and cations

Electrolytes are substances that, when in solution, separate (or dissociate) into electrically charged particles called *ions*. Some ions are positively charged; others, negatively charged. Anions are electrolytes that generate a negative charge; cations are electrolytes that produce a positive charge. An electrical charge makes cells function normally. Chloride, phosphorus, and bicarbonate are anions; sodium, potassium, calcium, and magnesium are cations.

> **Memory jogger**
>
> To remind yourself about the difference between anions and cations, remember that the T in "cation" looks like the positive symbol, "+."

Electrolyte balance

Sodium and chloride, the major electrolytes in ECF, exert most of their effects outside the cell. Calcium and bicarbonate are two other electrolytes found in ECF. Potassium, phosphate, and magnesium are among the most abundant electrolytes inside the cell.

Although electrolytes are concentrated in one compartment or another, they aren't locked or frozen in these areas. Like fluids, electrolytes move about trying to maintain balance and electroneutrality.

Fluid and electrolyte movement

Just as the heart beats constantly, fluids and solutes move constantly within the body. That movement allows the body to maintain homeostasis, the constant state of balance the body seeks.

Compartmentalize

Solutes within the body's intracellular, interstitial, and intravascular compartments move through the membranes separating those compartments in different ways. The membranes are semipermeable, meaning that they allow some solutes to pass through, but not others. Fluids and solutes move through membranes at the cellular level by diffusion, active transport, and osmosis and through the capillaries by capillary filtration and reabsorption.

Diffusion goes with the flow

In diffusion, solutes move from an area of higher concentration to an area of lower concentration, which eventually results in an equal distribution of solutes within the two areas. Diffusion is a form of passive transport because no energy is required to make it happen; it just happens. Like fish swimming downstream, the solutes simply go with the flow. (See *Diffusion*.)

> Diffusion is our favorite way to move through the body. We just go with the flow.

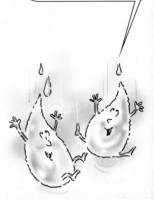

Diffusion

In diffusion, solutes move from areas of higher concentration to areas of lower concentration until their concentration is equal in both areas.

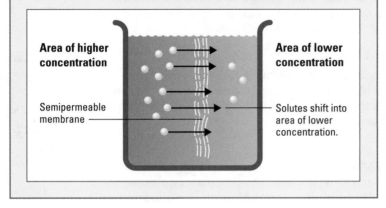

Area of higher concentration

Area of lower concentration

Semipermeable membrane

Solutes shift into area of lower concentration.

Actively transporting

In active transport, solutes move from an area of lower concentration to an area of higher concentration. Like fish swimming upstream, active transport requires energy to make it happen.

The energy required for a solute to move against a concentration gradient comes from a substance called *adenosine triphosphate* (ATP). Stored in all cells, ATP supplies energy for solute movement in and out of cells.

Some solutes, such as sodium and potassium, use ATP to move in and out of cells in a form of active transport called the *sodium-potassium pump*. With the help of this pump, sodium ions move from ICF (an area of lower concentration) to ECF (an area of higher concentration). With potassium, the reverse happens: A large amount of potassium in intracellular fluid causes an electrical potential at the cell membrane. As ions rapidly shift in and out of the cell, electrical impulses are conducted. These impulses are essential for maintaining life.

Other solutes that require active transport to cross cell membranes include calcium ions, hydrogen ions, amino acids, and certain sugars.

Sodium and potassium keep things pumping.

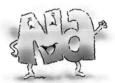

Osmosis lets fluids through

Osmosis refers to the passive movement of fluid across a membrane from an area of lower solute concentration and comparatively more fluid into an area of higher solute concentration and comparatively less fluid. Osmosis stops when enough fluid has moved through the membrane to equalize the solute concentration on both sides of the membrane. (See *Osmosis.*)

Boy, these walls are thin

Within the vascular system, only capillaries have walls thin enough to let solutes pass through. The movement of fluids and solutes through the walls of the body's capillaries plays a critical role in fluid balance.

The pressure is on

The movement of fluids through capillaries — a process called *capillary filtration* — results from blood pushing against the walls of the capillary. That pressure, called *hydrostatic* (or "fluid-pushing") *pressure*, forces fluids and solutes through the capillary wall.

When the hydrostatic pressure inside a capillary is greater than the pressure in the surrounding interstitial space, fluids and solutes inside the capillary are forced out into the interstitial space. When the pressure inside the capillary is less than the pressure outside of it, fluids and solutes move back into the capillary.

> Sometimes, the pressure just gets to me and I can't contain myself...I gotta let it out!

Osmosis

In osmosis, fluid moves passively from areas with more fluid (and fewer solutes) to areas with less fluid (and more solutes). Remember that in osmosis fluid moves, whereas in diffusion solutes move.

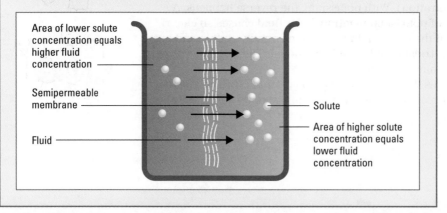

Area of lower solute concentration equals higher fluid concentration

Semipermeable membrane

Fluid

Solute

Area of higher solute concentration equals lower fluid concentration

Keeping the fluid in

A process called *reabsorption* prevents too much fluid from leaving the capillaries no matter how much hydrostatic pressure exists within the capillaries. When fluid filters through a capillary, the protein albumin remains behind in the diminishing volume of water. Albumin is a large molecule that usually can't pass through capillary membranes. As the concentration of albumin inside a capillary increases, fluid begins to move back into the capillaries through osmosis.

Think of albumin as a "water magnet." The osmotic, or pulling, force of albumin in the intravascular space is referred to as the *plasma colloid osmotic pressure*. The plasma colloid osmotic pressure in capillaries averages about 25 mm Hg. (See *Albumin*.)

You're free to leave the capillaries

As long as capillary blood pressure (the hydrostatic pressure) exceeds plasma colloid osmotic pressure, water and solutes can leave the capillaries and enter the interstitial fluid. When capillary blood pressure falls below plasma colloid osmotic pressure, water and diffusible solutes return to the capillaries.

Normally, blood pressure in a capillary exceeds plasma colloid osmotic pressure in the arteriole end and falls below it in the venule end. As a result, capillary filtration occurs along the first half of the vessel; reabsorption, along the second half. As long as capillary blood pressure and plasma albumin levels remain normal, the amount of water that moves into the vessel equals the amount that moves out.

Occasionally, extra fluid filters out of the capillary. When that happens, the excess fluid shifts into the lymphatic vessels located just outside the capillaries and eventually returns to the heart for recirculation.

Albumin

Albumin, a large protein molecule, acts like a magnet to attract water and hold it inside the blood vessel.

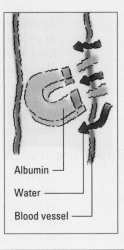

Albumin —
Water —
Blood vessel —

> Maintaining the fluid-electrolyte system is a real balancing act.

Maintaining the balance

Various elements and processes in the body work together to maintain fluid and electrolyte balance. Because one problem can affect the entire fluid-electrolyte maintenance system, it's important to keep all problems in check. Here's a closer look at what makes this balancing act possible.

Kidneys

The kidneys play a vital role in fluid and electrolyte balance. If the kidneys don't work properly, the body has great difficulty controlling fluid balance. The work-horse of the kidney is the nephron, which forms urine. The body puts the nephrons through their paces every day.

A nephron consists of a glomerulus and a tubule. The tubule, sometimes convoluted, ends in a collecting duct. The glomerulus is a cluster of capillaries that filters blood. Like a vascular cradle, Bowman's capsule surrounds the glomerulus.

Capillary blood pressure forces fluid through the capillary walls and into Bowman's capsule at the proximal end of the tubule. Along the length of the tubule, water and electrolytes are either excreted or retained according to the body's needs. If the body needs more fluid, for instance, it retains more. If it needs less fluid, less is re-absorbed and more is excreted. Electrolytes, such as sodium and potassium, are either filtered or reabsorbed throughout the same area. The resulting filtrate, which eventually becomes urine, flows through the tubule into the collecting ducts and eventually into the bladder as urine.

Superabsorbent

Nephrons filter about 125 ml of blood every minute, or about 180 L/day. That rate, called the *glomerular filtration rate*, leads to the production of 1 to 2 L of urine per day. The nephrons reab-sorb the remaining 178 L or more of fluid, an amount equivalent to more than 30 oil changes for the family car!

A strict conservationist

If the body loses even 1% to 2% of its fluid, the kidneys take steps to conserve water. Perhaps the most important step involves reabsorbing more water from the filtrate, which pro-duces a more concentrated urine.

The kidneys must continue to excrete at least 20 ml of urine every hour (500 ml/day) to eliminate body wastes. A urine ex-cretion rate that's less than 20 ml/hour usually indicates renal pathology. The minimum excretion rate varies with age.

The kidneys respond to fluid excesses by excreting a more dilute urine, which rids the body of fluid and conserves electrolytes.

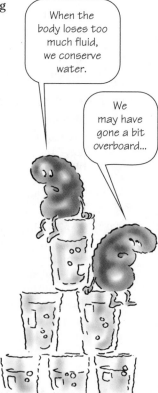

When the body loses too much fluid, we conserve water.

We may have gone a bit overboard...

Other organs and glands

In addition to the kidneys, other organs and glands are essential to maintaining fluid and electrolyte balance. Sodium, potassium, chloride, and water are lost from the GI tract; however, electro-lytes and fluid are also absorbed from the GI tract.

The parathyroid glands also play a role in electrolyte balance, specifically the balance of calcium and phosphorus. The thyroid gland is also involved by balancing the body's calcium level.

Antidiuretic hormone

Several hormones affect fluid balance, among them a water retainer called *antidiuretic hormone* (ADH). (You may also hear this hormone called *vasopressin*.) The hypothalamus produces ADH, but the posterior pituitary gland stores and releases it. If you can remember what ADH stands for, you can remember its job: to restore blood volume by reducing diuresis and increasing water retention.

> Like a dam on a river, the body holds water when fluid levels drop and releases it when fluid levels rise. Just right for keeping the body afloat!

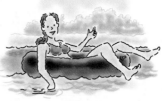

Sensitive to changes

Increased serum osmolality or decreased blood volume can stimulate the release of ADH, which in turn increases the kidneys' reabsorption of water. The increased reabsorption of water results in more concentrated urine.

Likewise, decreased serum osmolality or increased blood volume inhibits the release of ADH and causes less water to be reabsorbed, making the urine less concentrated. The amount of ADH released varies throughout the day, depending on the body's needs.

This up-and-down cycle of ADH release keeps fluid levels in balance all day long. Like a dam on a river, the body holds water when fluid levels drop and releases it when fluid levels rise.

Renin and angiotensin

To help maintain a balance of sodium and water in the body as well as to maintain a healthy blood volume and blood pressure, special cells (juxtaglomerular cells) near each glomerulus secrete an enzyme called *renin*. Through a complex series of steps, renin leads to the production of angiotensin II, a powerful vasoconstrictor.

Angiotensin II causes peripheral vasoconstriction and stimulates the production of aldosterone. Both actions raise blood pressure. (See *Aldosterone production*, page 38.)

As soon as the blood pressure reaches a normal level, the body stops releasing renin and this feedback cycle of renin to angiotensin to aldosterone stops.

The ups and downs of renin

The amount of renin secreted depends on blood flow and the level of sodium in the bloodstream. If blood flow to the kidneys diminishes, as happens in a patient who's hemorrhaging, or if the amount of sodium reaching the glomerulus drops, the juxtaglomerular cells secrete more renin. The renin causes vasoconstriction and a subsequent increase in blood pressure.

Aldosterone production

The illustration shows the steps involved in the production of aldosterone (a hormone that helps to regulate fluid balance) through the renin-angiotensin-aldosterone system.

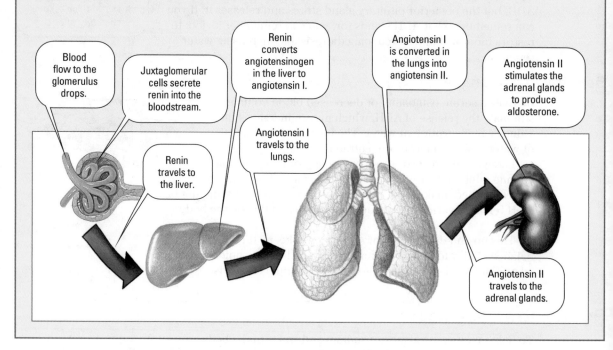

Blood flow to the glomerulus drops.

Juxtaglomerular cells secrete renin into the bloodstream.

Renin converts angiotensinogen in the liver to angiotensin I.

Angiotensin I is converted in the lungs into angiotensin II.

Angiotensin II stimulates the adrenal glands to produce aldosterone.

Renin travels to the liver.

Angiotensin I travels to the lungs.

Angiotensin II travels to the adrenal glands.

Conversely, if blood flow to the kidneys increases, or if the amount of sodium reaching the glomerulus increases, juxtaglomerular cells secrete less renin. A drop-off in renin secretion reduces vasoconstriction and helps to normalize blood pressure.

Aldosterone

The hormone aldosterone also plays a role in maintaining blood pressure and fluid and electrolyte balance. Secreted by the adrenal cortex, aldosterone regulates the reabsorption of sodium and water within the nephron.

Triggering active transport

When blood volume drops, aldosterone initiates the active transport of sodium from the distal tubules and the collecting ducts into the bloodstream. That active transport forces sodium back into the bloodstream. When sodium is forced into the bloodstream, more water is reabsorbed and blood volume expands.

Atrial natriuretic peptide

The renin-angiotensin system isn't the only factor at work balancing fluids in the body. A cardiac hormone called *atrial natriuretic peptide* (ANP) also helps keep that balance. Stored in the cells of the atria, ANP is released when atrial pressure increases. The hormone opposes the renin-angiotensin system by decreasing blood pressure and reducing intravascular blood volume.

This powerful hormone:
- suppresses serum renin levels
- decreases aldosterone release from the adrenal glands
- increases glomerular filtration, which increases urine excretion of sodium and water
- decreases ADH release from the posterior pituitary gland
- reduces vascular resistance by causing vasodilation.

Thirst

Perhaps the simplest mechanism for maintaining fluid balance is the thirst mechanism. Thirst occurs as a result of even small losses of fluid. Losing body fluids or eating highly salty foods leads to an increase in ECF osmolality. This increase leads to the drying of mucous membranes in the mouth, which in turn stimulates the thirst center in the hypothalamus.

Quenching that thirst

Usually, when a person is thirsty, he drinks fluid. The ingested fluid is absorbed from the intestine into the bloodstream, where it moves freely between fluid compartments. This movement leads to an increase in the amount of fluid in the body and a decrease in the concentration of solutes, thus balancing fluid levels throughout the body.

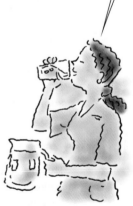

Drinking when you're thirsty — it's the simplest way to maintain fluid balance. Who knew?

Fluid and electrolyte imbalances

Fluid and electrolyte balance is essential for health. Many factors, such as illness, injury, surgery, and treatments, can disrupt a patient's fluid and electrolyte balance. Even a patient with a minor illness is at risk for fluid and electrolyte imbalance. (See *Understanding electrolyte imbalances.*)

Dehydration

The body loses water all the time. A person responds to the thirst reflex by drinking fluids and eating foods that contain water. However, if water isn't adequately replaced, the body's cells can lose water. This causes dehydration, or fluid volume deficit. Dehydration refers to a fluid loss of 1% or more of body weight.

Signs and symptoms of dehydration include:
- dizziness
- fatigue
- weakness
- irritability
- delirium
- extreme thirst
- dry skin and mucous membranes
- poor skin turgor
- increased heart rate
- falling blood pressure
- decreased urine output
- seizures and coma (in severe dehydration).

Laboratory values may include a serum sodium level above 150 mEq/L and serum osmolality above 305 mOsm/kg. The patient may also have an increase in his blood urea nitrogen and hemoglobin levels.

Treatment of dehydration involves determining its cause (such as diarrhea or decreased fluid intake) and replacing lost fluids — either orally or I.V. Most patients receive hypotonic, low-sodium fluids such as dextrose 5% in water (D_5W).

Hypervolemia

Hypervolemia refers to an excess of isotonic fluid (water and sodium) in ECF. The body has compensatory mechanisms to deal with hypervolemia. However, if these fail, signs and symptoms develop.

Hypervolemia can occur if a person consumes more fluid than needed, if fluid output is impaired, or if too much sodium is retained. Conditions that may lead to hypervolemia include kidney failure, cirrhosis, heart failure, and steroid therapy.

Depending on the severity of hypervolemia, signs and symptoms may include:
- edema
- weight gain

If the body's compensatory mechanisms fail, so can I. Gulp!

(*Text continues on page 45.*)

Understanding electrolyte imbalances

This chart summarizes the causes, signs and symptoms (with defining characteristic in italics), and nursing care related to electrolyte imbalances. For all imbalances, treatment goals include diagnosis and correction of the underlying cause, restoring normal electrolyte levels, and preventing complications and recurrence of the imbalance.

Cause	Signs and symptoms	Nursing care
Hypocalcemia • Hypoparathyroidism, infusion of citrated blood, acute pancreatitis, hyperphosphatemia, inadequate dietary intake of vitamin D, or continuous or long-term use of laxatives • Magnesium deficiency, medullary thyroid carcinoma, low serum albumin levels, or alkalosis • Use of aminoglycosides, caffeine, calcitonin, corticosteroids, loop diuretics, nicotine, phosphates, radiographic contrast media, or aluminum-containing antacids	• *Calcium level below 4.5 mEq/L* • Tingling around the mouth and in the fingertips and feet, numbness, painful muscle spasms, and tetany • Positive Trousseau's and Chvostek's signs • Bronchospasm, laryngospasm, and airway obstruction • Seizures • Changes in cardiac conduction • Depression, impaired memory, confusion, and hallucinations • Dry or scaling skin, brittle nails, dry hair, and cataracts • Skeletal fractures resulting from osteoporosis	• Identify patients at risk for hypocalcemia. • Assess the patient for signs and symptoms of hypocalcemia, especially changes in cardiovascular and neurologic status and in vital signs. • Administer I.V. calcium as prescribed. • Administer a phosphate-binding antacid. • Review the procedure for eliciting Trousseau's and Chvostek's signs. • Take seizure or emergency precautions as needed. • Encourage a patient with osteoporosis to perform weight-bearing exercise regularly. • Encourage the patient to increase his intake of foods that are rich in calcium and vitamin D. • Teach the patient and his family how to prevent, recognize, and treat hypocalcemia.
Hypercalcemia • Malignant neoplasms, metastatic bone cancer, hyperparathyroidism, immobilization and loss of bone mineral, or thiazide diuretic use • High calcium intake • Hyperthyroidism or hypothyroidism	• *Calcium level above 5.5 mEq/L* • Muscle weakness and lack of co-ordination • Anorexia, constipation, abdominal pain, nausea, vomiting, peptic ulcers, and abdominal distention • Confusion, impaired memory, slurred speech, and coma • Polyuria and renal colic • Cardiac arrest	• Identify patients at risk for hypercalcemia. • If the patient is receiving digoxin (Lanoxin), assess him for signs of digoxin toxicity. • Assess the patient for signs and symptoms of hypercalcemia. • Encourage ambulation. • Move the patient carefully to prevent fractures. • Take safety or seizure precautions as needed. • Have emergency equipment available. • Administer phosphate to inhibit GI absorption of calcium. • Administer a loop diuretic to promote calcium excretion. • Force fluids with a high acid-ash concentration, such as cranberry juice, to dilute and absorb calcium. • Reduce dietary calcium. • Teach the patient and his family how to prevent, recognize, and treat hypercalcemia, especially if the patient has metastatic cancer.

(continued)

Understanding electrolyte imbalances (continued)

Cause	Signs and symptoms	Nursing care
Hypokalemia • GI losses from diarrhea, laxative abuse, prolonged gastric suctioning, prolonged vomiting, ileostomy, or colostomy • Renal losses related to diuretic use, renal tubular acidosis, renal stenosis, or hyperaldosteronism • Use of certain antibiotics, including penicillin G sodium, carbenicillin, or amphotericin B (Abelcet) • Steroid therapy • Severe perspiration • Hyperalimentation, alkalosis, or excessive blood insulin levels • Poor nutrition	• *Potassium level under 3.5 mEq/L* • Fatigue, muscle weakness, and paresthesia • Prolonged cardiac repolarization, decreased strength of myocardial contraction, orthostatic hypotension, reduced sensitivity to digoxin, increased resistance to antiarrythmics, and cardiac arrest • Flat ST segment and Q wave on electrocardiogram (ECG) • Decreased bowel motility • Suppressed insulin release and aldosterone secretion • Inability to concentrate urine and increased renal phosphate excretion • Respiratory muscle weakness • Metabolic alkalosis, low urine osmolality, slightly elevated glucose level, and myoglobinuria	• Identify patients at risk for hypokalemia. • Assess the patient's diet for a lack of potassium. • Assess the patient for signs and symptoms of hypokalemia. • Administer a potassium replacement as prescribed. • Encourage intake of high-potassium foods, such as bananas, dried fruit, and orange juice. • Monitor the patient for complications. • Have emergency equipment available for cardiopulmonary resuscitation and cardiac defibrillation. • Teach the patient and his family how to prevent, recognize, and treat hypokalemia.
Hyperkalemia • Decreased renal excretion related to oliguric renal failure, potassium-sparing diuretic use, or adrenal steroid deficiency • High potassium intake related to the improper use of oral supplements, excessive use of salt substitutes, or rapid infusion of potassium solutions • Acidosis, tissue damage, or malignant cell lysis after chemotherapy	• *Potassium level above 5 mEq/L* • Cardiac conduction disturbances, ventricular arrhythmias, prolonged depolarization, decreased strength of contraction, and cardiac arrest • Tall, tented T wave; prolonged QRS complex and PR interval on ECG • Muscle weakness and paralysis • Nausea, vomiting, diarrhea, intestinal colic, uremic enteritis, decreased bowel sounds, abdominal distention, and paralytic ileus	• Identify patients at risk for hyperkalemia. • Assess the patient's diet for excess use of salt substitutes. • Assess for signs and symptoms of hyperkalemia. • Assess arterial blood gas studies for metabolic alkalosis. • Take precautions when drawing blood samples. A falsely elevated potassium level can result from hemolysis or prolonged tourniquet application. • Have emergency equipment available. • Administer calcium gluconate to decrease myocardial irritability. • Administer insulin and I.V. glucose to move potassium back into cells. Carefully monitor serum glucose levels. • Administer sodium polystyrene sulfonate (Kayexalate) with 70% sorbitol to exchange sodium ions for potassium ions in the intestine.

Understanding electrolyte imbalances (continued)

Cause	Signs and symptoms	Nursing care
Hyperkalemia (continued)		• Perform hemodialysis or peritoneal dialysis to remove excess potassium. • Teach the patient and his family how to prevent, recognize, and treat hyperkalemia.
Hypomagnesemia • Alcoholism, protein-calorie malnutrition, I.V. therapy without magnesium replacement, gastric suctioning, malabsorption syndromes, laxative abuse, bulimia, anorexia, intestinal bypass for obesity, diarrhea, or colonic neoplasms • Hyperaldosteronism or renal disease that impairs magnesium reabsorption • Use of osmotic diuretics or antibiotics, such as gentamicin • Overdose of vitamin D or calcium, burns, pancreatitis, sepsis, hypothermia, exchange transfusion, hyperalimentation, or diabetic ketoacidosis	• *Magnesium level under 1.5 mEq/L* • Muscle weakness, tremors, tetany, and clonic or focal seizures • Laryngeal stridor • Decreased blood pressure, ventricular fibrillation, tachyarrhythmias, and increased susceptibility to digoxin toxicity • Apathy, depression, agitation, confusion, delirium, and hallucinations • Nausea, vomiting, and anorexia • Decreased calcium level • Positive Chvostek's and Trousseau's signs	• Identify patients at risk for hypomagnesemia. • Assess the patient for signs and symptoms of hypomagnesemia. • Administer I.V. magnesium as prescribed. • Encourage the patient to consume magnesium-rich foods. • If the patient is confused or agitated, take safety precautions. • Take seizure precautions as needed. • Have emergency equipment available. Calcium gluconate is used to treat tetany. • Teach the patient and his family how to prevent, recognize, and treat hypomagnesemia.
Hypermagnesemia • Renal failure, excessive antacid use (especially in a patient with renal failure), adrenal insufficiency, or diuretic abuse • Excessive magnesium replacement or excessive use of milk of magnesia or other magnesium-containing laxative	• *Magnesium level above 2.5 mEq/L* • Peripheral vasodilation with decreased blood pressure, facial flushing and sensations of warmth and thirst • Lethargy or drowsiness, apnea, and coma • Loss of deep tendon reflexes, paresis, and paralysis • Cardiac arrest	• Identify patients at risk for hypermagnesemia. • Review all medications for a patient with renal failure. • Assess the patient for signs and symptoms of hypermagnesemia. • Assess reflexes; if absent, notify the practitioner. • Administer calcium gluconate. • Have emergency equipment available. • Prepare the patient for hemodialysis if prescribed. • If the patient is taking an antacid, a laxative, or another drug that contains magnesium, instruct him to stop. • Teach the patient and his family how to prevent, recognize, and treat hypermagnesemia.

(continued)

Understanding electrolyte imbalances (continued)

Cause	Signs and symptoms	Nursing care
Hyponatremia *Dilutional* • Excessive water gain caused by inappropriate administration of I.V. solutions, syndrome of inappropriate antidiuretic hormone, oxytocin use for labor induction, water intoxication, heart failure, renal failure, or cirrhosis	• *Sodium level under 136 mEq/L* • Confusion • Nausea, vomiting • Weight gain • Edema • Muscle spasms, convulsions	• Identify patients at risk for hyponatremia. • Assess fluid intake and output. • Assess the patient for signs and symptoms of hyponatremia. • If the patient has dilutional hyponatremia, restrict his fluid intake. • If the patient has true hyponatremia, administer isotonic I.V. fluids. • Teach the patient and his family dietary measures that ensure appropriate fluid and sodium intake.
True • Excessive sodium loss due to GI losses, excessive sweating, diuretic use, adrenal insufficiency, burns, lithium (Lithobid) use, or starvation	• *Sodium level under 136 mEq/L* • Orthostatic hypotension • Tachycardia • Dry mucous membranes • Weight loss • Nausea, vomiting • Oliguria	• If the patient is receiving lithium, teach him how to prevent alterations in his sodium levels. • If the patient has adrenal insufficiency, teach him how to prevent hyponatremia. • Teach the patient and his family how to prevent, recognize, and treat hyponatremia.
Hypernatremia • Sodium gain that exceeds water gain related to salt intoxication (resulting from sodium bicarbonate use in cardiac arrest), hyperaldosteronism, or use of diuretics, vasopressin, corticosteroids, or some antihypertensives • Water loss that exceeds sodium loss related to profuse sweating, diarrhea, polyuria resulting from diabetes insipidus or diabetes mellitus, high-protein tube feedings, inadequate water intake, or insensible water loss	• *Sodium level above 145 mEq/L* • Thirst; rough, dry tongue; dry sticky mucous membranes; flushed skin, oliguria; and low-grade fever that returns to normal when sodium levels return to normal • Restlessness, disorientation, hallucinations, lethargy, seizures, and coma • Muscle weakness and irritability • Serum osmolality above 295 mOsm/kg and urine specific gravity above 1.015	• Identify patients at risk for hypernatremia. • Assess the patient for fluid losses and gains. • Assess the patient for signs and symptoms of hypernatremia. • Consult with a nutritionist to determine the amount of free water needed with tube feedings. • Encourage the patient to increase his fluid intake but decrease his sodium intake. • If the patient is agitated or is experiencing a seizure, take safety precautions. • Teach the patient and his family how to prevent, recognize, and treat hypernatremia.

Understanding electrolyte imbalances (continued)

Cause	Signs and symptoms	Nursing care
Hypophosphatemia • Glucose administration or insulin release, nutritional recovery syndrome, overzealous feeding with simple carbohydrates, respiratory alkalosis, alcohol withdrawal, diabetic ketoacidosis, or starvation • Malabsorption syndromes, diarrhea, vomiting, aldosteronism, diuretic therapy, or use of drugs that bind with phosphate, such as aluminum hydroxide (Amphojel) or magnesium salts (milk of magnesia)	• *Phosphorus level below 2.5 mg/dl* • Irritability, apprehension, confusion, decreased level of consciousness, seizures, and coma • Weakness, numbness, and paresthesia • Congestive cardiomyopathy • Respiratory muscle weakness • Hemolytic anemia • Impaired granulocyte function, elevated creatine kinase level, hyperglycemia, and metabolic acidosis	• Identify patients at risk for hypophosphatemia. • Assess the patient for signs and symptoms of hypo-phosphatemia, especially neurologic and hematologic ones. • Administer phosphate supplements as prescribed. • Note calcium and phosphorus levels because calcium and phosphorus have an inverse relationship. • Gradually introduce hyperalimentation as prescribed. • Teach the patient and his family how to prevent, recognize, and treat hypophosphatemia.
Hyperphosphatemia • Renal disease • Hypoparathyroidism or hyperthyroidism • Excessive vitamin D intake • Muscle necrosis, excessive phosphate intake, or chemotherapy	• *Phosphorus level above 4.5 mg/dl* • Soft-tissue calcification (chronic hyperphosphatemia) • Hypocalcemia, possible with tetany • Increased red blood cell count	• Identify patients at risk for hyperphosphatemia. • Assess the patient for signs and symptoms of hyperphosphatemia and hypocalcemia, including tetany and muscle twitching. • Advise the patient to avoid foods and medications that contain phosphorus. • Administer phosphorus-binding antacids. • Prepare the patient for possible dialysis. • Teach the patient and his family how to prevent, recognize, and treat hyperphosphatemia.

• distended neck and hand veins
• heart failure
• initially, rising blood pressure and cardiac output; later, falling values.

Laboratory tests may reveal a serum sodium level above 135 mEq/L and serum osmolality below 275 mOsm/kg.

Treatment involves determining the cause and treating the underlying condition. Typically, patients require fluid and sodium restrictions and diuretic therapy.

Water intoxication

Water intoxication occurs when excess fluid moves from the ECF to the ICF. Excessive low-sodium fluid in the ECF is hypotonic to cells; cells are hypertonic to the fluid. As a result, fluids shift into the cells, which have comparatively less fluid and more solutes. The fluid shift, in turn, balances the concentrations of fluid between the two spaces.

Acting inappropriately

Water intoxication may occur in a patient with syndrome of inappropriate antidiuretic hormone, which can result from central nervous system or pulmonary disorders, head trauma, tumors, or the use of certain drugs. Other causes of water intoxication include:
• rapid infusion of hypotonic solutions
• excessive use of tap water as a nasogastric tube irrigant or enema
• psychogenic polydipsia, a psychological disturbance in which a person drinks large amounts of fluid even when they aren't needed.

I.V. fluid replacement

To maintain health, the balance of fluids and electrolytes in the intracellular and extracellular spaces must remain relatively constant. Whenever a person experiences an illness or a condition that prevents normal fluid intake or causes excessive fluid loss, I.V. fluid replacement may be necessary.

Quick and predictable

I.V. therapy that provides the patient with life-sustaining fluids, electrolytes, and medications offers the advantages of immediate and predictable therapeutic effects. The I.V. route is, therefore, the preferred route — especially for administering fluids, electrolytes, and drugs in an emergency.

This route also allows for fluid intake when a patient has GI malabsorption. I.V. therapy permits accurate dosage titration for analgesics and other medications. Potential disadvantages associated with I.V. therapy include drug and solution incompatibility, adverse reactions, infection, and other complications.

To the rescue! I offer immediate and predictable therapy for fluid imbalance.

Types of solutions

Solutions used for I.V. fluid replacement fall into the broad categories of crystalloids (which may be isotonic, hypotonic, or hypertonic) and colloids (which are always hypertonic).

Crystalloids

Crystalloids are solutions with small molecules that flow easily from the bloodstream into cells and tissues. Isotonic crystalloids contain about the same concentration of osmotically active particles as ECF, so fluid doesn't shift between the extracellular and intracellular areas.

Hypotonic crystalloids are less concentrated than ECF, so they move from the bloodstream into the cell, causing the cell to swell. In contrast, hypertonic crystalloids are more highly concentrated than ECF, so fluid is pulled into the bloodstream from the cell, causing the cell to shrink. (See *Comparing fluid tonicity*.)

Isotonic solutions

Isotonic solutions, such as D_5W, have an osmolality (or concentration) of 275 to 295 mOsm/kg. The dextrose metabolizes quickly, however, acting like a hypotonic solution and leaving water behind. Large amounts of the solution may cause hyperglycemia.

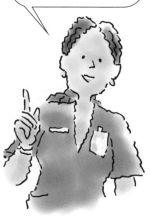

Crystalloids are solutions with small molecules that flow easily from the bloodstream into cells and tissues.

Comparing fluid tonicity

These illustrations show the effects of different types of I.V. fluids on fluid movement and cell size.

Isotonic
Isotonic fluids, such as normal saline solution, have a concentration of dissolved particles, or tonicity, equal to that of intracellular fluid (ICF). Osmotic pressure is therefore the same inside and outside the cells, so they neither shrink nor swell with fluid movement.

Hypertonic
Hypertonic fluid has a tonicity greater than that of ICF, so osmotic pressure is unequal inside and outside the cells. Dehydration or a rapidly infused hypertonic fluid, such as 3% saline or 50% dextrose, draws water out of the cells into the more highly concentrated extracellular fluid (ECF).

Hypotonic
Hypotonic fluids, such as half-normal saline solution, have a tonicity less than that of ICF, so osmotic pressure draws water into the cells from the ECF. Severe electrolyte losses or inappropriate use of I.V. fluids can make body fluids hypotonic.

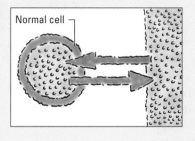

Normal cell

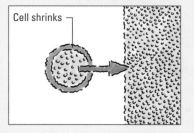

Cell shrinks

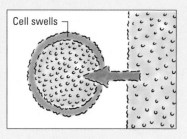

Cell swells

Did someone ring for more isotonic solutions?

Normal saline solution, another isotonic solution, contains only the electrolytes sodium and chloride. Other isotonic fluids are more similar to ECF. For instance, Ringer's solution contains sodium, potassium, calcium, and chloride. Lactated Ringer's solution contains those electrolytes plus lactate, which the liver converts to bicarbonate.

Hypotonic fluids

Hypotonic fluids are those fluids that have an osmolality less than 275 mOsm/kg. Examples of hypotonic fluids include:
- half-normal saline solution
- 0.33% sodium chloride solution
- dextrose 2.5% in water.

It makes a cell swell

Hypotonic solutions should be given cautiously because fluid then moves from the extracellular space into cells, causing them to swell. That fluid shift can cause cardiovascular collapse from vascular fluid depletion. It can also cause increased intracranial pressure (ICP) from fluid shifting into brain cells.

Hypotonic solutions shouldn't be given to a patient at risk for increased ICP — for example, those who have had a stroke, head trauma, or neurosurgery. Signs of increased ICP include a change in the patient's level of consciousness, motor or sensory deficits, and changes in the size, shape, or response to light in the pupils. Hypotonic solutions also shouldn't be used for patients who suffer from abnormal fluid shifts into the interstitial space or the body cavities — for example, as a result of liver disease, a burn, or trauma.

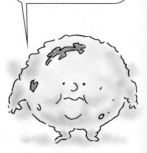

Yes, I'm swell, but too much of a good thing can be bad. Administer hypotonic solutions cautiously, please.

Hypertonic solutions

Hypertonic solutions are those that have an osmolality greater than 295 mOsm/kg. Examples include:
- dextrose 5% in half-normal saline solution
- dextrose 5% in normal saline solution
- dextrose 5% in lactated Ringer's solution
- dextrose 10% in water.

The incredible shrinking cell

A hypertonic solution draws fluids from the intracellular space, causing cells to shrink and the extracellular space to expand. Patients with cardiac or renal disease may be unable to tolerate extra fluid. Watch for fluid overload and pulmonary edema.

Because hypertonic solutions draw fluids from cells, patients at risk for cellular dehydration (patients with diabetic ketoacidosis, for example) shouldn't receive them.

Colloids

The practitioner may prescribe a colloid (plasma expander) if your patient's blood volume doesn't improve with crystalloids. Examples of colloids that may be given include:
• albumin (available in 5% solutions, which are osmotically equal to plasma, and 25% solutions, which draw about four times their volume in interstitial fluid into the circulation within 15 minutes of administration)
• plasma protein fraction
• dextran
• hetastarch.

Flowing into the stream

Colloids pull fluid into the bloodstream. The effects of colloids last several days if the lining of the capillaries is normal. The patient needs to be closely monitored during a colloid infusion for increased blood pressure, dyspnea, and bounding pulse, which are all signs of hypervolemia.

If neither crystalloids nor colloids are effective in treating the imbalance, the patient may require a blood transfusion or other treatment.

> The choice of I.V. therapy delivery depends on several factors, including the condition of the patient's veins. As you can see, I'm in top condition.

Delivery methods

The choice of I.V. therapy delivery is based on the purpose of the therapy and its duration; the patient's diagnosis, age, and health history; and the condition of the patient's veins. I.V. solutions can be delivered through a peripheral or a central vein. Catheters are chosen based on the therapy and the site to be used. Here's a look at how to choose a site — peripheral or central — and which equipment you'll need for each.

Peripheral lines

Peripheral I.V. therapy is administered for short-term or intermittent therapy through a vein in the arm, hand, leg or, rarely, foot. Potential I.V. sites include the metacarpal, cephalic, basilic, median cubital, and greater saphenous veins. Using veins in the leg or foot is unusual because of the risk of thrombophlebitis. Also keep in mind that dextrose concentrations greater than 10% shouldn't be administered peripherally because of the risk of vein irritation.

Central lines

Central venous therapy involves administering solutions through a catheter placed in a central vein, typically the subclavian or internal jugular vein, less commonly the femoral vein.

Central venous therapy is used for patients who:
• have inadequate peripheral veins
• need access for blood sampling
• require a large volume of fluid
• need a hypertonic solution to be diluted by rapid blood flow in a larger vein
• need to receive vessel-irritating drugs
• need a high-calorie nutritional supplement.

Types of central venous catheters include the traditional multilumen catheter for short-term therapy and a peripherally inserted central catheter or a vascular access device (such as a Broviac or Hickman catheter) for long-term therapy.

Complications of I.V. therapy

Caring for a patient with an I.V. line requires careful monitoring as well as a clear understanding of the possible complications, what to do if they arise, and how to deal with flow issues.

Infiltration

During infiltration, fluid may leak from the vein into surrounding tissue. This occurs when the access device dislodges from the vein. Look for coolness at the site, pain, swelling, leaking, and lack of blood return. Also look for a sluggish flow that continues even if a tourniquet is applied above the site. If you see infiltration, stop the infusion, elevate the extremity, and apply warm soaks.

Smaller is better

To prevent infiltration, use the smallest catheter that will accomplish the infusion, avoid placement in joint areas, and secure the catheter in place.

Infection

I.V. therapy involves puncturing the skin, one of the body's barriers to infection. Look for purulent drainage at the site, tenderness, erythema, warmth, or hardness on palpation. Signs and symptoms that the infection has become systemic include fever, chills, and an elevated white blood cell count.

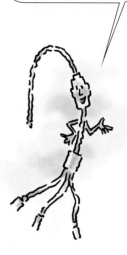

I can be spunky. Be sure to secure me in place to prevent infiltration.

This monitoring is vital

Nursing actions for an infected I.V. site include monitoring vital signs and notifying the practitioner. Swab the site for culture and remove the catheter as ordered. Always maintain sterile technique to prevent this complication.

Phlebitis and thrombophlebitis

Phlebitis is inflammation of a vein. Thrombophlebitis is an irritation of the vein along with the formation of a clot; it's usually more painful than phlebitis. Poor insertion technique or the pH or osmolality of the infusing solution or medication can cause these complications. Look for pain, redness, swelling, or induration at the site; a red line streaking along the vein; fever; or a sluggish flow of the solution.

Prevention begins with big veins

When phlebitis or thrombophlebitis occurs, remove the I.V. line, monitor the patient's vital signs, notify the practitioner, and apply warm soaks to the site. To prevent these complications, choose large veins and change the catheter according to your facility's policy when infusing a medication or solution with high osmolality.

Extravasation

Extravasation, similar to infiltration, is the leakage of fluid into surrounding tissues. It results when medications, such as dopamine, calcium solutions, and chemotherapeutic agents, seep through veins and can produce blistering and necrosis. Initially, the patient may experience discomfort, burning, or pain at the site. Also, look for skin tightness, blanching, and lack of blood return. Delayed reactions include inflammation and pain within 3 to 5 days and ulcers or tissue necrosis within 2 weeks.

> Before you administer a medication that may extravasate, make sure you know your facility's policy.

Review policy

When administering medications that may extravasate, know your facility's policy. Nursing actions include stopping the infusion, notifying the practitioner, removing the catheter, applying ice early and warm soaks later, and elevating the extremity. The doctor may inject an antidote into the site. Assess the circulation and nerve function of the limb.

Air embolism

An air embolism occurs when air enters the vein. It can cause a decrease in blood pressure, an increase in the pulse rate, respiratory distress, an increase in ICP, and a loss of consciousness.

Problems in the air

If the patient develops an air embolism, notify the practitioner and clamp off the I.V. line. Place the patient on his left side and lower his head to allow the air to enter the right atrium, where it can disperse more safely by way of the pulmonary artery. Monitor the patient and administer oxygen. To avoid this serious complication, prime all tubing completely, tighten all connections securely, and use an air detection device on an I.V. pump.

How you intervene

Nursing care for the patient with an I.V. line includes the following actions:
• Check the I.V. order for completeness and accuracy. Most I.V. orders expire after 24 hours. A complete order should specify the amount and type of solution, specific additives and their concentrations, and the rate and duration of the infusion. If the order is incomplete or confusing, clarify the order with the prescriber before proceeding.
• Measure intake and output carefully at scheduled intervals. The kidneys attempt to restore fluid balance during dehydration by reducing urine production. Urine output less than 30 ml/hour signals retention of metabolic wastes. Notify the practitioner if your patient's urine output falls below 30 ml/hour.
• Monitor daily weights to document fluid retention or loss. A 2% increase or decrease in body weight is significant. A 2.2-lb (1-kg) change corresponds to 1 qt (1 L) of fluid gained or lost.
• Always carefully monitor the infusion of solutions that contain medication because rapid infusion and circulation of the drug can be dangerous.
• Note the pH of the I.V. solution. The pH can alter the effect and stability of drugs mixed in the I.V. bag. Consult medication literature, the pharmacist, or the prescriber if you have questions.
• Using sterile technique, change the site, dressing, and tubing as often as facility policy requires. Solutions should be changed at least every 24 hours.
• When changing I.V. tubing, be sure not to move or dislodge the I.V. catheter. If you have trouble disconnecting the used tubing, use a hemostat to hold the I.V. hub while twisting the tubing. Don't clamp the hemostat shut because doing so may crack the hub.

Memory jogger

To remember the correlation of daily weights to fluid gains or losses, think in terms of picking up a quart of reduced-fat milk on the way home from work. A 2% change in fluid status is significant and a 2.2 lb (1 kg) change corresponds to 1 qt (1 L) of fluid gained or lost. That's a lot of milk!

Keep in mind, most I.V. orders expire after 24 hours.

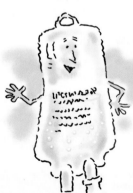

• Always report needle-stick injuries immediately so that treatment can be initiated. Exposure to a patient's blood increases the risk of infection with blood-borne viruses, such as human immunodeficiency virus (HIV), hepatitis B virus, hepatitis C virus, and cytomegalovirus. About 1 out of 300 people with occupational needle-stick injuries become HIV-seropositive.

• Always follow standard precautions when inserting, caring for, or discontinuing an I.V. line.

Focus on the patient

• Always listen to your patient carefully. Subtle statements such as "I just don't feel right" may be your clue to the beginning of an allergic reaction.

• Provide appropriate patient teaching. (See *Teaching about I.V. therapy.*)

• Keep in mind that a candidate for home I.V. therapy must have a family member or friend who can safely and competently administer the I.V. fluids as well as a backup helper, a suitable home environment, a telephone, available transportation, adequate reading skills, and the ability to prepare, handle, store, and dispose of equipment properly. Procedures for caring for the I.V. line are the same at home as in a health care facility, except at home the patient uses clean technique instead of sterile technique.

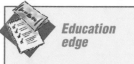

Education edge

Teaching about I.V. therapy

Make sure you cover the following points with your patient and then evaluate his learning:

• what to expect before, during, and after the I.V. procedure

• signs and symptoms of complications and when to report them

• activity or diet restrictions

• how to care for an I.V. line at home.

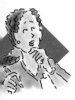

Quick quiz

1. Hydrostatic pressure, which pushes fluid out of the capillaries, is opposed by colloid osmotic pressure, which involves:

    A.   reduced renin secretion.

    B.   the pulling power of albumin to reabsorb water.

    C.   an increase in ADH secretion.

    D.   aldosterone production.

Answer: B. Albumin in capillaries draws water toward it, a process called *reabsorption.*

2. When a person's blood pressure drops, the kidneys respond by:

    A.   secreting renin.

    B.   producing aldosterone.

    C.   slowing the release of ADH.

    D.   increasing urine output.

Answer: A. Juxtaglomerular cells in the kidneys secrete renin in response to low blood flow or a low sodium level. The eventual effect of renin secretion is an increase in blood pressure.

3.   The main extracellular cation is:
    A.   calcium.
    B.   potassium.
    C.   magnesium.
    D.   sodium.

Answer: D. Sodium is the main extracellular cation. Among other things, it helps regulate fluid balance in the body.

4.   Hypertonic solutions cause fluids to move from the:
    A.   interstitial space to the intracellular space.
    B.   intracellular space to the extracellular space.
    C.   extracellular space to the intracellular space.
    D.   extracellular space to the interstitial space.

Answer: B. Hypertonic solutions, because of their increased osmolality, draw fluids out of the cells and into the extracellular space.

5.   Extravasation of I.V. fluid is associated with administration of which solution?
    A.   Hypertonic fluid
    B. D_5W
    C.   An antineoplastic
    D.   Normal saline solution

Answer: C. Antineoplastics are highly irritating to the veins and are typically administered using a steel needle. Extravasation is common in those situations.

Scoring

✩✩✩   If you answered all five questions correctly, great job! Your fluid and electrolyte knowledge is flowing smoothly.

✩✩   If you answered four questions correctly, nice going! You'll have fluid and electrolyte imbalances on the run in no time.

✩   If you answered fewer than four questions correctly, relax! With a little more active transport of this chapter, it will all balance out.

Perioperative care

Just the facts

In this chapter, you'll learn:

♦ perioperative nursing measures

♦ the effects of anesthesia

♦ techniques for preventing and managing postoperative complications

♦ steps in planning patient discharge.

A look at perioperative care

Many technological advances have made operations quicker, safer, and more effective. Even so, surgery remains one of the most stressful experiences a patient can undergo. Before the patient enters the operating room, you must fully address his psychological and physiologic needs. If prepared properly with careful teaching, a surgical patient will experience less pain, fewer postoperative complications, and shorter hospitalization.

Preoperative care

Careful, considerate preoperative care will help prevent future complications for the patient and ease anxiety felt by the patient and his family.

Preoperative assessment

A thorough preoperative assessment helps systematically identify and correct problems before surgery and establishes a baseline for postoperative comparison. Begin by confirming the patient's identity using two identifiers, according to your facility's policy. Then verify the surgical procedure and surgical site with the patient. Next, focus on problem areas suggested by the patient's history and on any body system that will be directly affected by the surgery. (See *History lesson.*) Consider your findings in relation to the specific age-group norms. Don't forget to include the patient's psychological status in your assessment because depression and anxiety can significantly interfere with recovery from surgery.

Patient teaching

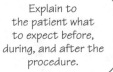

Explain to the patient what to expect before, during, and after the procedure.

Your teaching can help the patient cope with the physical and psychological stress of surgery. Preadmission and preoperative teaching are more important than ever in these days of shorter hospital stays and same-day surgeries.

Evaluate, adapt, and consider

Evaluate the patient's understanding and tell him what to expect before, during, and after the procedure. Adapt your teaching to fit the patient's age, understanding, and cultural background. Also, consider the needs of the patient's family or caregivers.

What to teach

Be sure to include these topics in your preoperative patient teaching:
• diagnostic tests
• the need to abstain from food and fluids for a period of time before surgery
• what type of anesthesia is planned, such as general, regional, or balanced
• airway management
• placement of other tubes, such as nasogastric tubes or drains
• operating room procedure
• I.V. therapy
• what to expect on the postanesthesia care unit (PACU)
• pain control
• postoperative care, including diet, mobility, and treatments.

Prepare for postop

Before surgery, teach the patient early postoperative mobility and ambulation techniques and leg exercises. In addition, teach coughing and deep-breathing exercises, including how to use an incentive spirometer. Make it clear that the patient will have to repeat these maneuvers several times after surgery. (See *Teaching coughing and deep-breathing exercises*, page 58.)

History lesson

Finding out about the patient's history is very important, but doing so requires you to ask a lot of questions. To conduct a thorough history, ask about:
• allergies to drugs, food, and environmental factors
• family history of problems with anesthesia
• the patient's regular use of medications or herbal preparations (it's important to know how often these medications are taken and if any were taken before admission).

Don't stop there
Also ask the patient about alcohol and drug use. A patient using recreational drugs or alcohol has a higher tolerance for anesthesia and pain medications. A patient in substance withdrawal may exhibit behavioral changes and may be more difficult to manage in the operating room and postoperatively. Determine the frequency of substance use to assess the likelihood of postoperative substance withdrawal.

Before surgery, also ask patients if they:
• have any loose teeth
• wear dentures or a partial plate
• wear glasses or contact lenses
• use a hearing aid
• are wearing jewelry (especially body jewelry)
• have joint implants, metal implants, or a pacemaker.

For the gals
Ask female patients about pregnancy. Some facilities routinely check pregnancy status of all females age 10 and older. Be considerate when asking adolescent girls about being sexually active or about pregnancy in the presence of family members.

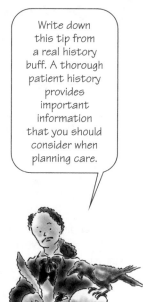

Write down this tip from a real history buff. A thorough patient history provides important information that you should consider when planning care.

Tell the patient that postoperative exercises help prevent such complications as:
• atelectasis
• hypostatic pneumonia
• thrombophlebitis
• constipation
• abdominal distention
• venous pooling.

Have the patient perform postoperative exercises to assess whether further teaching is necessary and to support the teaching plan.

Getting ready

To prepare the patient for surgery, you may have to perform skin and bowel preparations and administer drugs.

Education edge

Teaching coughing and deep-breathing exercises

These exercises will speed your patient's recovery and reduce his risk of respiratory complications.

Coughing exercises

Patients who risk developing excess secretions should practice coughing exercises before surgery. However, patients about to undergo ear or eye surgery or repair of hiatal or large abdominal hernias won't need to practice coughing. Also, patients undergoing neurosurgery shouldn't cough postoperatively because intracranial pressure will rise. Tell the patient to practice coughing exercises, as follows:

• If the patient's condition permits, instruct him to sit on the edge of his bed (as shown at right). Provide a stool if his feet don't touch the floor. Tell him to bend his legs and lean slightly forward.

• If the patient is scheduled for chest or abdominal surgery, teach him how to splint his incision before he coughs.

• Instruct the patient to take a slow, deep breath; he should breathe in through his nose and concentrate on fully expanding his chest. Then he should breathe out through his mouth and concentrate on feeling his chest sink downward and inward. Then he should take a second breath in the same manner.

• Next, tell him to take a third deep breath and hold it. He should then cough two or three times in a row (once isn't enough). This will clear his breathing passages. Encourage him to concentrate on feeling his diaphragm force out all the air in his chest. Then he should take three to five normal breaths, exhale slowly, and relax.

• Have the patient repeat this exercise at least once. After surgery, he'll need to perform it at least every 2 hours to help keep his lungs free from secretions. Re-assure the patient that his stitches are very strong and won't split during coughing.

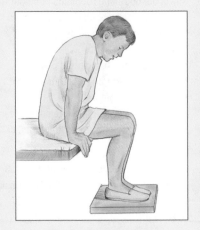

Deep-breathing exercises

Advise the patient that performing deep-breathing exercises several times per hour helps keep lungs fully expanded. To deep-breathe correctly, he must use his diaphragm and abdominal muscles, not just his chest muscles. Tell the patient to practice deep-breathing exercises two or three times per day before surgery, as follows:

• Have him lie on his back in a comfortable position with one hand placed on his chest and the other over his upper abdomen (as shown at right). Instruct him to relax and bend his legs slightly.

• Instruct him to exhale normally. He should then close his mouth and inhale deeply through his nose, concentrating on feeling his abdomen rise. His chest shouldn't expand. Have him hold his breath and slowly count to five.

• Next, have the patient purse his lips as though about to whistle, then exhale completely through his mouth, without letting his cheeks puff out. His ribs should sink downward and inward.

• After resting several seconds, the patient should repeat the exercise five to ten times. He should also do this exercise while lying on his side, sitting, standing, or while turning in bed.

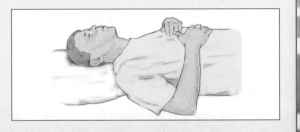

Skin preparation

In most facilities, skin preparation is carried out during the intra-operative phase. However, making sure the skin is as free from microorganisms as possible reduces the risk of infection at the incision site. The patient may be asked to bathe, shower, or scrub a local skin area with an antiseptic the evening before or the morning of surgery. The surgeon will usually specify the site for a local skin scrub if indicated.

Make it big, real big

To reduce the number of microorganisms in areas near the incision site, prepare a much larger area than the expected incision site. Doing so also helps prevent contamination during surgical draping. Document skin preparation, including the area prepared and any unexpected outcomes.

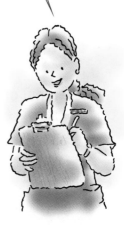

Document skin preparation, including the area prepared and unexpected outcomes.

Bowel preparation

The extent of bowel preparation depends on the type and site of surgery. A patient scheduled for several days of postoperative bed rest who hasn't had a recent bowel movement may receive a mild laxative or sodium phosphate enema. On the other hand, a patient scheduled for GI, pelvic, perianal, or rectal surgery will undergo more extensive intestinal preparation.

After three, make the call

If enemas are ordered until the bowel is clear and the third enema still hasn't removed all stool, notify the practitioner because repeated enemas may cause fluid and electrolyte imbalances. Elderly patients, children, and patients who are allowed nothing by mouth and haven't received I.V. fluids are at particularly high risk for these imbalances.

Preoperative drugs

The practitioner may order preoperative or preanesthesia drugs to:
• ease anxiety
• permit a smoother induction of anesthesia
• decrease the amount of anesthesia needed
• create amnesia for the events preceding surgery
• minimize the flow of pharyngeal and respiratory secretions
• minimize gastric secretions
• reduce the risk of infection.

Discussing drugs

Expect to administer ordered drugs 30 to 75 minutes before induction of anesthesia. Teach the patient about ordered drugs, their desired effects, and their possible adverse effects. These drugs include:
- anticholinergics (vagolytic or drying agents)
- sedatives
- antianxiety drugs
- opioid analgesics
- neuroleptanalgesic agents
- histamine-2 receptor antagonists
- antibiotics.

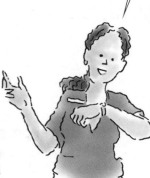

The patient should have no solid food for at least 6 hours and no water for at least 2 hours before surgery.

Final check

Before surgery, follow these important steps:
- Make sure the patient has had no solid food for at least 6 hours and no water for at least 2 hours before surgery.
- Make sure the chart contains all necessary information, such as signed surgical consent, diagnostic test results, health history, and physical examination. Patient allergies should be easily visible.
- Tell the patient to remove jewelry (including body piercings), makeup, and nail polish. Ask the patient to shower with antimicrobial soap, if ordered, and to perform mouth care. Warn against swallowing water.
- Instruct him to remove dentures or partial plates. Note on the chart if he has dental crowns, caps, or braces. Also have him remove contact lenses, glasses, or prostheses (such as an artificial eye). You may remove his hearing aid to make sure it doesn't become lost. However, if the patient wishes to keep his hearing aid in place, inform operating room and PACU staff of this decision.
- Have the patient void.
- Put on a surgical cap and gown.
- Take and record vital signs.
- Make sure the informed consent form is signed by the patient or a responsible family member.
- If the surgical site involves a right or left distinction, multiple structures (such as fingers or toes), or multiple levels (such as the spine), the site should be marked with a permanent marker by the person doing the procedure. The site should be marked before the patient is taken to the area where the procedure will be done, and the marking should be visible after the patient is prepped and draped.
- Administer preoperative medication as ordered.

Intraoperative care

The intraoperative period begins with the transfer of the patient to the operating room bed and ends with his admission to the PACU. No matter what kind of surgery your patient needs, he'll receive an anesthetic during this time.

Anesthesia

To induce loss of the pain sensation, the anesthesiologist or nurse-anesthetist will use some form of anesthesia. (See *Types of anesthesia*.)

Types of anesthesia

The three types of anesthesia are general, regional, and balanced. This chart describes each type.

Type	Description
General	• Blocks awareness centers in the brain • Produces unconsciousness, body relaxation, and loss of sensation • Is administered by inhalation or I.V. infusion
Regional	• Inhibits excitatory processes in nerve endings or fibers • Provides analgesia over a specific body area • Doesn't produce unconsciousness • Can be applied topically or be injected (nerve infiltration or epidural or spinal administration)
Balanced	• Combines opioid analgesics, sedative-hypnotics, nitrous oxide, and muscle relaxants • Induces rapid anesthesia with minimal cardiac depression and decreased postoperative adverse effects (such as nausea and pain) • Produces sleep and analgesia, eliminating certain reflexes and providing good muscle relaxation

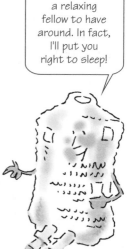

I'm quite a relaxing fellow to have around. In fact, I'll put you right to sleep!

What OR nurses do

Operating room responsibilities are divided between the scrub nurse and the circulating nurse. The scrub nurse scrubs before the operation, sets up the sterile table, prepares sutures and special equipment, and provides help to the surgeon and his assistants throughout the operation. The circulating nurse manages the operating room and monitors cleanliness, humidity, lighting, and safety of equipment. She also coordinates activities of operating room personnel, monitors aseptic practices, assists in monitoring the patient, and acts as a patient safety advocate.

Other nursing responsibilities during the intraoperative period may include positioning the patient, preparing the incision site, draping the patient, and documenting information (such as surgical team information, assessment, the care and handling of specimens, and the count sheet).

Time out for safety

Just before the procedure begins, the entire operative team stops and performs a final verification of the correct patient, procedure, and surgical site. Called a *time out*, this final step helps prevent serious errors from occurring.

Postoperative care

The patient's recovery from the anesthesia is monitored in the PACU. His ongoing recovery is managed on either an intensive care unit (ICU) or medical-surgical unit. The postoperative period extends from the time the patient leaves the operating room until the last follow-up visit with the surgeon.

What the PACU nurse does

The postoperative period begins when the patient arrives in the PACU, accompanied by the anesthesiologist or nurse-anesthetist. The PACU nurse's main goal is to meet the patient's physical and emotional needs, thereby minimizing the development of postoperative complications. Such factors as pain, lack of oxygen, and sudden movement may threaten his physiologic equilibrium.

Thanks to the use of short-acting anesthetics, the average PACU stay lasts less than 1 hour. The patient is assessed every 10 to 15 minutes initially and then as his condition warrants.

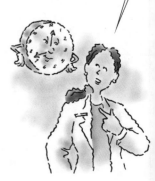

Thanks to technological advances, the average PACU stay is less than 1 hour.

Discharge

Whether the patient is discharged from the PACU to the medical-surgical unit, the ICU, or to the short-procedure unit, safety remains the major consideration. The patient should:
• demonstrate quiet and unlabored respirations
• be awake or easily aroused to answer simple questions
• have stable vital signs with a patent airway and spontaneous respirations
• have a gag reflex
• feel minimal pain

- have return of movement and partial return of sensation to all anesthetized areas if a regional anesthetic was administered.

If the patient had major surgery or has a concurrent serious illness or if complications occurred during or immediately after surgery, he may be discharged to the ICU. Appropriate documentation should accompany the patient on discharge, according to facility policy.

Medical-surgical unit

When assessing the patient after he returns to the medical-surgical unit, be systematic yet sensitive to his needs. Compare your findings with intraoperative and preoperative assessment findings, and report significant changes immediately.

Have a system

Follow a systematic approach to your physical assessment in order to make easier comparisons. Facilities typically have protocols for assessing patients postoperatively. Some facilities require assessments every 15 minutes until the patient stabilizes, every hour for the next 4 hours, and then every 4 hours after that.

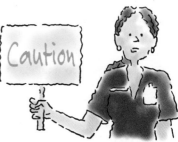

Immediately report postoperative findings that significantly differ from preoperative or intraoperative assessment findings.

Caution

Assessing postoperative status

Pay special attention to the patient's breathing. Make sure the patient has a patent airway and check his respiratory rate, rhythm, and depth. Additional assessment measures include:
- assessing the patient's level of consciousness by testing his ability to follow commands
- observing for tracheal deviation from the midline
- noting chest symmetry, lung expansion, or use of accessory muscles
- obtaining the patient's blood pressure (systolic pressure shouldn't vary more than 15% from the preoperative reading except in patients who experience preoperative hypotension)
- taking the patient's apical pulse rate for 1 minute and assessing the rate and quality of radial and pedal pulses, noting any dependent edema
- taking the patient's temperature, which may be low (due to slowing of basal metabolism associated with anesthesia or to the cold operating room or I.V. solution) or high (due to the body's response to the trauma of surgery).

Encourage deep breathing to promote elimination of the anesthetic and optimal gas exchange and acid-base balance.

Assessing for respiratory distress

You should assess for signs of respiratory distress as part of your postoperative assessment. Contact the doctor if your findings include the following signs.

The blues
Cyanosis is a major indicator of respiratory distress. Circumoral, nail bed, or sublingual cyanosis indicates an arterial oxygen saturation level of less than 90%. Earlobe cyanosis, usually accompanying chronic obstructive pulmonary disease, may be exacerbated by anesthesia.

Other signs
Also, assess for other signs of respiratory distress, including:
• nasal flaring
• inspiratory or expiratory grunts
• changes in posture to ease breathing
• progressive disorientation.

A little help from your friends
You may use a pulse oximeter to supplement your assessment. Report a saturation level of 90% or less.

Encourage coughing if the patient has secretions. Excessive sedation from analgesics or a general anesthetic can cause respiratory depression. Respiratory depression can also occur if reversal agents wear off. (See *Assessing for respiratory distress.*)

Examining the surgical wound

When examining the surgical wound, follow the practitioner's orders. Don't remove dressings from a surgical wound without permission. Some dressings provide pressure to the wound; others keep skin grafts intact. If the dressing is stained by drainage, estimate the quantity and note its color and odor. Reinforce wet dressings with additional sterile dressings. If the patient has a drainage device, record the amount and color of drainage. Make sure the device is secure and free from kinks. If the patient has an ileostomy or colostomy, describe output. If the wound isn't dressed, note the wound's location and describe its length, width, and type (horizontal, transverse, or puncture). Describe the sutures, staples, or adhesive strips used to close the wound and assess approximation of wound edges.

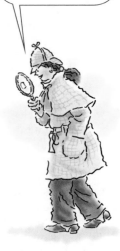

Closely examining surgical wounds can help minimize complications.

Assessing the abdomen

When assessing the abdomen, first observe for changes in abdominal contour. Abdominal dressings, tubes, or other devices may operating room and monitors cleanliness, humidity, lighting, and safety of equipment. She also coordinates activities of operating room personnel, monitors aseptic practices, assists in monitoring the patient, and acts as a patient safety advocate.

Other nursing responsibilities during the intraoperative period may include positioning the patient, preparing the incision site, draping the patient, and documenting information (such as surgical team information, assessment, the care and handling of specimens, and the count sheet).

Time out for safety

Just before the procedure begins, the entire operative team stops and performs a final verification of the correct patient, procedure, and surgical site. Called a *time out*, this final step helps prevent serious errors from occurring.

Postoperative care

The patient's recovery from the anesthesia is monitored in the PACU. His ongoing recovery is managed on either an intensive care unit (ICU) or medical-surgical unit. The postoperative period extends from the time the patient leaves the operating room until the last follow-up visit with the surgeon.

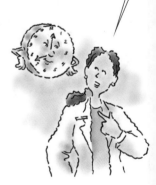

Thanks to technological advances, the average PACU stay is less than 1 hour.

What the PACU nurse does

The postoperative period begins when the patient arrives in the PACU, accompanied by the anesthesiologist or nurse-anesthetist. The PACU nurse's main goal is to meet the patient's physical and emotional needs, thereby minimizing the development of postoperative complications. Such factors as pain, lack of oxygen, and sudden movement may threaten his physiologic equilibrium.

Thanks to the use of short-acting anesthetics, the average PACU stay lasts less than 1 hour. The patient is assessed every 10 to 15 minutes initially and then as his condition warrants.

Discharge

Whether the patient is discharged from the PACU to the medical-surgical unit, the ICU, or to the short-procedure unit, safety remains the major consideration. The patient should:
• demonstrate quiet and unlabored respirations
• be awake or easily aroused to answer simple questions
• have stable vital signs with a patent airway and spontaneous respirations
• have a gag reflex
• feel minimal pain

Intraoperative care

The intraoperative period begins with the transfer of the patient to the operating room bed and ends with his admission to the PACU. No matter what kind of surgery your patient needs, he'll receive an anesthetic during this time.

Anesthesia

To induce loss of the pain sensation, the anesthesiologist or nurse-anesthetist will use some form of anesthesia. (See *Types of anesthesia.*)

Types of anesthesia

The three types of anesthesia are general, regional, and balanced. This chart describes each type.

Type	Description
General	• Blocks awareness centers in the brain • Produces unconsciousness, body relaxation, and loss of sensation • Is administered by inhalation or I.V. infusion
Regional	• Inhibits excitatory processes in nerve endings or fibers • Provides analgesia over a specific body area • Doesn't produce unconsciousness • Can be applied topically or be injected (nerve infiltration or epidural or spinal administration)
Balanced	• Combines opioid analgesics, sedative-hypnotics, nitrous oxide, and muscle relaxants • Induces rapid anesthesia with minimal cardiac depression and decreased postoperative adverse effects (such as nausea and pain) • Produces sleep and analgesia, eliminating certain reflexes and providing good muscle relaxation

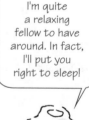

I'm quite a relaxing fellow to have around. In fact, I'll put you right to sleep!

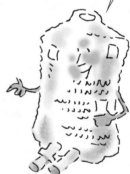

What OR nurses do

Operating room responsibilities are divided between the scrub nurse and the circulating nurse. The scrub nurse scrubs before the operation, sets up the sterile table, prepares sutures and special equipment, and provides help to the surgeon and his assistants throughout the operation. The circulating nurse manages the distort this contour. To detect asymmetry, view the abdomen from the foot of the patient's bed. Also, observe for Cullen's sign, a bluish hue around the umbilicus that commonly accompanies intra-abdominal or peritoneal bleeding.

Auscultation station

Auscultate bowel sounds for at least 1 minute in each of the four quadrants. You probably won't be able to detect bowel sounds for 6 hours or more after surgery because general anesthetics slow peristalsis. If the surgeon handled the patient's intestines during surgery, bowel sounds will be absent even longer.

Patent patient

If the patient has a nasogastric tube, regularly check its patency. Confirm proper tube placement by checking the pH of gastric aspirate (normal pH is from 1 to 4), or by X-ray. Document findings for a baseline assessment and for future reference.

Providing comfort

The postsurgical patient may be unable to assume a comfortable position because of incisional pain, activity restrictions, immobilization devices, or an array of tubes and monitoring lines. Assess the patient's pain by having him rate his pain on a scale of 0 to 10 (with 0 being no pain and 10 being the worst pain imaginable) and offer analgesics as ordered. Although most patients will tell you when they experience severe pain, some may suffer silently. Increased pulse rate and blood pressure may provide the only clues to their condition.

Support, promote, and discuss

Although emotional support can do much to relieve pain, it doesn't replace adequate analgesia. Physical measures, such as positioning, back rubs, and creating a comfortable environment in the patient's room, can also promote comfort and enhance the effectiveness of analgesics. (See *Reducing pain after surgery*.)

Discuss specific measures the patient can take to prevent or reduce incisional pain. (See *Tips for reducing incisional pain*, page 66.) Encourage the patient to request analgesics or use patient-controlled analgesia before pain is severe.

Recording intake and output

Measure postoperative intake of food and fluids, including ice chips, I.V. fluids, blood products, and irrigation fluid. Measure postoperative output of urine, tube drainage, and wound drainage.

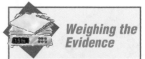

Weighing the Evidence

Reducing pain after surgery

In a recent study, researchers assessed 517 patients who underwent abdominal surgery and received patient-controlled analgesia for pain control. The study looked at the effect of two additional interventions for managing postoperative pain: patient teaching and relaxation with music.

Conclusion

The study found that patient teaching didn't result in a significant reduction in pain. In contrast, relaxation with music resulted in patients reporting a statistically significant decrease in pain. The researchers concluded that adding music with relaxation to analgesics can help ease pain with no adverse effects.

Good, M., et al. (2010). Supplementing relaxation and music for pain after surgery. *Nursing Research*, 59(4), 259-69.

Education edge

Tips for reducing incisional pain

Teach the postoperative patient these techniques to reduce pain when he moves, coughs, or breathes deeply.

Proper movement
Instruct the patient to use the bed's side rails for support when he moves and turns. He should move slowly and smoothly, without sudden jerks. Advise him to wait to move until after his pain medication has taken effect, whenever possible.

The patient should frequently move parts of his body not affected by surgery to prevent them from becoming stiff and sore. Make sure the patient is medicated so that he can move comfortably. If moving alone proves difficult for the patient, urge him to ask a staff member to help.

Splinting the incision
Following chest or abdominal surgery, splinting the incision may help the patient reduce pain when he coughs or moves.

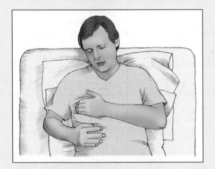

Splinting with the hands
Have the patient place one hand above and the other hand below his incision, as shown, then press gently and breathe normally when he moves.

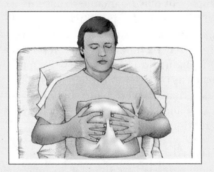

Splinting with a pillow
Alternatively, the patient may place a small pillow over his incision. As he holds the pillow in place with his hands and arms, he should press gently, as shown, breathe normally, and move to a sitting or standing position.

Acting like an adult

An adult should have a minimum urine output of 0.5 to 1 ml/kg/ hour. Report an output of less than 30 ml/hour for more than 2 consecutive hours. After surgery, the patient may have difficulty voiding; this occurs when medications, such as atropine, depress parasympathetic stimulation. In order to assess for catheterization, monitor the patient's intake and palpate his bladder or use a bladder scanner regularly. Because some anesthetics slow peristalsis, the patient may not defecate until his bowel sounds return.

Ordinary output

When documenting output, note the source of output; its quantity, color, and consistency; and the duration over which the output occurred. Notify the practitioner of significant changes, such as a change in the color and consistency of nasogastric contents from dark green to "coffee grounds" or a larger volume of output than expected.

Postoperative complications

After surgery, take steps to avoid complications. Be ready to recognize and manage them if they occur.

Reducing the risk of complications

To avoid extending the patient's hospital stay and to speed his recovery, perform these measures to prevent postoperative complications.

Turn and reposition the patient

Turn and reposition the patient every 2 hours to promote circulation and reduce the risk of skin breakdown, especially over bony prominences. When the patient is in a lateral recumbent position, tuck pillows under bony prominences to reduce friction and promote comfort. Each time you turn the patient, carefully inspect the skin to detect redness or other signs of breakdown.

Don't turn 'em all

Keep in mind that turning and repositioning may be contraindicated in some patients such as those who have undergone neurologic or musculoskeletal surgery that demands immobilization postoperatively.

Encourage coughing and deep breathing

Deep breathing promotes lung expansion, which helps clear anesthetics from the body. Coughing and deep breathing also lower the risk of

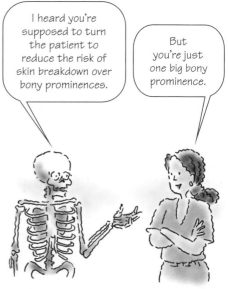

I heard you're supposed to turn the patient to reduce the risk of skin breakdown over bony prominences.

But you're just one big bony prominence.

pulmonary and fat emboli and of hypostatic pneumonia associated with secretion buildup in the airways.

Encourage the patient to deep-breathe and cough every hour while he's awake. (Deep breathing doesn't increase intracranial pressure.) Also, show him how to use an incentive spirometer. (See *Using spirometers*.)

Monitor nutrition and fluids

Adequate nutrition and fluid intake is essential to ensure proper hydration, promote healing, and provide energy to match the increased basal metabolism associated with surgery. If the patient has a protein deficiency or compromised immune function pre-operatively, expect to deliver supplemental protein via parenteral nutrition to promote healing. If he has renal failure, this treatment would be contraindicated because his inability to break down pro-tein could lead to dangerously high blood urea nitrogen levels.

Promote exercise and ambulation

Early postoperative exercise and ambulation can significantly reduce the risk of thromboembolism. They can also improve ven-tilation and brighten the patient's outlook.

Passive, okay; active, better

Perform passive range-of-motion (ROM) exercises — better yet, encourage active ROM exercises — to prevent joint contractures and muscle atrophy and to promote circulation. These exercises can also help you assess the patient's strength and tolerance.

Tolerance test

Before encouraging ambulation, have the patient sit and dangle his legs over the side of the bed and perform deep-breathing exer-cises. How well the patient tolerates this step is usually a key predictor of out-of-bed tolerance. Document frequency of movement, the patient's tolerance, use of analgesics, and any other relevant information.

Despite your best efforts, complications sometimes occur.

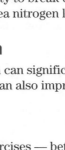

Detecting and managing complications

Despite your best efforts, complications sometimes occur. These may include atelectasis, pneumonia, and pulmonary embolism and thrombophlebitis. By knowing how to recog-nize and manage them, you can limit their effects. (See *Detect-ing and managing postoperative complications*, pages 70 and 71.)

Using spirometers

Although all spirometers encourage slow, sustained maximal inspiration, they can be divided into two types: flow incentive and volume incentive.

Differences between the two

A flow incentive spirometer measures the patient's inspiratory effort (flow rate) in cubic centimeters per second (cc/second). A volume incentive spirometer goes one step further. From the patient's flow rate, it calculates the volume of air the patient inhales. Because of this extra step, many volume incentive spirometers are larger, more complicated, and more expensive than flow incentive spirometers.

Volume incentive

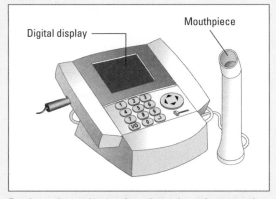

Flow incentive

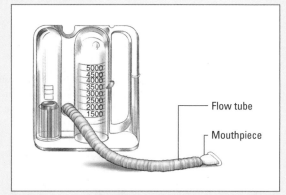

For the patient using a volume incentive spirometer, the practitioner or respiratory therapist will order a "goal volume" (in cubic centimeters) for the patient to reach. This will be the amount of air the patient should inspire when he takes a deep breath.

One type of volume incentive spirometer includes a display of the goal volume. As the patient inhales, the volume of air he takes into his lungs is also shown, climbing a scale until he reaches or surpasses the goal volume. This not only helps him fully expand his lungs, but also provides immediate feedback as to how well he's doing.

The patient usually does this exercise five times each day. Between exercises he should rest. Each morning, he should reset the goal-volume-achieved display so he can try to do even better.

With another smaller and easier-to-use volume incentive spirometer, the patient inhales slowly and deeply as a piston inside a cylinder rises to meet the preset volume. The number of exercises the patient should do each day remains the same.

Flow incentive spirometers have no preset volume. These spirometers contain plastic floats that rise according to how much air the patient pulls through the device with inhalation. The cylinder that encloses the floats is graduated so the patient can monitor his progress. The number of exercises the patient should do each day is the same as with volume incentive spirometers.

Choosing the right type

The right type of spirometer depends on the patient's condition. For a low-risk patient, a flow incentive spirometer is probably better. Lightweight and durable, it can be left at the bedside for the patient to use even when you aren't there to supervise.

A patient who faces high risk of developing atelectasis may require a volume incentive spirometer. Because it measures lung inflation more precisely, this type of spirometer helps you determine whether your patient is inhaling adequately.

What do I do?

Detecting and managing postoperative complications

This chart will help you recognize some postoperative complications and know how to intervene appropriately.

Complication	What to look for	What to do
Septicemia and septic shock	*For septicemia* • Fever, chills, rash, abdominal distention, prostration, pain, headache, nausea, or diarrhea	*For septicemia* • Obtain specimens (blood, wound, and urine) for culture and sensitivity tests. • Administer antibiotics as ordered. • Monitor vital signs and level of consciousness to detect septic shock.
	For septic shock • Early stages: warm, dry, flushed skin; slightly altered mental status; increased pulse and respiratory rates; decreased or normal blood pressure; and reduced urine output • Late stage: pale, moist, cold skin; significant decrease in mentation, pulse and respiratory rates, blood pressure, and urine output	*For septic shock* • Administer I.V. antibiotics as ordered. • Monitor serum peak and trough levels. • Administer I.V. fluids and blood or blood products.
Paralytic ileus	• Severe abdominal distention and possibly vomiting • Severe constipation, or passage of flatus and small, liquid stools	• Encourage ambulation and keep the patient on nothing by mouth status. • Insert a nasogastric tube as ordered; keep the tube patent and functioning properly. • Monitor for nausea and vomiting. If nausea occurs, administer an antiemetic to prevent vomiting.
Urine retention	• Absence of voided urine • Distended bladder above the level of the symphysis pubis on palpation • Discomfort or pain, restlessness, anxiety, diaphoresis, or hypertension	• Help the patient ambulate as soon as possible after surgery unless contraindicated. • Assist the patient to a normal voiding position and, if possible, leave him alone. • Turn on the water so the patient can hear it and pour warm water over his perineum. • Prepare for urinary catheterization if the patient can't void despite other interventions.
Wound infection, dehiscence, and evisceration	*For wound infection* • Increased tenderness, deep pain, and edema at wound site • Increased pulse rate and temperature • Elevated white blood cell count	*For wound infection* • Obtain a wound culture and sensitivity test as ordered. • Administer antibiotics as ordered. • Irrigate the wound with an appropriate solution as ordered, and monitor wound drainage.

Detecting and managing postoperative complications *(continued)*

Complication	What to look for	What to do
Wound infection, dehiscence, and evisceration *(continued)*	*For dehiscence* • Gushes of serosanguineous fluid from the wound • Patient reports a "popping sensation" after retching or coughing *For evisceration* • Protruding contents; visible coils of intestine	*For dehiscence or evisceration* • Stay with the patient; have a colleague notify the practitioner. • If an abdominal wound dehisces, help the patient to low Fowler's position, with knees bent in. This will decrease abdominal tension. • Cover the extruding wound contents with warm, sterile normal saline soaks. • Monitor the patient's vital signs.
Altered body image	• Comments from the patient that indicate depression or insecurity • Inability to look at or talk about his incision or stoma	• Encourage verbalization and offer support. • Refer to appropriate support group and counseling. • Encourage participation in care.
Postoperative psychosis	• Change in behavior from baseline	• Reorient the patient frequently to person, place, and time. • Place a clock and calendar in his room where he can see them. • Keep changes in his environment to a minimum. • Provide familiar objects close by. • Encourage family participation in postoperative care. • Use sedatives and restraints only if necessary.

Discharge planning

Begin planning for the patient's discharge at your first contact with him. Include his family or other caregivers in your planning to ensure proper home care. The discharge plan should include:
• medication
• diet
• activity
• home care procedures and referrals
• potential complications
• return appointments.

Problem potential

Recognizing potential problems early on will help your discharge plan succeed. The initial nursing history and preoperative

assessment as well as subsequent assessments can provide useful information. Tailor the contents of your plan to the patient's individual needs. Assess the strengths and limitations of the patient and his family. Consider several factors, including:
• physiologic factors — general physical and functional abilities, current medications, and general nutritional status
• psychological factors — self-concept, motivation, and learning abilities
• social factors — duration of care needed, types of services available, and family involvement in the patient's care.

Can I get that in writing?

Provide written materials as a reference for the patient at home. Assess your patient's reading and comprehension level and always make sure that readings are reinforced by personal teaching. Include information on these topics:
• Medications—Teach the patient the purpose of drug therapy, proper dosages and routes, special instructions, potential adverse effects, and when to notify the practitioner. Try to establish a medication schedule that fits in with the patient's lifestyle.

> Medications... diet...activities... home care.... Yep! I've got hand-outs for all of them!

• Diet—Teach the patient and, if appropriate, the family member or caregiver who will prepare his meals. Refer the patient to a dietitian if appropriate.
• Activity—After surgery, the patient is commonly advised not to lift a heavy weight such as a basket of laundry. Restrictions usually last 4 to 6 weeks after surgery. Let him know when he can return to work, drive, and resume sexual activity.
• Home care procedures—After the patient watches you demonstrate a procedure, have him (or his caregiver) perform a return demonstration. If the patient needs to rent or purchase special equipment, such as a hospital bed or walker, give him a list of suppliers in the area.

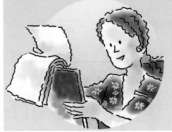

• Wound care—Teach the patient about changing his wound dressing. Tell him to keep the incision clean and dry, and teach proper hand-washing technique.
• Potential complications—Make sure the patient can recognize signs and symptoms of wound infection and other potential complications, and provide this information in writing. Advise the patient to call the practitioner with any questions.
• Return appointments—Stress the importance of the follow-up appointment in your teaching, and make sure the patient has the practitioner's office telephone number. If the patient has no means of transportation, refer him to an appropriate community resource.
• Referrals—Reassess whether the patient needs referral to a home care agency or other community resource. In some hospitals, the responsibility for making referrals falls to a home care coordinator, discharge planning nurse, or case manager.

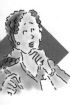

Quick quiz

1. What is the purpose of a thorough preoperative assessment?
    A. To identify and correct problems before surgery and establish a baseline for postoperative comparison
    B. To save time doing an assessment after the patient returns from surgery
    C. To save the practitioner time before the procedure begins
    D. To ensure that postoperative complications don't occur

Answer: A. A thorough preoperative assessment helps systematically identify and correct problems before surgery and establish a baseline for postoperative comparison. During the assessment, the nurse should focus on problem areas suggested by the history and body systems that will be directly affected by surgery.

2. In teaching about pain management, a nurse-educator should discuss:
    A. the need to use pain medication only when absolutely necessary.
    B. that pain medication will be ordered and given according to the patient's needs.
    C. how the method of pain medication administration can't be altered after surgery.
    D. the need to limit narcotics to avoid addiction.

Answer: B. The patient should be aware that pain medication will be ordered and given according to his needs. Because each patient responds differently to pain and medication, dosage and administration is individualized.

3. What is balanced anesthesia?
    A. Medication that enhances certain reflexes and provides good muscle tone
    B. The use of opioid analgesic medication preoperatively, intraoperatively, and postoperatively
    C. A combination of opioid analgesics, sedative-hypnotics, nitrous oxide, and muscle relaxants
    D. The use of both local and general anesthesia

Answer: C. Balanced anesthesia is a combination of opioid analgesics, sedative-hypnotics, nitrous oxide, and muscle relaxants.

4.   The reason that patients are sent to a PACU after surgery is:
    A. to be monitored while recovering from anesthesia.
    B. to remain near the surgeon immediately after surgery.
    C. to allow the medical-surgical unit time to prepare for transfer.
    D. to provide time for the patient to cope with the effects of surgery.

Answer: A. Patients are sent to a PACU to be monitored while they're recovering from anesthesia.

5.   To help prevent postoperative complications, the nurse should:
    A. have the patient rest quietly for the first 24 hours with minimal exertion.
    B. have the patient splint his incision and take deep, rapid breaths before moving.
    C. encourage the patient to begin exercising as soon as possible after surgery.
    D. encourage the patient to drink increased fluids beginning immediately after surgery.

Answer: C. Early postoperative exercises and ambulation can significantly improve circulation, ventilation, and psychological outlook.

6.   Discharge planning should begin on:
    A. the day of admission.
    B. the day after surgery.
    C. the day of discharge.
    D. the day of surgery.

Answer: A. Although the day of admission may also be the day of surgery, planning for the patient's discharge should begin on admission and first contact with the patient.

Scoring

☆☆☆ If you answered all six questions correctly, wowee! You're perioperative perfection!

☆☆ If you answered four or five questions correctly, gadzooks! You're perilously close to perfect in perioperative care!

☆ If you answered fewer than four questions correctly, perk up! Follow this perioperative teaching plan: Review the chapter and try again!

Pain management

Just the facts

In this chapter, you'll learn:

♦ types of pain and theories that explain them

♦ ways in which opioid and nonopioid analgesics control pain

♦ interventions to help alleviate pain.

A look at pain

Pain is a complex, subjective phenomenon that involves biological, psychological, cultural, and social factors. To put it succinctly, pain is whatever the patient says it is, and it occurs whenever she says it does. The only true authority on any given pain is the person experiencing it. Therefore, health care professionals must understand and rely on the patient's description of her pain when developing a pain management plan. The Joint Commission requires that all patients be assessed for pain.

Each patient reacts to pain differently because pain thresholds and tolerances vary. Pain threshold is a physiologic attribute that denotes the smallest intensity of a painful stimulus required to perceive pain. Pain tolerance is a psychological attribute that describes the amount of stimulus (duration and intensity) that the patient can endure before stating that she's in pain.

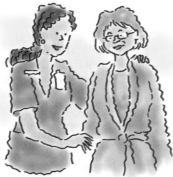

Pain is whatever the patient says it is and occurs whenever she says it does.

Theories about pain

Three theories attempt to explain the mechanisms of pain:

☝ specificity

✌ pattern

🤟 gate control.

Let's get specific

The specificity theory maintains that individual specialized periph-eral nerve fibers are responsible for pain transmission. This bio-logically oriented theory doesn't explain pain tolerance, nor does it allow for social, cultural, or empirical factors that influence pain.

Pain pattern

The pattern theory suggests that excessive stimulation of all nerve endings produces a unique pattern interpreted by the cerebral cortex as pain. Although this theory addresses the brain's ability to determine the amount, intensity, and type of sensory input, it doesn't address nonbiological influences on pain perception and transmission.

Opening the gate

The gate control theory asserts that some sort of gate mechanism in the spinal cord allows nerve fibers to receive pain sensations. (See *Understanding the gate control theory*.) This theory has encouraged a more holistic approach to pain management and research by taking into account the nonbiological components of pain. Pain management techniques, such as cutaneous stimulation, distraction, and acupuncture are, in part, based on this theory.

Categorizing pain by duration

There are two fundamental pain types that are classified accord-ing to their duration: acute and chronic.

Acute pain

Acute pain commonly accompanies tissue damage from injury or disease. It varies from mild to severe in intensity and typically lasts for a brief period (less than 6 months). Acute pain is consid-ered a protective mechanism, alerting the individual to tissue dam-age or organ disease. A patient can get relief from acute pain, and the pain itself dissipates as the underlying disorder heals.

Relief and healing

Treatment goals for acute pain include relieving pain and healing the underlying injury or disease responsible for the pain. Palliative treatment may include surgery, drug therapy, application of heat or cold, or psychological and behavioral techniques to control pain.

A closer look

Understanding the gate control theory

Intensive research into the pathophysiology of pain has yielded several theories about pain perception, including the Melzack-Wall gate control theory. According to this theory, pain and thermal impulses travel along small-diameter, slow-conducting afferent nerve fibers to the spinal cord's dorsal horns. There, they terminate in an area of gray matter called the *substantia gelatinosa.*

Open or close the gate
When sensory stimulation reaches a critical level, a theoretical "gate" in the substantia gelatinosa opens, allowing nearby transmission cells to send the pain impulse to the brain along the interspinal neurons to the spinothalamic tract, and then to the thalamus and cerebral cortex (see

illustration below, left). The small size of the fibers enhances pain transmission.

In contrast, large-diameter fibers inhibit pain transmission. Stimulation of these large, fast-conducting afferent nerve fibers counters the input of the smaller fibers, thereby closing the theoretical gate in the substantia gelatinosa and blocking the pain transmission (see illustration below, right).

Keys to the gate
Descending (efferent) impulses along various tracts from the brain and brain stem can enhance or reduce pain transmission at the gate. For example, triggering specific brain processes, such as attention, emotions, and memory of pain, can intensify pain by opening the gate.

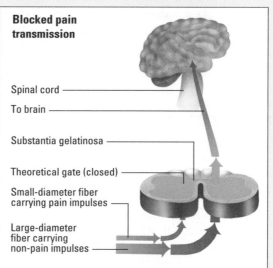

Pain impulse transmission

Spinal cord

To brain

Substantia gelatinosa

Theoretical gate (open)

Small-diameter fiber carrying pain impulses

How we perceive pain
This diagram shows how pain impulses traveling along a small-diameter nerve fiber pass through an open gate in the substantia gelatinosa, and then travel to the brain for interpretation.

Blocked pain transmission

Spinal cord

To brain

Substantia gelatinosa

Theoretical gate (closed)

Small-diameter fiber carrying pain impulses

Large-diameter fiber carrying non-pain impulses

How pain transmission is blocked
Impulses carried by a large-diameter fiber can close the gate to small-fiber impulses, blocking the transmission of pain.

Chronic pain

The cause of chronic pain isn't always clear. Chronic pain can stem from prolonged disease or dysfunction, as in cancer and arthritis, or it can be associated with a mental disorder such as posttraumatic stress syndrome. It can be intermittent, limited, or persistent and usually lasts 6 months or longer. Instead of stemming from an easily identifiable location, chronic pain is typically generalized. It's also strongly influenced by the patient's emotions and environment.

Not the pain next door

Patients with chronic pain often have difficulty describing what they're feeling. Different patients also react to the pain in different ways. One may cry out or moan; another may simply withdraw. Changes in appetite and sleep may occur, and patients may become anxious or irritable, but vital signs frequently don't change.

If you can't beat it, work with it

With many patients unable to find complete relief, chronic pain can become a life-altering condition, making long-term pain management challenging. The main goal is to help patients participate as fully as possible in desired daily activities and to get adequate rest, which can improve emotional well-being. Treatments include the use of analgesic medications supplemented with such therapies as massage, heat or ice packs, exercise, meditation, and distraction.

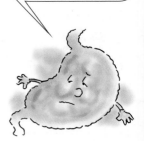

Visceral pain comes from organs, like the stomach. That doesn't make me feel too well.

Categorizing pain by physiologic source

Pain can be classified not just by its duration but also by its physiologic source.

Nociceptive pain

In *nociceptive pain*, injury or inflammation stimulates special injury-sensing receptors in the peripheral nervous system. The receptors then communicate this information to the brain, resulting in the sensation of pain. The two types of nociceptive pain are *somatic pain*, which comes from skin, musculoskeletal structures, or connective tissue, and *visceral pain*, which initiates in organs and the lining of body cavities.

Neuropathic pain

Damage to peripheral nerves or to the central nervous system can result in *neuropathic pain*. Patients describe this poorly localized type of pain as tingling, burning or fiery, or shooting. Types of neuropathic pain include phantom limb pain that occurs after a limb amputation as well as the peripheral extremity pain that diabetics often experience.

Assessing pain

The only way to get an accurate understanding of the patient's pain is to ask him. Begin by asking the patient to describe his pain. Where does it hurt? What exactly does it feel like? When does it start, how long does it last, and how often does it recur? What provokes it? What makes it feel better? There are a variety of assessment tools that can help. Use one to obtain a more accurate and consistent description of pain intensity and relief — two important measurements. The key to effective pain management is an accurate baseline assessment and continual reassessment of the pain. (See *Pain assessment tools*.)

Where does it hurt?

Find out how the patient responds to pain. Does his pain interfere with eating? Sleeping? Working? His sex life? His relationships? Ask the patient to point to the area where he feels pain, keeping in mind that:
- localized pain is felt only at its origin
- projected pain travels along the nerve pathways
- radiated pain extends in several directions from the point of origin
- referred pain occurs in places remote from the site of origin.

Nature's source

Factors that influence the nature of a patient's pain include duration, severity, and source. The source may be:
- cutaneous, originating in the skin or subcutaneous tissue
- deep somatic, which includes nerve, bone, muscle, and supporting tissue
- visceral, which includes the body organs.

Watch for physiologic responses to pain (nausea, vomiting, changes in vital signs) and behavioral responses to pain (facial expression, movement and positioning, what the patient says or doesn't say). Also note psychological responses, such as anger, depression, and irritability.

All about attitude

Assess the patient's attitude about pain. Ask him how he usually handles pain. Does he tell others when he hurts, or does he try to hide it? Does his family understand his pain and try to help him deal with it? Does he accept their help?

Pain assessment tools

Several easy-to-use tools can help you better understand the patient's pain:
- A *rating scale* is a quick method of determining the patient's perception of pain intensity. Ask him to rate his pain on a scale from 0 to 10, with 0 representing pain-free and 10 representing the most pain imaginable.
- A *face rating scale* uses illustrations of five or more faces with expressions that range from happy to very unhappy. The patient chooses the face that represents how he feels at the moment. It's particularly useful with a young child or a patient with language difficulty.
- A *body diagram* allows the patient to draw the location and radiation of pain on an illustration of the body.
- A *questionnaire* provides the patient with key questions about the pain's location, intensity, quality, onset, and factors that relieve and aggravate pain.

Managing pain

Pain management can involve drug therapy with opioid or nonopioid analgesics, including patient-controlled analgesia (PCA) and adjuvant analgesics; neurosurgery; transcutaneous electrical nerve stimulation (TENS); cognitive-behavioral strategies; and intrathecal drug delivery via a pain-control pump.

Opioid analgesics

Opioid analgesics are prescribed to relieve moderate to severe pain. Opioids can be natural or synthetic. Natural opium alkaloids and their derivatives are called opiates. Morphine (Duramorph) is the prototype for both natural and synthetic opioid analgesics.

The agony and the ecstasy

Opioid analgesics are classified as full agonists, partial agonists, or mixed agonist-antagonists. Agonists are drugs that produce analgesia by binding to central nervous system (CNS) opiate receptors. These drugs are the drugs of choice for severe chronic pain. They include:

- codeine
- hydromorphone (Dilaudid)
- hydrocodone
- fentanyl transdermal system (Duragesic)
- methadone (Dolophine)
- morphine.

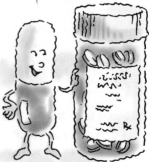

Agonists are the drugs of choice for severe chronic pain.

Up the anti

Agonist-antagonists also produce analgesia by binding to CNS receptors. However, they're of limited use for patients with chronic pain because many have a ceiling effect or upper dosing limit. As the dosage increases, they also can cause hallucinations and other psychotomimetic effects and, in opioid-dependent patients, can produce withdrawal symptoms. This class of drugs includes:

- buprenorphine (Buprenex)
- butorphanol (Stadol)
- nalbuphine
- pentazocine (Talwin).

Any route you choose

Opioid analgesics can be given by many routes, including oral, sublingual, buccal, intranasal, rectal, transdermal, I.M., I.V., epidural, intrathecal, and PCA device. For most patients, oral administration is preferred. I.M. administration, though effective, can result in erratic absorption, especially in debilitated patients.

For severe pain, such as the pain caused by an angina attack, I.V. administration may be preferred because it allows the drug to take effect quickly and permits precise dosage control. Be aware that sudden profound respiratory depression and hypotension can occur with this route. Continuous I.V. infusion using a PCA system allows lower dosing. (See *Understanding patient-controlled analgesia,* page 82.)

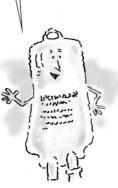

I.V. administration is preferred for severe pain because it allows the drug to take effect quickly and permits precise dosing.

Caution is the key

Opioids can produce severe adverse effects; therefore, caution is the key. They're contraindicated in patients with severe respiratory depression and should be used cautiously in patients with:
• chronic obstructive pulmonary disease
• hepatic or renal impairment because they're metabolized by the liver and excreted by the kidneys
• head injuries or any condition that raises intracranial pressure (ICP) because they increase ICP and can induce miosis (which can mask pupil dilation, an indicator of increased ICP).

But wait, there's more...

Other possible adverse effects include drowsiness, dizziness, nausea, vomiting, itching, constipation, and urine retention. Prolonged use of opioids can cause physical dependency, an expected consequence of long-term opioid use that shouldn't be confused with addiction.

I'll pencil you in

Analgesic schedules are commonly used in managing chronic pain. This approach may call for a single medication (usually an opioid) or a combination of medications to be administered on a set schedule. If breakthrough or acute pain occurs, additional medications may be added.

Monitoring

Before giving an opioid analgesic, make sure the patient isn't already taking a CNS depressant such as a barbiturate. Concurrent

Understanding patient-controlled analgesia

A patient-controlled analgesia (PCA) system provides optimal opioid dosing while maintaining a constant serum concentration of the drug.

How it works

A PCA system consists of a syringe injection pump piggybacked into an I.V. or subcutaneous infusion port. When the patient presses a button, he receives a preset bolus dose of medication. The prescriber orders the bolus dose and the "lock-out" time between boluses, thus preventing overdose. The device automatically records the number of times the patient presses the button, helping the prescriber adjust the dosage.

In some cases, the PCA system allows a reduction in drug dosage, possibly because the patient feels more control over his pain relief and knows that, if he's in pain, analgesia is quickly available. This tends to reduce the patient's level of stress and anxiety, which can exacerbate pain.

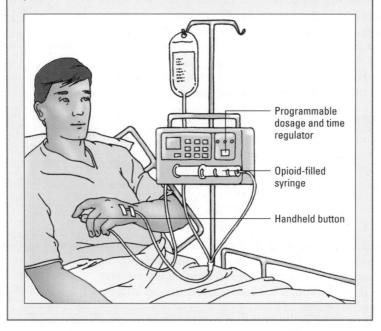

Programmable dosage and time regulator

Opioid-filled syringe

Handheld button

use of another CNS depressant enhances drowsiness, sedation, and disorientation.

During administration, check the patient's vital signs and watch for respiratory depression. If his respiratory rate declines to 10 breaths/minute or less, call his name, touch him, and tell him to breathe deeply. If he can't be aroused or if he's confused or restless, notify the practitioner and prepare to administer oxygen. If ordered, administer an opioid antagonist such as naloxone.

Countering adverse effects

Opioids may have several adverse effects. To prevent or manage them, follow these recommendations:
• If the patient experiences persistent nausea and vomiting during therapy, ask the practitioner about changing medications and give the patient an antiemetic, such as promethazine (Phenergan), as ordered.
• To help prevent constipation, administer a stool softener together with a mild laxative. Also, provide a high-fiber diet, and encourage fluids, as ordered. Regular exercise may also promote motility.
• Encourage the patient to practice coughing and deep-breathing. These exercises promote ventilation and prevent pooling of secretions, which can cause respiratory difficulty.
• Because opioid analgesics can cause postural hypotension, take measures to avoid accidents. For example, keep the bed at the lowest level with its side rails raised. If the patient is able to move around, help him in and out of bed and walk with him to provide support if necessary.

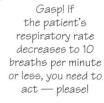

Gasp! If the patient's respiratory rate decreases to 10 breaths per minute or less, you need to act — please!

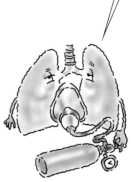

Evaluate for effect

Evaluate the effectiveness of the drug. Is the patient experiencing relief? Does his dosage need to be increased because of persistent or worsening pain? Is he developing a tolerance to the drug? Remember that the patient should receive the smallest effective dose over the shortest period. At the same time, a dosage that's too low to be effective is pointless. Opioid analgesics are safe and effective; they simply require close monitoring to ensure the most effective dosage. Physical and psychological dependence are rare. In fact, psychological dependence occurs in less than 1% of hospitalized patients.

Getting worse instead of better?

Not all patients develop a tolerance to opioids. If a patient has been taking an opioid long-term and suddenly doesn't have pain relief, check for worsening of the patient's condition. Don't assume he has developed tolerance.

Patient teaching

Teach the patient about his drug therapy and ways to avoid or resolve adverse effects. Tell him to:
• take the prescribed drug before the pain becomes intense to maximize its effectiveness and talk with the practitioner if the drug seems less effective over time

- not increase the dose or frequency of administration and take a missed dose as soon as he remembers, while maintaining the interval between doses
- skip the missed dose if it's just about time for the next dose to avoid serious complications of a double dose
- refrain from drinking alcohol while taking the drug to avoid pronounced CNS depression
- talk with his practitioner if he decides to stop taking the drug because the practitioner can suggest an appropriate gradual dosage reduction to avoid withdrawal symptoms
- avoid postural hypotension by getting up slowly when getting out of bed or a chair
- eat a high-fiber diet, drink plenty of fluids, and take a stool softener, if prescribed.

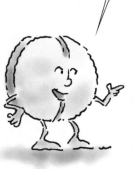

When opioid and nonopioid analgesics are used together, they relieve moderate to severe pain...

Watch out for O.D.

Teach the patient's family the signs of overdose: cold, clammy skin; confusion; severe drowsiness or restlessness; slow or irregular breathing; pinpoint pupils; or unconsciousness. Tell them to notify the practitioner immediately if they notice these signs. Teach them how to maintain the patient's respiration in an emergency until help arrives.

Weighing the evidence

Addressing addiction fears

One barrier to effective pain management is the fear many health care providers have that patients may become addicted to opium analgesics. To study this fear of patient addiction, researchers looked at the usual practices of 145 nurses providing care to patients considered to be at high risk for addiction who were receiving treatment for pain.

Experience and confidence pay off

The researchers found that one third of the nurses were reluctant to discuss addiction with their patients; those most likely to talk about addiction with their patients were more experienced, independent, and confident. The researchers concluded that pain management facilities should retain staff members experienced in pain assessment and develop strategies to improve the confidence and skills of less experienced nurses.

Goebel, J.R., et al. (2010). Addressing patients' concerns about pain management and addiction risks. *Pain Management Nursing, 11*(2), 92-8.

Avoiding addiction

A concern many health care workers have when caring for patients taking opioid analgesics is the risk of addiction. Discussing the possibility with at-risk patients can help reduce that risk. (See *Addressing addiction fears*.)

Nonopioid analgesics

Nonopioid analgesics are prescribed to manage mild to moderate pain. When used with an opioid analgesic, they help relieve moderate to severe pain and also allow lower dosing of the opioid agent. These drugs include acetaminophen (Tylenol) and NSAIDs, such as aspirin, ibuprofen (Advil), indomethacin (Indocin), naproxen (Naprosyn), naproxen sodium (Aleve), and ketorolac.

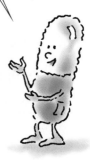

...plus, they allow lower dosing of the opioid — which is always a good thing!

Special effects

NSAIDs and acetaminophen produce antipyretic and analgesic effects. In addition, as their name suggests, NSAIDs have an anti-inflammatory effect. Because these drugs all differ in chemical structure, they vary in their onset of action, duration of effect, and method of metabolism and excretion.

In most cases, the analgesic regimen includes a nonopioid drug even if the patient's pain is severe enough to warrant treatment with an opioid. They're commonly used to treat postoperative and postpartum pain, headache, myalgia, arthralgia, dysmenorrhea, and cancer pain.

Not so special effects

The chief adverse effects of NSAIDs include:
- inhibited platelet aggregation (rebounds when drug is stopped)
- GI irritation
- hepatotoxicity
- nephrotoxicity
- headache.

NSAIDs shouldn't be used in patients with aspirin sensitivity, especially those with allergies, asthma, and aspirin-induced nasal polyps, due to the increased risk of bronchoconstriction or anaphylaxis. Also, NSAIDs are contraindicated in patients with thrombocytopenia, and should be used cautiously in neutropenic patients because antipyretic activity may mask the only sign of infection. Some NSAIDs are contraindicated in patients with renal dysfunction, hypertension, GI inflammation, or ulcers.

Just call me in the morning

Aspirin increases prothrombin and bleeding times; consequently, it's contraindicated in a patient with a bleeding disorder. Don't administer aspirin with anticoagulants or ulcer-causing drugs such as corticosteroids. Avoid aspirin use in a patient scheduled for surgery within 1 week.

Acetaminophen may be used in place of aspirin and other NSAIDs in patients with peptic ulcer or a bleeding disorder. High doses of acetaminophen may lead to hepatic damage, however.

Monitoring

Before administering nonopioid analgesics, check the patient's history for a previous hypersensitivity reaction, which may indicate hypersensitivity to a related drug in this group. If the patient is already taking an NSAID, ask him if he has experienced GI irritation. If he has, the practitioner may choose to reduce the dosage or discontinue the drug.

Always report any abnormalities in renal and liver function studies. Also, monitor hematologic studies and evaluate complaints of nausea or gastric burning. Watch for signs of iron deficiency anemia, such as pallor, unusual fatigue, and weakness.

Patient teaching

For a patient taking an NSAID, teach him the signs and symptoms of overdose, hypersensitivity, and GI bleeding, such as rash, dyspnea, confusion, blurred vision, nausea, bloody vomitus, and black, tarry stools. Tell him to report any of these signs to his practitioner immediately.

If the patient is taking acetaminophen, teach him that nausea, vomiting, abdominal cramps, or diarrhea may indicate an overdose and that he should notify his practitioner immediately.

Understanding adverse effects

To help the patient respond to adverse effects, teach him to:
• take his medication with food or a full glass of water to minimize the GI upset
• remain upright for 15 to 30 minutes after taking his medication if he experiences esophageal irritation
• notify the practitioner if he experiences gastric burning or pain
• take special care to avoid injury that could cause bleeding because NSAIDs can increase bleeding time
• talk to the practitioner about persistent tinnitus (a reversible, dose-related adverse effect)
• exercise caution when driving or using machinery when taking ibuprofen, naproxen, or sulindac (which may cause dizziness)
• get periodic blood tests to detect nephritis or hepatotoxicity.

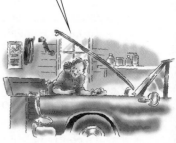

Tell the patient taking NSAIDs to be careful when driving. Of course, if you can't get your car running, that may not be a problem...

Adjuvant analgesics

Adjuvant analgesics are drugs that have other primary indications but are used as analgesics in some circumstances. Adjuvants may be given in combination with opioids or used alone to treat chronic pain. Patients receiving adjuvant analgesics should be reevaluated periodically to monitor their pain level and check for adverse reactions.

A real potpourri

Drugs used as adjuvant analgesics include certain anticonvulsants, local and topical anesthetics, muscle relaxants, tricyclic antidepressants, selective serotonin reuptake inhibitors, benzodiazepines, psychostimulants, and cholinergic blockers. (See *Understanding adjuvant analgesics*.)

Understanding adjuvant analgesics

Adjuvant analgesics are drugs that have other primary indications but are used as analgesics in some circumstances. The major types are discussed here.

Anticonvulsants
Anticonvulsants may be used to treat neuropathic pain (pain generated by peripheral nerves). Carbamazepine (Tegretol) and gabapentin (Neurontin) are the anticonvulsants most commonly used as adjuvant analgesics; others include clonazepam (Klonapin), phenytoin (Dilantin), and valproic acid (Depakene).

Local anesthetics
Local anesthetics may be used to help manage neuropathic pain or as an alternative to general anesthesia. These drugs include:
• amide drugs, such as bupivacaine (Marcaine), lidocaine (Xylocaine), mepivacaine, prilocaine, and ropivacaine
• ester drugs, such as benzocaine, cocaine, chloroprocaine, and procaine.

Topical anesthetics
Topical anesthetics are applied directly to the skin or mucous membranes to prevent or relieve minor pain. These agents include:
• amide drugs, such as lidocaine
• ester drugs, such as benzocaine, cocaine, pramoxine, and tetracaine.

This drug category also includes topical combinations of local anesthetics, such as:
• Aerocaine — a mixture of benzocaine and benzethonium
• Cetacaine — a mixture of benzocaine, butamben, dyclonine, lidocaine, and tetracaine
• EMLA (eutectic mixture of local anesthetics), which contains lidocaine and prilocaine.

Muscle relaxants
Muscle relaxants can be classified as:
• neuromuscular agents (such as pancuronium), used primarily as adjuncts to general anesthesia (and secondarily to induce muscle relaxation and promote relaxation in patients on mechanical ventilation)
• antispasmodic agents, used to relieve spasticity associated with central nervous system disorders, such as baclofen (Lioresal), dantrolene (Dantrium), and diazepam (Valium)
• agents used for short-term pain relief and muscle spasms, such as carisoprodol (Soma), chlorzoxazone, cyclobenzaprine (Flexeril), and tizanidine (Zanaflex).

Tricyclic antidepressants (TCAs)
Of the various types of antidepressants, TCAs have the longest history in managing pain — particularly

(continued)

Understanding adjuvant analgesics (continued)

neuropathic pain. TCAs include amitriptyline, amoxapine; desipramine (Norpamin); doxepin (Silenor); imipramine (Tofranil); nortriptyline (Aventyl); and protriptyline (Vivactil).

Selective serotonin reuptake inhibitors (SSRIs)
A well-known class of antidepressants, SSRIs are being investigated for pain relief as well. These agents include fluoxetine (Prozac); paroxetine (Paxil); and sertraline (Zoloft).

Benzodiazepines
Benzodiazepines are used primarily to ease anxiety. Although they aren't effective in treating acute pain, they have some value in easing muscle spasms. Benzodiazepines include alprazolam (Xanax), diazepam, and lorazepam (Ativan).

Psychostimulants
Psychostimulants are used mainly to treat such disorders as Parkinson's disease and attention deficit hyperactivity disorder. In pain management, they may be used adjunctively to manage acute or chronic pain disorders. Psychostimulants include caffeine, dextroamphetamine, and methylphenidate.

Cholinergic blockers
Cholinergic blockers are used to treat spastic or hyperactive conditions of the GI tract. They relax muscles and decrease GI secretions. Major cholinergic blockers are the belladonna alkaloids, which include belladonna and scopolamine hydrobromide (Scopace).

Neurosurgery

Neurosurgery is an extreme form of pain management and is rarely needed. However, there are a number of procedures, such as rhizotomy and cordotomy, that can control pain by surgically modifying critical points in the nervous system. (See *Surgical interventions for pain.*)

TENS

TENS relieves acute and chronic pain by using a mild electrical current that stimulates nerve fibers to block the transmission of pain impulses to the brain. The current is delivered through electrodes placed on the skin at points determined to be related to the pain. TENS is used to treat:
- chronic pain
- postoperative pain
- dental pain
- labor or pelvic pain
- pain from peripheral neuropathy or nerve injury
- postherpetic neuralgia
- reflex sympathetic dystrophy
- musculoskeletal trauma
- phantom limb pain.

Surgical interventions for pain

Surgery is typically considered to manage pain only when pharmacologic therapies fail. More and more, however, these techniques are being used earlier with excellent effect. Surgical procedures used to treat pain include neurectomy, rhizotomy, cordotomy, cryoanalgesia, radio-frequency lesioning, and percutaneous electrical nerve stimulation.

Neurectomy

Neurectomy involves the resection or partial or total excision of a spinal or cranial nerve. This procedure is relatively quick and only requires local or regional anesthesia. Unfortunately, loss of motor sensation is a possible adverse effect, and pain relief may only be temporary. Peripheral neurectomy is considered when all standard pain management therapies have failed.

Rhizotomy

Rhizotomy involves cutting a nerve to relieve pain. Rhizotomy of the dorsal nerve root may produce analgesia for localized severe pain, such as on the trunk, abdomen, or limb. Motor function is usually unaffected if one dorsal nerve root for the area is left intact.

Cordotomy

Cordotomy can be performed as an open surgery or percutaneously. A unilateral cordotomy is performed to relieve somatic pain on one side of the body. A bilateral cordotomy is performed to relieve visceral pain on both sides of the body.

Cryoanalgesia

Cryoanalgesia deactivates a nerve using a cooled probe that causes temporary nerve injury. Nerve function returns over time and the procedure can be repeated. Cryoanalgesia can provide effective pain relief for the patient with pain from a surgical scar, a neuroma trapped in scar tissue, and occipital neuralgia.

Radio-frequency lesioning

Radio-frequency lesioning may affect the nerve from the heat generated, the magnetic field created by the radio waves, or both. Nerve function is stopped for a prolonged period. If it does return, the procedure can be repeated. The most frequent use of this technology is to treat pain related to the facet joint and lumbar sympathetic and peripheral nerves. Because it's a focused therapy, it's used when specific nerves can be targeted.

Percutaneous electrical nerve stimulation

This technique uses implanted leads and a surface stimulator or implanted generator to block pain impulses by delivering electrical current to a target nerve.

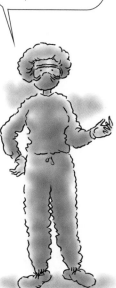

When all pharmacologic therapies fail, surgery may be your patient's best chance for pain relief.

Can't touch this

Although TENS therapy presents few risks, the electrodes should never be placed over the carotid sinus nerves or over laryngeal or pharyngeal muscles. Similarly, the electrodes should never be placed on the eyes or over the uterus of a pregnant patient because this treatment's safety during pregnancy has yet to be determined.

TENS is contraindicated if the patient has a pacemaker. The current may also interfere with electrocardiography or cardiac monitoring. Furthermore, TENS shouldn't be used when the etiology of the pain is unknown because it might mask a new pathology.

Patient preparation

Make sure that the skin beneath the electrode sites is intact. Clean it with an alcohol wipe and dry well. Clip the hair in the area if necessary. Next, if electrodes aren't pregelled, apply a small amount of electrode gel to the bottom of each to improve conductivity. Place the electrodes on the skin. If they aren't self-adhering, secure them with tape, leaving at least 2″ (5 cm) between the electrodes.

Turn that off!

Make sure the controls on the control box are turned to the OFF position. Attach the leadwires to the electrodes, and plug them into the control box. Set the pulse width and rate as recommended. Turn on the unit, and adjust the intensity to the prescribed setting or to the setting most comfortable for the patient. Now secure the unit to the patient. After the prescribed duration of treatment, turn the unit off and remove the electrodes. Wash and dry the patient's skin. Then clean the unit and replace the battery pack.

Monitoring

Assess the patient for signs of excessive or inadequate stimulation. Muscle twitching may indicate overstimulation, whereas an inability to feel any tingling sensation may mean that the current is too low. If the patient complains of pain or intolerable paresthesia, check the settings, connections, and electrode placements. Adjust the settings if necessary. If you must relocate the electrodes during treatment, first turn off the TENS unit. Evaluate the patient's response to each TENS treatment and compare the results. Also, use your baseline assessment to evaluate the effectiveness of the procedure.

Patient teaching

If the patient will use the TENS unit at home, have him demonstrate the procedure, including electrode placement, the setting of the unit's controls, electrode removal, and proper care of the equipment. Explain that he should strictly follow the prescribed settings and electrode placements.

Warn against using high voltage, which can increase pain, or using the unit to treat pain for which he doesn't know the cause. Also, tell the patient to notify the practitioner if pain worsens or develops at another site.

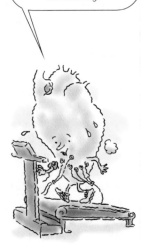

Keep in mind that TENS can interfere with cardiac monitoring.

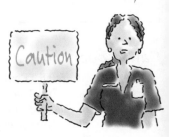

If you must relocate electrodes, first turn off the TENS unit.

Caution

It's electric

If skin irritation occurs, instruct the patient to keep the area clean and apply a soothing lotion. However, if skin breakdown occurs, he should notify the practitioner. Make sure the patient understands that he should remove the unit before bathing or swimming.

Cognitive-behavioral techniques

Behavior modification and relaxation techniques can be used to help the patient reduce the suffering associated with pain. These techniques include biofeedback, distraction, guided imagery, hypnosis, and meditation. These "mind-over-pain" techniques allow the patient to exercise a degree of control over his pain. In addition, they have the added benefit of being virtually risk-free with few contraindications. Even so, if the patient has a significant psychiatric problem, a psychotherapist should teach him the relaxation techniques.

> Behavior modification and relaxation techniques can help reduce pain.

Patient preparation

Because all of these techniques require concentration, try to choose a time when the patient isn't feeling pain or when pain is at its lowest ebb. However, if pain is persistent, begin with short, simple exercises and build on the patient's abilities.

First, relaxxxxx...

Choose a quiet location and dim the lights. Have the patient remove or loosen restrictive clothing. To help the patient lessen muscle tension, tell him to alternately tighten and relax a specific group of muscles — for example, muscles in his neck — while concentrating on tension and relaxation. Repeat the exercise for all muscles groups. If a particular muscle group is painful, move on to the next group.

Good feedback

Biofeedback requires the use of a special machine that allows the patient to see how his body reacts to his efforts. When the patient is connected to the machine, he performs the relaxation technique that he finds most beneficial. The equipment provides feedback regarding his progress with tones, lights, or a digital readout. In this way, the patient can determine which techniques work best to promote relaxation and reduce pain.

Forgetting to feel the pain

Distraction is a technique that involves focusing on music, a book or magazine, or the television or a movie instead of pain and related health issues. If the patient listens to music, suggest that he use a headset to help him focus on the music or imagery produced by the music. Keeping time to the beat or increasing the volume can help if the pain worsens. Other distraction strategies include singing, rhythmic breathing, and meditation.

I have a dream

In *guided imagery*, the patient concentrates on visualizing the calm and peaceful images described by the leader, either you or a recording. Many recordings are available, so the patient should experiment to find imagery that helps him most. Quiet and peaceful nature imagery — for example, the smell of spring grass, the sound of rolling ocean surf, or the burbling of a forest brook — seems to be most effective.

Look into my eyes

Hypnosis is performed by a qualified therapist. During the session, the therapist may use techniques such as symptom suppression, which helps block the patient's awareness of pain, or symptom substitution, which encourages a positive interpretation of pain.

Acting differently

In *behavior modification* therapy, the patient is encouraged to identify behaviors that reinforce or exacerbate pain, suffering, and disability, such as being overly dependent on others or using a cane when it isn't medically indicated. With the therapist's help, the patient defines specific goals, such as reducing his dependence on others, and then uses positive and negative reinforcement to shed old behaviors and promote new, beneficial patterns of behavior.

Monitoring

Remember to be consistent when working with the patient, and make sure that all staff members are aware of the patient's choices for cognitive pain reduction. If the patient becomes frustrated with his progress with any of these techniques, calmly have him stop and try again later. End each session on a positive note by pointing out improvements; even small improvements show progress.

Even small improvements show progress. You're doing great!

Patient teaching

If the patient has overwhelming psychosocial problems, recommend that he seek therapy. Provide him with referrals to appropriate professionals. Any gains in pain management may be quickly lost unless he deals with these factors.

For all others, help develop a plan for using the cognitive-behavioral strategies at home. A plan will increase the likelihood that the patient will continue to benefit from these strategies after he's home again.

Nursing care of the patient in pain

These nursing interventions are appropriate for a patient in pain:
• Assess the pain's location and ask the patient to rate the pain using a pain scale.
• Ask the patient to describe the pain's quality and pattern, including any precipitating or relieving factors.

Making faces

• Monitor the patient's vital signs and note subjective responses to pain, such as facial grimacing and guarding the affected part of the body.
• Administer pain medication around-the-clock, as ordered. This schedule is preferred to as-needed dosing because it avoids major peaks and valleys of pain and relief. Teach the patient the importance of taking the prescribed analgesics before the pain becomes severe.
• Provide comfort measures, such as back massage, positioning, linen changes, and oral or skin care.
• Teach noninvasive techniques to control pain, such as relaxation, guided imagery, distraction, and cutaneous stimulation.
• Explain the role of sleep and the importance of being well rested.

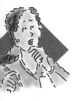

Quick quiz

1.   The person who knows the most about the patient's pain is the:
A.   practitioner.
B.   nurse.
C.   patient.
D.   physical therapist.

Answer: C. The person who experiences the pain—the patient—is the only true authority on that pain.

2. What does the pain threshold reflect?
   A. The frequency of pain that the patient experiences in 24 hours
   B. The duration or intensity of pain the patient can tolerate before openly expressing pain
   C. The location of the pain and the areas to which it radiates
   D. Smallest intensity of a painful stimulus required to perceive pain

Answer: D. A person's pain threshold is a physiologic component that reflects the intensity of stimulus needed to cause painful sensation.

3. The best type of pain assessment tool to use with an adult who has difficulty communicating due to stroke is the:
   A. 0-to-10 number scale.
   B. face rating scale.
   C. body diagram.
   D. questionnaire.

Answer: B. The face rating scale would be best for this patient because he can simply point to the face that illustrates how he's feeling.

4. What should you monitor in a patient taking high doses of acetaminophen over a prolonged period?
   A. Prothrombin time
   B. GI irritation
   C. Liver function
   D. Kidney function

Answer: C. Prolonged use of high doses of acetaminophen increases the risk of liver damage.

5. What makes techniques, such as relaxation, distraction, and guided imagery, effective tools in managing pain?
   A. Drug interaction
   B. Electrical stimulation
   C. Surgical intervention
   D. Power of the mind

Answer: D. The power of the mind makes cognitive-behavioral pain control techniques effective.

Scoring

☆☆☆ If you answered all five questions correctly, bravo! No need for a hypnotist…you've got this pain topic under control.

☆☆ If you answered three or four questions correctly, nicely done! We'd say you just missed a perfect TENS on this quiz.

☆ If you answered fewer than three questions correctly, don't suffer needlessly. A quick review will alleviate your pain.

Neurologic disorders

Just the facts

In this chapter, you'll learn:
♦ neurologic structures and functions
♦ components of a neurologic assessment
♦ diagnostic tests, nursing diagnoses, and treatments for common neurologic disorders.

A look at neurologic disorders

Complex and infinitely diverse, the nervous system is the body's internal communication network. It coordinates all body functions and all adaptations to changes in the body's internal and external environments. Because of the intricacy and complexity of the nervous system, neurologic impairments can manifest in many ways.

Anatomy and physiology

The nervous system is divided into the central nervous system (CNS), the peripheral nervous system, and the autonomic nervous system. Through complex and coordinated interactions, these three parts integrate all physical, intellectual, and emotional activities.

Central nervous system

The CNS includes the brain and the spinal cord, the two structures that collect and interpret voluntary and involuntary motor and sensory stimuli. (See *The CNS*, page 96.)

There's no disguising the fact that I'm the brains of this operation.

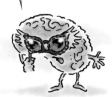

A closer look

The CNS

This illustration shows a cross section of the brain and spinal cord, which together make up the central nervous system (CNS). The brain joins the spinal cord at the base of the skull and ends near the second lumbar vertebra. Note the H-shaped mass of gray matter in the spinal cord.

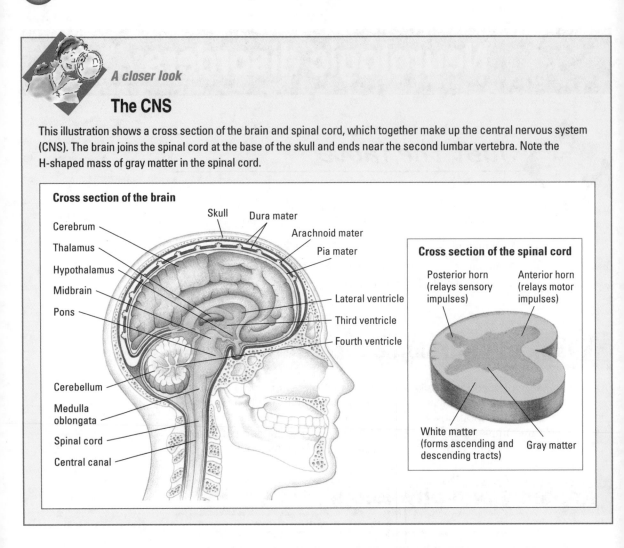

Cross section of the brain

- Cerebrum
- Thalamus
- Hypothalamus
- Midbrain
- Pons
- Cerebellum
- Medulla oblongata
- Spinal cord
- Central canal

Skull
Dura mater
Arachnoid mater
Pia mater

Lateral ventricle
Third ventricle
Fourth ventricle

Cross section of the spinal cord

Posterior horn (relays sensory impulses)
Anterior horn (relays motor impulses)

White matter (forms ascending and descending tracts)
Gray matter

Brain

The brain consists of the cerebrum (cerebral cortex), the brain stem, and the cerebellum. It collects, integrates, and interprets all stimuli; in addition, it initiates and monitors voluntary and involuntary motor activity.

I think; therefore, I am

The cerebrum gives us the ability to think and reason. Within the skull, it's enclosed in three membrane layers called *meninges*. If blood or fluid accumulates between these layers, pressure builds inside the skull and compromises brain function.

The cerebrum has four lobes and two hemispheres. The right hemisphere controls the left side of the body, and the left

A closer look

The lobes of the cerebrum

The cerebrum's four lobes — the parietal, occipital, temporal, and frontal lobes — are discerned by anatomic landmarks and functional differences. The name of each lobe is derived from the overlying cranial bone. This illustration shows the locations of the cerebral lobes and explains their functions. It also shows the location of the cerebellum.

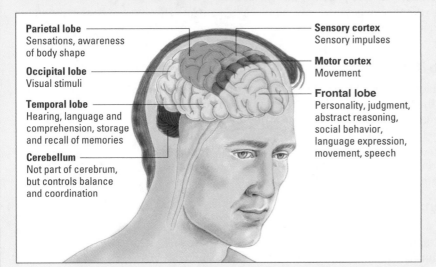

Parietal lobe
Sensations, awareness of body shape

Occipital lobe
Visual stimuli

Temporal lobe
Hearing, language and comprehension, storage and recall of memories

Cerebellum
Not part of cerebrum, but controls balance and coordination

Sensory cortex
Sensory impulses

Motor cortex
Movement

Frontal lobe
Personality, judgment, abstract reasoning, social behavior, language expression, movement, speech

hemisphere controls the right side of the body. Each lobe controls and coordinates specific functions. (See *The lobes of the cerebrum*.)

Regulatory affairs

A part of the cerebrum called the *diencephalon* contains the thalamus and hypothalamus. The thalamus relays sensory impulses and plays an important part in conscious pain awareness. The hypothalamus regulates many body functions, including temperature control, pituitary hormone production, appetite, thirst, and water balance.

Motoring up the path

The brain stem is beneath the diencephalon and is divided into the midbrain, pons, and medulla. The brain stem contains the nuclei for cranial nerves III through XII. It relays messages between the cerebrum and diencephalon and the spinal cord; it also regulates automatic body functions, such as heart rate, breathing, swallowing, and coughing.

Darn! My hypothalamus must be on the fritz again!

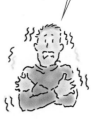

At the back of the brain

The cerebellum is located below the occipital lobes at the back of the brain and consists of two hemispheres. It facilitates smooth, coordinated muscle movement and equilibrium.

Spinal cord

The spinal cord is the primary pathway for nerve impulses traveling between peripheral areas of the body and the brain. It also contains the sensory-to-motor pathway known as the *reflex arc*. A reflex arc is the route followed by nerve impulses to and from the CNS in the production of a reflex action. (See *Understanding the reflex arc*.)

Where it is and what it's got

The spinal cord extends from the upper border of the first cervical vertebra to the lower border of the first lumbar vertebra. It's encased by meninges, the same membrane structure as the brain, and is protected by the bony vertebrae of the spine. The spinal cord is made up of an H-shaped mass of gray matter, divided into the dorsal (posterior) and ventral (anterior) horns. White matter surrounds the horns.

What matter, white matter?

Dorsal white matter contains ascending tracts that transmit impulses up the spinal cord to higher sensory centers. Ventral white matter contains descending motor tracts that transmit motor impulses down from the higher motor centers to the spinal cord.

Mapping the nerves

Sensory (afferent) nerve fibers originate in the nerve roots along the spine — cervical, thoracic, lumbar, or sacral — and supply specific areas of the skin. These areas, known as *dermatomes*, provide a nerve "map" of the body and help when testing sensation to determine the location of a lesion.

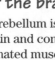

Nerve maps? Sure, we got a ton of them behind the counter. Help yourself! You fellas lost?

Peripheral nervous system

The peripheral nervous system includes the peripheral and cranial nerves. Peripheral sensory nerves transmit stimuli from sensory receptors in the skin, muscles, sensory organs, and viscera to the dorsal horn of the spinal cord. The upper motor neurons of the brain and the lower motor neurons of cell bodies in the ventral horn of the spinal cord carry impulses that affect movement. The 12 pairs of cranial nerves are the primary motor and sensory paths

A closer look

Understanding the reflex arc

The reflex arc is a response system that bypasses the brain and provides a rapid reflex (or response) to a given stimulus. Spinal nerves have sensory and motor portions and control deep tendon and superficial reflexes. A simple reflex arc requires a sensory (afferent) neuron and a motor (efferent) neuron. The knee-jerk or patellar reflex illustrates the sequence of events in a normal reflex arc.

First, a sensory receptor detects the mechanical stimulus produced by the reflex hammer striking the patellar tendon. The sensory neuron carries the impulse along its axon by way of the spinal nerve to the dorsal root, where it enters the spinal column.

Next, in the anterior horn of the spinal cord, shown here, the sensory neuron joins with a motor neuron, which carries the impulse along its axon by way of a spinal nerve to the muscle. The motor neuron transmits the impulse to the muscle fibers through stimulation of the motor end plate. This triggers the muscle contraction that extends the leg. *Don't stand directly in front of a patient when testing this reflex!*

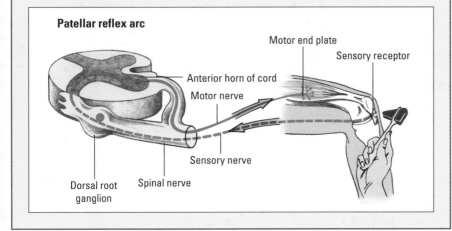

Patellar reflex arc

Motor end plate

Sensory receptor

Anterior horn of cord

Motor nerve

Sensory nerve

Dorsal root ganglion

Spinal nerve

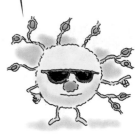

My friends and I make up the autonomic nervous system and help control visceral organs as well as some muscles and glands — which makes us pretty cool dudes.

in the brain, head, and neck. (See *Identifying cranial nerves*, page 100.)

Autonomic nervous system

The autonomic nervous system contains motor neurons that regulate visceral organs and innervate (supply nerves to) smooth and cardiac muscles and the glands. This nervous system has two parts:

Identifying cranial nerves

Each cranial nerve (CN) has sensory function, motor function, or both. Although each cranial nerve has a name, it's also identified by Roman numerals, which are written this way: CN I, CN II, CN III, and so forth. The illustration here shows the location and functions of each cranial nerve.

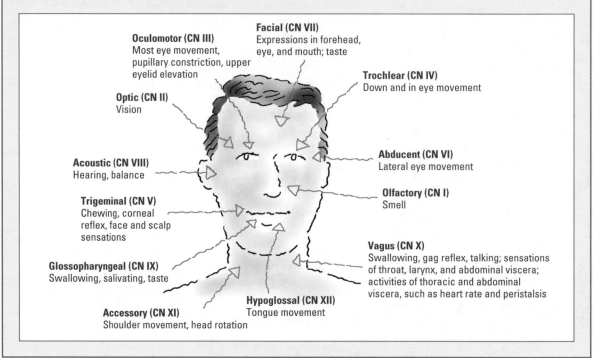

Oculomotor (CN III)
Most eye movement, pupillary constriction, upper eyelid elevation

Facial (CN VII)
Expressions in forehead, eye, and mouth; taste

Optic (CN II)
Vision

Trochlear (CN IV)
Down and in eye movement

Acoustic (CN VIII)
Hearing, balance

Abducent (CN VI)
Lateral eye movement

Trigeminal (CN V)
Chewing, corneal reflex, face and scalp sensations

Olfactory (CN I)
Smell

Glossopharyngeal (CN IX)
Swallowing, salivating, taste

Vagus (CN X)
Swallowing, gag reflex, talking; sensations of throat, larynx, and abdominal viscera; activities of thoracic and abdominal viscera, such as heart rate and peristalsis

Accessory (CN XI)
Shoulder movement, head rotation

Hypoglossal (CN XII)
Tongue movement

- the sympathetic portion, which controls fight-or-flight responses
- the parasympathetic portion, which maintains baseline body functions (rest and digest).

Assessment

Conducting an assessment for possible neurologic impairment includes a thorough health history and an investigation of physical signs of impairment.

History

Begin by asking the patient what brings him to seek care at this time. Gather details about his current health, previous health, family health, and lifestyle. Also, perform a complete systems review. It's best to include members of the patient's family in the assessment process, if they're available, or a close friend. If the patient does have neurologic impairment, he may have trouble remembering or remembering accurately. Family or friends can help corroborate or correct the details.

Current health status

Discover the patient's chief complaint by asking such questions as, "What brings you to the hospital?" or "What has been bothering you lately?" Using his words, document his reasons for seeking care. If he's suffering a neurologic disorder, you can expect reports of headaches, motor disturbances (including weakness, paresis, and paralysis), seizures, sensory deviations, or an altered level of consciousness (LOC).

Ask and you shall perceive

Encourage the patient, or a family member, to elaborate on his current condition by asking such questions as:
• Do you have headaches? If so, how often? What triggers or causes them to occur?
• Do you feel dizzy from time to time? If so, how often and what seems to trigger the episodes?
• Do you ever feel a tingling or prickling sensation or numbness? If so, where?
• Have you ever had seizures or tremors? How about weakness or paralysis in your arms or legs?
• Do you have trouble urinating? Walking?
• How's your memory and ability to concentrate?
• Have you ever had trouble speaking or understanding others?
• Do you have trouble reading or writing?

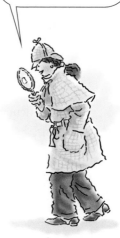

Chronic diseases can affect the neurologic system, so investigate the patient's previous health problems and any medications he may be taking.

Previous health status

Many chronic diseases can affect the neurologic system, so ask the patient what medications, if any, he's taking as well as questions about his past health. Specifically, ask if he has had any:
• major illnesses
• recurrent minor illnesses
• accidents or injuries
• surgical procedures
• allergies.

Family health status

Information about the patient's family may reveal a hereditary disorder. Ask if anyone in his family has had diabetes, cardiac or renal disease, high blood pressure, cancer, a bleeding disorder, a mental disorder, or a stroke.

Lifestyle patterns

The patient's cultural and social background will affect decisions about his care, so ask questions about these facets of his life. Also, note the patient's education level, occupation, drug use, and hobbies. As you gather this information, assess the patient's self-image as well.

Physical examination

A complete neurologic examination is so long and detailed that — as a medical-surgical nurse — you'll probably never perform one in its entirety. Instead, you'll rely on a brief neurologic assessment of key neurologic status indicators, including:
- LOC
- pupil size and response
- verbal responsiveness
- extremity strength and movement
- vital signs.

When baseline values are established, regular reevaluation of these indicators, called *neuro checks*, will reveal trends in the patient's neurologic function and help detect the transient changes that may signal pending problems.

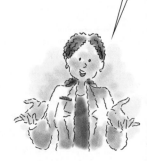

Because a complete neurologic assessment is so long, you'll most likely perform an abbreviated assessment called a neuro-check.

In more detail

If the initial assessment suggests that the patient has an existing neurologic problem, a more detailed assessment is warranted. Always examine the patient's neurologic system in an orderly fashion. Begin with the highest levels of neurologic function and proceed to the lowest, covering these five areas:

mental status (cerebral function)

cranial nerve function

sensory function

motor function

reflexes.

Mental status

Develop a sense of the patient's mental status as you talk with him during the health history. Listen and watch for clues to his orientation and memory. If you have doubts about his mental status, perform a brief screening examination. (See *Quick check of mental status*, page 104.)

Stop, look, and listen

Assessing mental status involves evaluating the patient's LOC, appearance, behavior, speech, cognitive function, and constructional ability:

• *Level of consciousness*—A change in LOC is the earliest and most sensitive indicator that neurologic status has changed. The Glasgow Coma Scale is one objective way to assess the patient's LOC. (See *Using the Glasgow Coma Scale*, page 105.)

• *Appearance and behavior*—Note the patient's behavior, dress, and grooming. Even subtle changes in behavior can signal the onset of chronic disease or an acute change involving the frontal lobe.

• *Speech*—Listen to how well the patient expresses himself. His ability to follow instructions and cooperate with the examination will provide clues about his level of comprehension.

• *Cognitive function*—Evaluate the patient's memory, orientation, attention span, thought content, ability to perform simple calculations, capacity for abstract thought, judgment, and emotional status.

• *Constructional ability*—Assess the patient's ability to perform simple tasks and use common objects.

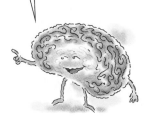

An alteration in the patient's LOC is the earliest sign of a change in his neurologic status.

Cranial nerves

Cranial nerve assessment provides valuable information about the status of the CNS, particularly the brain stem.

Getting on your nerves

Due to their location, the optic, oculomotor, trochlear, and abducens nerves are more vulnerable to an increase in intracranial pressure (ICP) than other cranial nerves. For this reason, assessment and screening focuses on these four nerves. However, if the patient's history or symptoms indicate a potential cranial nerve disorder, or a complete nervous system assessment is ordered, assess all cranial nerves.

Quick check of mental status

You can get a quick idea of how well the patient organizes his thoughts by asking the questions below. An incorrect answer to any question may indicate the need for a more thorough examination of mental status. Be sure you know the correct answers before asking the questions.

Question	Function screened
What's your name?	Orientation to person
What's today's date?	Orientation to time
What year is it?	Orientation to time
Where are you now?	Orientation to place
How old are you?	Memory
Where were you born?	Remote memory
What did you have for breakfast?	Recent memory
Who's the current U.S. president?	General knowledge
Can you count backward from 20 to 1?	Attention and calculation skills
Why are you here?	Judgment

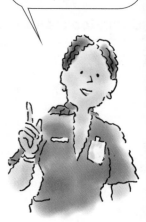

Uh, just one quick suggestion... make sure you know the right answers before you ask the questions.

Sensory function

Sensory function assessment helps reveal problems related to:
• stimuli detection by sensory receptors
• sensory impulse transmission to the spinal cord by afferent nerves
• sensory impulse transmission to the brain by sensory tracts in the spinal cord.

Few and light

Typically, screening consists of evaluating light-touch sensation in all extremities and comparing arms and legs for symmetry of sensation. Most experts also recommend evaluating the patient's sense of pain and vibration in the hands and feet and his ability to recognize objects by touch alone, usually with both eyes closed (stereognosis). Because the sensory system becomes fatigued

Using the Glasgow Coma Scale

The Glasgow Coma Scale provides an easy way to describe a patient's baseline mental status and to help detect and interpret changes from baseline findings. To use the scale, test the patient's ability to respond to verbal, motor, and sensory stimulation and grade your findings according to the scale. If a patient is alert, can follow simple commands, and is oriented to person, place, and time, his score will total 15 points, the highest possible score. A low score in one or more categories may signal an impending neurologic crisis. A total score of 7 or less indicates severe neurologic damage.

Test	Score	Patient's response
Eye opening response		
Spontaneously	4	Opens eyes spontaneously
To speech	3	Opens eyes when told to
To pain	2	Opens eyes only on painful stimulus
Never	1	Doesn't open eyes in response to stimulus
Motor response		
Obeys commands	6	Shows two fingers when asked
Localizes pain	5	Reaches toward painful stimulus and tries to remove it
Withdraws	4	Moves away from painful stimulus
Abnormal flexion	3	Assumes a decorticate posture (in which the hands are toward the cord, shown below) 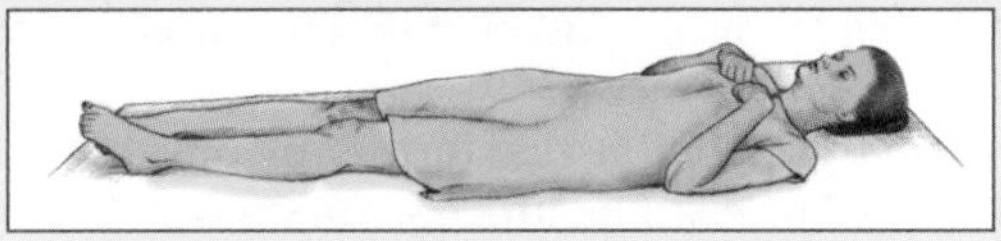

Test	Score	Patient's response
Abnormal extension	2	Assumes a decerebrate posture (shown below) 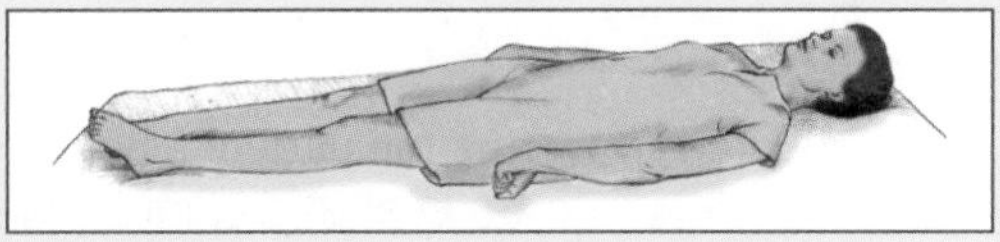

Test	Score	Patient's response
None	1	No response; just lies flaccid (an ominous sign)
Verbal response		
Oriented	5	Tells correct date
Confused conversation	4	Tells incorrect year
Inappropriate words	3	Replies randomly with incorrect words
Incomprehensible	2	Moans or screams
None	1	No response

Total score [ ]

with repeated stimulation, complete sensory system testing in all dermatomes tends to yield unreliable results. Usually, a few screening procedures are sufficient to reveal dysfunction.

Motor function

Assessing the motor system includes inspecting the muscles and testing muscle tone and strength. Cerebellar testing is also done because the cerebellum plays a role in smooth-muscle movements, such as tics, tremors, or fasciculations.

Tone up

Muscle tone represents muscular resistance to passive stretching. To test arm muscle tone, move the shoulder through passive range-of-motion (ROM) exercises. You should feel a slight resistance. Then let the arm drop to the patient's side. It should fall easily.

To test muscle tone in a leg, guide the hip through passive ROM exercises; then let the leg fall to the bed. If it falls into an externally rotated position, this is an abnormal finding.

Strength and symmetry

To perform a general examination of muscle strength, observe the patient's gait and motor activities. To evaluate muscle strength, ask the patient to move major muscles and muscle groups against resistance. For instance, to test shoulder girdle strength, have him extend his arms with his palms up and maintain this position for 30 seconds.

If he can't maintain this position, test further by pushing down on his outstretched arms. If he lifts both arms equally, look for pronation of the hand and downward drift of the arm on the weaker side.

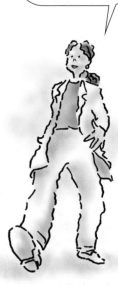

Being able to walk heel to toe demonstrates balance and coordination.

Heel to toe for the cerebellum

Cerebellar function is evaluated by testing the patient's balance and coordination. Ask the patient to walk heel to toe, and observe his balance. Then perform Romberg's test. (See *Romberg's test*.)

Reflexes

Reflex assessment is usually performed as part of a comprehensive neurologic assessment. It evaluates deep tendon and superficial reflexes to determine:
• the integrity of the sensory receptor organ
• how effective afferent nerves are in relaying sensory impulses to the spinal cord

Romberg's test

Romberg's test detects a person's inability to maintain a steady posture with his eyes closed. To perform this test:
• Observe the patient's balance as he stands with his eyes open, feet together, and arms at his sides.
• Ask the patient to close his eyes.
• Hold your arms out on either side of the patient to protect him and observe whether he begins to sway or fall.
   Swaying or falling to one side is considered a positive test result.

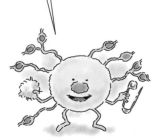

A light, rapid tactile stimulation can elicit a superficial reflex. Don't worry; I'll use the cotton ball, not the pin!

• how effectively the lower motor neurons transmit impulses to the muscles
• how well the muscles respond to the motor impulses.

Deep or superficial?

Deep tendon reflexes (muscle-stretch reflexes) occur when deep muscles stretch in response to a sudden stimulus. Superficial reflexes (cutaneous reflexes) can be elicited by light, rapid tactile stimulation, such as stroking or scratching the skin. Sometimes called *primitive reflexes*, pathologic superficial reflexes usually occur in early infancy and then disappear as time passes. When present in adults, they usually indicate an underlying neurologic disease.

Diagnostic tests

A complete nervous system evaluation typically includes imaging studies, angiography, and electrophysiologic studies. Keep in mind that while these tests may be routine for you, they can be frightening for the patient. It's important to fully explain each procedure and carefully prepare him because stress and anxiety can affect test results.

Imaging studies

The most common imaging studies used to detect neurologic disorders include:
• computed tomography (CT) scan
• isotope brain scan
• magnetic resonance imaging (MRI)

- positron emission tomography (PET)
- skull and spinal X-rays.

Computed tomography scan

CT scanning combines radiology and computer analysis of tissue density (determined by contrast dye absorption) to study intracranial structures. Although CT doesn't show blood vessels as well as an angiogram, it carries less risk of complications and causes less trauma than cerebral angiography.

A scan for all seasons

A CT scan of the spine helps the practitioner to assess spinal disorders, such as a herniated disk, spinal cord tumors, and spinal stenosis. A CT scan of the brain can help detect:
- brain contusion
- brain calcifications
- cerebral atrophy
- hydrocephalus
- inflammation
- space-occupying lesions (tumors, hematomas, abscesses)
- vascular anomalies (arteriovenous malformations [AVMs], infarctions, blood clots, hemorrhage). (See *CT scans and strokes.*)

Nursing considerations
- Confirm that the patient isn't allergic to iodine or shellfish. (A patient with these allergies may have an adverse reaction to the contrast medium and requires premedication with corticosteroids.)
- If the test calls for a contrast medium, explain that an I.V. catheter will be inserted for injection of the contrast medium.

Weighing the evidence

CT scans and strokes

According to the American Stroke Association, any patient suspected of having a stroke should have a CT of the head within 25 minutes after arriving in the emergency department; results of the test should be read within 45 minutes. The results of the CT scan help guide patient treatment during the crucial first 3 hours after the onset of a stroke.

Source: 2005 American Heart Association Guidelines for Cardiopulmonary Resuscitation and Emergency Cardiovascular Care, Part 9: Adult Stroke. (2005). *Circulation 112*(24 Suppl.), IV-111–IV-120.

- Explain to the patient that he may feel flushed or notice a metallic taste in his mouth when the contrast medium is injected (if used).
- Tell him that the CT scanner will circle around him for 10 to 30 minutes (depending on the procedure and type of equipment) and that he must lie still during the test.

Good to go

- Encourage the patient to resume normal activities and a regular diet after the test.
- Explain that the contrast medium may discolor his urine for 24 hours, and suggest that he drink more fluids to help flush this medium out of his system.

Isotope brain scan

In this procedure, a scanning device monitors the brain's uptake of a radioactive isotope, such as technetium-99m pertechnetate. Damaged brain tissue absorbs more of the isotope than healthy tissue (probably due to an abnormally permeable blood-brain barrier). Although the brain scan can locate cerebral lesions and determine their size, it doesn't reveal the cause — for example, whether it's caused by a tumor, cerebral edema, an infarction, a hematoma, or an abscess.

Nursing considerations

- Withhold medications, as ordered.
- Confirm that the patient isn't allergic to iodine or shellfish. (A patient with these allergies may have an adverse reaction to the contrast medium.)
- Explain that an I.V. catheter will be inserted for injection of the contrast medium.
- Tell him that he'll be asked to change position several times during the procedure while a technician takes pictures of his brain.
- Unless contraindicated, encourage the patient to drink more fluids to help flush the contrast medium out of his system.

> Encourage the patient to drink fluids to help flush the contrast medium out of his system.

Magnetic resonance imaging

MRI generates detailed pictures of body structures. The test may involve the use of a contrast medium such as gadolinium.

Feeling superior

Compared with conventional X-rays and CT scans, MRI provides superior contrast of soft tissues, sharply differentiating healthy, benign, and cancerous tissue and clearly revealing blood vessels. In addition, MRI permits imaging in multiple planes, including sagittal and coronal views in regions where bones normally hamper visualization. MRI is especially useful for studying the CNS because it can detect the structural and biochemical abnormalities associated with such conditions as transient ischemic attacks (TIAs), tumors, multiple sclerosis (MS), cerebral edema, and hydrocephalus.

Nursing considerations

• Explain to the patient that the procedure can take up to $1^1/2$ hours and that he'll have to remain still for intervals of 5 to 20 minutes.
• Have the patient remove all metallic items, such as hair clips, bobby pins, jewelry (including body piercing jewelry), watches, eyeglasses, hearing aids, or dentures.
• Ask the patient if he feels claustrophobic in confined spaces. Obtain an order for an antianxiety medication as needed.
• Explain that the test is painless, but the machinery may seem loud and frightening and the tunnel confining. Tell the patient that he'll receive earplugs for the noise, but he'll be in constant communication with the technician.
• Provide sedation, as ordered, to promote relaxation during the test.
• Encourage the patient to resume normal activities, as ordered.

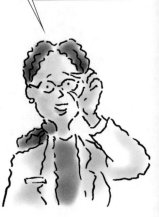

Before an MRI, have the patient remove all metal items, such as hair clips, bobby pins, and jewelery. And don't forget the glasses!

Positron emission tomography

PET provides colorimetric information about the brain's metabolic activity by detecting how quickly tissues consume radioactive isotopes. This technology can help reveal cerebral dysfunction associated with tumors, seizures, TIAs, head trauma, some mental illnesses, Alzheimer's disease, Parkinson's disease, and MS. (See *Neuroimaging and Alzheimer's disease.*) In addition, a PET scan can help evaluate the effect of drug therapy and neurosurgery.

Inject, scan, and translate

In PET, a technician administers a radioactive gas or an I.V. injection of glucose (or another biochemical substance) tagged with isotopes, which act as tracers. The isotopes emit positrons that combine with negatively charged electrons in tissue cells to create gamma rays. After the scanner registers the gamma rays, a computer translates the information into patterns that reflect cerebral blood flow, blood volume, and neuron and neurotransmitter metabolism.

Weighing the evidence

Neuroimaging and Alzheimer's disease

The Alzheimer's Disease Neuroimaging Initiative is a multisite prospective study that's examining the potential cerebrospinal fluid and imaging markers of Alzheimer's disease and their relationship to cognitive changes. Results from the first 12 months of study—which included 210 control subjects, 357 subjects with mild cognitive impairment, and 162 subjects diagnosed with Alzheimer's disease—strongly support the hypothesis that measurable changes in cerebrospinal fluid, positron emission tomography, and magnetic resonance imaging occur well before an actual diagnosis of Alzheimer's disease is made.

Beckett, L.A., et al. (2010). The Alzheimer's disease neuroimaging initiative: Annual change in biomarkers and clinical outcomes. *Alzheimer's & Dementia, 6*(3), 257-64.

Nursing considerations
- Assure the patient that the test won't expose him to dangerous levels of radiation.
- Explain that the test may require insertion of an I.V. catheter.
- Encourage the patient to resume normal activities, as ordered.

Skull and spinal X-rays

Typically, the skull X-ray is taken from two angles: anteroposterior (AP) and lateral. The practitioner may also order other angles, including Waters' view to examine the frontal and maxillary sinuses, facial bones, and eye orbits and Towne's view to examine the occipital bone. Skull X-rays help detect:
- fractures
- bony tumors or unusual calcifications
- pineal displacement (indicates a space-occupying lesion)
- skull or sella turcica erosion (indicates a space-occupying lesion)
- vascular abnormalities.

Is your spine fine?

If the practitioner suspects spinal disease or an injury to the cervical, thoracic, lumbar, or sacral vertebral segments, he may order AP and lateral spinal X-rays. Depending on the patient's condition, he may also order special angles such as the open-mouth view (to confirm odontoid fracture). Spinal X-rays help detect:
- spinal fracture
- displacement and subluxation (partial dislocation)

- destructive lesions (such as primary and metastatic bone tumors)
- arthritic changes or spondylolisthesis
- structural abnormalities (such as kyphosis, scoliosis, and lordosis)
- congenital abnormalities.

Nursing considerations
- Reassure the patient that X-rays are painless.
- Administer an analgesic before the procedure, as ordered, if the patient has existing pain so he'll be more comfortable.
- Remove a cervical collar if cervical X-rays reveal that no fracture is present and the practitioner orders it.
- Encourage the patient to resume normal activities, as ordered.

Angiographic studies

Angiographic studies include cerebral angiography and digital subtraction angiography (DSA).

Cerebral angiography

For cerebral angiography, the radiologist injects a radiopaque contrast medium, usually into the brachial artery (through retrograde brachial injection) or the femoral artery (through catheterization). This procedure highlights cerebral vessels, making it easier to:
- detect stenosis or occlusion associated with thrombi or spasms
- identify aneurysms and arteriovenous malformations (AVMs)
- locate vessel displacement associated with tumors, abscesses, cerebral edema, hematoma, or herniation
- assess collateral circulation.

Nursing considerations
- Explain the procedure to the patient and answer his questions.
- Confirm that he isn't allergic to iodine or shellfish. (A patient with these allergies may have an adverse reaction to the contrast medium and require premedication with corticosteroids.)
- Tell him that he'll need to lie still during the procedure.

Feel the burn
- Explain to the patient that he'll probably feel a flushed sensation in his face as the dye is injected.
- Maintain bed rest, as ordered, and monitor his vital signs and LOC.

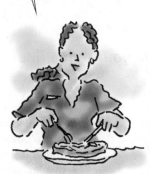

My shellfish allergy means I may have an adverse reaction to contrast media—and means I'm better off ordering steak rather than shrimp for dinner!

- Monitor the catheter injection site for signs of bleeding.
- Monitor vital signs frequently for signs of internal bleeding.
- As ordered, maintain pressure over the injection site.
- Monitor the patient's peripheral pulse in the arm or leg used for catheter insertion (mark the site).
- Unless contraindicated, encourage the patient to drink more fluids to help flush the dye from his system.
- Monitor the patient for neurologic changes and such complications as hemiparesis, hemiplegia, aphasia, and impaired LOC.
- Monitor for an adverse reaction to the contrast medium, which may include restlessness, tachypnea and respiratory distress, tachycardia, facial flushing, urticaria, and nausea and vomiting.

Digital subtraction angiography

Like cerebral angiography, DSA highlights cerebral blood vessels. Using a special type of computerized fluoroscopy, a technician takes an image of the selected area, which is then stored in the computer's memory. After administering a contrast medium, the technician takes several more images. By manipulating the two sets of images, the computer produces high-resolution images for interpretation. Although arterial DSA requires more contrast medium than cerebral angiography, because it's injected I.V., DSA doesn't increase the patient's risk of stroke and can be performed on an outpatient basis.

Nursing considerations

- Confirm that the patient isn't allergic to iodine or shellfish. (A patient with these allergies may have an adverse reaction to the contrast medium and require premedication with corticosteroids.)
- Determine if the patient is taking any anticoagulant or antiplatelet medications; he'll need to stop taking these drugs for a period of time before the procedure.
- Restrict the patient's consumption of solid foods for 4 hours before the test.
- Explain that the test requires insertion of an I.V. catheter.
- Tell him that he must remain still during the test.
- Explain that he'll probably feel a flush or have a metallic taste in his mouth as the contrast medium is injected.
- Tell the patient to alert the doctor immediately if he feels discomfort or shortness of breath.
- After the catheter is removed, encourage the patient to resume his normal activities.
- Encourage him to drink more fluids for the rest of the day to help flush the contrast medium out of his system.

Electrophysiologic studies

Electrophysiologic studies are commonly performed and include EEG and electromyography.

Electroencephalography

By recording the brain's continuous electrical activity, EEG can help identify seizure disorders, head injuries, intracranial lesions (such as abscesses and tumors), TIAs, stroke, or brain death. In EEG, electrodes attached to standard areas of the patient's scalp record a portion of the brain's activity. These electrical impulses are transmitted to an electroencephalogram, which magnifies them 1 million times and records them as brain waves on moving strips of paper.

Nursing considerations

• Tell the patient that during the EEG, he'll be positioned comfortably in a reclining chair or on a bed.
• Explain that a technician will apply paste and attach electrodes to areas of skin on the patient's head and neck after these areas have been lightly abraded to ensure good contact.
• Explain that he must remain still throughout the test.
• Discuss any specific activity that the patient will be asked to perform, such as hyperventilating for 3 minutes or sleeping, depending on the purpose of the EEG.
• Use acetone to remove any remaining paste from the patient's skin.
• Encourage him to resume his normal activities, as ordered.

> A patient may be asked to perform a specific activity for an EEG, such as sleeping. I think the patient is ready...

Electromyography

Electromyography records a muscle's electrical impulses to help distinguish lower motor neuron disorders from muscle disorders — for example, amyotrophic lateral sclerosis (ALS) from muscular dystrophy. It also helps evaluate neuromuscular disorders such as myasthenia gravis. In this test, a needle electrode is inserted percutaneously into a muscle. The muscle's electrical discharge is then displayed and measured on an oscilloscope screen.

Nursing considerations

• Tell the patient that the test may take 1 hour to complete and that he may be asked to sit or lie down during the procedure.
• Warn him that he'll probably feel some discomfort when the doctor inserts a needle attached to an electrode into his muscle and when a mild electrical charge is delivered to the muscle.

• Explain that he must remain still during the test except when asked to contract or relax a muscle.
• Explain that an amplifier may emit crackling noises whenever his muscle moves.
• Encourage him to resume his normal activities, as ordered.
• Explain why he shouldn't take any stimulants, depressants, or sedatives for 24 hours before the test.

Treatments

The most common treatments for neurologic disorders are drug therapy and surgery.

Drug therapy

Drug therapy is a common and important treatment for neurologic disorders. When caring for a patient undergoing drug therapy, you'll need to be alert for severe adverse reactions and for interactions with other drugs. Some drugs, such as barbiturates, also carry a high risk of toxicity.

Keep in mind that drug therapy's success hinges on the patient's strict adherence to his medication schedule. Compliance is especially critical for drugs that require steady-state blood levels for therapeutic effectiveness, such as anticonvulsants, or for drugs used prophylactically such as beta-adrenergic blockers. (See *Drugs used to treat neurologic disorders*, page 116.)

Surgery

Surgical procedures typically used to treat neurologic disorders include cerebral aneurysm repair, craniotomy, and intracranial hematoma aspiration. As a medical-surgical nurse, you should prepare to handle the patient's preoperative assessment and preparation and postoperative care.

Questions, concerns, fears

When confronted with surgery, the patient and his family usually have questions, concerns, and fears that require compassionate attention. Keep in mind that a patient requiring surgery to address a neurologic disorder may be left with deficits that can be frustrating for him and his family. A positive, caring attitude and support can help them cope with their ordeal.

A patient facing surgery usually has questions, concerns, and fears that require your compassionate attention.

Drugs used to treat neurologic disorders

This chart lists the most common classes of drugs used to treat neurologic disorders and includes several examples of each.

Drug classification	Examples
Adrenergic blockers	Dihydroergotamine mesylate (Migranal), ergotamine tartrate
Anticoagulants	Heparin, low-molecular-weight heparin (Lovenox), warfarin (Coumadin)
Anticonvulsants	Carbamazepine (Tegretol), diazepam (Valium), fosphenytoin (Cerebyx), gabapentin (Neurotin), phenytoin (Dilantin)
Antiparkinson agents	Benztropine (Cogentin), carbidopa-levodopa, pramipexole (Mirapex), ropinirole (Requip)
Calcium channel blockers	Nimodipine
Corticosteroids	Dexamethasone, prednisone
Diuretics	Mannitol (Osmitrol), bumetanide, furosemide (Lasix)
Immune-modulating agents	Glatiramer acetate (Copaxone), interferon beta-1a (Avonex), inteferon beta-1b (Betaseron)
Opioid analgesics	Codeine, meperidine (Demerol), morphine
Skeletal muscle relaxants	Baclofen (Lioresal), dantrolene (Dantrium)

Cerebral aneurysm repair

Surgical intervention is the standard method for preventing rupture or rebleeding of a cerebral aneurysm. First, a craniotomy is performed to expose the aneurysm. Then, there are several corrective techniques the surgeon may use, depending on the shape and location of the aneurysm. He can clamp the affected artery, wrap the aneurysm wall with a biological or synthetic material, or clip or ligate the aneurysm. (See *Clipping a cerebral aneurysm.*)

Newer surgical approaches use a combination of therapies to repair an aneurysm. For instance, interventional radiology may be used in conjunction with endovascular balloon therapy to occlude

Clipping a cerebral aneurysm

Clipping is one method of surgical repair for a cerebral aneurysm.

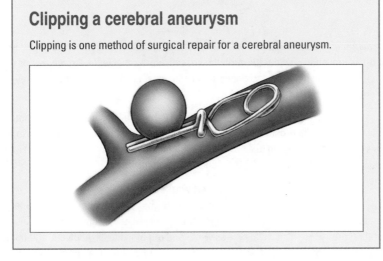

the aneurysm or vessel and treat arterial vasospasm with cerebral angiography.

Don't flip your lid yet

Another less invasive technique that has been successful for some patients is electrothrombosis, or coiling. This endovascular technique doesn't require open surgery; instead, the surgeon uses a catheter to thread a platinum coil into the aneurysm sac and, through electrolysis, seal off the aneurysm to prevent further bleeding. (See *Electrothrombosis*, page 118.)

Patient preparation

Before the procedure, take these steps:
• Tell the patient and his family that he'll be monitored in the intensive care unit (ICU) after surgery, where he'll be observed for signs of vasospasm, bleeding, and elevated intracranial pressure.
• Explain that he'll return to the medical-surgical unit for further care when his condition is stable.

Monitoring and aftercare

After the procedure, take these steps:
• Gradually increase the patient's level of activity, as ordered.
• Monitor the incision for signs of infection or drainage.
• Monitor the patient's neurologic status and vital signs, and report acute changes immediately. Watch for increased ICP: pupil changes, weakness in extremities, headache, and a change in LOC.
• Provide the patient and his family with emotional support as they cope with residual neurologic deficits.

Electrothrombosis

For some patients, open surgical repair of a cervical aneurysm isn't the best option, or even an option at all. In these cases, the doctor may decide to take an endovascular (through the vessel) approach. *Electrothrombosis,* or *coiling,* is one technique that's gaining popularity, proving to be especially successful at sealing off small-necked aneurysms and those with no significant intrafundal thrombosis.

What's electrothrombosis?

Electrothrombosis is a relatively noninvasive fluoroscopic procedure that uses electrolysis and coils of platinum to plug an aneurysm, thereby inducing thrombosis and sealing off the aneurysm to prevent rebleeding or rupture.

How it's done

• The doctor inserts a catheter into the femoral artery and advances it to the affected cerebral artery.
• Soft platinum coils are soldered to a stainless steel delivery wire, then positioned within the fundus of the aneurysm through a microcatheter.
• A tiny electrical current is applied to the delivery wire and the wire is removed, leaving the platinum coil in place.

• Additional wires are introduced one at a time. This process is continued until the aneurysm is densely packed with platinum and no longer opacifies when injected with a contrast medium.

How it works

The positively charged platinum left in the aneurysm theoretically attracts negatively charged blood elements, such as white and red blood cells, platelets, and fibrinogen. This induces intra-aneurysmal thrombosis.

The coils provide immediate protection against further hemorrhage by reducing blood pulsations in the fundus and sealing the hole or weak portion of the artery wall. Eventually, clots form, and the aneurysm separates from the parent vessel by the formation of new connective tissue.

Home care instructions

Before discharge, give the patient these instructions:
• Teach the patient or family member proper dressing change and wound care techniques and how to evaluate the incision regularly for redness, warmth, or tenderness, and to report any occurrence to the practitioner immediately.

Dazed and confused

• Remind the patient to continue taking prescribed anticonvulsant medications to minimize the risk of seizures. Depending on the type of surgery performed, he may need to continue anticonvulsant therapy for up to 12 months after surgery. Also, tell him to notify his practitioner of any adverse drug reactions such as excessive drowsiness or confusion.
• Emphasize the importance of returning for scheduled follow-up examinations and tests.
• Refer the patient and his family for appropriate home care or support groups.

Craniotomy

Craniotomy involves creation of a surgical incision into the skull to expose the brain for various treatments, such as ventricular shunting, excision of a tumor or abscess, hematoma aspiration, and aneurysm clipping. Craniotomy has many potential complications, including infection, hemorrhage, respiratory compromise, and increased ICP. The degree of risk depends on the patient's condition and the surgery's complexity.

Patient preparation

Before the procdedure, take these steps:
• Answer questions the family may have about the procedure to help reduce confusion and anxiety and help them cope.
• Explain to the patient that his hair will be clipped or shaved.
• Discuss the recovery period so the patient understands what to expect. Explain that he'll awaken with a dressing on his head to protect the incision and may have a surgical drain as well.
• Tell him to expect a headache and facial swelling for 2 to 3 days after surgery, and reassure him that he'll receive pain medication.
• Perform and document a baseline neurologic assessment.
• Explain that the patient will go to the ICU after surgery for close monitoring.

Monitoring and aftercare

After the procedure, take these steps:
• Gradually increase the patient's level of activity, as ordered.
• Monitor the incision site for signs of infection or drainage.
• Monitor the patient's neurologic status and vital signs, and report any acute change immediately. Watch for signs of increased ICP, such as pupil changes, weakness in extremities, headache, and change in LOC.
• Provide the patient and his family with emotional support as they cope with residual neurologic deficits.

Home care instructions

Before discharge, take these steps:
• Teach the patient or family member proper wound care techniques and how to evaluate the incision regularly for redness, warmth, or tenderness and report occurrences to the practitioner.
• Remind the patient to continue taking prescribed anticonvulsant medications to minimize the risk of seizures. Depending on the type of surgery performed, he may need to continue anticonvulsant therapy for up to 12 months after surgery. Also, remind him to report any adverse drug reactions, such as excessive drowsiness or confusion.

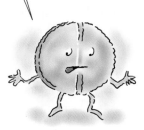

Depending on surgery type, the patient may need to continue anticonvulsants for up to 12 months after surgery.

What do I do?

Emergency intracranial hematoma aspiration

An intracranial hematoma (epidural, subdural, or intracerebral) commonly requires immediate, lifesaving surgery to lower intracranial pressure. Even if the patient's life isn't in immediate danger, timely surgery remains the only viable option for preventing irreversible damage from cerebral or brain stem ischemia.

When emergency aspiration is necessary, tailor your patient preparation to the time available. Start with a brief, succinct description of the procedure. As time allows, cover these additional points:

• Clarify the surgeon's explanation, if necessary, and ask the patient if he has any questions. Provide clear, concise answers.
• Tell the patient that his hair will be clipped or shaved for the procedure.
• Explain that after surgery, he'll awaken with a dressing on his head to protect the incision and may have a surgical drain in place.
• Tell him he'll probably have a headache and swollen face for 2 to 3 days after surgery.
• Reassure him that he'll receive pain medication.
• Explain that he'll be in the intensive care unit after surgery for close monitoring.
• Perform a baseline neurologic assessment.

• Emphasize the importance of returning for scheduled follow-up examinations and tests.
• Refer the patient and his family for home care or support groups as appropriate.
• Provide written copies of home care instructions and a list of medications for the patient and family members.

Intracranial hematoma aspiration

In intracranial hematoma aspiration, an epidural, subdural, or intracerebral hematoma is aspirated with a small suction tip. This suction tip is inserted through burr holes in the skull (for a fluid hematoma) or through a craniotomy (for a solid clot or a liquid one that can't be aspirated through burr holes).

It's complicated

Patients undergoing hematoma aspiration risk severe infection and seizures as well as physiologic problems associated with immobility during the prolonged recovery period. Even if hematoma removal proves successful, associated head injuries and other complications, such as cerebral edema, can produce permanent neurologic deficits, coma, or even death. (See *Emergency intracranial hematoma aspiration*.)

What you can do

Patient preparation, monitoring and aftercare, and home care instructions are the same as those for cerebral aneurysm repair.

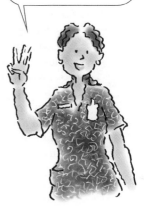

Keep in mind the three most common complications in patients with neurologic disorders: respiratory infection, UTI, and infected pressure ulcers.

Nursing diagnoses

When caring for patients with neurologic disorders, certain nursing diagnoses are commonly used. When developing your care plan, keep in mind interventions to prevent the three most common complications in patients with neurologic disorders: respiratory infection, urinary tract infection (UTI), and infected pressure ulcers. See *NANDA-I taxonomy II by domain*, page 936, for the complete list of NANDA diagnoses.

Impaired physical mobility

Impaired physical mobility can occur in ALS, cerebral palsy, stroke, MS, muscular dystrophy, myasthenia gravis, Parkinson's disease, poliomyelitis, or spinal cord injury.

Expected outcomes

• The patient will show no evidence of complications, such as contractures, venous stasis, thrombus formation, or skin breakdown.
• The patient will achieve the highest level of mobility possible.
• The patient will maintain muscle strength and joint ROM.

Nursing interventions and rationales

• Have the patient perform ROM exercises at least once every shift, unless contraindicated. Progress from passive to active exercises, as tolerated. This prevents joint contractures and muscular atrophy.
• Turn and position the dependent patient every 2 hours. Establish a turning schedule, post this schedule at the bedside, and monitor the frequency of turning. Turning prevents skin breakdown by relieving pressure.
• Place joints in functional positions (use hand splints if needed and available), use a trochanter roll along the thigh, abduct the thighs, use high-top sneakers, and put a small pillow under the patient's head. These measures maintain joints in a functional position and prevent musculoskeletal deformities.
• Identify the patient's level of functioning using a functional mobility scale. Communicate the patient's skill level to all staff members to provide continuity and preserve a specific level of independence.

• Encourage mobility independence by helping the patient use a trapeze and side rails to reposition himself; use his good leg to move his affected leg; and perform self-care activities, such as feeding and dressing, to increase muscle tone and build self-esteem.

Declaration of independence

• If one-sided weakness or paralysis is present, place items within reach of the patient's unaffected arm to promote independence.
• Monitor and record evidence of immobility complications (such as contractures, venous stasis, thrombus, pneumonia, skin breakdown, and UTI) each day. The patient with a history of a neuromuscular disorder or dysfunction may be prone to complications.
• Promote progressive mobilization to the degree possible in light of the patient's condition (bed mobility to chair mobility to ambulation) to maintain muscle tone and prevent complications.
• Refer the patient to physical and occupational therapists for development of a mobility regimen to help rehabilitate the patient's musculoskeletal deficits. Request written mobility plans and use these as references.
• Teach the patient and his family how to perform ROM exercises, transfers, and skin inspection and explain the mobility regimen to prepare the patient for discharge.
• Demonstrate the mobility regimen, and have the patient and his caregivers do a return demonstration and note the dates of both. This ensures continuity of care and correct completion.
• Help identify resources that will help the patient carry out the mobility regimen, such as Strokesurvivors International, the United Cerebral Palsy Associations, and the National Multiple Sclerosis Society, to help provide a comprehensive approach to rehabilitation.

Impaired skin integrity

Impaired skin integrity is a potential (and common) problem for anyone with a lower than normal level of activity. However, it can be deadly for a patient who can't turn or move by himself. Infected pressure ulcers are one of the primary causes of death in a patient with neurologic disease. Even when not infected, pressure ulcers still cause prolonged distress and adversely affect the patient's ability to function and his quality of life.

Expected outcomes

- The patient will maintain intact skin integrity.
- The patient won't develop complications, should skin break-down occur.
- The patient will maintain the optimal nutrition needed to pre-vent skin breakdown.

Nursing interventions and rationales

- Turn and move the patient at least every 2 hours if he's unable to do so. Teach wheelchair patients to shift position several times each hour; provide help if needed. Pressure reduces skin circulation very quickly, which is a precursor to breakdown.

Steering clear of breakdowns

- Use appropriate support surfaces, such as 4″ convoluted foam mattresses or gelmats. If the patient develops pres-sure ulcers, consult established guidelines and protocols to determine the proper supportive surfaces for the patient. Repositioning and proper support surfaces reduce pressure on skin and help prevent skin breakdown.
- Consult with an enterostomal therapist and published guidelines to determine preventive measures and interven-tions.
- Encourage optimal food and fluid intake to maintain skin health.

To help a wheelchair-bound patient prevent pressure ulcers, teach her to shift position several times each hour.

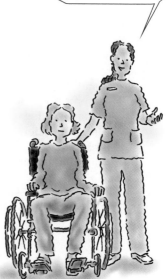

Impaired urinary elimination

Impaired urinary elimination is another of the major complica-tions affecting patients with neurologic disorders. Many of these patients have bladder spasticity or are unable to empty their bladders fully or properly. UTIs are common and can lead to pro-longed hospitalization or even death.

Expected outcomes

- The patient will empty his bladder completely and regularly.
- The patient won't develop a UTI.

Nursing interventions and rationales

• Use appropriate strategies for assessing adequacy of output and bladder emptying. Although regular emptying is essential to urinary tract health, the patient may be unable to do so or may be unable to sense whether or not he's completely emptying his bladder.
• Encourage the patient to drink plenty of fluids each day. Fluid intake is essential to the production of urine to clean the urinary tract and bladder.
• If the patient can't empty his bladder alone, use the least invasive strategies to improve bladder emptying. Start with such techniques as Credé's maneuver, in which the patient bends forward and presses on the bladder while urinating. Intermittent self-catheterization is more invasive, but less likely to cause infection than an indwelling urinary catheter.
• If the patient voids adequately but is incontinent, a condom catheter will help keep his skin dry, while being less likely than intermittent or indwelling urinary catheterization to cause infection.

Impaired gas exchange

Impaired gas exchange relates to the third most common complication for patients with neurologic disorders: respiratory infection.

Expected outcomes

• The patient won't develop a respiratory infection.
• The patient will maintain optimal oxygen saturation levels.

Nursing interventions and rationales

• If the patient is immobile or has impaired respiratory muscle function, encourage the use of incentive spirometry, deep breathing, and coughing several times per day. Deep breathing and coughing help prevent atelectasis, which can become a respiratory infection as secretions accumulate.
• Encourage fluid intake. Fluids keep respiratory secretions thin and easy to cough up.
• Discourage smoking and exposure to second-hand smoke that impair respiration and the body's ability to clear the lungs.
• Encourage adequate rest, exercise, and nutrition, which will help maintain the strength of respiratory muscles.

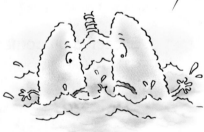

I know increased fluid intake can help keep respiratory secretions thin and easy to cough up, but this is ridiculous!

Common neurologic disorders

Below are several common neurologic disorders, along with their causes, pathophysiology, signs and symptoms, diagnostic test findings, treatments, and nursing interventions.

Alzheimer's disease

Alzheimer's disease is a progressive neurologic disorder that affects the brain and results in cognitive impairments, such as impaired thinking, memory loss, and bizarre behavior. Alzheimer's disease is the most common form of dementia and the fourth leading cause of death in adults.

What causes it

The cause of Alzheimer's disease isn't known; however, several factors appear to have some association with the disease. These include:
• deficiencies in the neurotransmitters acetylcholine, somatostatin, substance P, and norepinephrine
• repeated head trauma
• abnormalities on chromosomes 14 or 21
• deposits of beta amyloid protein.

Pathophysiology

The brain tissue of patients with Alzheimer's disease has three distinguishing features:

neurofibrillatory tangles (fibrous proteins)

amyloid plaques (composed of degenerating axons and dendrites)

granulovacuolar degeneration.

Autopsy commonly reveals an atrophic brain that can weigh 1,000 g or less. Normal brain weight is 1,380 g. (See *Brain tissue changes in Alzheimer's disease*, page 126.)

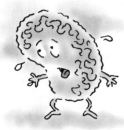

You don't have to be a brain to know that *atrophic* doesn't sound good!

What to look for

The onset of Alzheimer's disease is insidious. Initial changes are almost imperceptible, but gradually progress to serious problems. Initial signs and symptoms include:
• forgetfulness and short-term memory loss
• difficulty learning and remembering new information

A closer look

Brain tissue changes in Alzheimer's disease

The brain tissue of patients with Alzheimer's disease exhibits three characteristic features:
• *neurofibrillatory tangles,* which are bundles of filaments (in neurons) that twist abnormally around one another. They're most numerous in areas of the brain associated with memory and learning, fear and aggression, and thinking.
• *amyloid plaques,* also known as senile plaques, are deposits found outside neurons in the extracellular space of the cerebral cortex and hippocampus. Amyloid plaques contain a core of beta amyloid protein surrounded by abnormal nerve endings, or neurites.
• *granulovacuolar degeneration,* or degeneration of neurons in the hippocampus, is a process in which fluid-filled spaces called *vacuoles* enlarge the cell body, resulting in neuron malfunction or death.

• deterioration in personal hygiene and appearance
• inability to concentrate.
    Later signs and symptoms include:
• difficulty with abstract thinking and activities that require judgment
• progressive difficulty communicating
• severe deterioration in memory, language, and motor function
• repetitive actions or perseveration (a classic sign)
• nocturnal wakening, disorientation, and personality changes, such as restlessness and irritability.

What tests tell you

• Psychometric testing and neurologic examination can help establish the diagnosis.
• A PET scan measures the metabolic activity of the cerebral cortex and may help confirm an early diagnosis.
• EEG, CT scan, and MRI may help diagnose later stages of Alzheimer's disease.
• Testing for soluble amyloid beta protein precursor helps assess the extracellular deposits of amyloid beta-peptide, which is a major neuropathic sign of Alzheimer's disease.
• Additional tests may help rule out other causes of dementia, such as vitamin B_{12} deficiency and hypothyroidism.

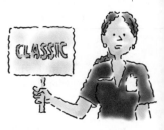

Perseveration, or inappropriate repetition of a thought or act, is a classic sign of Alzheimer's disease.

CLASSIC

How it's treated

Although there's no known cure for Alzheimer's disease, donepezil, tacrine, and rivastigmine have proven partially effective in improving mental performance. Drug therapy is also used to treat behavioral symptoms, such as aggression, paranoia, depression, and delusions. These drugs include:
• antipsychotics, such as haloperidol (Haldol), olanzapine (Zyprexa), quetiapine (Seroquel), and risperidone (Risperdal)
• anxiolytics, such as alprazolam (Xanax), buspirone (BuSpar), diazepam (Valium), and lorazepam (Ativan)
• antidepressants, such as amitriptyline, bupropion (Wellbutrin), fluoxetine (Prozac), and paroxetine (Paxil).

What to do

• Establish an effective communication system with the patient and his family to help them adjust to his altered cognitive abilities.

Returning to a safe haven

• Protect the patient from injury by providing a safe, structured, and supervised environment.
• Encourage the patient to exercise, as ordered, to help maintain mobility.
• Refer family members to appropriate social service agencies that can help the family assess its needs.
• Evaluate the patient. He should be free from injury; have an established, adequate sleep pattern; and have adequate nutrition.
• Assess the patient's family to determine if they have sufficient support systems to help them cope with this crisis.
• Encourage the patient and his family to express their feelings of loss. (See *Alzheimer's disease teaching tips*.)

Amyotrophic lateral sclerosis

ALS causes progressive physical degeneration while leaving the patient's mental status intact. Thus, the patient is keenly aware of each new physical change. The most common motor neuron disease of muscular atrophy, ALS results in degeneration of upper motor neurons in the medulla oblongata and lower motor neurons in the spinal cord.

Onset typically occurs between ages 40 and 70, and most patients die within 3 to 10 years, usually due to aspiration pneumonia or respiratory failure.

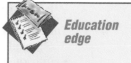

Education edge

Alzheimer's disease teaching tips

• Teach the patient and his family about Alzheimer's disease — what's known, what's suspected, and the degenerative nature of the disorder. Listen to their concerns and answer all questions honestly and with compassion.
• Refer the family to local and national support groups for additional information and coping strategies. Family members commonly find a degree of solace in knowing that other families are going through the same devastating experience. To locate support groups in your area, contact the Alzheimer's Disease and Related Disorders Association.
• Encourage the family to allow the patient as much independence as possible while keeping him safe.
• Explain how proper diet, regular daily routines, and normal sleep patterns can help.

What causes it

The cause of ALS isn't known; however, factors associated with ALS include:
- autosomal dominant inheritance
- a slow-acting virus
- a nutritional deficiency in motor neurons related to a disturbance in enzyme metabolism
- metabolic interference in nucleic acid production by the nerve fibers
- an autoimmune disorder.

Precipitating factors for acute deterioration include trauma, viral infections, and physical exhaustion.

Pathophysiology

In ALS, motor neurons located in the anterior horns of the spinal column and motor nuclei located in the lower brain stem die. As they die, the muscles they served begin to atrophy. The loss of motor neurons may occur in the upper and lower motor neuron systems. Signs and symptoms vary according to the motor neurons affected because specific neurons activate specific muscle fibers.

What to look for

The patient with ALS develops fasciculations (twitching, involuntary muscle contractions) accompanied by atrophy and weakness, especially in the muscles of the forearms and hands. Other signs and symptoms include:
- impaired speech
- difficulty chewing and swallowing
- difficulty breathing
- depression
- choking
- excessive drooling.

What tests tell you

- Electromyography and muscle biopsy help determine if the disease is affecting the nerves rather than the muscles.
- In one-third of all patients with ALS, cerebrospinal fluid (CSF) examination reveals an increased protein level.

How it's treated

No effective treatment exists for ALS. Management focuses on controlling symptoms and providing the patient and his family with the emotional, psychological, and physical support they

> Loss of motor neurons may occur in the upper and lower motor neuron systems.

need. Care begins with a complete neurologic assessment, which functions as a baseline for future evaluations. Collectively, these assessments will reveal the progression of ALS over time.

What to do

• Implement a rehabilitation program that maintains as much independence for the patient for as long as possible.
• Help the patient obtain equipment that will help him move about, such as a walker or a wheelchair. Arrange for a visiting nurse to oversee home care and provide ongoing support, and to teach the family about the illness.
• Depending on the patient's muscular ability, help with bathing, personal hygiene, and transfers from wheelchair to bed, as needed. Encourage a regular bowel and bladder routine.
• Provide meticulous skin care if the patient is bedridden, to prevent skin breakdown. Also, turn him often, keep his skin clean and dry, and use pressure-relieving devices to preserve skin integrity.
• If the patient has trouble swallowing, give him soft, solid foods and position him upright during meals. He'll need gastrostomy and nasogastric (NG) tube feedings when he's no longer able to swallow.
• Provide the patient and family with information on support groups.

Making informed decisions

• Provide the patient and his family with emotional support and the information they need to make informed decisions regarding end-of-life care and help them prepare for the eventual death of the patient. Encourage all concerned to start the grieving process. The patient with ALS may benefit from a hospice program.
• Evaluate the patient. Intervene as needed to maintain adequate respiratory function with a patent airway, clear lungs, and acceptable results from pulmonary function studies. Help maintain a system of communication and as much physical mobility as possible for as long as possible. Note whether the patient expresses feelings of loss. (See *ALS teaching tips*.)

Arteriovenous malformation

In AVM, a tangled array of dilated vessels forms an abnormal network of communication between the arterial and venous systems. AVMs are usually located in the cerebral hemispheres. Spontaneous bleeding from these lesions into the subarachnoid space or brain tissue causes the patient's signs and symptoms.

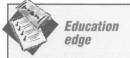

Education edge

ALS teaching tips

• Teach one or more family members the proper way to suction the patient. This will help the patient cope with the increasing accumulation of secretions and dysphagia.
• Explain that he must eat slowly at mealtime and always sit upright. If he develops swallowing difficulties, refer him to the dysphagia team for further evaluation and treatment.
• If the patient is still able to feed himself, teach him (and a family member) how to administer gastrostomy feedings.
• When verbal communication becomes too difficult, teach the patient an alternate method of communicating with those around him.

AVMs range in size from a few millimeters to large malformations extending from the cerebral cortex to the ventricles. Most are present at birth; however, symptoms rarely occur before ages 10 to 30. AVMs are more common in men than in women.

What causes it

Most AVMs are caused by congenital defects in capillary development. Traumatic injury is another possible cause of AVM.

Pathophysiology

AVMs lack the structural characteristics typical of normal blood vessels. The vessels of an AVM are very thin; when more than one artery feeds into the AVM, it appears dilated and tortuous. Because vessels are thin, there's a risk that an aneurysm will develop. If the AVM is large enough, shunting can deprive surrounding tissue of adequate blood flow. In addition, the thin-walled vessels may ooze small amounts of blood or they may rupture, causing hemorrhage into the brain or subarachnoid space.

What to look for

- Seizures that are initially focal but become generalized
- Headache that doesn't respond to treatment

Mind games

- Transient episodes of syncope, dizziness, motor weakness, or sensory deficits
- Tingling, aphasia, dysarthria, visual deficits (usually hemianopsia)
- Mental confusion
- Intellectual impairment

What tests tell you

- Cerebral angiography provides the most definitive diagnostic information by localizing the AVM and enabling visualization of large feeding arteries and large drainage veins.
- A CT scan can help differentiate an AVM from a clot or tumor, especially when a contrast medium is used.
- EEG may help localize the AVM.
- Brain scan immediately after isotope injection will reveal an uptake in the AVM.
- MRI-magnetic resonance angiography (especially with gadolinium) may provide information that supports a diagnosis of AVM.

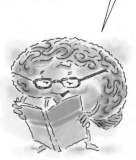

Says here that cerebral angiography provides the most definitive diagnostic information for an AVM.

How it's treated

The choice of treatment depends on the size and location of the AVM, the feeder vessels supplying it, and the age and general health of the patient. Possible methods include embolization, proton-beam radiation, Nd:YAG laser surgery, surgical excision, and a combination of embolization and surgery.

What to do

- Prevent bleeding if hemorrhage hasn't occurred.
- Control hypertension and seizure activity, and reduce activities and eliminate stressors that raise the patient's systemic blood pressure.
- Maintain a quiet, therapeutic environment.
- Monitor and control associated hypertension with drug therapy, as ordered.
- Establish a baseline and then conduct ongoing neuro checks.
- Monitor the patient's vital signs frequently.
- Assess and monitor characteristics of headache, seizure activity, or bruit, as needed.
- Provide emotional support.
- Evaluate the patient's LOC, body temperature, heart rate, respiratory rate, and blood pressure.
- Assess whether he continues to experience pain or seizures.
- Provide appropriate pain management.
- Note whether the patient has expressed feelings of loss to members of the staff, his friends, or his family. Similarly, note whether his family or friends have expressed their understanding of the disease process, treatment options, and outcome. (See *AVM teaching tips.*)

> ### *Education edge*
> ## AVM teaching tips
> - Tailor your teaching to the surgical procedure chosen by the surgeon.
> - Describe the surgical procedure and all preoperative tests and assessments. Answer all of the patient's questions, and those of his family, directly and honestly.
> - Describe what the patient can expect upon awakening after surgery.
> - After surgery, focus teaching on helping the patient develop the highest level of independence possible.

Bell's palsy

Bell's palsy blocks conduction of impulses along the facial nerve (CN VII), which is the nerve responsible for motor innervation of the facial muscles. This block results from an inflammatory reaction around the nerve (usually at the internal auditory meatus).

Bell's palsy affects all age-groups, but occurs most commonly in patients under age 60. Onset is rapid and, in 80% to 90% of all patients, it subsides spontaneously, with complete recovery in 1 to 8 weeks. Recovery can take longer in elderly patients. If patients experience only partial recovery, contractures may develop on the paralyzed side of the face. Bell's palsy may recur on the same or opposite side of the face.

What causes it

Bell's palsy can be caused by:
• infection
• hemorrhage
• tumor
• meningitis
• local traumatic injury.

Pathophysiology

Inflammation around CN VII where it leaves bony tissue blocks conduction along the nerve. As a consequence, CN VII can't adequately stimulate the muscle fibers, and unilateral or bilateral facial weakness or paralysis is the result.

What to look for

Patients may experience incomplete eye closure and Bell's phenomenon (eye rolling upward as eye is closed). Other signs and symptoms of Bell's palsy include:
• unilateral facial weakness or paralysis, with aching at the jaw angle
• drooping mouth, causing drooling on the affected side
• distorted taste perception over the affected anterior portion of the tongue
• markedly impaired ability to close the eye on the weak side
• inability to raise the eyebrow, smile, show the teeth, or puff out the cheek on the affected side.

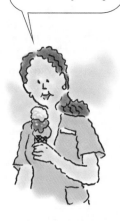

When ice cream tastes like chalk, something is definitely wrong.

What tests tell you

Electromyography helps predict recovery by distinguishing temporary conduction defects from a pathologic interruption of nerve fibers.

How it's treated

Prednisone, an oral corticosteroid, reduces facial nerve edema and improves nerve conduction and blood flow. Specific antiviral agents can also be helpful. After the 14th day of prednisone therapy, electrotherapy may help prevent atrophy of facial muscles.

What to do

• Apply moist heat to the affected side of the face to reduce pain, taking care not to burn the skin.

• Massage the patient's face with a gentle upward motion two to three times daily for 5 to 10 minutes, and teach him how to perform this massage.
• Apply a facial sling to improve lip alignment.

Residual effects

• Give the patient frequent and complete mouth care. Remove residual food that collects between the cheeks and gums.
• Provide support, and reassure the patient that recovery is likely within 1 to 8 weeks.
• Assess the effectiveness of pain medications.
• Assess the patient's nutritional status. Bell's palsy shouldn't interfere with the patient's ability to maintain adequate nutrition.
• Note whether the patient has expressed feelings of loss or fear to staff, friends, or family. (See *Bell's palsy teaching tips.*)

Cerebral aneurysm

Cerebral aneurysm, a localized dilation of a cerebral artery, results from a weakness in the arterial wall. (See *Common sites of cerebral aneurysm*, page 134.) The incidence is slightly higher in women than in men, especially those in their late 40s to mid-50s, but cerebral aneurysm may occur at any age.

Prognosis is uncertain because cerebral aneurysms can rupture and cause subarachnoid hemorrhage; one-half of all patients suffering subarachnoid hemorrhages die immediately. However, with new and better treatment, the prognosis is improving.

What causes it

Cerebral aneurysm results from congenital vascular disease, infection, or atherosclerosis.

Pathophysiology

Blood flow exerts pressure against a congenitally weak area of arterial wall, causing it to stretch and thin, somewhat like an overblown balloon. At this point, the risk of rupture is high. A rupture is followed by a subarachnoid hemorrhage, in which blood spills into the space normally occupied by CSF. In some cases, blood also spills into brain tissue, where a clot can damage brain tissue or cause a life-threatening increase in ICP.

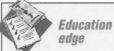

Education edge

Bell's palsy teaching tips

• Advise the patient to protect the eye on the affected side by covering it with an eye patch, especially when outdoors. The eyelid must be taped shut at night using a small piece of hypoallergenic tape. Tell him to keep warm and to avoid exposure to dust and wind. If exposure is unavoidable, instruct him to cover his face.
• To prevent excessive weight loss, teach the patient how to cope with eating and drinking difficulties. Tell him to chew on the unaffected side of his mouth. Provide a nutritionally balanced diet of soft foods. Eliminate hot foods and fluids (soups, sauces, and purees, for example). Arrange for privacy at mealtimes to minimize embarrassment.
• When the patient is ready, teach him to exercise facial muscles by grimacing in front of a mirror.

Common sites of cerebral aneurysm

A cerebral aneurysm usually arises at arterial bifurcations in the circle of Willis and its branches. The shaded areas in the illustration below indicate the most common sites for aneurysm.

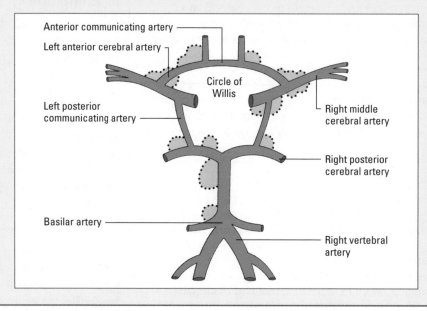

Anterior communicating artery

Left anterior cerebral artery

Circle of Willis

Left posterior communicating artery

Right middle cerebral artery

Right posterior cerebral artery

Basilar artery

Right vertebral artery

What to look for

Most patients are asymptomatic until the time of bleeding. Premonitory symptoms resulting from oozing of blood into the subarachnoid space include:
• headache, intermittent nausea
• nuchal rigidity
• stiff back and legs.
    Rupture usually occurs abruptly and may cause:
• sudden severe headache
• nausea and projectile vomiting
• altered LOC, including deep coma
• meningeal irritation, resulting in nuchal rigidity, back and leg pain, fever, restlessness, irritability, seizures, photophobia, and blurred vision
• hemiparesis, hemisensory defects, dysphagia, and visual defects
• diplopia, ptosis, dilated pupils, and an inability to rotate the eye.

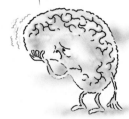

Preliminary symptoms of an aneurysm include headache and intermittent nausea.

What tests tell you

• Angiography can confirm an unruptured cerebral aneurysm. Unfortunately, diagnosis usually follows the rupture.
• A CT scan may help detect subarachnoid hemorrhage.
• MRI may detect vasospasm.

How it's treated

To reduce the risk of rebleeding, the surgeon may attempt to repair the aneurysm. Usually, surgical repair (by clipping, ligating, wrapping the aneurysm neck with muscle, or using electrothrombosis) takes place within several days after the initial bleed.

More conservative

The patient may receive conservative treatment if surgical correction poses too great a risk (common with elderly patients and those with heart, lung, or other serious diseases), the aneurysm is in a particularly dangerous location, or vasospasm necessitates a delay in surgery.

Commonly, treatment for the patient who isn't a good candidate for surgery includes bed rest in a quiet, darkened room for as long as 4 to 6 weeks. The patient must avoid stimulants (including caffeine) and aspirin. He may receive codeine or another analgesic, hydralazine or another antihypertensive (if he's hypertensive), corticosteroids to reduce edema, and phenobarbital or another sedative. Nimodipine may be prescribed to limit possible neurologic deficits. If the patient is hypotensive, he may receive dopamine to ensure adequate brain perfusion.

An accurate neurologic assessment, good patient care, patient and family teaching, and psychological support can speed recovery and reduce complications. The medical-surgical nurse assumes care for the patient recovering from an aneurysm repair when he's transferred from the ICU.

What to do

• Assess neurologic status to screen for changes in the patient's condition.
• Administer medications, as ordered.
• Maintain adequate nutrition.
• Promote activity based on the patient's ability.
• Provide support to the patient and his family, especially if neurologic deficits have occurred.
• Refer the patient to appropriate health care team members, such as a social services representative and home care organization.

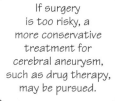

If surgery is too risky, a more conservative treatment for cerebral aneurysm, such as drug therapy, may be pursued.

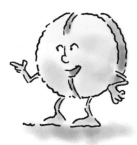

• Check for a patent airway, normal breath sounds, consistent LOC with no additional neurologic deficits, and adequate hydration and nutrition. (See *Cerebral aneurysm teaching tips*.)

Guillain-Barré syndrome

An acute, rapidly progressive, and potentially fatal form of polyneuritis, Guillain-Barré syndrome causes muscle weakness and mild distal sensory loss. About 95% of patients experience spontaneous and complete recovery, although mild motor or reflex deficits in the feet and legs may persist.

What causes it

The precise cause of this syndrome is unknown, but it may be a cell-mediated immunologic attack on peripheral nerves in response to a virus. Precipitating factors may include:
• mild febrile or viral illness
• surgery
• rabies or swine influenza vaccination
• Hodgkin's disease or some other cancer
• systemic lupus erythematosus.

Pathophysiology

The major pathologic manifestation of Guillain-Barré syndrome is segmental demyelination of the peripheral nerves, which prevents normal transmission of electrical impulses. Because this syndrome causes inflammation and degenerative changes in the posterior (sensory) and anterior (motor) nerve roots, signs of sensory and motor loss occur simultaneously. Additionally, autonomic nerve transmission may be impaired. (See *Phases of Guillain-Barré syndrome.*)

What to look for

Symmetrical muscle weakness usually appears in the legs first (ascending type) and then extends to the arms and facial nerves within 24 to 72 hours. Other signs and symptoms may include:
• facial diplegia, possibly with ophthalmoplegia (ocular paralysis)
• dysphagia, dysarthria
• hypotonia, areflexia.

What tests tell you

• Protein levels in CSF begin to rise several days after onset of signs and symptoms and peak in 4 to 6 weeks. White blood cell

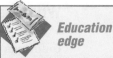

Education edge

Cerebral aneurysm teaching tips

• The amount of teaching you'll do depends on the extent of the neurologic deficit.
• If the patient can't speak, set up a simple means of communication; try using cards or a slate.
• Tell the patient's family to talk to him in a normal tone, even if he doesn't seem to respond.
• Provide the patient and his family with information about local support groups and other applicable services.

count in the CSF remains normal but, in severe disease, CSF pressure may rise above normal.
• Complete blood count (CBC) shows leukocytosis and immature forms early in the illness, but blood studies soon return to normal.
• Electromyography may show repeated firing of the same motor unit instead of widespread sectional stimulation. Nerve conduction velocities are slowed soon after paralysis develops.

How it's treated

At the onset of symptoms, the patient should be hospitalized. Monitor respiratory function several times daily because the ascending pathology can lead to respiratory failure. Mechanical ventilation may be necessary. The other key treatment is plasmapheresis, which temporarily reduces circulating antibodies. Patients need less ventilator support if plasmapheresis begins within 2 weeks of onset. High-dose immune globulins and steroids are also used.

What to do

• Watch for ascending motor loss. Commonly, sensation isn't lost; in fact, the patient may be hypersensitive to pain and touch.
• Monitor the patient's vital signs and LOC.

Take a deep breath

• Assess respiratory function. Watch for signs of increasing partial pressure of arterial carbon dioxide ($Paco_2$), such as confusion and tachypnea. Auscultate breath sounds, turn and position the patient, and encourage coughing and deep breathing. If respiratory failure becomes imminent, establish an emergency airway and assist with endotracheal intubation.
• Provide meticulous skin care to prevent skin breakdown.

Tanks, I needed that

• Perform passive ROM exercises within the patient's pain limits, perhaps using a Hubbard tank to prevent contractures. When the patient's condition stabilizes, change to gentle stretching and active assistance exercises.
• Evaluate the patient's gag reflex. If he has no gag reflex, administer NG feedings, as ordered. If it's present, position the patient to prevent aspiration.
• As the patient regains strength and can tolerate a vertical position, be alert for hypotension; prevent it with slow position changes.

Phases of Guillain-Barré syndrome

The clinical course of Guillain-Barré syndrome has three phases:

🖐 *acute phase,* which begins when the first definitive symptom develops and ends 1 to 3 weeks later, when no further deterioration is noted

✌ *plateau phase,* which lasts for several days to 2 weeks

🖖 *recovery phase,* which is believed to coincide with remyelination and axonal process regrowth and can last from 4 months to 3 years.

• Inspect the patient's legs regularly for signs of thrombophlebitis, a common complication of Guillain-Barré syndrome. To prevent thrombophlebitis, apply antiembolism stockings and a sequential compression device and give prophylactic anticoagulants, as ordered.

• Provide eye and mouth care every 4 hours if the patient has facial paralysis.

• Watch for urine retention. Measure and record intake and output every 8 hours, and offer the bedpan every 3 to 4 hours. Encourage adequate fluid intake (2 qt [2 L]/day), unless contraindicated. If urine retention develops, the patient may need to use manual pressure over the bladder (Credé's maneuver) to urinate. Use intermittent catheterization, if necessary.

Bulking up

• To prevent or relieve constipation, offer prune juice and a high-bulk diet. If necessary, give daily or alternate-day suppositories (docusate sodium [Colace] or bisacodyl [Dulcolax]), or enemas, as ordered.

• Refer the patient for physical therapy, as needed.

• Evaluate the patient for adequate respiratory function with a patent airway and clear lungs, adequate nutritional status, and optimal activity level.

• Note whether the patient has expressed his feelings about his illness to members of the staff, his friends, or his family. (See *Guillain-Barré syndrome teaching tips.*)

Headache

Muscle contraction, tension, and vascular changes cause 90% of headaches. Occasionally, however, a headache indicates an underlying intracranial, systemic, or psychological disorder.

Throbbing, vascular headaches — migraine headaches — affect up to 10% of Americans. Migraines usually begin in childhood or adolescence and recur throughout adulthood. Migraine headaches tend to run in families and are more common in women than in men.

What causes it

Most chronic headaches result from muscle tension caused by:
• emotional stress or fatigue
• menstruation
• environmental stimuli (noise, crowds, bright lights).
    Other possible causes include:
• glaucoma
• inflammation of the eyes or of the nasal or paranasal sinus mucosa

Education edge

Guillain-Barré syndrome teaching tips

• Before discharge, prepare a home care plan and review it thoroughly with the patient and his family.

• Reinforce the physical and occupational therapist's teaching about how to transfer from bed to wheelchair and from wheelchair to toilet or tub as well as how to walk short distances with a walker or a cane.

• Teach the family how to help the patient eat, compensate for facial weakness, and prevent skin breakdown.

• Stress the need for a regular bowel and bladder routine. Explain Credé's maneuver, if complete urinary emptying is a problem.

• Provide the patient and his family with appropriate referrals to support organizations and public service agencies in the area.

- diseases of the scalp, teeth, extracranial arteries, or external or middle ear
- vasodilators (nitrates, alcohol, histamine)
- systemic disease
- hypertension
- head trauma or tumor
- intracranial bleeding, abscess, or aneurysm.

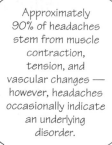

Approximately 90% of headaches stem from muscle contraction, tension, and vascular changes — however, headaches occasionally indicate an underlying disorder.

Pathophysiology

Headache pain may emanate from the pain-sensitive structures of the skin, scalp, muscles, arteries, and veins; from cranial nerves V, VII, IX, and X; or from cervical nerves 1, 2, and 3. Intracranial mechanisms of headache include traction or displacement of arteries, venous sinuses, or venous tributaries and inflammation or direct pressure on the cranial nerves with afferent pain fibers.

The cause of migraine headaches isn't known, but researchers associate the disorder with constriction and dilation of intracranial and extracranial arteries.

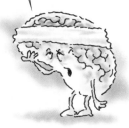

What to look for

Signs and symptoms depend on the type or cause of the headache: migraine headache, muscle contraction and traction-inflammatory vascular headache, intracranial bleeding, or tumor.

Migraine headache

- Unilateral pulsating pain, which becomes more generalized over time, lasting up to 2 days
- Premonitory aura of scintillating scotoma, hemianopsia, unilateral paresthesia, or a speech disorder
- Irritability, anorexia, nausea, vomiting, photophobia

Muscle contraction and traction-inflammatory vascular headache

- Dull, persistent ache or severe, unrelenting pain
- Tender spots on the head or neck
- Feeling of tightness around the head with a characteristic "hatband" distribution

Intracranial bleeding

- Neurologic deficits, such as paresthesia and muscle weakness
- Pain unrelieved by opioids

Tumor

- Pain that's most severe when the patient wakes

What tests tell you

Skull X-rays (including cervical spine and sinus), EEG, MRI, CT scan (performed before lumbar puncture to rule out increased ICP), brain scan, and lumbar puncture may help determine the cause.

How it's treated

Depending on the type of headache, analgesics ranging from aspirin to codeine or meperidine (Demerol) may provide symptomatic relief. A tranquilizer, such as diazepam, may help during acute attacks, as could identification and elimination of causative factors and, possibly, psychotherapy for headaches caused by emotional stress. Chronic tension headaches may require muscle relaxants.

Taking a coffee break

For migraine headache, ergotamine (Ergomar) alone or with caffeine provides the most effective treatment. Sumatriptan (Imitrex), which binds with serotonin receptors, is also effective in aborting migraine headaches. These drugs and others, such as metoclopramide (Reglan) or naproxen (Naprosyn), work best when taken early in the course of an attack. Antiemetics, such as promethazine (Phenergan), may be prescribed to control nausea and vomiting. Drugs that can help prevent migraine headache include propranolol (Inderal); calcium channel blockers, such as verapamil (Calan) and diltiazem (Cardizem); and antiseizure medications such as valproic acid.

What to do

Unless the headache is caused by a serious underlying disorder, hospitalization is rarely required. In these rare cases, direct your attention to treating the primary problem. The patient with migraine usually needs to be hospitalized only if nausea and vomiting are severe enough to induce dehydration and possible shock.

Finding a sea of tranquility

Evaluate the patient to determine the effectiveness of prescribed analgesics, tranquilizers, or muscle relaxants and document your findings. Help the patient understand the possible causes and remedies for the headaches. (See *Headache teaching tips*.)

Huntington's disease

Huntington's disease (Huntington's chorea) is a hereditary disease that causes degeneration in the cerebral cortex and basal ganglia.

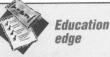
Education edge

Headache teaching tips

• Help the patient understand the reason for headaches so that he can avoid exacerbating factors. Use his history and diagnosis as a guide.
• Advise him to lie down in a dark, quiet room during an attack and to place ice packs on his forehead or a cold cloth over his eyes, or use other measures that are helpful for him.
• Instruct the patient to take prescribed medication at the onset of migraine symptoms, prevent dehydration by drinking plenty of fluids after nausea and vomiting subside, and use other headache-relief measures.

This degeneration leads to chronic progressive chorea and mental deterioration that ends in dementia.

What causes it

The cause of Huntington's disease isn't known. However, it's transmitted as an autosomal dominant trait.

Pathophysiology

Huntington's disease involves a disturbance in neurotransmitter substances, primarily gamma aminobutyric acid (GABA) and dopamine. GABA neurons in the basal ganglia, frontal cortex, and cerebellum are destroyed and replaced with glial cells. The deficiency of GABA (an inhibitory neurotransmitter) causes an excess of dopamine and abnormal neurotransmission along the affected pathways.

What to look for

• Severe choreic movements (involuntary, rapid, usually violent, and purposeless movements), initially unilateral and more prominent in the face and arms than in the legs
• Dementia, typically mild at first and then growing more severe until it disrupts the personality
• Loss of musculoskeletal control

What tests tell you

• PET scan and deoxyribonucleic acid analysis can detect Huntington's disease.
• CT scan and MRI reveal brain atrophy.

How it's treated

Huntington's disease has no known cure. Therefore, treatment focuses on supporting and protecting the patient, treating symptoms, and providing emotional support to the patient and his family. Tranquilizers and drugs, such as chlorpromazine, haloperidol, and imipramine (Tofranil), can help control choreic movement and alleviate discomfort and depression. However, they can't stop mental deterioration. In addition, tranquilizers increase rigidity.

What to do

• Attend to the patient's basic needs, such as hygiene, skin care, bowel and bladder care, and nutrition. Increase support as his mental and physical deterioration becomes more pronounced.
• Provide emotional support. The patient and his family can feel overwhelming despondency due to the degenerative and irreversible course of the disease. An extremely depressed patient may attempt suicide. Be alert for signs, and make sure the patient's environment is free from instruments that could permit self-inflicted injury.

Maintaining high levels

• Evaluate the patient's mobility and level of function. Plan interventions that help him maintain the highest level of mobility and independence possible for as long as possible.
• Keep the patient free from injury.
• Help the family identify resources that can help them cope with the patient's illness. (See *Huntington's disease teaching tips*.)

Meningitis

In meningitis, infection (bacterial or otherwise) causes inflammation of the brain and spinal meninges that can involve all three meningeal membranes: dura mater, arachnoid, and pia mater.

What causes it

• Bacteremia, especially due to pneumonia, empyema, osteomyelitis, or endocarditis
• Other infections, such as sinusitis, otitis media, encephalitis, or myelitis
• Brain abscess, usually caused by *Neisseria meningitidis, Haemophilus influenzae, Streptococcus pneumoniae,* or *Escherichia coli*
• Head injury, such as skull fracture, penetrating head wound, or neurosurgery
• Virus or other organism (aseptic meningitis) (See *Recognizing aseptic meningitis*, page 145.)

What to look for

• Fever, chills, malaise
• Headache, vomiting
• Signs of meningeal irritation, such as nuchal rigidity, positive Brudzinski's and Kernig's signs (see *Important signs of meningitis*), exaggerated and symmetrical deep tendon reflexes, or opisthotonos
• Seizures
• Delirium, deep stupor, and coma

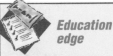

Education edge

Huntington's disease teaching tips

• Talk with the patient and family about the disease. Listen to their concerns and fears, and provide clear answers to questions.
• Keep in mind the patient's dysarthria and allow him time to express his thoughts.
• Teach the family appropriate patient care measures, and help them assume a greater role as the patient's condition deteriorates.
• Explain that children have a 50% chance of inheriting the disease and that genetic counseling is a good idea before starting a family.
• Refer the patient and family to organizations that can help them cope with the disease, such as a visiting nurse service, social services, psychiatric counseling, and long-term care facilities.

Important signs of meningitis

A positive response to these tests helps establish a diagnosis of meningitis.

Brudzinski's sign
Place the patient in a dorsal recumbent position, and then put your hands behind his neck and bend it forward. Pain and resistance may indicate neck injury or arthritis. However, if the patient also flexes the hips and knees, chances are that he has meningeal irritation and inflammation, a sign of meningitis.

Kernig's sign
Place the patient in a supine position. Flex his leg at the hip and knee, and then straighten the knee. Pain or resistance suggests meningitis.

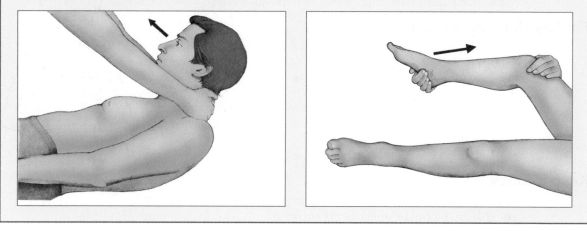

What tests tell you

Typically, CSF testing and positive Brudzinski's and Kernig's signs establish the diagnosis:
• Look for elevated CSF pressure, high CSF protein levels and, possibly, low glucose levels.
• CSF culture and sensitivity tests usually identify the infecting organism unless it's a virus. The Xpert EV test identifies the enterovirus in CSF.

How it's treated

Treatment includes antibiotic therapy (if the cause is bacterial) and vigorous supportive care. Usually, the patient receives I.V. antibiotics for 2 or more weeks, followed by oral antibiotics. Other prescribed drugs may include:
• digoxin (Lanoxin) to control arrhythmias
• mannitol (Osmitrol) to decrease cerebral edema
• an anticonvulsant or a sedative to reduce restlessness
• acetaminophen (Tylenol) to relieve headache and fever.

Oh no! Culture and sensitivity tests usually give me away in meningitis.

Culture club

Supportive measures include bed rest and measures to prevent dehydration. If nasal cultures are positive, isolation is necessary. Any coexisting conditions, such as endocarditis and pneumonia, are treated as well.

What to do

• Assess the patient's neurologic function often and watch for deterioration. Be especially alert for a temperature increase up to 102° F (38.9° C), deteriorating LOC, onset of seizures, and altered respirations, all of which may signal an impending crisis.

Finding fluid equilibrium

• Monitor the patient's fluid balance. Make sure he consumes enough fluids to prevent dehydration, but avoids fluid overload to decrease the risk of cerebral edema. Measure his central venous pressure, and record intake and output accurately.
• Position the patient carefully to prevent joint stiffness and neck pain. Turn him often, according to a planned positioning schedule. Help with ROM exercises.
• Maintain adequate nutrition and elimination.

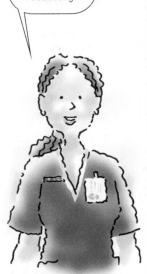

If nasal cultures are positive, isolation is necessary.

Keep it quiet...

• Maintain a quiet, comfortable environment. If necessary, darkening the room can help reduce photophobia.
• Relieve headache with a nonopioid analgesic, such as acetaminophen, as ordered. (Opioids interfere with accurate neurologic assessment.)

...and strictly aseptic

• Use strict aseptic technique when treating the patient with a head wound or skull fracture.
• Provide reassurance and support. The patient may be frightened by his illness and the need for frequent lumbar punctures. If he's disoriented or confused, calm and reorient him as often as needed. Reassure the family that the delirium and changes in behavior caused by meningitis usually disappear during recovery. However, if a severe neurologic deficit appears permanent, refer the patient to a rehabilitation program as soon as the acute phase of the illness has passed.
• Evaluate the patient's progress. If treatment is succeeding, the patient will be pain-free and his LOC will be normal. He'll maintain adequate hydration and nutrition and his blood pressure, heart

Recognizing aseptic meningitis

Aseptic meningitis, a benign syndrome, is characterized by headache, fever, vomiting, and meningeal symptoms. It results from infection by enteroviruses (most common), arboviruses, herpes simplex virus, mumps virus, or lymphocytic choriomeningitis virus.

First, a fever
Aseptic meningitis begins suddenly with a fever up to 104° F (40° C), alterations in level of consciousness (drowsiness, confusion, stupor), and neck or spine stiffness (slight at first) when bending forward. Other signs and symptoms include headache, nausea, vomiting, abdominal pain, poorly defined chest pain, and sore throat.

What virus is this anyway?
Patient history of recent illness and knowledge of seasonal epidemics are essential in differentiating among the many forms of aseptic meningitis. Negative bacteriologic cultures and cerebrospinal fluid (CSF) analysis that show pleocytosis and increased protein levels suggest the diagnosis. Isolation of the virus from the CSF confirms it.

Begin with bed rest
Supportive measures include bed rest, maintenance of fluid and electrolyte balance, analgesics for pain, and exercises to combat residual weakness. Isolation isn't necessary. Careful handling of excretions and good hand-washing technique prevent spreading the disease.

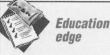

Education edge

Meningitis teaching tips

- Teach the patient and his family about the illness and expected recovery. The family may need to receive prophylactic antibiotics.
- Teach the patient and his family how to help prevent meningitis by seeking proper medical treatment for chronic sinusitis or other chronic infections.

rate, and respiratory rate will remain within normal limits. (See *Meningitis teaching tips.*)

Multiple sclerosis

MS is a major cause of chronic disability in young adults. It results from progressive demyelination of the white matter of the brain and spinal cord and is characterized by exacerbations and remissions. The prognosis varies. MS may progress rapidly, disabling patients by early adulthood or causing death within months of onset. Fortunately, however, 70% of all patients lead active, productive lives with long periods of remission.

What causes it

The exact cause is unclear; however, current theories suggest that it may be caused by an autoimmune response to a slow-acting or latent viral infection or by environmental or genetic factors.

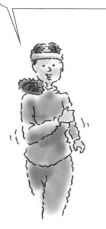

Fortunately, 70% of patients with MS lead active, productive lives with long periods of remission.

Pathophysiology

In MS, axon demyelination and nerve fiber loss occur in patches throughout the CNS, inducing widely disseminated and varied neurologic dysfunction.

What to look for

Accurate diagnosis requires evidence of multiple neurologic exacerbations and remissions. Signs and symptoms, which can vary considerably, include:
• vision disturbances, such as optic neuritis, diplopia, ophthalmoplegia, and blurred vision
• sensory impairment such as paresthesia
• muscle dysfunction, such as weakness, paralysis ranging from monoplegia to quadriplegia, spasticity, hyperreflexia, intention tremor, and gait ataxia
• urinary disturbances, such as incontinence, frequency, urgency, and frequent infections
• emotional lability, such as mood swings, irritability, and euphoria
• associated signs, such as poorly articulated speech and dysphagia.

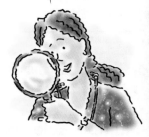

Because diagnosing MS is difficult, some patients undergo years of testing and close observation.

What tests tell you

Because of the difficulty inherent in establishing a diagnosis, some patients may undergo years of periodic testing and close observation. These tests may help diagnose MS:
• In one-third of all patients, EEG shows nonspecific abnormalities.
• Lumbar puncture reveals CSF with elevated gamma globulin fraction of immunoglobulin G, but normal total protein levels. An elevated CSF gamma globulin level is significant only when serum gamma globulin levels are normal. It reflects hyperactivity of the immune system due to chronic demyelination. Oligoclonal bands of immunoglobulin can be detected when CSF gamma globulin is examined by electrophoresis.

Evoking a reaction

• Evoked potential studies demonstrate slowed conduction of nerve impulses in 80% of patients.
• A CT scan may reveal lesions within the brain's white matter.

Legions with lesions

• MRI is the most sensitive method of detecting lesions and is also used to evaluate disease progression. Lesions are present in more than 90% of all patients undergoing this test.

How it's treated

The aim of treatment is to shorten exacerbations and relieve neurologic deficits to help the patient maintain as normal a lifestyle as possible. Drug therapy and other measures can achieve these goals.

Medicate, don't exacerbate

Methylprednisolone (Medrol) is commonly prescribed during acute exacerbations to reduce CNS inflammation. Other typically used corticosteroids include dexamethasone, prednisone, betamethasone (Celestone), and prednisolone (Prelone). For relapsing MS, glatiramer acetate (Copaxone) may be prescribed to reduce the frequency of attacks. Interferon beta-1a (Avonex) or interferon beta-1b (Betaseron) are effective in reducing disability progression and in decreasing the frequency of exacerbations.

In conjunction with corticosteroids, the practitioner may prescribe:
- fluoxetine to combat depression
- baclofen (Lioresal) or dantrolene (Dantrium) to relieve spasticity
- oxybutynin (Ditropan) to relieve urine retention and minimize frequency and urgency.

Support to cut short

During acute exacerbation, treatment routinely calls for:
- bed rest
- physical therapy and massages
- measures to prevent fatigue
- meticulous skin care to prevent pressure ulcers
- bowel and bladder training (if necessary)
- antibiotic treatment of bladder infection
- counseling.

What to do

- Nursing interventions focus on maintaining mobility, ensuring proper nutrition, and controlling pain during exacerbations.
- Form a care plan based on the patient's abilities and symptoms.
- Help with physical therapy and provide massages, relaxing baths, and other measures that promote comfort.
- Assist with active, resistive, and stretching exercises to maintain muscle tone and joint mobility, reduce spasticity, improve coordination, and boost morale.
- Encourage emotional stability by helping the patient establish a daily routine that maintains optimal functioning. Let the patient's tolerance regulate the level of daily activity. Encourage daily physical exercise and regular rest periods to prevent fatigue.
- Watch for drug therapy adverse effects. (See *MS teaching tips.*)

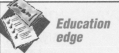

Education edge

MS teaching tips

- Teach the patient and family about the chronic course of the disease. Explain that exacerbations are unpredictable and will require physical and emotional adjustments.
- Emphasize the need to avoid stress, infections, and fatigue and to maintain independence by finding new ways to perform daily activities.
- Explain the value of a well-balanced, nutritious diet that contains sufficient fiber.
- Evaluate the need for bowel and bladder training and provide instruction, as needed.
- Encourage adequate fluid intake and regular urination.
- Teach the patient the correct use of suppositories to help establish a regular bowel schedule.
- Refer the patient and family to the National Multiple Sclerosis Society for more information.

Myasthenia gravis

Myasthenia gravis produces sporadic but progressive weakness and abnormal fatigue in striated (skeletal) muscles. This weakness and fatigue are exacerbated by exercise and repeated movement but improved by anticholinesterase drugs. Usually, myasthenia gravis affects muscles innervated by the cranial nerves (face, lips, tongue, neck, and throat), but it can affect any muscle group.

Hard to predict

Myasthenia gravis has an unpredictable course that includes periods of exacerbation and remission. There's no known cure. Drug treatment has improved the prognosis and allows patients to lead relatively normal lives, except during exacerbations. However, if the disease involves the respiratory system, it can be life-threatening. Myasthenia gravis affects 2 to 20 people per 100,000. It's most common in women between ages 18 and 25 and in men between ages 50 and 60.

What causes it

The cause of myasthenia gravis isn't known; however, it commonly accompanies autoimmune and thyroid disorders. In fact, 15% of all patients with myasthenia gravis have thymomas.

Pathophysiology

The patient's blood cells and thymus gland produce antibodies that block, destroy, or weaken the neuroreceptors that transmit nerve impulses, causing a failure in transmission of nerve impulses at the neuromuscular junction. (See *What happens in myasthenia gravis.*)

What to look for

Common signs of myasthenia gravis include:
- gradual, progressive skeletal muscle weakness and fatigue that worsens during the day
- weak eye closure, ptosis, and diplopia
- blank, masklike facial expression
- difficulty chewing and swallowing
- a hanging jaw
- bobbing motion of the head
- symptoms of respiratory failure if respiratory muscles are involved.

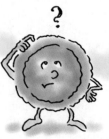

In myasthenia gravis, blood cells produce antibodies that ultimately cause nerve impulse transmission failure. Can you tell me why we do that?

A closer look

What happens in myasthenia gravis

During normal neuromuscular transmission, a motor nerve impulse travels to a motor nerve terminal, stimulating the release of a chemical neurotransmitter called acetylcholine (ACh). When ACh diffuses across the synapse, receptor sites in the motor end plate react and depolarize the muscle fiber. The depolarization spreads through the muscle fiber, causing muscle contraction.

Those darned antibodies
In myasthenia gravis, antibodies attach to the ACh receptor sites. They block, destroy, and weaken these sites, leaving them insensitive to ACh, thereby blocking neuromuscular transmission.

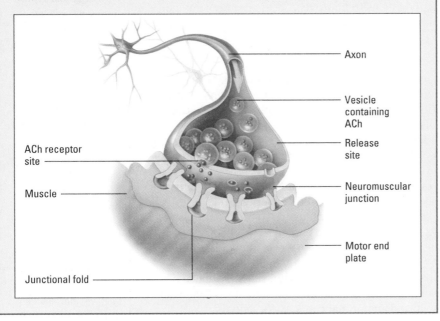

Axon

Vesicle containing ACh

Release site

ACh receptor site

Neuromuscular junction

Muscle

Motor end plate

Junctional fold

What tests tell you

- The Tensilon test confirms the diagnosis by temporarily improving muscle function after an I.V. injection of edrophonium or neostigmine. Long-standing ocular muscle dysfunction, however, may not respond. This test also differentiates a myasthenic crisis from a cholinergic crisis.
- Electromyography helps differentiate nerve disorders from muscle disorders.
- Nerve conduction studies test for receptor antibodies.

How it's treated

Treatment is symptomatic. Anticholinesterase drugs, such as pyridostigmine (Mestinon), counteract fatigue and muscle weakness and enable about 80% of normal muscle function. However, these measures become less effective as the disease worsens. Corticosteroids may help to relieve symptoms. A patient may undergo plasmapheresis. One with thymomas requires thymectomy, which may lead to remission in adult-onset myasthenia gravis.

In a crisis

Acute exacerbations that cause severe respiratory distress necessitate emergency treatment. Tracheotomy, positive-pressure ventilation, and vigorous suctioning to remove secretions usually yield improvement in a matter of days. Anticholinesterase drugs aren't effective during myasthenic crisis, so they're discontinued until respiratory function begins to improve. A crisis requires immediate hospitalization and vigorous respiratory support.

What to do

• Establish an accurate neurologic and respiratory baseline. Help remove secretions as they accumulate. Be alert for signs of an impending crisis (increased muscle weakness, respiratory distress, and difficulty talking or chewing).
• For the best results, administer drugs at evenly spaced intervals and on time, as ordered. Be prepared to give atropine for anticholinesterase overdose or toxicity.
• Plan periods of exercise, meals, patient care, and daily activities to take advantage of peaks in the patient's energy level.
• Provide soft, solid foods instead of liquids to reduce the risk of choking. Always sit the patient up to eat.
• Encourage the patient to take an active role in deciding about his care.
• Evaluate the patient. Look for normal vital signs, evidence of adequate hydration and normal elimination, skin that's free from sores or problems, and an optimal capacity for activity.
• Encourage the patient and his family to discuss their feelings, especially feelings of frustration, grief, or loss. Listen and provide emotional support. (See *Myasthenia gravis teaching tips*.)

Parkinson's disease

Parkinson's disease, a slowly progressive and degenerative disorder, is one of the most common neurologic disorders in the United States. Parkinson's disease may appear at any age; however, it's

Education edge

Myasthenia gravis teaching tips

• Help the patient plan daily activities to coincide with energy peaks. Stress the need for frequent rest periods throughout the day. Emphasize that periodic remissions, exacerbations, and day-to-day fluctuations are common.
• Teach the patient how to recognize adverse effects and signs of toxicity of anticholinesterase drugs (headaches, weakness, sweating, abdominal cramps, nausea, vomiting, diarrhea, excessive salivation, bronchospasm) and corticosteroids. Warn him to avoid strenuous exercise, stress, infection, and unnecessary exposure to the sun or cold weather. Caution him to avoid taking other medications without consulting his primary health care provider.
• Refer the patient to the Myasthenia Gravis Foundation for more information.

rare in people younger than age 30 and risk increases with age. Parkinson's disease most commonly affects men, and strikes 1 out of every 100 people older than age 60.

What causes it

In most instances, the cause of Parkinson's disease isn't known. However, some cases result from exposure to toxins, such as manganese dust and carbon monoxide, that destroy cells in the substantia nigra of the brain.

Pathophysiology

Parkinson's disease affects the extrapyramidal system, which influences the initiation, modulation, and completion of movement. The extrapyramidal system includes the corpus striatum, globus pallidus, and substantia nigra.

Parkinson's disease most commonly affects men, and the risk increases with age.

In Parkinson's disease, a dopamine deficiency occurs in the basal ganglia, the dopamine-releasing pathway that connects the substantia nigra to the corpus striatum. Reduction of dopamine in the corpus striatum upsets the normal balance between the dopamine (inhibitory) and acetylcholine (excitatory) neurotransmitters. Symptoms occur when affected brain cells can no longer perform their normal inhibitory function within the CNS.

What to look for

• Insidious tremor that begins in the fingers (unilateral pill-roll tremor), increases during stress or anxiety, and decreases with purposeful movement and sleep
• Muscle rigidity that resists passive muscle stretching; it may be uniform (lead-pipe rigidity) or jerky (cogwheel rigidity)
• Difficulty walking (gait lacks normal parallel motion and may be retropulsive or propulsive)
• Bradykinesia or slowing of muscle movements
• High-pitched monotone voice
• Drooling and dysphagia
• Masklike facial expression, poor blink reflex, and wide-open eyes
• Loss of postural control (body bent forward while walking)
• Slowed, monotonous, slurred speech that may become severely dysarthric
• Oculogyric crises (eyes are fixed upward, with involuntary tonic movements) and, occasionally, blepharospasm

What tests tell you

Laboratory test results rarely identify Parkinson's disease. Consequently, diagnosis depends on the patient's age, health history, and presence of characteristic signs of disease. However, urinalysis may reveal decreased dopamine levels, and CT scan or MRI may help rule out other disorders such as an intracranial tumor.

How it's treated

There's no known cure for Parkinson's disease. Treatment focuses on relieving symptoms and maintaining as high a level of function as possible for as long as possible. Drug therapy and physical therapy are the modes of treatment. In severe disease, stereotactic neurosurgery may be used.

Levodopa — with or without the carbs

Typical drug therapy includes levodopa (Dopar), a dopamine replacement that's most effective in the early stages. Levodopa can cause significant adverse reactions, so it's frequently given in combination with carbidopa, which halts peripheral dopamine synthesis. If carbidopa/levodopa (Sinemet) proves ineffective or too toxic, alternative drug therapy may include:
• dopamine agonists, such as bromocriptine (Parlodel), pramipexole (Mirapex), or ropinirole (Requip)
• anticholinergics such as trihexyphenidyl
• antihistamines such as diphenhydramine (Benadryl)
• amantadine (Symmetrel), an antiviral agent
• selegiline, an enzyme inhibitor.

A class by itself

A new class of drugs, catechol-O-methyltransferase (COMT) inhibitors (tolcapone [Tasmar]), which are combined with levodopa, are achieving some measure of success in prolonging relief from symptoms. These drugs block the enzyme that breaks down levodopa before it enters the brain. This enhances and prolongs the effect of levodopa. In younger patients, dopamine agonists may be used before COMT inhibitors. Unfortunately, prolonged use of any drug tends to reduce its effectiveness.

> A new class of drugs called COMT inhibitors are helping to prolong relief from symptoms.

In stereo

If drug therapy fails, stereotactic neurosurgery may offer a viable alternative. This procedure interrupts the function of the subthalamic nucleus, the pallidum, or the ventrolateral nucleus of the thalamus to prevent involuntary movement. This treatment is most effective in younger and otherwise healthy patients who have unilateral tremor or muscle rigidity. Neurosurgery is a palliative measure that can only relieve symptoms, not reverse the disease.

One deep brain

In some cases, deep brain stimulation is used to stop uncontrolled movements. The surgeon places electrodes in the thalamus or globus pallidus. Leads connect the electrodes to a device that the patient can activate when symptoms occur.

Get physical

Physical therapy complements drug treatment and neurosurgery to maintain normal muscle tone and function. Typically, physical therapy includes active and passive ROM exercises, routine daily activities, walking, and baths and massage to help relax muscles.

What to do

• If the patient has had surgery, monitor his LOC and vital signs closely for hemorrhage or increased ICP.
• Encourage independence. A patient with excessive tremor may have better control if he sits in a chair and uses the chair's arms to steady himself. Remember that fatigue can exacerbate symptoms and, in turn, increase the patient's dependence on others.
• Establish a regular bowel routine by encouraging the patient to drink 2 qt (2 L) of liquid daily and eat high-fiber foods. An elevated toilet seat can make it easier to transition from standing to sitting.
• Encourage the patient to remain as active as possible. The disease progresses more slowly in those who stay active.
• Encourage the patient and his family to ask questions. Listen to their concerns and provide succinct, accurate answers.
• Evaluate the patient. Optimal oxygen saturation levels will indicate adequate respiratory function. He should have normal urinary function and be free from UTI. In addition, he should perform normal daily activities within the limits imposed by his condition. The patient and his family should understand Parkinson's disease and its treatment. (See *Parkinson's disease teaching tips*.)

Seizure disorder

Patients with seizure disorders rarely have just one seizure. They're susceptible to recurrent seizures — paroxysmal events associated with abnormal electrical discharge of neurons in the brain. These discharges may be focal or diffuse, and the sites of the discharges determine the clinical manifestations that occur during the attack.

Seizures are among the most commonly observed neurologic dysfunctions in children and can occur with widely varying CNS conditions. The onset of seizures in adults should lead health care providers to suspect brain tumor or head injury.

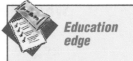

Education edge

Parkinson's disease teaching tips

• Teach the patient and family about the disease, its possible progressive stages, therapeutic management, and prevention of complications and injuries.
• Instruct the patient on his drug therapy and the relationship of drug administration to diet and food intake if he's taking levodopa. Caution him that drugs for Parkinson's disease commonly interact with medications taken for many other conditions.
• Encourage exercise, maximal independence in activities of daily living, and physical and occupational therapy to maintain muscle strength.
• Refer the patient and family to the National Parkinson Foundation or the United Parkinson Foundation for more information.

What causes it

Seizures are idiopathic (cause unknown) in about one-half of all cases. For the other half, possible causes include:
• genetic disorders or degenerative disease, such as phenylketonuria or tuberous sclerosis
• birth trauma (inadequate oxygen supply to the brain, blood incompatibility, or hemorrhage)
• infectious diseases (meningitis, encephalitis, or brain abscess)
• ingestion of toxins (mercury, lead, or carbon monoxide)
• brain tumors, head injury or trauma
• stroke (hemorrhage, thrombosis, or embolism).

Pathophysiology

Although the cause of seizures remains unclear, it's thought that a group of neurons may lose afferent stimulation (ability to transmit impulses from the periphery toward the CNS) and function as a seizure focus. These neurons are hypersensitive and easily activated. In response to changes in the cellular environment, the neurons become hyperactive and fire abnormally.

Fighting fire with fire

Upon stimulation, the seizure focus fires and spreads electrical current toward the synapse and surrounding cells. These cells fire in turn, and the impulse cascades to one side of the brain (a partial seizure), both sides of the brain (a generalized seizure), or toward the cortical, subcortical, or brain stem areas. A continuous seizure state known as *status epilepticus* can cause respiratory distress and even death. (See *Treating status epilepticus.*)

What to look for

There are generally six types of seizures:

    simple partial

    complex partial

    absence

    myoclonic

    generalized tonic-clonic

    atonic.

Simple partial seizure
- Sensory symptoms (flashing lights, smells, auditory hallucinations)
- Autonomic symptoms (sweating, flushing, pupil dilation)
- Psychic symptoms (dream states, anger, fear)

Complex partial seizure
- Altered LOC
- Amnesia

Absence seizure
- A brief change in LOC indicated by blinking or rolling of the eyes, a blank stare, and slight mouth movements

Myoclonic seizure
- Brief involuntary muscular jerks of the body or extremities

Generalized tonic-clonic seizure
- Typically beginning with a loud cry
- Change in LOC
- Body stiffening, alternating between muscle spasm and relaxation
- Tongue biting, incontinence, labored breathing, apnea, cyanosis
- Upon wakening, possible confusion and difficulty talking
- Drowsiness, fatigue, headache, muscle soreness, weakness

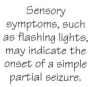

> Sensory symptoms, such as flashing lights, may indicate the onset of a simple partial seizure.

What do I do?

Treating status epilepticus

Status epilepticus is a continuous seizure that must be interrupted using emergency measures. It can occur during all types of seizures. For example, generalized tonic-clonic status epilepticus is a continuous generalized tonic-clonic seizure without an intervening return to consciousness.

Always an emergency
Status epilepticus is accompanied by respiratory distress and can be life-threatening. It can result from withdrawal of antiseizure medications (anticonvulsants or antiepileptics), hypoxic or metabolic encephalopathy, acute head trauma, or septicemia secondary to encephalitis or meningitis.

Acting fast
Typically, emergency treatment consists of diazepam (Valium), lorazepam (Ativan), fosphenytoin (Cerebyx), or phenobarbital; 50% dextrose I.V. when seizures are secondary to hypoglycemia; and thiamine I.V. in patients with chronic alcoholism or those undergoing withdrawal.

Atonic seizure
- General loss of postural tone
- Temporary loss of consciousness

What tests tell you

Primary diagnostic tests include:
- CT scan and MRI, which provide density readings of the brain and may indicate structural abnormalities
- EEG, which may show paroxysmal abnormalities that confirm the diagnosis of seizure disorder by providing evidence of the continuing tendency to have seizures. (A negative EEG doesn't rule out seizure disorder because the paroxysmal abnormalities occur intermittently.)

   Other informative tests include:
- serum glucose, electrolyte, drug, and calcium levels
- lumbar puncture
- brain scan
- PET scan
- cerebral angiography.

How it's treated

Typically, treatment consists of drug therapy. The most commonly prescribed drugs are phenytoin (Dilantin), carbamazepine (Tegretol), phenobarbital, and primidone (Mysoline) for generalized tonic-clonic seizures and complex partial seizures. Valproic acid (Depakene), clonazepam (Klonopin), and ethosuximide (Zarontin) are commonly prescribed for absence seizures.

   If drug therapy fails, the surgeon may choose to surgically remove a demonstrated focal lesion in an attempt to bring an end to seizures. Emergency treatment for status epilepticus usually consists of diazepam, lorazepam, fosphenytoin (Cerebyx), or phenobarbital; 50% dextrose I.V. (when seizures are secondary to hypoglycemia); and thiamine I.V. (in chronic alcoholism or withdrawal). Rectal preparations of diazepam and oral solutions of diazepam and lorazepam are concentrated and fast-acting.

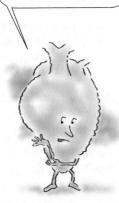

Make sure you monitor the patient's vital signs and cardiac status when you administer phenytoin.

What to do

- Monitor the patient for signs and symptoms of medication toxicity, such as nystagmus, ataxia, lethargy, dizziness, drowsiness, slurred speech, irritability, nausea, and vomiting.
- Administer phenytoin according to guidelines (not more than 50 mg/minute), and monitor the patient's vital signs and cardiac status often.

Education edge

Seizure disorder teaching tips

• Encourage the patient and his family to express their feelings about the patient's condition. Answer their questions honestly, and help them cope by dispelling some of the myths about seizures.

• Assure the patient and his family that following a prescribed regimen of medication will help in controlling seizures and maintaining a normal lifestyle.

• Stress the need for compliance with the prescribed drug schedule.

• Assure the patient that antiseizure medications are safe when taken as ordered. Reinforce dosage instructions, and find methods to help the patient remember to take his medication. Caution him to monitor the amount of medication left so he doesn't run out of it. It shouldn't be discontinued abruptly. He shouldn't take nonprescription drugs or herbs without consulting his practitioner.

• Describe the signs that may inadicate an adverse reaction, such as drowsiness, lethargy, hyperactivity, confusion, and vision and sleep disturbances. Tell the patient to report these signs to his practitioner immediately as they may indicate the need for a dosage adjustment.

• Phenytoin (Dilantin) therapy may lead to hyperplasia of the gums, which can be relieved by conscientious oral hygiene.

• Emphasize the importance of having antiseizure medication blood levels checked at regular intervals, even if the seizures are under control. Also, warn the patient against drinking alcoholic beverages.

Generalized tonic-clonic seizures

Generalized tonic-clonic seizures may necessitate first aid. Teach the patient's family how to give such aid correctly. Include these teaching points:

• Teach the family to provide safety measures if a seizure occurs by helping the patient to a lying position, loosening any tight clothing, and placing something flat and soft, such as a pillow, jacket, or hand, under his head. Advise them to clear the area of hard objects and not to force anything into the patient's mouth if his teeth are clenched. However, if his mouth is open, they can place a soft object (such as a folded cloth) between his teeth to protect his tongue.

• Know which social agencies in the patient's community can help. Refer the patient to the Epilepsy Foundation of America for general information and to the state motor vehicle department for information about his driver's license.

• Evaluate the patient to determine the effectiveness of the medication; seizure activity should decrease or stop. Note whether the patient has expressed his feelings regarding his illness to his friends or family. (See *Seizure disorder teaching tips*.)

Stroke

Stroke is the sudden interruption of circulation in one or more of the blood vessels supplying the brain. During a stroke, brain tissue fails to receive adequate oxygenation, resulting in serious tissue damage or necrosis. The speed with which circulation is restored determines the patient's chances for complete recovery.

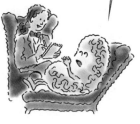

I hear that during a stroke the brain doesn't get enough oxygen. The whole idea makes me very anxious...

Not the back stroke

Strokes are classified by their course of progression. The least severe type, called *transient ischemic attack*, results from a temporary interruption of blood flow. (See *Understanding TIA*.) A progressive stroke, or stroke-in-evolution (thrombus-in-evolution), begins with a slight neurologic deficit that worsens over a day or two. In a complete stroke, the patient experiences maximum neurologic impairment immediately.

Factor this in

Stroke is the third most common cause of death in the United States and the most common cause of neurologic disability. Risk factors include a history of TIAs, atherosclerosis, hypertension, arrhythmias, lack of exercise, use of hormonal contraceptives, smoking, and a family history of cerebrovascular disease.

What causes it

• Thrombosis of the cerebral arteries that supply the brain or the intracranial vessels, occluding blood flow
• Embolism from a thrombus that formed outside the brain — for example, in the heart, aorta, or common carotid artery
• Hemorrhage from an intracranial artery or vein, possibly due to hypertension, ruptured aneurysm, AVM, trauma, hemorrhagic disorder, or septic embolism

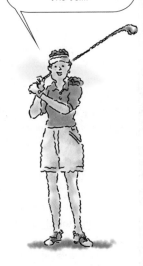

Thrombosis, embolus, and hemorrhage are the major causes of stroke. The main cause of a missed stroke in golf is not keeping your eye on the ball.

Understanding TIA

A transient ischemic attack (TIA) is a recurrent episode of neurologic deficit, lasting from seconds to hours, that clears within 12 to 24 hours. It's usually considered a warning sign of an impending thrombotic stroke. In fact, TIAs have been reported in 50% to 80% of patients who have had a cerebral infarction from thrombosis. The age of onset varies, but incidence rises dramatically after age 50 and is highest among blacks and men.

Interrupting blood flow

In a TIA, microemboli released from a thrombus may temporarily interrupt blood flow, especially in the small distal branches of the brain's arterial tree. Small spasms in those arterioles may precede the TIA and also impair blood flow.

A transient experience

The most distinctive characteristics of TIAs are the transient duration of neurologic deficits and the complete return of normal function. The signs and symptoms of a TIA correlate with the location of the affected artery. They include double vision, unilateral blindness, staggering or uncoordinated gait, unilateral weakness or numbness, falling because of weakness in the legs, dizziness, and speech deficits, such as slurring and thickness.

Preventing a complete stroke

During an active TIA, treatment aims to prevent a complete stroke and consists of aspirin or anticoagulants to minimize the risk of thrombosis. After or between attacks, preventive treatment includes treating the underlying cause (such as arrhythmias) and restoring adequate blood flow through the carotid arteries with carotid endarterectomy.

Pathophysiology

Thrombosis, embolus, and hemorrhage act in different ways.
• Thrombosis causes blockage and edema in the affected vessel and ischemia in the tissues supplied by the vessel.
• Embolus cuts off circulation in the cerebral vasculature by lodging in a narrow portion of the artery, causing ischemia and edema. If the embolus is septic and the infection extends beyond the vessel wall, an aneurysm may form, which increases the risk of a sudden rupture and cerebral hemorrhage.
• In hemorrhage, an artery in the brain leaks, rapidly reducing the blood supply to tissues served by the artery. Blood accumulates deep within the brain, causing even greater damage by further compromising neural tissue.

What to look for

When assessing signs of stroke, "sudden" is the key word. Signs typically include the sudden onset of:
• headache with no known cause
• numbness or weakness of the face, arm, or leg, especially on one side of the body
• confusion, trouble speaking or understanding
• trouble seeing or walking, dizziness, loss of coordination.

What tests tell you

• MRI or a CT scan shows evidence of thrombotic or hemorrhagic stroke, tumor, or hydrocephalus.
• Brain scan reveals ischemia, but may not be positive for up to 2 weeks after the stroke.
• In hemorrhagic stroke, lumbar puncture may reveal blood in the CSF.
• Carotid ultrasound may detect a blockage, stenosis, or reduced blood flow.
• Ophthalmoscopy may detect signs of hypertension and atherosclerosis in retinal arteries.
• Angiography can help pinpoint the site of occlusion or rupture.
• EEG may help localize the area of damage.
• Other laboratory studies, such as urinalysis, coagulation studies, CBC, serum osmolality, and electrolyte, glucose, lipid profile, antinuclear antibody, creatinine, and blood urea nitrogen levels, help establish baseline organ function.

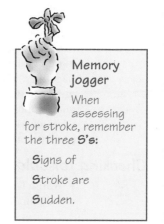

Memory jogger

When assessing for stroke, remember the three **S's**:

Signs of

Stroke are

Sudden.

How it's treated

Medical management of stroke commonly includes physical rehabilitation, diet and drug regimens to help reduce risk factors, possibly surgery, and care measures to help the patient adapt to specific deficits, such as motor impairment and paralysis.

Surgery possibilities

Depending on the stroke's cause and extent, the patient may undergo craniotomy to remove a hematoma, endarterectomy to remove atherosclerotic plaques from an arterial wall, placement of stents to reduce blockages, or extracranial bypass to circumvent a blocked artery. Ventricular shunts may be needed to drain CSF.

Take two

Drug therapy for stroke includes:
• low-dose aspirin (Ecotrin) or clopidogrel (Plavix) as an antiplatelet agent to prevent recurrent stroke (but not in hemorrhagic stroke)
• benzodiazepines, such as lorazepam and diazepam, to treat seizures
• anticonvulsants to treat or prevent seizures after the patient's condition has stabilized
• thrombolytics, such as alteplase (Activase) for emergency treatment of embolic stroke (typically within 3 hours of onset), or aspirin or heparin for patients with embolic or thrombotic stroke who aren't candidates for alteplase
• stool softeners, such as bisacodyl, to prevent straining, which increases ICP
• antihypertensives and antiarrhythmics to reduce risks associated with recurrent stroke
• corticosteroids, such as dexamethasone, to minimize cerebral edema
• analgesics to relieve headache following a hemorrhagic stroke.

What to do

• Maintain a patent airway and oxygenation. Loosen constricting clothes. Watch the patient's cheeks. If one side "balloons" with respiration, that's the side the stroke affected. If unconscious, the patient may aspirate saliva; keep him in a lateral position to promote drainage, or suction as needed. Insert an artificial airway and start mechanical ventilation or supplemental oxygen if needed.
• Check the patient's vital signs and neurologic status. Record observations and report any significant changes, such as changes in pupil dilation, signs of increased ICP, and nuchal rigidity or flaccidity. Monitor blood pressure, LOC, motor function (voluntary and involuntary movements), senses, speech, skin color, and temperature. A subsequent stroke may be imminent if blood pressure rises suddenly, the pulse is rapid and bounding, and the patient complains of a sudden headache.

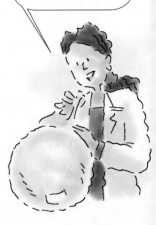

If one of the patient's cheeks "balloons" with respiration, that's the side the stroke affected.

Checking for color changes

• Watch for signs and symptoms of pulmonary emboli, such as chest pain, shortness of breath, dusky color, tachycardia, fever,

and changed sensorium. If the patient is unresponsive, monitor his arterial blood gas levels often, and alert the practitioner to increased $Paco_2$ or decreased partial pressure of arterial oxygen.
• Maintain fluid and electrolyte balance. If the patient can drink fluids, offer them as often as fluid limitations permit. Give I.V. fluids as ordered; yet, never give a large volume rapidly as this can increase ICP. Offer the bedpan or help the patient to the bathroom every 2 hours. If incontinent, the patient may need an indwelling urinary catheter; however, this increases the risk of infection.
• Ensure adequate nutrition. Check for gag reflex before offering small amounts of semisolid foods. Place the food tray within the patient's visual field. If the patient can't eat, insert an NG tube.
• Manage GI problems. Be alert for signs of straining as this increases ICP. Modify the patient's diet and administer a stool softener, as ordered. If the patient is nauseous, position him on his side to prevent aspiration of vomit. Provide antacids to reduce the risk of ulcer formation.
• Clean and irrigate the patient's mouth or dentures to remove food particles.

Keeping a watchful eye

• Provide meticulous eye care. Remove secretions with a gauze pad and sterile normal saline solution. Instill eyedrops, as ordered. If he's unable to close his eye, cover it with a patch.
• Position the patient. High-top sneakers, splints, or a footboard will help prevent footdrop and contracture. To prevent pressure ulcers, reposition the patient often or use a special mattress. Turn the patient at least once every 2 hours to prevent pneumonia. Raise the hand on the affected side to control dependent edema.
• Help the patient exercise. Perform ROM exercises for the affected and unaffected sides. Show him how to use his unaffected limbs to exercise his affected limbs.
• Administer medications, as ordered, and monitor the patient for adverse reactions.

Speak no evil

• Maintain communication with the patient. If he's aphasic, set up a simple method of communicating. Remember that an unresponsive patient may be able to hear. Don't say anything in his presence that you wouldn't want him to hear.
• Provide emotional support and establish a rapport. Spend time with the patient. Set realistic short-term goals and get the patient's family involved in his care when possible.
• Evaluate the patient. Look for a patent airway, normal breath sounds, adequate mobility, stable or improving LOC, and proper nutrition. Encourage the patient and his family as they cope with the disorder. (See *Stroke teaching tips*.)

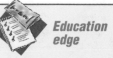

Education edge

Stroke teaching tips

• Teach the patient to comb his hair, dress, and wash, if needed. Obtain appliances, such as walkers, grab bars for the bathtub and toilet, and ramps, as needed.
• Encourage the patient to begin speech therapy, and follow through with the speech pathologist's suggestions.
• Involve the patient's family in all aspects of rehabilitation.
• If aspirin has been prescribed to minimize the risk of embolic stroke, tell the patient to watch for GI bleeding related to ulcer formation. Make sure the patient realizes that he can't substitute acetaminophen for aspirin.
• Warn the patient and family to report symptoms of stroke, such as severe headache, drowsiness, confusion, and dizziness. Emphasize the importance of regular follow-up visits.

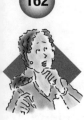

Quick quiz

1. The most common cause of dementia is:
A.   Alzheimer's disease.
B.   stroke.
C.   Parkinson's disease.
D.   aging.

Answer: A. Alzheimer's disease is the most common cause of dementia and the fourth leading cause of death in adults.

2. Brudzinski's sign and Kernig's sign are two tests that help diagnose:
A.   stroke.
B.   seizure disorder.
C.   meningitis.
D.   Parkinson's disease.

Answer: C. A positive response to one or both tests indicates meningeal irritation and helps diagnose meningitis.

3. MS is characterized by:
A.   progressive demyelination in the CNS.
B.   impaired cerebral circulation.
C.   deficiency of the neurotransmitter dopamine.
D.   deterioration of the spinal column.

Answer: A. Patches of demyelination cause widespread neurologic dysfunction.

4. Drug therapy for seizure disorder typically includes:
A.   antibiotics.
B.   anticonvulsants.
C.   antihypertensives.
D.   antiparkinson agents.

Answer: B. Anticonvulsants are commonly prescribed to control seizures. Adhering to the prescribed drug treatment plan and obtaining follow-up care to evaluate drug effectiveness are very important in controlling seizure activity.

Scoring

☆☆☆   If you answered all four questions correctly, yowza! Your neurons are firing at hyperspeed!

☆☆   If you answered three questions correctly, what an achievement! Hope you didn't strain a cranial nerve.

☆   If you answered fewer than three questions correctly, never fear. A review will restore your knowledge of neurologic disorders.

7

Eye disorders

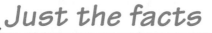

Just the facts

In this chapter, you'll learn:

♦ structures and functions of the eyes

♦ techniques for assessing the eyes

♦ appropriate nursing diagnoses for eye disorders

♦ common eye disorders and treatments.

A look at eye disorders

About 70% of all sensory information reaches the brain through the eyes. Disorders in vision can interfere with a patient's ability to function independently, perceive the world, and enjoy beauty.

No matter where you practice nursing, you're likely to encounter patients with eye problems. Some patients may report an eye problem as their chief complaint; others may tell you of a problem while you're evaluating another complaint or performing routine care.

Anatomy and physiology

The eye is the sensory organ of sight. It's a hollow ball filled with fluid (vitreous humor) and consists of three layers:

fibrous outer layer — sclera, bulbar conjunctiva, and cornea

vascular middle layer — iris, ciliary body, and choroid

inner layer — retina.

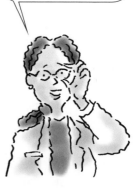

Some patients may seek care for an eye problem, and others may tell you of a problem during routine care.

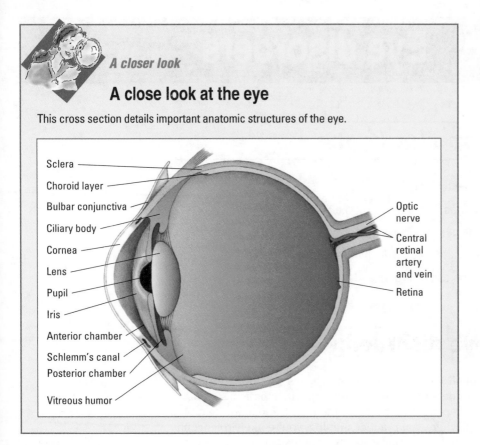

A closer look

A close look at the eye

This cross section details important anatomic structures of the eye.

Sclera
Choroid layer
Bulbar conjunctiva
Ciliary body
Cornea
Lens
Pupil
Iris
Anterior chamber
Schlemm's canal
Posterior chamber
Vitreous humor

Optic nerve
Central retinal artery and vein
Retina

Lens and liquids

Between the iris and retina lies the lens, suspended by ligaments from the ciliary body. The vitreous and aqueous humors are separated by the lens. The vitreous humor lies behind the lens, and the aqueous humor, in front of the lens.

Muscles for movement

Six extraocular muscles, innervated by the cranial nerves, control the movement of the eyes. The coordinated actions of those muscles allow the eyes to move in tandem, ensuring clear vision.

Lashes and lacrimals

Outside the eye, the bony orbits protect the eye from trauma. Eyelids (palpebrae), lashes, and the lacrimal apparatus protect it from injury, dust, and foreign bodies. (See *A close look at the eye.*)

> Eyelids, lashes, and the lacrimal apparatus protect the eye. I'm always glad to have help in the protection deparment!

Sclera, bulbar conjunctiva, and cornea

The sclera is the white coating on the outside of the eyeball. Together with the vitreous humor on the inside, the sclera helps maintain the retina's placement and the eyeball's nearly spherical shape. The bulbar conjunctiva, a thin, transparent membrane that lines the eyelid, covers and protects the anterior portion of the white sclera. The cornea is a smooth, avascular, transparent tissue located in front of the iris that refracts (bends) light rays entering the eye. A film of tears coats the cornea, keeping it moist. The cornea merges with the sclera at the corneal limbus.

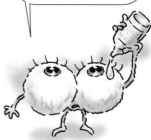

Pardon me while I freshen up the tears coating my cornea...

Here's mud in your eye

The ophthalmic branch of cranial nerve V (trigeminal nerve) innervates the cornea. Stimulation of this nerve initiates a protective blink called the *corneal reflex*.

Iris and pupil

The iris is a circular, contractile diaphragm that contains smooth and radial muscles and is perforated in the center by the pupil. Varying amounts of pigment granules within the iris's smooth muscle fibers give it color. Its posterior portion contains involuntary muscles that control pupil size to regulate the amount of light entering the eye.

Grand opening

The pupil, the iris's central opening, is normally round and equal in size to the opposite pupil. The pupil permits light to enter the eyes. Depending on the patient's age, pupil diameter can range from 3 to 5 mm.

The lens of the eye refracts and focuses light onto the retina.

Ciliary body and choroid

Suspensory ligaments attached to the ciliary body control the lens's shape for close and distant vision. The pigmented, vascular choroid supplies the outer retina's blood supply, then drains blood through its remaining vasculature.

Lens and vitreous chamber

Located behind the iris at the pupillary opening, the lens consists of avascular, transparent fibrils in an elastic membrane called the *lens capsule*. The lens refracts and focuses light onto the retina. The vitreous chamber, located behind the lens, makes up four-fifths of the eyeball. This chamber is filled with vitreous humor,

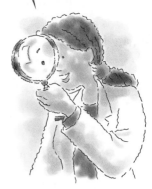

the gelatinous substance that, along with the sclera, maintains the shape of the eyeball.

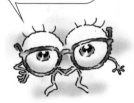

I keep in close touch with the brain.

Posterior and anterior chambers

The posterior chamber, which lies right in front of the lens, is filled with a watery fluid called *aqueous humor.* As it flows through the pupil into the anterior chamber, this fluid bathes the lens capsule. The amount of aqueous humor in the anterior chamber varies to maintain pressure in the eye. Fluid drains from the anterior chamber through collecting channels (trabecular meshwork) into Schlemm's canal.

Retina

The retina is the innermost layer of the eyeball. It receives visual stimuli and transmits images to the brain for processing. Vision of any kind depends on the retina and its structures. The retina contains the retinal vessels, the optic disk, the physiologic cup, rods and cones, the macula, and the fovea centralis.

The retina has four sets of retinal vessels. Each of the four sets contains a transparent arteriole and vein that nourish the inner areas of the retina. As these vessels leave the optic disk, they become progressively thinner, intertwining as they extend to the periphery of the retina.

No light here

The optic disk is a well-defined, round or oval area measuring less than ⅛" (0.3 cm) within the retina's nasal portion. The ganglion nerve fibers (axons) exit the retina through this area to form the optic nerve. This area is called the *blind spot* because it contains no light-sensitive cells (photoreceptors). The physiologic cup is a light-colored depression within the temporal side of the optic disk where blood vessels enter the retina. It covers a quarter to a third of the disk.

It doesn't take very much light to make a rod respond.

Now I see the light!

Photoreceptor neurons called *rods and cones* make vision possible. Rods respond to low-intensity light and shades of gray. Cones respond to bright light and are responsible for sharp, color vision.

Look sharp!

Located near the center of the retina lateral to the optic disk, the macula is slightly darker than the rest of the retina. The macula provides the sharpest

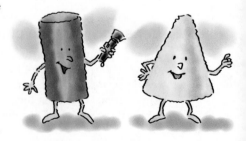

vision, allowing us to read and recognize faces, for example. The fovea centralis, a slight depression within the macula, contains the heaviest concentration of cones and provides the clearest vision and color perception.

Assessment

Now that you're familiar with the anatomy and physiology of the eyes, you're ready to assess them.

History

To obtain an accurate and complete patient history, adjust your questions to the patient's specific complaint and compare the answers with the results of the physical assessment.

Current health status

Begin by asking the patient some basic questions about his vision:
• Do you have any problems with your eyes?
• Do you wear or have you ever worn corrective lenses? If so, for how long? Are they glasses or hard or soft contact lenses?
• For what eye condition do you wear corrective lenses? Do you wear them all the time or just for certain activities, such as reading or driving?

Previous health status

To gather information about the patient's past eye health, ask these questions:
• Have you ever had blurred vision or lost your vision in one eye temporarily? Have you ever seen spots, floaters, or halos around lights?
• Have you ever had eye surgery or an eye injury?
• Do you have a history of high blood pressure or diabetes?
• Are you taking prescription medications for your eyes or other conditions? If so, which medications and how much and how often do you take them?

Family health status

Next, ask the patient if anyone in his family has an eye disorder. Also ask if anyone in the patient's family has ever been treated for myopia, cataracts, glaucoma, retinal detachment, or loss of vision.

Lifestyle patterns

To explore daily habits that might affect the patient's eyes, ask these questions:
• Does your occupation require intensive use of your eyes, such as long-term reading or prolonged use of a video display terminal?
• Does the air where you work or live contain anything that causes you to have eye problems?
• Do you wear goggles when working with power tools, or when engaging in sports that might irritate or endanger the eye, such as swimming, fencing, or playing racquetball?

> Ask your patient about daily routines that may affect eye health, such as prolonged computer use.

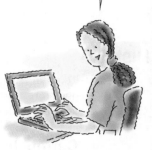

Physical examination

An eye assessment involves inspecting the conjunctivae, assessing the pupils, assessing eye muscle function, and examining intraocular structures with an ophthalmoscope.

Inspecting the conjunctivae

To inspect the conjunctivae, ask the patient to look up. Gently pull the lower eyelid down to inspect the bulbar conjunctiva. It should be clear and shiny. Note excessive redness or exudate. Also observe the sclera's color, which should be white to buff. In black patients, you may see flecks of tan.

In the pink

To examine the palpebral conjunctiva (the membrane that lines the eyelids), have the patient look down. Then lift the upper lid, holding the upper lashes against the eyebrow with your finger. The palpebral conjunctiva should be uniformly pink.

Assessing the pupils

The pupils should be equal in size, round, and reactive to light. In normal room light, the pupil will be about one-fourth the size of the iris. Unequal pupils generally indicate neurologic damage, iritis, glaucoma, or therapy with certain drugs.

The direct approach

Test the pupils for direct and consensual response. In a slightly darkened room, hold a penlight about 20″ (51 cm) from the patient's eyes, and direct the light at one eye from the side. Note the reaction of the pupil you're testing (direct response) and the opposite pupil (consensual response). They should both react the same way. Also note sluggishness or inequality in the response.

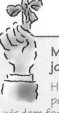

Memory jogger

Here's a pearl of wisdom for you: When examining the patient's pupils, remember the acronym **PERRL:**

Pupils

Equal

Round and

Reactive to

Light.

A pupil that doesn't react to light (a "fixed" pupil) can be an ominous neurologic sign. Repeat the test with the other pupil.

So accommodating

To test the pupils for accommodation, place your finger approximately 4″ (10 cm) from the bridge of the patient's nose. Ask the patient to look at a fixed object in the distance and then to look at your finger. His pupils should constrict and his eyes converge as he focuses on your finger.

Assessing eye muscle function

Testing the six cardinal positions of gaze evaluates the function of each of the six extraocular muscles and the cranial nerves responsible for their movement (cranial nerves III, IV, and VI).

Roving eyes

To perform the test, ask the patient to remain still while you hold a pencil or other small object directly in front of his nose at a distance of about 18″ (46 cm). Ask him to follow the object with his eyes without moving his head. Then move the object to each of the six cardinal positions, returning to the midpoint after each movement. The patient's eyes should remain parallel as they move. (See *Cardinal positions of gaze.*)

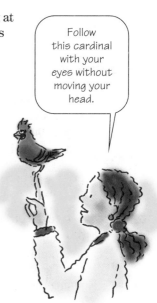

Follow this cardinal with your eyes without moving your head.

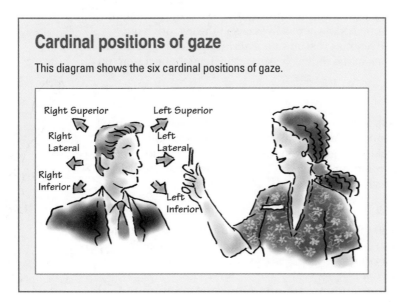

Cardinal positions of gaze

This diagram shows the six cardinal positions of gaze.

Right Superior
Left Superior
Right Lateral
Left Lateral
Right Inferior
Left Inferior

Examining intraocular structures

The ophthalmoscope allows you to directly observe internal structures of the eye. To see those structures properly, you should adjust the lens disc several times during your examination. Use the black, positive numbers on the disc to focus on near objects, such as the patient's cornea and lens. Use the red, negative numbers to focus on distant objects such as the retina. (See *Seeing eye to eye.*)

Looking at the lens

First, set the ophthalmoscope's lens disc to zero and hold the ophthalmoscope about 4″ (10 cm) from the patient's eye. Direct the light through the pupil to elicit the red reflex, a reflection of light off the choroid.

Now, move the ophthalmoscope closer to the eye. Adjust the lens disc so you can focus on the eye's anterior chamber and lens. If the lens is opaque, indicating cataracts, you may not be able to complete the examination.

Rotating to the retinal structures

To examine the retinal structures, start with the dial turned to zero. Rotate the lens-power disc to keep the retinal structures in focus. The first retinal structures you'll see are the blood vessels. Rotating the dial into the negative numbers will bring the blood vessels into focus. The arteries will look thinner and brighter than the veins.

Follow one of the vessels along its path toward the nose until you reach the optic disk, where all vessels in the eye originate. Examine arteriovenous crossings for arteriovenous nicking (localized constrictions in the retinal vessels), which might be a sign of hypertension.

Diggin' the disk

The optic disk is a creamy pink to yellow-orange structure with clear borders and a round-to-oval shape. The disk may fill or exceed your field of vision. If you don't see it, follow a blood vessel toward the center until you do. The nasal border of the disk may look somewhat blurred.

Riveted on the retina

Completely scan the retina by following four blood vessels from the optic disk to different peripheral areas. As you scan, note lesions or hemorrhages. (See *A close look at the retina.*)

Seeing eye to eye

This illustration shows how to correctly hold an ophthalmoscope when examining the internal structures of the eye.

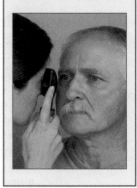

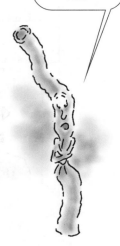

Constrictions in the retinal vessels may be a sign of hypertension. Ack!

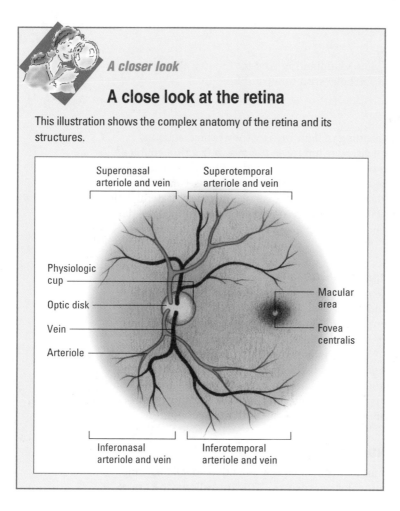

A closer look

A close look at the retina

This illustration shows the complex anatomy of the retina and its structures.

Superonasal arteriole and vein

Superotemporal arteriole and vein

Physiologic cup

Optic disk

Vein

Arteriole

Macular area

Fovea centralis

Inferonasal arteriole and vein

Inferotemporal arteriole and vein

Movin' in on the macula

Finally, move the light laterally from the optic disk to locate the macula, the part of the eye most sensitive to light. It appears as a darker structure, free from blood vessels. If you locate it, ask the patient to shift his gaze into the light.

Diagnostic tests

Tests to determine the presence of eye disorders include direct evaluation techniques as well as radiologic and imaging studies.

Direct evaluation

Refraction, slit-lamp examination, and tonometry allow direct evaluation of various eye structures and functions.

Refraction

Defined as the bending of light rays by the cornea, aqueous humor, lens, and vitreous humor in the eye, refraction enables images to focus on the retina and directly affects visual acuity. This test is done routinely during a complete eye examination or whenever a patient complains of a change in vision. It defines the degree of impairment (refractive error) and determines the degree of correction required to improve visual acuity with glasses or contact lenses.

Nursing considerations
• Explain to the patient the test is painless and safe and that it takes about 30 minutes.
• Tell the patient he shouldn't use any eyedrops, including prescription eyedrops, for at least 24 hours before the test.
• Explain that eyedrops may be instilled to dilate the pupils and inhibit accommodation by the lens. Ask the patient whether he has had a hypersensitivity reaction to eyedrops, has angle-closure glaucoma, or has an intraocular lens implant. Dilating eyedrops shouldn't be administered to anyone with those conditions.

Slit-lamp examination

The slit lamp is an instrument equipped with a special lighting system and a binocular microscope. This tool allows the practitioner to visualize in detail the anterior segment of the eye, which includes the eyelids, eyelashes, conjunctiva, sclera, cornea, tear film, anterior chamber, iris, lens, and anterior portion of the vitreous humor (vitreous face). If abnormalities are noted, special devices may be attached to the slit lamp to allow more detailed investigation.

Nursing considerations
• If the patient is wearing contact lenses, have him remove them before the test, unless the test is being performed to evaluate the fit of the contact lenses.
• When instilling dilating drops, tell the patient that his near vision will be blurred for 40 minutes to 2 hours. Advise him to wear dark glasses in bright sunlight until his pupils return to normal diameter.

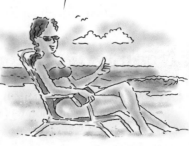

Tell the patient taking dilating eyedrops to wear dark glasses in bright sunlight.

• Don't administer dilating eyedrops to the patient who has angle-closure glaucoma, is hypersensitive to mydriatics, or has an intraocular lens implant.

Tonometry

Tonometry allows noninvasive measurement of intraocular pressure (IOP) to detect glaucoma, a common cause of blindness, at an early stage in the disease. In the early stages of glaucoma, increased IOP causes the eyeball to harden and become more resistant to extraocular pressure. Pneumotonometry uses a puff of air to the eye to measure pressure; applanation tonometry provides the same information by measuring the amount of force required to flatten a known corneal area.

Nursing considerations

• Because an anesthetic is instilled before the test, tell the patient not to rub his eyes for at least 20 minutes after the test, to prevent corneal abrasion.
• If the patient wears contact lenses, tell him not to reinsert them for at least 30 minutes after the test.
• If the tonometer moved across the cornea during the test, tell the patient that he may feel a slight scratching sensation in the eye when the anesthetic wears off. Explain that this sensation could be the result of a corneal abrasion and should disappear within 24 hours; however, the practitioner may prescribe prophylactic antibiotic drops.

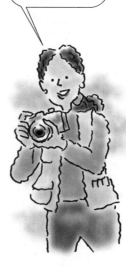

Show me that beautiful retinal circulation. Work it, work it!

Radiologic and imaging studies

Radiologic and imaging studies include fluorescein angiography, ocular ultrasonography, and orbital computed tomography (CT).

Fluorescein angiography

Fluorescein angiography records the appearance of blood vessels inside the eye through rapid-sequence photographs of the fundus (posterior inner part of the eye).

Picture perfect

The photographs, which are taken with a special camera, follow the I.V. injection of sodium fluorescein. This contrast medium enhances the visibility of microvascular structures of the retina and choroid, allowing evaluation of the entire retinal vascular bed, including retinal circulation.

Nursing considerations

• Check the patient's history for an intraocular lens implant, glaucoma, and hypersensitivity reactions, especially reactions to contrast media and dilating eyedrops.
• If miotic eyedrops are ordered, tell the patient with glaucoma not to use them on the day of the test.
• Explain to the patient that eyedrops will be instilled to dilate his pupils and that a dye will be injected into his arm. Remind him to maintain his gaze position and fixation as the dye is injected. Tell him that he may briefly experience nausea and a feeling of warmth. Reassure him as necessary.
• Observe the patient for hypersensitivity reactions to the dye, such as vomiting, dry mouth, metallic taste, sudden increased salivation, sneezing, light-headedness, fainting, and hives. Rarely, anaphylactic shock may result.
• Remind the patient that his skin and urine will be a yellow color for 24 to 48 hours after the test and that his near vision will be blurred for up to 12 hours.

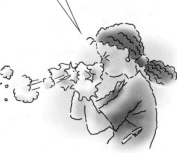

Hypersensitivity reactions to the dye include dry mouth, metallic taste, light-headedness, and... and...AH-CHOO! sneezing...

Ocular ultrasonography

Ocular ultrasonography measures high-frequency sound waves that pass through the eye and reflect off ocular structures, providing an illustration of the eye's structures. This method especially helps to evaluate a fundus clouded by an opaque medium such as a cataract. In such a patient, this test can identify pathologies that ophthalmoscopy can't normally detect. The practitioner may also order this test before such surgery as cataract removal or intraocular lens implantation. Ocular ultrasonography may also be performed before such surgery as cataract removal or implantation of an intraocular lens.

Nursing considerations

• Tell the patient that a small transducer will be placed on his closed eyelid and that the transducer will transmit high-frequency sound waves that will reflect off the structures in the eye.
• Inform him that he may be asked to move his eyes or change his gaze during the procedure; explain that his cooperation will help to ensure accurate results.
• After the test, remove the water-soluble jelly that was placed on the patient's eyelids.

Orbital computed tomography

Orbital CT allows visualization of abnormalities that standard X-rays don't readily show. For instance, orbital CT can delineate the size, position, and relationship of an abnormality to adjoining structures. Contrast media may be used to define ocular tissues and help confirm a suspected circulatory disorder, hemangioma, or subdural hematoma. Orbital CT does more than just evaluate orbital and adjoining structures; it also permits precise diagnosis of many intracranial lesions that affect vision.

Nursing considerations

• If a contrast medium will be administered, withhold food and fluids from the patient for 4 hours before the test. Check his history for hypersensitivity reactions to iodine, shellfish, or radiographic dyes.
• Tell the patient that he'll be positioned on an X-ray table and that the head of the table will move into the scanner, which will rotate around his head and make a whirring noise.
• If a contrast medium will be used for the procedure, tell the patient that he may feel flushed and warm and may experience a transient headache, a salty taste, and nausea or vomiting after injection of the medium. Reassure him that these reactions to the contrast medium are typical.

Treatments

For eye disorders, treatments consist of drug therapy and surgery.

Drug therapy

Topical medications are commonly used to treat eye disorders; however, the practitioner may also prescribe systemic medications. These medications include anti-infectives, anti-inflammatories, miotics, mydriatics, vasoconstrictors, and other medications. It's essential to provide proper patient teaching on instillation of these topical agents. (See *Instilling eye ointment and eyedrops.*)

Surgery

Surgical treatments for eye disorders include cataract removal, iridectomy, laser surgery, scleral buckling, and trabeculectomy.

Cataract removal

Two techniques allow the removal of cataracts: intracapsular cataract extraction (ICCE) and extracapsular cataract extraction (ECCE).

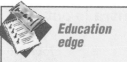

Education edge

Instilling eye ointment and eyedrops

To teach the patient how to instill eye ointment, tell him to follow these steps:
• Hold the tube for several minutes to warm the ointment.
• Squeeze a small amount of ointment $1/4''$ to $1/2''$ (0.5 to 1.5 cm) inside the lower lid.
• Gently close the eye and roll the eyeball in all directions.
• Wait 10 minutes before instilling other ointments.

To teach the patient how to instill eyedrops, tell him to follow these steps:
• Tilt the head back and pull down on the lower eye lid.
• Drop the medication into the conjunctival sac.
• Apply pressure to the inner canthus for 1 minute after administration of drops to prevent systemic absorption.
• Wait 5 minutes before instilling a second drop.

Intra is out

In ICCE, the entire lens is removed, most commonly with a cryo-probe. However, this technique isn't widely used today.

In ECCE, the patient's anterior capsule, cortex, and nucleus are removed, leaving the posterior capsule intact. This is the primary treatment for congenital and traumatic cataracts.

In with the implant

Immediately after removal of the natural lens, many patients receive an intraocular lens implant. An implant works especially well for elderly patients who can't use eyeglasses or contact lenses (because of arthritis or tremors, for example). (See *Bilateral cataract surgery: Simultaneous or staggered?*)

> Wearing an eye patch will prevent injury and infection after surgery — and you can pretend you're a pirate. Aaargh!

Patient preparation

Tell the patient he'll need to:
• temporarily wear an eye patch after surgery to prevent traumatic injury and infection
• get help when getting out of bed
• sleep on the unaffected side to reduce IOP.

Monitoring and aftercare

After the patient returns from surgery, follow these important steps:

Weighing the evidence

Bilateral cataract surgery: Simultaneous or staggered?

Because many patients develop cataracts in both eyes, surgery is typically performed on both eyes to remove the cataracts. That raises a question: Is it better for the patient to have surgery on both eyes simultaneously or to stagger the surgeries on different days?

A safe and satisfying option

To answer that question, researchers compared 94 patients who had simultaneous bilateral cataract removal with 100 patients who had bilateral cataract surgeries staggered by 2 days. The researchers found no differences in the clinical outcomes between the two groups. They concluded that bilateral simultaneous cataract surgery is not only safe and effective but has a high degree of patient satisfaction.

Chung, J.K., et al. (2009). Bilateral cataract surgery: A controlled clinical trial. *Japanese Journal of Ophthalmology, 53*(2), 107–13.

• Notify the practitioner if the patient has severe pain. Also, report increased IOP.
• Because of the change in the patient's depth perception, assist him with ambulation and observe other safety precautions.
• Make sure the patient wears the eye patch for 24 hours, except when instilling eyedrops as ordered, and have him wear an eye shield, especially when sleeping.
• Instruct the patient to continue wearing the shield at night or whenever he sleeps for several weeks, as ordered.

Home care instructions

Before discharge, teach the patient:
• how to administer eyedrops or ointments
• to contact the practitioner immediately if sudden eye pain, red or watery eyes, photophobia, or sudden vision changes occur
• to avoid activities that raise IOP, including heavy lifting, straining during defecation, and vigorous coughing and sneezing
• not to exercise strenuously for 6 to 10 weeks
• to wear dark glasses to relieve glare
• that changes in his vision can present safety hazards if he wears eyeglasses
• how to use up-and-down head movements to judge distances to help compensate for loss of depth perception
• how to insert, remove, and care for contact lenses, if appropriate, or how to arrange to visit a practitioner routinely for removal, cleaning, and reinsertion of extended-wear lenses
• when to remove the eye patch and when to begin using his eyedrops.

Iridectomy

Performed by laser or standard surgery, an iridectomy reduces IOP by easing the drainage of aqueous humor. This procedure makes a hole in the iris, creating an opening through which the aqueous humor can flow to bypass the pupil. An iridectomy is commonly performed to treat acute angle-closure glaucoma.

Another angle

Because glaucoma usually affects both eyes eventually, patients commonly undergo preventive iridectomy on the unaffected eye. It may also be indicated for a patient with an anatomically narrow angle between the cornea and iris. An iridectomy is also used for chronic angle-closure glaucoma, with excision of tissue for biopsy or treatment, and sometimes with other eye surgeries, such as cataract removal, keratoplasty, and glaucoma-filtering procedures.

Patient preparation

Make it clear to the patient that an iridectomy doesn't restore vision loss caused by glaucoma but that it may prevent further loss.

Monitoring and aftercare

After an iridectomy, take the following steps:
• Watch for hyphema (hemorrhaging into the anterior chamber of the eye) with sudden, sharp eye pain or the presence of a small half-moon-shape blood speck in the anterior chamber when checked with a flashlight. If either occurs, have the patient rest quietly in bed, with his head elevated, and notify the practitioner.
• Administer a topical corticosteroid to decrease inflammation and medication to dilate the pupil.
• Administer a stool softener to prevent constipation and straining during bowel movements, which increases venous pressure in the head, neck, and eyes. This increased pressure can led to increased IOP or strain on the suture line or blood vessels in the affected area.

Home care instructions

Before discharge, teach the patient to:
• report sudden, sharp eye pain immediately, because it may indicate increased IOP
• refrain from strenuous activity for 3 weeks
• refrain from coughing, sneezing, and vigorous nose blowing, which raise venous pressure
• move slowly, keep his head raised, and sleep with two pillows under his head.

Laser surgery

The treatment of choice for many ophthalmic disorders is laser surgery because it's relatively painless and especially useful for elderly patients, who may be poor surgical risks. Depending on the type of laser, the finely focused, high-energy beam shines at a specific wavelength and color to produce various effects. Laser surgery can be used to treat retinal tears, diabetic retinopathy, macular degeneration, and glaucoma.

Patient preparation

Before the procedure, take these steps:
• Tell the patient he'll be awake and seated at a slit lamp–like instrument for the procedure.
• Explain that his chin will be supported and that he'll wear a special contact lens that will prevent him from closing his eye.

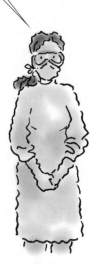

Laser surgery calls for safety precautions, including eye protection for everyone in the room.

- Explain that laser use requires safety precautions, including eye protection for everyone in the room.

Monitoring and aftercare

After the procedure, the patient may occasionally have eye pain. Apply ice packs as needed to help decrease the pain. The patient may be discharged after this office procedure.

Home care instructions

Instruct the patient to receive follow-up care as scheduled. Tell him that ice packs may ease eye discomfort.

Scleral buckling

Used to repair retinal detachment, scleral buckling involves applying external pressure to the separated retinal layers to bring the choroid into contact with the retina. Indenting (or buckling) brings the layers together so that an adhesion can form. It also prevents vitreous fluid from seeping between the detached layers of the retina, which could lead to further detachment and possible blindness. (See *Scleral buckling for retinal detachment.*)

Scleral buckling for retinal detachment

In scleral buckling, cryothermy (cold therapy), photocoagulation (laser therapy), or diathermy (heat therapy) creates a sterile inflammatory reaction that seals the retinal hole and causes the retina to readhere to the choroid. The surgeon then places a silicone plate or sponge — called an *explant* — over the site of reattachment and holds it in place with a silicone band. The pressure exerted on the explant indents (buckles) the eyeball and gently pushes the choroid and retina closer together.

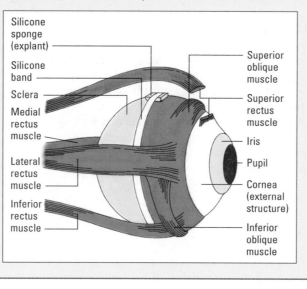

- Silicone sponge (explant)
- Silicone band
- Sclera
- Medial rectus muscle
- Lateral rectus muscle
- Inferior rectus muscle
- Superior oblique muscle
- Superior rectus muscle
- Iris
- Pupil
- Cornea (external structure)
- Inferior oblique muscle

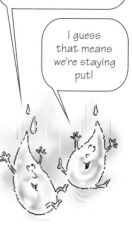

Scleral buckling also prevents vitreous fluid from seeping between layers of the retina.

I guess that means we're staying put!

A frigid look

Another method of reattaching the retina is pneumatic retinopexy. This procedure involves sealing the tear or hole with cryotherapy and introducing gas to provide a tamponade of the retina and the layer beneath it.

Patient preparation

Depending on the patient's age and the surgeon's preference, advise him whether he'll receive a local or general anesthetic.

Monitoring and aftercare

After the procedure, take these steps:
• Notify the practitioner immediately if you observe eye discharge or if the patient experiences fever or sudden, sharp, or severe eye pain.
• As ordered, administer mydriatic and cycloplegic eyedrops to keep the pupil dilated, an antibiotic to prevent infection, and a corticosteroid to reduce inflammation.
• For swelling of the eyelids, apply ice packs.
• Because the patient will probably have binocular patches in place for several days, institute safety precautions while he's hospitalized. Raise the side rails of his bed, and help him when he walks.
• Advise the patient to avoid activities that increase IOP, such as hard coughing or sneezing, or straining during defecation. If he's nauseated, administer an antiemetic, because vomiting increases IOP.

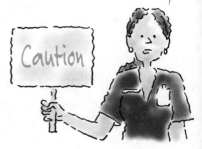

Tell the patient to avoid strenuous activity that increases IOP.

Home care instructions

Before discharge, instruct the patient to:
• notify the practitioner of signs of recurring detachment, including floating spots, flashing lights, and progressive shadow
• report fever, persistent excruciating eye pain, or drainage
• avoid activity that risks eye injury
• avoid heavy lifting, straining, or any strenuous activity that increases IOP
• use dilating, antibiotic, or corticosteroid drops as prescribed
• avoid rapid eye movements.

Trabeculectomy

Trabeculectomy is a surgical filtering procedure that removes part of the trabecular meshwork to allow aqueous humor to bypass blocked outflow channels and flow safely away from the eye. This procedure creates an opening under the conjunctiva. An iridectomy is then performed to prevent the iris from prolapsing into the new opening and obstructing the flow of aqueous humor. A trabeculectomy helps treat glaucoma that doesn't respond to drug therapy.

> Trabeculectomy will probably prevent further vision problems but won't restore the vision you've already lost.

Patient preparation

Inform the patient that this procedure will probably prevent further vision impairment but that it won't restore vision that's already lost.

Monitoring and aftercare

After a trabeculectomy:
• Report excessive bleeding from the affected area.
• Observe for nausea; if necessary, administer an antiemetic because vomiting can raise IOP.
• Administer eyedrops (usually a miotic such as pilocarpine [Carpine]).
• Immediately instill a cycloplegic such as atropine. If ordered, give a corticosteroid to reduce iritis, an analgesic to relieve pain, and a beta-adrenergic blocker to reduce pressure.
• Continue previously prescribed eyedrops — a miotic such as pilocarpine or a beta-adrenergic blocker — in the unaffected eye.
• Remind the patient that he should avoid all activities that increase IOP, including trying to avoid hard coughing or sneezing as well as straining during defecation.

Home care instructions

Instruct the patient to:
• immediately report sudden onset of severe eye pain, photophobia, excessive tearing, inflammation, or vision loss
• understand that glaucoma isn't curable but can be controlled by taking prescribed drugs regularly to treat this condition
• avoid constrictive clothing, coughing, sneezing, or straining because they can increase IOP
• anticipate changes in his vision that present safety hazards and that to overcome the loss of peripheral vision, he should turn his head fully to view objects at his side.

Nursing diagnoses

When caring for patients with eye disorders, you'll find that several nursing diagnoses may be used over and over. These diagnoses are listed here, along with nursing interventions and rationales. See *NANDA-I taxonomy II by domain*, page 936, for the complete list of NANDA diagnoses.

Disturbed sensory perception (visual)

Related to a vision impairment, *Disturbed sensory perception (visual)* refers to the patient's deprivation of environmental stimuli. It's associated with near-sightedness, far-sightedness, diabetes mellitus, cataracts, detached retina, glaucoma, hemianopsia, macular degeneration, optic nerve damage, and blindness.

Expected outcomes
• Patient performs self-care activities safely and within limits.
• Patient uses adaptive and assistive devices.

Nursing interventions and rationales
• Allow the patient to express his feelings about his vision loss. Allowing him to voice his fears helps him to accept vision loss.
• Remove excess furniture or equipment from the patient's room, and orient him to his surroundings. If appropriate, allow him to direct the arrangement of the room. This promotes patient safety while allowing him to maintain an optimal level of independence.

Skip the fine print
• Modify the patient's environment to maximize any vision the patient may have. Place objects within his visual field, and make sure he's aware of them. Provide large-print books. Modifying the environment helps the patient meet his self-care needs.
• Always introduce yourself or announce your presence when entering the patient's room, and let him know when you're leaving. Familiarizing the patient with his caregivers helps reality orientation.
• Provide nonvisual sensory stimulation, such as talking books, audiotapes, and the radio, to help compensate for the patient's vision loss. Nonvisual sensory stimulation helps the patient adjust to his vision loss.

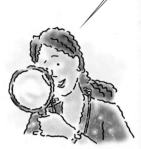

Teach the patient about adaptive devices that can help him cope better with his vision loss.

- Teach the patient about adaptive devices, such as eyeglasses, magnifying glasses, and contact lenses. A knowledgeable patient will be better able to cope with vision loss.
- Refer the patient to appropriate support groups, community resources, or organizations such as the American Foundation for the Blind. Postdischarge support will help the patient and his family cope better with vision loss.

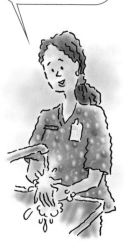

Hand hygiene is the best way to minimize infection risk.

Risk for infection

Related to eye surgery, *Risk for infection* refers to the patient's risk of contracting an infection.

Expected outcomes

- Patient has a normal temperature.
- Patient develops no infection postoperatively.
- Patient states that he understands postoperative care and the signs and symptoms of infection.

Nursing interventions and rationales

- Minimize the patient's risk of infection by performing hand hygiene before and after providing care and by wearing gloves when providing direct care. Hand hygiene is the single best way to avoid spreading pathogens, and gloves offer protection when handling wound dressings or carrying out various treatments.
- Monitor the patient's temperature. Report elevations immediately. An elevated temperature lasting longer than 24 hours after surgery may indicate ocular infection.

Keeping it clean

- Use strict aseptic technique when suctioning the lower airway, inserting indwelling urinary catheters, providing wound care, and providing I.V. care. This technique helps prevent the spread of pathogens.
- Teach the patient about good hand hygiene, factors that increase infection risk, and the signs and symptoms of infection. These measures allow the patient to participate in his care and help the patient modify his lifestyle to maintain optimal health.

Common eye disorders

Cataracts, glaucoma, retinal detachment, and vascular retinopathies are common eye disorders.

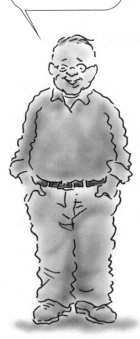

Cataracts are most prevalent in patients over age 70, but surgery improves vision in 95% of cases. Phew!

Cataracts

A common cause of vision loss, a cataract is a gradually developing opacity of the lens or lens capsule of the eye. Cataracts commonly occur bilaterally, with each progressing independently. Exceptions are traumatic cataracts, which are usually unilateral, and congenital cataracts, which may remain stationary. Cataracts occur most frequently in patients over age 70. Prognosis is usually good, with surgery improving vision in 95% of cases.

What causes it

• The cause of a cataract depends on its type:
• Senile cataracts develop in elderly people, probably because of changes in the chemical state of lens proteins.
• Congenital cataracts occur in neonates as a result of genetic defects or maternal rubella during the first trimester.
• Traumatic cataracts develop after a foreign body injures the lens with sufficient force to allow aqueous or vitreous humor to enter the lens capsule.

It gets complicated

• Complicated cataracts can occur secondary to uveitis, glaucoma, retinitis pigmentosa, or detached retina. They may also occur in the course of a systemic disease (such as diabetes, hypoparathyroidism, or atopic dermatitis) or can result from ionizing radiation or infrared rays.
• Toxic cataracts result from drug or chemical toxicity with ergot, naphthalene, phenothiazine and, in patients with galactosemia, from galactose.

Pathophysiology

Pathophysiology may vary with each form of cataract. However, cataract development typically goes through these four stages:
• immature — partially opaque lens
• mature — completely opaque lens; significant vision loss
• tumescent — water-filled lens, which may lead to glaucoma
• hypermature — deteriorating lens proteins and peptides that leak through the lens capsule, which may develop into glaucoma if intraocular outflow is obstructed.

What to look for

Signs and symptoms of a cataract include:
- painless, gradual blurring and loss of vision
- with progression, whitened pupil
- appearance of halos around lights
- blinding glare from headlights at night
- glare and poor vision in bright sunlight.

What tests tell you

- Ophthalmoscopy or slit-lamp examination confirms the diagnosis by revealing a dark area in the normally homogeneous red reflex.
- Shining a penlight on the pupil reveals the white area behind it (unnoticeable until the cataract is advanced).

How it's treated

Treatment consists of surgical extraction of the opaque lens and postoperative correction of vision deficits. The current trend is to perform the surgery as a 1-day procedure.

What to do

- For information on care of the patient undergoing cataract removal surgery, see "Cataract removal," page 175.
- For patient teaching topics on cataract removal, see *Cataract teaching tips*.

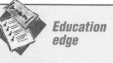

Education edge

Cataract teaching tips

- After surgery, tell the patient to wear sunglasses that filter out ultraviolet rays in bright sunshine.
- Explain that he should avoid activities that increase intraocular pressure, such as straining with coughing or bowel movements and lifting heavy objects.

Glaucoma

The term *glaucoma* refers to a group of disorders characterized by abnormally high IOP that can damage the optic nerve. It occurs in three primary forms: open-angle (primary), acute angle-closure, and congenital. It may also be secondary to other causes. In the United States, glaucoma affects 2% of the population over age 40 and accounts for 12.5% of all new cases of blindness. Its incidence is highest among blacks. Prognosis is good with early treatment.

What causes it

Risk factors for chronic open-angle glaucoma include genetics, hypertension, diabetes mellitus, aging, race (blacks are at increased risk), and severe myopia. Precipitating risk factors for acute angle-closure glaucoma include drug-induced mydriasis (extreme dilation of the pupil) and excitement or stress, which can lead to hypertension. Secondary glaucoma may result from uveitis, trauma, steroids, diabetes, infections, or surgery.

Pathophysiology

Chronic open-angle glaucoma results from overproduction of aqueous humor or obstruction of its outflow through the trabecular meshwork or Schlemm's canal, causing increased IOP and damage to the optic nerve. (See *How aqueous humor normally flows.*) In secondary glaucoma, such conditions as trauma and surgery increase the risk of intraocular fluid obstruction caused by edema or other abnormal processes.

Pressure's rising

Acute angle-closure glaucoma, also called *narrow-angle glaucoma*, results from obstruction to the outflow of aqueous humor from anatomically narrow angles between the anterior iris and the posterior corneal surface. It also results from shallow anterior chambers, a thickened iris that causes angle closure on pupil dilation, or a bulging iris that presses on the trabeculae, closing the angle (peripheral anterior synechiae). Any of these conditions may cause IOP to increase suddenly.

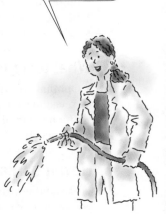

Regardless of the type of glaucoma, it's all about flow.

What to look for

Patients with IOP within the normal range of 8 to 21 mm Hg can develop signs and symptoms of glaucoma, and patients who have abnormally high IOP may have no clinical effects. Nonetheless, each type of glaucoma has specific signs and symptoms.

Slow but steady

Chronic open-angle glaucoma is usually bilateral and slowly progressive. Symptoms don't appear until late in the disease. These symptoms include:
- mild aching in the eyes
- gradual loss of peripheral vision
- seeing halos around lights
- reduced visual acuity, especially at night, that's uncorrectable with glasses.

Rapid reaction

The onset of acute angle-closure glaucoma is typically rapid, constituting an ophthalmic emergency. Unless treated promptly, this glaucoma produces permanent loss of or decreased vision in the affected eye. Signs and symptoms include:
- unilateral inflammation and pain
- pressure over the eye
- moderate pupil dilation that's nonreactive to light
- cloudy cornea and blurring and decreased visual acuity
- photophobia and seeing halos around lights
- nausea and vomiting.

How aqueous humor normally flows

Aqueous humor, a plasmalike fluid produced by the ciliary epithelium of the ciliary body, flows from the posterior chamber to the anterior chamber through the pupil. Here it flows peripherally and filters through the trabecular meshwork to Schlemm's canal and ultimately into venous circulation.

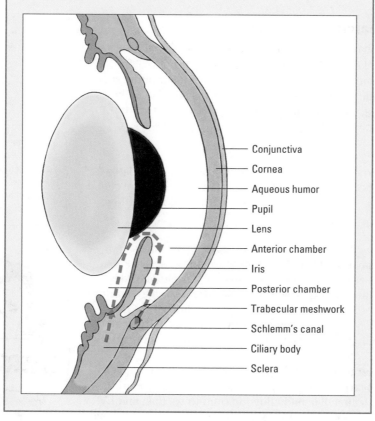

- Conjunctiva
- Cornea
- Aqueous humor
- Pupil
- Lens
- Anterior chamber
- Iris
- Posterior chamber
- Trabecular meshwork
- Schlemm's canal
- Ciliary body
- Sclera

What tests tell you

- Tonometry (using an applanation, Schiøtz', or pneumatic tonometer) measures the IOP and provides a reference baseline.
- Slit-lamp examination is used to assess the anterior structures of the eye, including the cornea, iris, and lens.
- Gonioscopy determines the angle of the eye's anterior chamber, enabling differentiation between chronic open-angle glaucoma and acute angle-closure glaucoma. The angle is normal in chronic open-angle glaucoma; however, in older patients with chronic

open-angle glaucoma, partial closure of the angle may also occur, so the two forms of glaucoma coexist.

• Ophthalmoscopy shows the fundus, where cupping and atrophy of the optic disk are apparent in chronic open-angle glaucoma. A pale disk appears in acute angle-closure glaucoma.

• Perimetry establishes peripheral vision loss in chronic open-angle glaucoma. Fundus photography recordings are used to monitor the optic disk for changes.

How it's treated

For open-angle glaucoma, patients initially receive a beta-adrenergic blocker (such as timolol [Timoptic] or betaxolol [Betoptic]), epinephrine, or a carbonic anhydrase inhibitor (such as acetazolamide) to decrease IOP. Drug treatment also includes miotic eyedrops, such as pilocarpine, to promote the outflow of aqueous humor.

Plan B

Patients who don't respond to drug therapy may be candidates for argon laser trabeculoplasty or a surgical filtering procedure called *trabeculectomy*, which creates an opening for aqueous outflow.

Emergency action

For acute angle-closure glaucoma — an ophthalmic emergency — drug therapy may lower IOP. When pressure decreases, the patient undergoes laser iridotomy or surgical peripheral iridectomy to maintain aqueous flow from the posterior to the anterior chamber. Iridectomy relieves pressure by excising part of the iris to reestablish aqueous humor outflow. The patient typically undergoes prophylactic iridectomy a few days later on the normal eye.

Medical emergency drug therapy includes acetazolamide to lower IOP; pilocarpine to constrict the pupil, forcing the iris away from the trabeculae and allowing fluid to escape; and I.V. mannitol (20%) or oral glycerin (50%) to force fluid from the eye by making the blood hypertonic. The patient with severe pain may need a opioid analgesic.

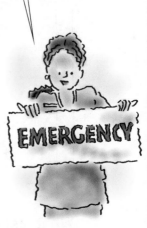

Onset of acute angle-closure glaucoma is typically an ophthalmic emergency.

EMERGENCY

What to do

• For the patient with acute angle-closure glaucoma, give medications, as ordered, and prepare him psychologically for laser iridotomy or surgery. (For care of the surgical patient, see "Iridectomy," page 177, and "Trabeculectomy," page 181.)

• Evaluate the patient. Make sure he follows the treatment regimen and obtains frequent IOP tests. Teach him how to recognize the signs and symptoms of elevated IOP and when to seek immediate medical attention. (See *Glaucoma teaching tips.*)

Retinal detachment

In retinal detachment, the retinal layers split, creating a subretinal space. This space then fills with fluid, called *subretinal fluid.* Retinal detachment usually involves only one eye but may involve the other eye later. Surgical reattachment is almost always successful. However, prognosis for good vision depends on the affected retinal area.

What causes it

Predisposing factors include high myopia and cataract surgery. The most common causes are degenerative changes in the retina or vitreous humor. Other causes include:
• trauma or inflammation
• systemic diseases such as diabetes mellitus
• rarely, retinopathy of prematurity or tumors.

Pathophysiology

Any retinal tear or hole allows the vitreous humor to seep between the retinal layers, separating the retina from its choroidal blood supply. Retinal detachment may also result from seepage of fluid into the subretinal space or from traction that's placed on the retina by vitreous bands or membranes. (See *Understanding retinal detachment*, page 190.)

What to look for

Symptoms of retinal detachment include:
• floaters
• light flashes
• sudden, painless vision loss the patient may describe as a curtain that eliminates a portion of the visual field.

What tests tell you

• Ophthalmoscopic examination through a well-dilated pupil confirms the diagnosis. In severe detachment, examination reveals folds in the retina and a ballooning out of the area.
• Indirect ophthalmoscopy is also used to search the retina for tears and holes.
• Ocular ultrasonography may be necessary if the lens is opaque or the vitreous humor is cloudy.

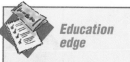

Glaucoma teaching tips

• Stress the importance of meticulous compliance with prescribed drug therapy to prevent increased intraocular pressure, which can lead to disk changes and vision loss.
• Tell him that vision he's already lost won't return, but treatment may prevent further loss.
• Explain the importance of glaucoma screening for early detection and prevention. Remind him that all persons over age 35, especially those with a family history of glaucoma, should have an annual tonometric examination.

A closer look

Understanding retinal detachment

Traumatic injury or degenerative changes cause retinal detachment by allowing the retina's sensory tissue layers to separate from the retinal pigment epithelium. This permits fluid — for example, from the vitreous — to seep into the space between the retinal pigment epithelium and the rods and cones of the tissue layers.

The pressure that results from the fluid entering the space balloons the retina into the vitreous cavity away from choroidal circulation. Separated from its blood supply, the retina can't function. Without prompt repair, the detached retina can result in permanent vision loss.

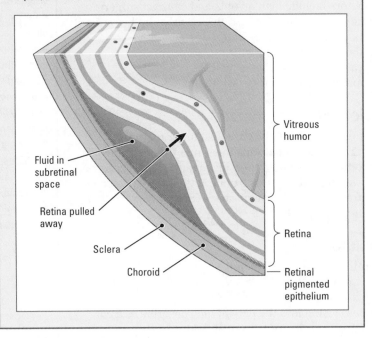

Fluid in subretinal space

Retina pulled away

Sclera

Choroid

Vitreous humor

Retina

Retinal pigmented epithelium

How it's treated

Depending on the location and severity of the detachment, treatment may include:

• Placing the patient on bed rest and sedation to restrict eye movements. If the patient's macula is threatened, he may need his head positioned so the tear or hole is below the rest of the eye.

• A hole in the peripheral retina can be treated with cryotherapy; a hole in the posterior portion, with laser therapy.

• Retinal detachment rarely heals spontaneously. Surgery — including scleral buckling, pneumatic retinopexy, or vitrectomy, or a combination of these procedures — can reattach the retina.

What to do

• Provide emotional support because the patient may be understandably distraught about his loss of vision.
• Position the patient face down if gas has been injected to maintain pressure on the retina.
• Evaluate the patient. With successful treatment, he'll experience restored vision without impairment. He should follow up as directed. (See *Retinal detachment teaching tips*.)

Vascular retinopathies

Vascular retinopathies are noninflammatory disorders that result from disruption of the eye's blood supply. The four distinct types of vascular retinopathy are central retinal artery occlusion, central retinal vein occlusion, diabetic retinopathy, and hypertensive retinopathy.

Backup on the central artery

Central retinal artery occlusion typically causes permanent blindness. However, some patients experience resolution within hours of treatment and regain partial vision.

What causes it

Central retinal artery occlusion may be idiopathic (no known cause) or result from:
• embolism, atherosclerosis, or infection (such as syphilis or rheumatic fever)
• conditions that retard blood flow, such as temporal arteritis, massive hemorrhage, or carotid blockages by atheromatous plaques.

In the same vein

Central retinal vein occlusion can result from:
• trauma or external compression of the retinal vein
• diabetes, phlebitis, thrombosis, atherosclerosis, glaucoma, polycythemia vera, or sickling hemoglobinopathies.

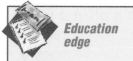
Education edge

Retinal detachment teaching tips

• If the patient will undergo laser surgery, explain that he may have blurred vision for several days afterward.
• Show the patient having scleral buckling surgery how to instill eyedrops properly. After surgery, remind him to lie in the position recommended by the doctor.
• Instruct the patient to rest and to avoid driving, bending, heavy lifting, and other activities that affect intraocular pressure for several days after eye surgery. Discourage activities that could cause the patient to bump the eye.
• Review early symptoms of retinal detachment, and emphasize the need for immediate treatment.

It's all in a name

The names of the two types of vascular retinopathy indicate their causes. Diabetic retinopathy can stem from diabetes, and hypertensive retinopathy can result from prolonged hypertension.

Pathophysiology

Central retinal artery occlusion and central retinal vein occlusion occur when a retinal vessel becomes obstructed. The diminished blood flow causes vision deficits.

Diabetes dysfunction

Diabetic retinopathy results from the microcirculatory changes that occur with diabetes. These changes occur more rapidly in poorly controlled diabetes. Diabetic retinopathy may be nonproliferative or proliferative; proliferative diabetic retinopathy produces fragile new blood vessels (neovascularization) on the disk and elsewhere in the fundus.

Hypertension havoc

In hypertensive retinopathy, prolonged hypertension produces retinal vasospasm and consequent damage to and narrowing of the arteriolar lumen.

What to look for

Signs and symptoms of vascular retinopathies depend on the cause:
• *central retinal artery occlusion* — sudden painless, unilateral loss of vision (partial or complete) that doesn't pass; this may follow transient episodes of unilateral loss of vision
• *central retinal vein occlusion* — reduced visual acuity that's painless except when it results in secondary neovascular glaucoma (uncontrolled proliferation of blood vessels)
• *diabetic retinopathy* — in nonproliferative form, possibly no signs or symptoms, or loss of central visual acuity and diminished night vision from fluid leakage into the macular region; in proliferative form, sudden vision loss from vitreous hemorrhage or macular distortion or retinal detachment from scar tissue formation
• *hypertensive retinopathy* — signs and symptoms dependent on the location of retinopathy (for example, blurred vision if located near the macula).

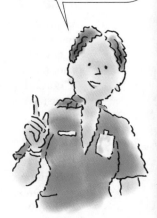

Symptoms of and tests for vascular retinopathies depend on the type.

Diagnostic tests for vascular retinopathies

In vascular retinopathies, diagnostic tests vary depending on the type of retinopathy: central retinal artery occlusion, central retinal vein occlusion, diabetic retinopathy, or hypertensive retinopathy.

Central retinal artery occlusion
• Ophthalmoscopy (direct or indirect) shows blockage of retinal arterioles during transient attack.
• Retinal examination within 2 hours of onset shows clumps or segmentation in artery. Later, a milky white retina is seen around the disk because of swelling and necrosis of ganglion cells caused by reduced blood supply. Also, a cherry red spot in macula is seen that subsides after several weeks.
• Color Doppler tests evaluate carotid occlusion without the need for arteriography.

Central retinal vein occlusion
• Ophthalmoscopy (direct or indirect) shows flame-shaped hemorrhages, retinal vein engorgement, white patches among hemorrhages, and edema around the disk.
• Color Doppler tests confirm or rule out occlusion of blood vessels.

Diabetic retinopathy
• Indirect ophthalmoscopic examination shows retinal changes, such as microaneurysms (earliest change), retinal hemorrhages and edema, venous dilation and beading, lipid exudates, fibrous bands in the vitreous, growth of new blood vessels, and infarcts of the nerve fiber layer.
• Fluorescein angiography shows leakage of fluorescein from weak-walled vessels and "lights up" microaneurysms, differentiating them from true hemorrhages.

Hypertensive retinopathy
• Ophthalmoscopy (direct or indirect) in early stages shows hard, shiny deposits; flame-shaped hemorrhages; silver wire appearance of narrowed arterioles; and nicking of veins where arteries cross them (arteriovenous nicking). In late stages, this test shows cotton wool patches, lipid exudates, retinal edema, papilledema due to ischemia and capillary insufficiency, hemorrhages, and microaneurysms in both eyes.

What tests tell you

Tests depend on the type of vascular retinopathy. (See *Diagnostic tests for vascular retinopathies.*)

How it's treated

Treatment depends on the cause of the retinopathy.

Central retinal artery occlusion

No known treatment exists, although the practitioner may attempt to release the occlusion into the peripheral circulation. To reduce IOP, therapy includes acetazolamide, eyeball massage using a Goldman-type gonioscope and, possibly, anterior chamber paracentesis. The patient may receive inhalation therapy of carbogen (95% oxygen and 5% carbon dioxide) to improve retinal oxygenation. The patient may also receive inhalation treatments hourly for 48 hours, so he should be hospitalized for careful monitoring.

Central retinal vein occlusion

Anticoagulant administration is the treatment of choice. The practitioner may also recommend laser photocoagulation for patients with widespread capillary nonperfusion to reduce the risk of neovascular glaucoma.

Diabetic retinopathy

Treatment includes controlling the patient's blood glucose levels and laser photocoagulation to cauterize weak, leaking blood vessels. If a vitreous hemorrhage occurs when one of these weak blood vessels breaks and it isn't absorbed in 3 to 6 months, the patient may undergo vitrectomy to restore partial vision.

Hypertensive retinopathy

Treatment consists of controlling the patient's blood pressure.

What to do

• Arrange for immediate ophthalmologic evaluation when a patient complains of sudden, unilateral loss of vision. A delay in treatment may result in permanent blindness.
• Administer acetazolamide I.M. or I.V. as ordered. During inhalation therapy, monitor vital signs carefully and discontinue if blood pressure fluctuates markedly or if the patient becomes arrhythmic or disoriented. Monitor the patient's blood pressure if he complains of occipital headache or blurred vision.
• Evaluate the patient. After successful therapy, the patient with a chronic illness should receive follow-up care as directed and comply with the treatment regimen.
• A patient with diabetes should understand the need for a stable blood glucose level.
• A patient with hypertension should keep his blood pressure in a safe range.
• If vision worsens, the patient should seek immediate medical attention and follow safety precautions to prevent injury. (See *Vascular retinopathy teaching tips.*)

Removing obstacles

• Maintain a safe environment for a patient with vision impairment, and teach him how to make his home safer (by removing obstacles and throw rugs, for instance).

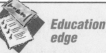

Education edge

Vascular retinopathy teaching tips

• Encourage the patient to comply with prescribed diet, exercise, and medication regimens to minimize the risk of diabetic retinopathy.
• Advise the patient to receive regular ophthalmologic examinations.
• For the patient with hypertensive retinopathy, stress the importance of complying with antihypertensive therapy.

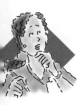

Quick quiz

1. Cone receptors are mainly responsible for sensing:
   A. light.
   B. shades of gray.
   C. shapes.
   D. color.

Answer: D. Cones aid in color recognition and are located in the fovea centralis.

2. A gradually developing opacity of the lens can be found when the patient has:
   A. cataracts.
   B. glaucoma.
   C. corneal abrasion.
   D. vascular retinopathy.

Answer: A. A gradually developing opacity of the lens is a characteristic of cataracts.

3. A patient complains of unilateral eye inflammation and pain, pressure over his eye, blurred and decreased visual acuity, seeing halos around lights, and nausea and vomiting. He most likely has:
   A. acute angle-closure glaucoma.
   B. chronic open-angle glaucoma.
   C. cataracts.
   D. retinal detachment.

Answer: A. These signs and symptoms are characteristics of acute angle-closure glaucoma.

4. The most common cause of retinal detachment is:
   A. diabetes mellitus.
   B. brain tumors.
   C. degenerative changes in the retina or vitreous.
   D. trauma.

Answer: C. Degenerative changes are the most common cause of retinal detachment.

5. Which statement about chronic open-angle glaucoma *isn't* true?

    A.   It results from overproduction of aqueous humor or obstruction of its outflow through the trabecular meshwork.

    B.   It's usually familial.

    C.   It results from obstruction to the outflow of aqueous humor from anatomically narrow angles between the anterior iris and the posterior corneal surface.

    D.   It affects 90% of patients with glaucoma.

Answer: C. Acute angle-closure glaucoma — not chronic open-angle glaucoma — results from obstruction to the outflow of aqueous humor from narrow angles between the anterior iris and the posterior corneal surface.

Scoring

☆☆☆ If you answered all five questions correctly, gadzooks! Your understanding of eye disorders is 20/20.

☆☆ If you answered three or four questions correctly, good job! You have a keen insight on eye disorders.

☆ If you answered fewer than three questions correctly, no tears! Focus in on the chapter and try again.

8

Ear, nose, and throat disorders

Just the facts

In this chapter, you'll learn:

♦ structures and functions of the ear, nose, and throat

♦ techniques for assessing the ear, nose, and throat

♦ nursing diagnoses appropriate for ear, nose, and throat disorders

♦ common ear, nose, and throat disorders and treatments.

A look at ear, nose, and throat disorders

Because ear, nose, and throat (ENT) conditions can cause pain and severely impair a patient's ability to communicate, they require careful nursing assessment and, in many cases, recommendations for follow-up treatment. For example, you may need to refer a patient with a hearing loss to an audiologist for further evaluation or refer a patient with rhinitis to a doctor for hypersensitivity testing.

Anatomy and physiology

To perform an accurate physical assessment, you'll need to understand the anatomy and physiology of the ear, nose, and throat. Let's look at each of them.

Ear

The ear, a sensory organ, enables hearing and maintains equilibrium. It's divided into three main parts — the external ear, the middle ear, and the inner ear.

Can you hear me now?

A close look at the ear

Use this illustration to review the structures of the ear.

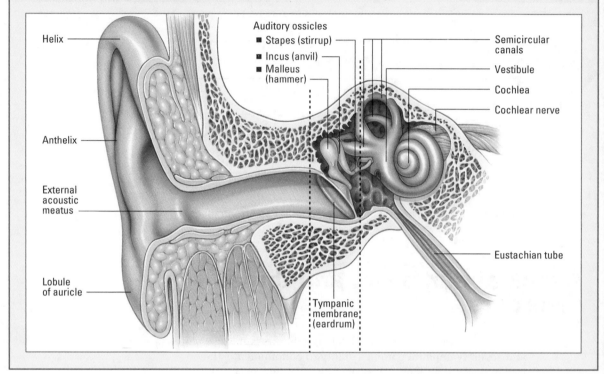

Helix

Anthelix

External acoustic meatus

Lobule of auricle

Auditory ossicles
- Stapes (stirrup)
- Incus (anvil)
- Malleus (hammer)

Semicircular canals

Vestibule

Cochlea

Cochlear nerve

Eustachian tube

Tympanic membrane (eardrum)

Let's start outside

The external ear is made up of the skin-covered cartilaginous auricle (pinna) and the external auditory canal. The tympanic membrane (eardrum) separates the external ear from the middle ear at the proximal portion of the auditory canal.

Three in the middle

The middle ear, a small, air-filled cavity in the temporal bone, contains three small bones — the malleus, the incus, and the stapes.

Enter the inner labyrinth

This cavity leads to the inner ear, a bony and membranous labyrinth, which contains the vestibule, the semicircular canals (the vestibular apparatus), and the cochlea. (See *A close look at the ear.*)

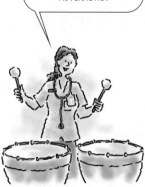

Sound waves strike the tympanic membrane, which starts all those vibrations.

How we hear here

The auricle picks up sound waves and channels them into the auditory canal. There, the waves strike the tympanic membrane, which vibrates and causes the handle of the malleus to vibrate too. These vibrations travel from the malleus, to the incus, to the stapes, through the oval window and the fluid in the cochlea, to the round window.

Hearing hair

The membrane covering the round window shakes the delicate hair cells in the organ of Corti, which stimulates the sensory endings of the cochlear branch of the acoustic nerve (cranial nerve VIII). The nerve sends the impulses to the auditory area of the temporal lobe in the brain, which then interprets the sound.

Nose, sinuses, and mouth

Not only is the nose the sensory organ for smell, but it also warms, filters, and humidifies inhaled air. The sinuses are hollow, air-filled cavities that lie within the facial bones. They include the frontal, sphenoidal, ethmoidal, and maxillary sinuses. The same mucous membrane lines the sinuses and the nasal cavity. Consequently, the same viruses and bacteria that cause upper respiratory tract infections also infect the sinuses. In addition to aiding voice resonance, the sinuses may also warm, humidify, and filter inhaled air, although this role hasn't been firmly established. (See *A close look at the nose and mouth*, page 200.)

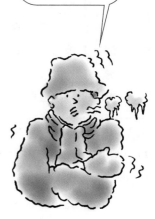

Sure, smelling is important, but the nose also helps warm inhaled air, which is pretty important right about now!

Open wide

The lips surround the mouth anteriorly. The soft palate and uvula (a small, cone-shaped muscle lined with mucous membrane that hangs from the soft palate) border it posteriorly. The mandibular bone, which is covered with loose, mobile tissue, forms the floor of the mouth; the hard and soft palates form the roof of the mouth.

Throat

Located in the anterior part of the neck, the throat includes the pharynx, epiglottis, and larynx (voice box). Food travels through the pharynx to the esophagus. Air travels through it to the larynx. The epiglottis diverts material away from the glottis during swallowing and helps prevent aspiration.

A close look at the nose and mouth

These illustrations show the anatomic structures of the nose and mouth.

Nose and mouth

Mouth and oropharynx

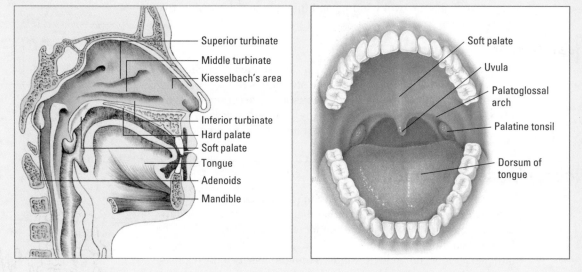

Nose and mouth labels: Superior turbinate, Middle turbinate, Kiesselbach's area, Inferior turbinate, Hard palate, Soft palate, Tongue, Adenoids, Mandible

Mouth and oropharynx labels: Soft palate, Uvula, Palatoglossal arch, Palatine tonsil, Dorsum of tongue

High jinx in the larynx

By vibrating exhaled air through the vocal cords, the larynx produces sound. Changes in vocal cord length and air pressure affect the voice's pitch and intensity. The larynx also stimulates the vital cough reflex when a foreign body touches its sensitive mucosa. The most important function of the larynx is to act as a passage for air between the pharynx and the trachea.

Assessment

Now that you're familiar with the anatomy and physiology of the ears, nose, and throat, you're ready to assess them.

History

Before the interview, determine whether the patient hears well. If not, use his preferred technique to communicate.

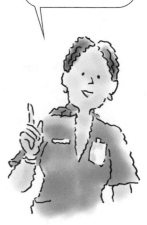

If your patient speech reads, look directly at him and speak clearly during your assessment.

Current health status

Document in the patient's own words his chief complaint. Ask relevant questions, such as:
• Have you recently noticed a difference in hearing in one or both ears?
• Do you have ear pain? Is it unilateral or bilateral?
• Do you have any drainage from one or both ears? What color is it? How often does it occur?
• Do you have frequent headaches, nasal discharge, or postnasal drip?
• Do you experience frequent or prolonged nosebleeds, difficulty swallowing or chewing, or hoarseness or changes in the sound of your voice?

Previous health status

To gather information about the patient's past ENT health, inquire about previous hospitalization, drug therapy, or surgery for an ENT disorder or other relevant condition. Also, be sure to ask these questions:
• Have you ever had an ear injury? Do you suffer from frequent ear infections?
• Have you experienced ringing or crackling in your ears?
• Have you had drainage from your ears or problems with balance, dizziness, or vertigo?
• Have you had sinus infections or tenderness, allergies that cause breathing difficulty, or sensations that your throat is closing?

Family health status

Next, question the patient about possible familial ENT disorders. Ask whether anyone in the patient's family has ever had hearing, sinus, or nasal problems.

Lifestyle patterns

To explore the patient's daily habits that might affect the ears, nose, or throat, ask these questions:
• Do you work around loud equipment, such as printing presses, air guns, or airplanes? If so, do you wear ear protectors?
• Do you listen to loud music with headphones?

• Do you smoke, chew tobacco, use cocaine, or drink alcohol? If so, to what extent?

Physical examination

You'll primarily use inspection and palpation to assess the ears, nose, and throat. If appropriate, you'll also perform an otoscopic examination.

Inspecting and palpating the ears

Examine ear color and size. The ears should be similarly shaped, colored the same as the face, sized in proportion to the head, and symmetrically placed. Look for drainage, nodules, and lesions. Cerumen is usually present and varies from gray-yellow to light brown and black.

Palpate pinna to process; then pull for pain

Palpate the external ear, including the pinna and the tragus, and the mastoid process to discover areas of tenderness, swelling, nodules, or lesions. Then gently pull the helix of the ear backward to determine whether the patient feels pain or tenderness.

Performing an otoscopic examination
Before examining the auditory canal and the tympanic membrane, become familiar with the function of the otoscope. (See *Using an otoscope.*)

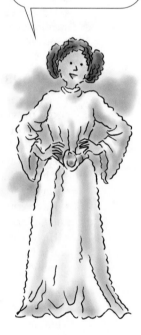

I know my hair is a little out of proportion to my head, but my ears are quite proportional, thank you!

Assessing the nose

Inspect the nose for midline position and proportion to other facial features. To assess nasal symmetry, ask the patient to tilt his head back; then observe the position of the nasal septum. The septum should be aligned with the bridge of the nose. With the head in the same position, use a nasal speculum to inspect the inferior and middle turbinates, the nasal septum, and the nasal mucosa. Note the color of the mucosa, evidence of bleeding, and the color and character of drainage. The nasal mucosa is normally redder than the oral mucosa. Identify abnormalities such as polyps.

Palpate me tender

Next, palpate the nose, checking for painful or tender areas, swelling, and deformities. Evaluate nostril patency by gently occluding one nostril with your finger and having the patient exhale through the other.

Using an otoscope

Here's how to use an otoscope to examine the ears.

Inserting the speculum

Before inserting the speculum into the patient's ear, straighten the ear canal by grasping the auricle and pulling it up and back in an adult as shown at right, or down and back in a child.

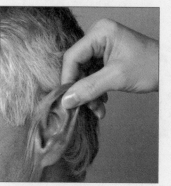

Positioning the scope

To examine the ear's external canal, hold the otoscope with the handle parallel to the patient's head, as shown at right. Bracing your hand firmly against his head keeps you from hitting the canal with the speculum.

Viewing the structures

Gently insert the speculum to inspect the canal and tympanic membrane. When the otoscope is positioned properly, you should see the tympanic membrane structures, as shown below. The tympanic membrane should be pearl gray, glistening, and transparent. The annulus should be white and denser than the rest of the membrane.

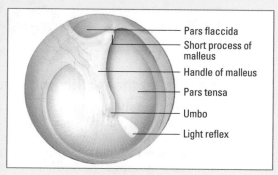

Pars flaccida
Short process of malleus
Handle of malleus
Pars tensa
Umbo
Light reflex

Assessing the sinuses

To assess the paranasal sinuses, inspect, palpate, and percuss the frontal and maxillary sinuses. (The ethmoidal and sphenoidal sinuses lie above the middle and superior turbinates of the lateral nasal walls and can't be assessed.) To assess the frontal and maxillary sinuses, first inspect the external skin surfaces above and to the side of the nose for inflammation or edema. Then palpate and percuss the sinuses. (See *Palpating the maxillary sinuses*, page 204.) If the nose and sinuses require more extensive assessment, use the techniques of direct inspection and transillumination.

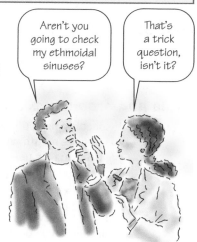

Aren't you going to check my ethmoidal sinuses?

That's a trick question, isn't it?

Palpating the maxillary sinuses

To palpate the maxillary sinuses, gently press your thumbs on each side of the nose just below the cheekbones, as shown. The illustration also shows the location of the frontal sinuses.

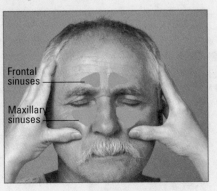

Frontal sinuses

Maxillary sinuses

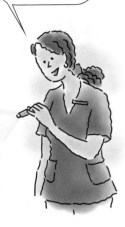

You'll need a tongue blade and a bright light to inspect the oral mucosa.

Assessing the mouth and throat

Use inspection and palpation to assess the mouth and throat. First, inspect the patient's lips. They should be pink, moist, symmetrical, and without lesions. Use a tongue blade and a bright light to inspect the oral mucosa. Have the patient open his mouth; then place the tongue blade on top of his tongue. The oral mucosa should be pink, smooth, moist, and free from lesions and unusual odors.

Past the teeth, past the gums

Next, observe the gums (gingivae). They should be pink and moist and should have clearly defined margins at each tooth. Inspect the teeth, noting their number and condition and whether any are missing or crowded.

Next stop, the tongue

Next, inspect the tongue. It should be midline, moist, pink, and free from lesions. It should move easily in all directions, and it should lie straight to the front at rest.

Uvula and oropharynx and tonsils — Oh, my!

Inspect the back of the throat (oropharynx) by asking the patient to open his mouth while you shine the penlight on the uvula and palate. You may need to insert a tongue blade into the mouth to depress the tongue. The uvula and oropharynx should be pink and moist, without inflammation or exudates. The tonsils should be pink and shouldn't be hypertrophied. Ask the patient to say "Ahhh." Observe for movement of the soft palate and uvula. The uvula should be centered at the midline.

Palpation station

Finally, wearing clean gloves, palpate the lips, tongue, and oropharynx. Note lumps, lesions, ulcers, or edema of the lips or tongue. Assess the patient's gag reflex by gently touching the back of the pharynx with a cotton-tipped applicator or the tongue blade. This should produce a bilateral response.

Diagnostic tests

Tests to determine the presence of ENT disorders should cause your patient little discomfort. These tests include auditory screening tests, audiometric tests, and cultures.

Auditory screening tests

Several tests can help you screen for hearing loss. The first test, the voice test, is a crude method and must be used with other auditory screening tests. Two other screening tests, the Weber and Rinne tests, help detect conductive or sensorineural hearing loss.

Voice test

For the voice test, have the patient occlude one ear with his finger. Test the other ear by standing behind the patient at a distance of 1' to 2' (30 to 60 cm) and whispering a word or phrase. A patient with normal acuity should be able to repeat what was whispered.

Weber test

The Weber test evaluates bone conduction. Perform the test by placing a vibrating tuning fork on top of the patient's head at midline or in the middle of the patient's forehead. The patient should perceive the sound equally in both ears.

Lateral means loss

If the patient has a conductive hearing loss, the sound will lateralize to the ear with the conductive loss because the sound is being conducted directly through the bone to the ear. With a sensorineural hearing loss in one ear, the sound will lateralize to the unimpaired ear because nerve damage in the impaired ear prevents hearing.

Normal is negative

Document a normal Weber test by recording a negative lateralization of sound — that is, sound heard with equal volume in both ears.

Rinne test

The Rinne test compares bone conduction to air conduction in both ears. To administer this test, strike the tuning fork against your hand and place it over the patient's mastoid process. Ask him to tell you when the tone stops, and note this time in seconds.

Tuning in

Next, move the still-vibrating tuning fork to the opening of his ear without touching the ear. Ask him to tell you when the tone stops. Note the time in seconds. (See *Positioning the tuning fork*.)

> Ask the patient to tell you when the tone stops, and note each time in seconds.

Positioning the tuning fork

These illustrations show how to hold a tuning fork to test a patient's hearing. Be sure to perform the Rinne test after you perform the Weber test.

Weber test
With the tuning fork vibrating lightly, position the tip on the patient's forehead at the midline, or place the tuning fork on the top of the patient's head, as shown.

Rinne test
Strike the tuning fork against your hand, and then hold it behind the patient's ear, as shown. When your patient tells you the tone has stopped, move the still-vibrating tuning fork to the opening of his ear.

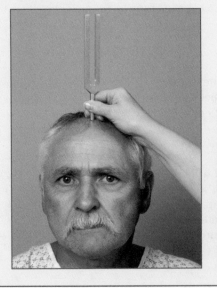

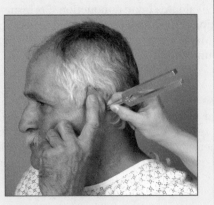

The patient should hear the air-conducted tone for twice as long as he hears the bone-conducted tone. If he doesn't hear the air-conducted tone longer than he hears the bone-conducted tone, he has a conductive hearing loss in the affected ear.

Audiometric tests

Audiometric tests include acoustic immittance tests and pure tone audiometry. Audiologists perform these tests to confirm hearing loss.

Acoustic immittance tests

Immittance tests help diagnose middle ear disorders, lesions in the seventh (facial) or eighth (acoustic) cranial nerve, and eustachian tube dysfunction. They also can help verify a labyrinthine fistula and identify nonorganic hearing loss. Acoustic immittance tests evaluate middle ear function by measuring sound energy's flow into the ear (admittance) and the opposition to that flow (impedance). Acoustic immittance tests include tympanometry and acoustic reflex testing.

Rising resistance

Tympanometry is the indirect measurement of mobility (compliance) and impedance (resistance of the tympanic membrane and ossicles of the middle ear). It's performed by subjecting the external auditory canal and tympanic membrane to positive and negative air pressure.

That's intense

Acoustic reflex testing measures the change in admittance produced by contraction of the stapedial muscle as it responds to an intense sound. A stimulation in one ear causes reaction in both ears.

Nursing considerations
• Instruct the patient not to move, speak, or swallow while admittance is being measured.
• Tell him not to startle during the loud tone, reflex-eliciting measurement.
• Ask him to report discomfort or dizziness (which occurs rarely).
• Explain that the probe forms an airtight seal in the ear canal and may cause discomfort but that it won't harm the ear.

Pure tone audiometry

Performed with an audiometer in a soundproof booth, pure tone audiometry provides a record of the thresholds (the lowest intensity levels) at which a patient can hear a set of test tones through earphones or a bone conduction (sound)

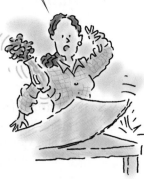

Tell your patient not to startle during the loud tone, reflex-eliciting measurement. Although not startling is easier said than done!

vibrator. Comparison of air and bone conduction thresholds can help identify a conductive, sensorineural, or mixed hearing loss but won't indicate the cause of the loss.

Nursing considerations

• Make sure the patient has had no exposure to unusually loud noises in the past 16 hours.
• For bone conduction testing, remove the earphones and place the vibrator on the mastoid process of the better ear (the auricle shouldn't touch the vibrator).
• It's important that the ear canals be free from cerumen before audiologic testing begins.

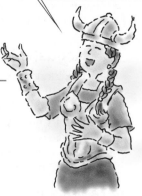

Make sure the patient hasn't been exposed to unusually loud noises in the past 16 hours. I don't think a night at the opera counts.

Cultures

Nasopharyngeal and throat cultures can identify various pathogens related to ENT disorders.

Nasopharyngeal culture

A nasopharyngeal culture isolates and identifies pathogens in nasopharyngeal secretions. For this test, a specimen is obtained, streaked onto a culture plate, and left alone for organisms to grow. Sensitivity testing of the cultured pathogens can then help to determine appropriate antibiotic therapy.

Nursing considerations

• Ask the patient to cough before you begin collecting the specimen. Then have him sit with his head tilted back.
• Using a penlight and a tongue blade, inspect the nasopharyngeal area.
• Next, gently pass the sterile swab through the nostril and into the nasopharynx, keeping the swab near the septum and floor of the nose. Rotate the swab quickly and remove it.
• Take care not to injure the nasal mucosa and cause bleeding.

Throat culture

A throat culture primarily isolates and identifies group A beta-hemolytic streptococci *(Streptococcus pyogenes)*. This allows early treatment of pharyngitis and can help prevent aftereffects, such as rheumatic heart disease and glomerulonephritis. A throat culture also screens for other pathogens.

Isolate and identify

This test involves swabbing the throat, streaking a culture plate, and allowing the organisms to grow so that pathogens can be isolated and identified.

Nursing considerations

- Before beginning ordered antibiotic therapy, obtain the throat specimen. With the patient in a sitting position, tell him to tilt his head back and close his eyes. With the throat well illuminated, check for inflamed areas using a tongue blade.
- Next, use a sterile swab to swab the tonsillar areas from side to side, including inflamed or purulent sites. Don't touch the tongue, cheeks, or teeth with the swab.
- Finally, you'll need to immediately place the swab in the culture tube. If you're using a commercial sterile collection and transport system, crush the ampule and force the swab into the medium to keep the swab moist.

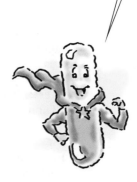

You help find the pathogen, and I'll help fight it off!

Treatments

Here's practical information about the most common drugs and surgical procedures used to treat ENT disorders.

Drug therapy

Drugs used to treat ENT disorders include antihistamines and decongestants as well as anti-infective agents and corticosteroids. The route of administration depends on the disorder:

- The nasal route is used for relief of seasonal or perennial rhinitis and nasal congestion.
- The systemic route is used for relief of inflammation and nasal congestion and to treat infection.
- The otic is the route of choice for external ear infections, cerumen removal, pain from otitis media, and inflammation of the external ear. Instruct the patient using eardrops to lie on his side with the affected ear up for 15 minutes to promote absorption.

Surgery

Surgical treatment of ENT disorders includes the Caldwell-Luc procedure and tonsillectomy and adenoidectomy.

Caldwell-Luc procedure

The Caldwell-Luc procedure, a surgical approach to the maxillary sinus, permits visualization of the antrum, promotes sinus drainage, and allows access to infected sinuses when an intranasal approach isn't possible because of suppuration or inflammation. It's usually used to treat chronic sinusitis that doesn't respond to other treatments. This procedure also halts persistent epistaxis, provides a tissue sample for histologic analysis, and supplements other treatments such as ethmoidectomy.

Patient preparation

Before the procedure, take these steps:
• Tell the patient to expect considerable swelling of his cheek and numbness and tingling on his upper lip.
• Explain that his maxillary sinus and nose may be packed. Let him know that nasal packing is removed after 24 hours and antral packing is removed after 48 to 72 hours.

Monitoring and aftercare

Immediately after surgery, take these steps:
• Check for facial edema, and advise the patient to report adverse reactions such as paresthesia of his upper lip.
• If the patient has packing in place, let him know how long it will be before the doctor removes it. If he has a drainage tube in place for irrigation, assist with irrigation and tell the patient that the tube will be removed in 3 to 4 days.
• Assess the patient's mouth frequently for bleeding.
• Remind the patient not to touch the incision with his tongue or finger.
• If the patient wears dentures, instruct him not to insert his upper plate for 2 weeks. Also, caution him not to brush his teeth, but rather to rinse his mouth gently with tepid saline solution or diluted mouthwash.
• Until the incision heals, avoid giving foods that require thorough chewing.

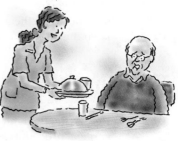

Until the incision heals, offer the patient foods that don't require thorough chewing.

Home care instructions

Before discharge, tell the patient to:
• expect some drainage from his nose for a few days after surgery and to monitor the amount, color, and odor
• call the practitioner if he notices bleeding or a foul smell or if drainage persists for more than 5 days
• avoid rubbing or bumping his incision
• avoid engaging in vigorous activity or blowing his nose forcefully for 2 weeks and to sniff gently if he needs to clear his nostrils.

Tonsillectomy and adenoidectomy

Tonsillectomy is the surgical removal of the palatine tonsils. Adenoidectomy is the surgical removal of the pharyngeal tonsils. These procedures were once routinely combined in an adenotonsillectomy to treat enlarged tonsils and adenoids.

However, these procedures aren't as common today. Instead, patients receive antibiotics to treat tonsils and adenoids enlarged by bacterial infection.

Still surgery sometimes

Even so, a patient may need either or both of these surgeries to resolve tonsillar tissue enlargement that obstructs the upper airway, causing hypoxia or sleep apnea. These procedures may also be used to relieve peritonsillar abscess, chronic tonsillitis, and recurrent otitis media.

Patient preparation

If a patient is scheduled for an adenoidectomy, evaluate whether he has nasal speech or difficulty articulating. If you note these problems, arrange for evaluation by a speech therapist.

Monitoring and aftercare

After surgery, take these steps:
• Monitor vital signs closely for 24 hours, and watch for hemorrhage. Use a flashlight to check the throat and assess for bleeding. Remember, blood can seep down the back of the patient's throat. Pay special attention to frequent swallowing; it may indicate excessive bleeding.
• Take care not to dislodge clots: Make sure the patient doesn't place straws or other utensils in his mouth. When ordered, start him on soft foods.
• Expect some vomiting; even coffee-ground vomitus is the normal result of swallowed blood. However, notify the practitioner if you see bright red blood; this indicates that vomiting has induced bleeding at the operative site.
• If the patient complains of a sore throat, provide cool compresses or an ice collar.

Home care instructions

Before discharge, instruct the patient to:
• immediately report bleeding; explain that the risk of bleeding is greatest 7 to 10 days after surgery, when the membrane formed at the operative site begins to slough off
• consume only liquids and soft foods for 1 to 2 weeks to avoid dislodging clots or precipitating bleeding
• practice good oral hygiene by gently brushing his teeth but avoiding vigorous brushing, gargling, and irritating mouthwashes for several weeks
• rest and avoid vigorous activity for 7 to 10 days after discharge
• avoid exposure to persons with colds or other contagious illnesses for at least 2 weeks.

Nursing diagnoses

When caring for a patient with an ENT disorder, you're likely to use several nursing diagnoses repeatedly. These commonly used diagnoses appear here, along with appropriate nursing interventions and rationales. See *NANDA-I taxonomy II by domain*, page 936, for the complete list of NANDA diagnoses.

Impaired swallowing

Related to pain and inflammation, *Impaired swallowing* may be associated with such conditions as pharyngitis, tonsillitis, and laryngitis.

Expected outcomes
- Patient can swallow.
- Patient maintains adequate hydration.
- Patient exhibits effective airway clearance.

Nursing interventions and rationales
- Elevate the head of the bed 90 degrees after food or fluid intake and at least 45 degrees at all other times to promote swallowing and prevent aspiration.
- Position the patient on his side while recumbent to decrease the risk of aspiration. Have suction equipment available in case aspiration occurs.
- Assess swallowing function frequently, especially before meals, to prevent aspiration.
- Administer pain medication before meals to enhance swallowing ability.
- Provide a liquid to soft diet, and consult with the dietitian as necessary to promote less painful swallowing.
- Provide mouth care frequently to remove secretions and enhance comfort and appetite.
- If the patient can't swallow fluids, notify the practitioner and administer I.V. fluids as ordered to maintain hydration.

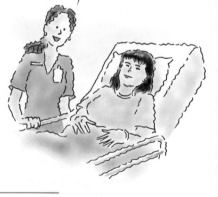

To promote swallowing and prevent aspiration, elevate the head of the bed at least 45 degrees — and 90 degrees after food or fluid intake.

Disturbed sensory perception (auditory)

Related to altered auditory reception or transmission, *Disturbed sensory perception (auditory)* may be associated with such conditions as otitis media, mastoiditis, otosclerosis, Ménière's disease, and labyrinthitis.

Expected outcomes

• Patient understands that progressive hearing loss is caused by the disease.
• Patient can communicate.

Nursing interventions and rationales

• Assess the patient's degree of hearing impairment, and determine the best way to communicate with him (for example, using gestures, lip reading, or written words) to ensure adequate patient care.
• When talking to a hearing-impaired person, speak clearly and slowly in a normal to deep voice and offer concise explanations of procedures to include the patient in his own care.
• Provide sensory stimulation by using tactile and visual stimuli to help compensate for hearing loss.
• Encourage the patient to express feelings of concern and loss for his hearing deficit, and be available to answer questions. This helps him accept his loss, clears up misconceptions, and reduces anxiety.
• Encourage the patient to use his hearing aid as directed to enhance auditory function.
• Upon discharge, teach him to watch for visual cues in the environment, such as traffic lights and flashing lights on emergency vehicles, to avoid injury.

Ineffective airway clearance

Related to nasopharyngeal obstruction, *Ineffective airway clearance* may be associated with such conditions as nasal papillomas, adenoid hyperplasia, nasal polyps, pharyngitis, and tonsillitis.

Expected outcomes

• Patient has clear nasal airways.
• Patient sleeps with normal oxygen saturation.
• Patient is free from infection.
• Patient is free from complications.

Nursing interventions and rationales

• Assess respiratory status (including rate, depth, and stridor) at least every 4 hours to detect early signs of compromise.
• Position the patient with the head of his bed elevated 45 to 90 degrees to promote drainage of secretions and aid breathing and chest expansion.

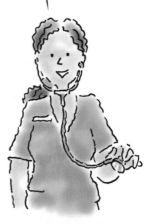

Assess respiratory status at least every 4 hours to detect early signs of compromise.

• Suction upper airways as needed to help remove secretions.
• Have emergency equipment at the bedside in case of airway obstruction.
• Encourage the patient to cough and deep-breathe every 2 hours to help loosen secretions in his lungs.
• Encourage the patient to drink at least 3 qt (3 L) of fluid per day to ensure adequate hydration and loosen secretions.

Common ENT disorders

Hearing loss, laryngitis, otitis externa, otitis media, and sinusitis are common ENT disorders.

Hearing loss

Impaired hearing, the most common disability in the United States, results from a mechanical or nervous system impediment to the transmission of sound waves. Hearing loss is further defined as an inability to perceive the range of sounds audible to an individual with normal hearing. Types of hearing loss include congenital hearing loss, sudden deafness, noise-induced hearing loss, and presbycusis (age-related hearing loss).

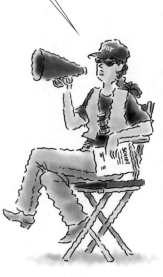

I said, "Impaired hearing is the most common disability in the United States."

What causes it

Causes of hearing loss depend on the type. (See *Causes of hearing loss.*)

Pathophysiology

The major forms of hearing loss are classified as:
• *conductive*, in which transmission of sound impulses from the external ear to the junction of the stapes and oval window is interrupted
• *sensorineural*, in which impaired cochlear or acoustic (CN VIII) nerve function prevents transmission of sound impulses within the inner ear or brain
• *mixed*, in which conductive and sensorineural transmission dysfunction combine.

What to look for

Although congenital hearing loss may produce no obvious signs of hearing impairment at birth, deficient response to auditory stimuli

Causes of hearing loss

Hearing loss falls into two main categories: conductive hearing loss (CHL) and sensorineural hearing loss (SNHL). Patients may also have mixed hearing loss that results from both conductive and sensorineural causes.

Conductive hearing loss

In CHL, a mechanical problem in the middle or outer ear prevents the tympanic membrane from vibrating or the ossicles from conducting sound properly; this type of hearing loss is often reversible. In older patients, CHL commonly results from cerumen impaction. Other causes include:
• otitis media, which causes fluid to build up in the middle ear
• sclerosis of the ossicles, which may be idiopathic or result from a genetic or infectious cause
• perforation of the tympanic membrane.

Sensorineural hearing loss

SNHL results from damage to the cochlea or vestibulo-cochlear nerve in the inner ear; unfortunately, it's usually not reversible. Causes include prolonged exposure to loud noise (greater than 85 dB) or exposure to a single, intensely loud noise (greater than 90 dB). Congenital SNHL can stem from a genetic trait, maternal exposure to rubella or ototoxic drugs, or prematurity. Other causes include:
• degeneration of the cochlea over time, particularly in the elderly
• loss of hair cells in the organ of Corti (presbycusis)
• use of ototoxic medications such as aminoglycoside antibiotics (gentamicin) or diuretics such as furosemide (Lasix)
• trauma to or tumors of the inner ear.

usually becomes apparent within 2 to 3 days. As the child grows older, hearing loss impairs speech development.

Loud and long

Noise-induced hearing loss causes sensorineural damage, the extent of which depends on the duration and intensity of the noise. Initially, the patient loses perception of certain frequencies (around 4,000 Hz) but, with continued exposure, he eventually loses perception of all frequencies.

What's that ringing?

Presbycusis usually produces tinnitus, with progressive decline in overall hearing and the ability to understand the spoken word.

What tests tell you

• Patient, family, and occupational histories and a complete audiologic examination usually provide ample evidence of hearing loss and suggest possible causes or predisposing factors.
• Weber and Rinne tests as well as specialized audiologic tests differentiate between conductive and sensorineural hearing loss.

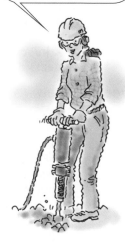

The degree of noise-induced hearing loss depends on the duration and intensity of the noise.

• Auditory evoked reponses, imaging studies, and electronystagmography help to evaluate disorders, such as vertigo, neuromas, and tinnitus.

How it's treated

To treat sudden deafness, the underlying cause must be promptly identified. Educating patients and health care professionals about the many causes of sudden deafness can greatly reduce the incidence of this problem.

Deafness and decibels

For individuals whose hearing loss was induced by noise levels greater than 90 dB for several hours, treatment includes:
• overnight rest, which usually restores normal hearing unless the patient was repeatedly exposed to such noise
• speech and hearing rehabilitation as the patient's hearing deteriorates, because hearing aids are rarely helpful.

What to do

• When talking to a patient with hearing loss who can read lips, stand directly in front of him, with the light on your face, and speak slowly and distinctly.
• Assess the degree of hearing impairment without shouting.
• Approach the patient within his visual range, and get his attention by raising your arm or waving; touching him may unnecessarily startle him.
• Write instructions on a tablet, if necessary, to make sure the patient understands.
• If the patient is learning to use a hearing aid, provide emotional support and encouragement.
• Inform other staff members and hospital personnel of the patient's disability and his established method of communication.

Seeing clues

• Make sure the patient is in an area where he can observe unit activities and persons approaching, because a patient with hearing loss depends on visual clues.
• Evaluate the patient. Make sure he expresses that his hearing loss has resolved or stabilized, is able to maintain communication with others, and exhibits decreased anxiety.
• Make sure the patient and his family understand the importance of wearing protective devices while in a noisy environment. (See *Hearing loss teaching tips.*)
• To prevent noise-induced hearing loss, the public must be educated about the dangers of noise exposure and come to insist on

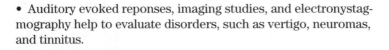

Memory jogger

When it comes to decibel levels, a "failing" grade passes the test. **Lower** levels won't harm hearing, and **higher** numbers signal greater risk:

60 dB—normal speech: no problem

85 dB—safe for a short time, but not too long

90 dB and up—dangerous decibels: Stop the noise!

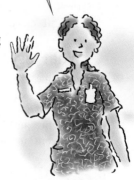

Approach a patient with hearing loss within his visual range, and get his attention by raising your arm or waving.

the use, as mandated by law, of protective devices, such as ear-plugs, during occupational exposure to noise.
• To help prevent congenital hearing loss, pregnant women need to understand the dangers of exposure to drugs, chemicals, and infection — especially rubella — during pregnancy.

Laryngitis

Laryngitis is an inflammation of the vocal cords. Acute laryngitis may occur as an isolated infection or as part of a generalized bacterial or viral upper respiratory tract infection. Repeated attacks of acute laryngitis cause inflammatory changes associated with chronic laryngitis.

What causes it

Acute laryngitis results from infection, excessive use of the voice, inhalation of smoke or fumes, or aspiration of caustic chemicals. Chronic laryngitis results from upper respiratory tract disorders (such as sinusitis, bronchitis, nasal polyps, or allergy), mouth breathing, smoking, gastroesophageal reflux, constant exposure to dust or other irritants, alcohol abuse, or cancer of the larynx.

Pathophysiology

Edema of the vocal cords caused by irritation (from an infection, lesion, or overuse of the voice or other cause) impairs the normal mobility of the vocal cords, causing an abnormal sound.

What to look for

Signs and symptoms of laryngitis include:
• hoarseness (persistent hoarseness in chronic laryngitis)
• changes in the character of the voice
• pain (especially when swallowing or speaking)
• a dry cough, fever, malaise, dyspnea, throat clearing, restlessness, or laryngeal edema.

What tests tell you

• Indirect laryngoscopy confirms the diagnosis by revealing exudate and red, inflamed, and occasionally hemorrhagic vocal cords, with rounded (not sharp) edges. Bilateral swelling that restricts movement but doesn't cause paralysis also may be apparent.
• Videostroboscopy shows the movement of the vocal cords.

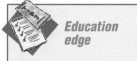

Education edge

Hearing loss teaching tips

• Explain the cause of hearing loss and the medical or surgical treatment options.
• Teach the patient who just received a hearing aid how it works and how to maintain it.
• Emphasize the danger of excessive exposure to noise, and encourage the use of protective devices in a noisy environment.

How it's treated

Treatment of laryngitis includes:
• resting the voice (primary treatment)
• symptomatic care, such as an analgesic and throat lozenges (for viral infection)
• antibiotic therapy (bacterial infection), usually with cefuroxime (Ceftin)
• identification and elimination of underlying cause (chronic laryngitis)
• possible hospitalization (in severe acute laryngitis)
• possible tracheotomy if laryngeal edema results in airway obstruction
• drug therapy, which may include antacids, histamine-2 blockers, antibiotics, and systemic steroids.

What to do

• Tell the patient to refrain from talking to avoid straining the vocal cords and allow vocal cord inflammation to decrease.
• If the patient is hospitalized, place a sign over his bed to remind others of talking restrictions and mark the intercom panel so other hospital personnel are aware that the patient can't answer.
• Provide a pad and pencil or a slate for communication.
• Provide an ice collar, a throat irrigant, and cold fluids for comfort.
• Evaluate the patient. Make sure he isn't hoarse or in pain; doesn't have a fever; doesn't need a tracheotomy; understands the need to stop smoking, maintain humidification, and complete his antibiotic therapy; and modifies his environment appropriately to prevent recurrence. (See *Laryngitis teaching tips*.)

Otitis externa

Otitis externa, or inflammation of the external ear canal skin and auricle, may be acute or chronic. It usually occurs in hot, humid summer weather and is also called *swimmer's ear*. With treatment, the acute form usually subsides within 7 days, although it may become chronic. Severe chronic otitis externa may reflect underlying diabetes mellitus, hypothyroidism, or nephritis.

What causes it

Causes may include:
• bacteria, such as *Pseudomonas*, *Proteus vulgaris*, streptococci, and *Staphylococcus aureus*

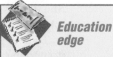
Education edge

Laryngitis teaching tips

• Suggest that the patient maintain adequate humidification by using a vaporizer or humidifier during the winter, avoiding air conditioning during the summer (because it dehumidifies), using medicated throat lozenges, and avoiding smoking and smoky environments.
• Teach the patient about prescribed medication, including dosage, frequency, and adverse effects.
• Instruct the patient to complete prescribed antibiotic therapy.
• If the patient has chronic laryngitis, obtain a detailed patient history to help determine the cause.
• Encourage modification of habits that can cause the disorder.
• Advise the patient to avoid crowds and people with upper respiratory tract infections.

- fungi, such as *Aspergillus niger* and *Candida albicans*
- dermatologic conditions, such as seborrhea or psoriasis.

Pathophysiology

Otitis externa usually results when a traumatic injury or an excessively moist ear canal predisposes the area to infection.

What to look for

Acute otitis externa is characterized by moderate to severe pain. The pain increases when manipulating the auricle or tragus, clenching the teeth, opening the mouth, or chewing. If palpating the tragus or auricle causes pain, the problem is otitis externa, not otitis media. Fungal otitis externa may be asymptomatic. However, *A. niger* produces a black or gray, blotting, paperlike growth in the ear canal.

And now for more

Other signs and symptoms of acute infection include:
- fever
- foul-smelling aural discharge
- regional cellulitis
- partial hearing loss
- scaling, itching, inflammation, or tenderness
- a swollen external ear canal and auricle, which can be seen on otoscopy
- periauricular lymphadenopathy (tender nodes in front of the tragus, behind the ear, or in the upper neck).

What tests tell you

- Otoscopic examination can determine the need for microscopic examination.
- Culture and sensitivity tests can identify the causative organism and help determine the appropriate antibiotic treatment.

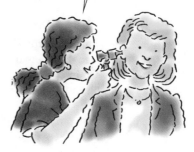

Check your patient's ear with an otoscope to see if she'll need culture and sensitivity tests.

How it's treated

Treatment for acute otitis externa consists of:
- heat application to the periauricular region (warm, damp compresses)
- drug therapy, including topical analgesics, such as otic antipyrine and benzocaine; antibiotic eardrops (with or without hydrocortisone) that are instilled after the ear is cleaned and debris removed; and, if fever persists or regional cellulitis develops, a systemic antibiotic

- careful ear cleaning (especially in fungal otitis externa), including application of a keratolytic or 2% salicylic acid in cream containing nystatin (for candidal organisms) or instillation of slightly acidic eardrops such as 0.5% neomycin (for most fungi and *Pseudomonas* organisms); performed only if the tympanic membrane is intact
- repeated cleaning of the ear canal with baby oil (for *A. niger* organisms).

The tonic for chronic

External ear infections are painful, and the patient with chronic otitis externa may require analgesia. Other treatments include:
- cleaning the ear and removing debris with antibiotic irrigations (primary)
- instilling antibiotic eardrops and applying antibiotic ointment or cream, such as neomycin, bacitracin, or polymyxin B, possibly combined with hydrocortisone (supplemental)
- for mild chronic otitis externa, instilling antibiotic eardrops once or twice weekly and wearing specially fitted earplugs while showering, shampooing, and swimming.

What to do

- Monitor vital signs, particularly temperature. Watch for and record the type and amount of aural drainage.
- Remove debris and gently clean the ear canal with 0.5% neomycin or polymyxin B. Place a wisp of cotton soaked with solution into the patient's ear, and apply a saturated compress directly to the auricle. Afterward, dry the ear gently but thoroughly. (If the patient has severe otitis externa, such cleaning may be delayed until after initial treatment with antibiotic eardrops.)

Traveling in the canal

- To instill eardrops in an adult, pull the pinna back to straighten the canal. To ensure that the drops reach the epithelium, insert a wisp of cotton moistened with eardrops, or have the patient lie on his side with the affected ear up for 15 minutes after instilling drops.
- If the patient has chronic otitis externa, clean the ear thoroughly. Use wet soaks intermittently on oozing or infected skin. If the patient has a chronic fungal infection, clean the ear canal well, and then apply an exfoliative ointment.
- Evaluate the patient. Make sure the patient is afebrile and pain-free, can administer his eardrops properly, and knows which risk factors to avoid. (See *Otitis externa teaching tips*.)

Otitis media

Otitis media, or inflammation of the middle ear, may be acute, chronic, or serous. The infection appears suddenly and typically lasts only a short time. Its incidence rises during the winter months, paralleling the seasonal rise in bacterial respiratory tract infections. It results from disruption of eustachian tube patency. (See *Sites of otitis media*, page 222.)

What causes it

Acute otitis media occurs as a result of pneumococci, beta-hemolytic streptococci, staphylococci, and gram-negative bacteria such as *Haemophilus influenzae*. Chronic otitis media results from inadequate treatment of acute infection as well as infection by resistant strains of bacteria.

Serious about serous

Serous otitis media occurs as a result of:
• viral upper respiratory tract infection, allergy, or residual otitis media
• enlarged lymphoid tissue
• barotrauma (pressure injury caused by an inability to equalize pressures between the environment and the middle ear).
    The causes of chronic serous otitis media are:
• adenoidal tissue overgrowth that obstructs the eustachian tube
• edema resulting from allergic rhinitis or chronic sinus infection
• inadequate treatment of acute suppurative otitis media.

Pathophysiology

With the acute form of otitis media, respiratory tract infection, allergic reaction, or positional changes (such as holding an infant in the supine position during feeding) allow reflux of nasopharyngeal flora through the eustachian tube and colonization in the middle ear.

With prompt treatment, the prognosis for acute otitis media is excellent; however, prolonged accumulation of fluid within the middle ear cavity causes chronic otitis media.

With serous otitis media, obstruction of the eustachian tube results in negative pressure in the middle ear that promotes transudation of sterile serous fluid from blood vessels in the membrane of the middle ear.

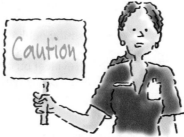

Prolonged accumulation of fluid within the middle ear cavity can lead to chronic otitis media.

Caution

Sites of otitis media

Middle ear inflammation may be suppurative or secretory. In the suppurative form, nasopharyngeal flora reflux through the eustachian tube and colonize in the middle ear. In the secretory form, obstruction of the eustachian tube promotes transudation of sterile serous fluid from blood vessels in the membrane lining the middle ear.

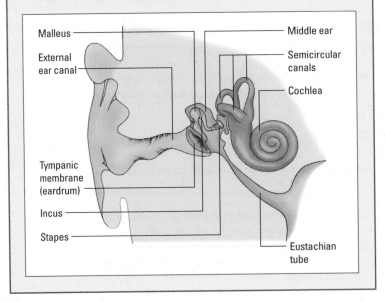

Malleus

External ear canal

Tympanic membrane (eardrum)

Incus

Stapes

Middle ear

Semicircular canals

Cochlea

Eustachian tube

What to look for

Although the patient with acute otitis media may be asymptomatic, typical signs and symptoms include:
- severe, deep, throbbing pain
- upper respiratory tract infection with a mild to high fever
- hearing loss, usually mild and conductive
- lack of response or inattention to spoken word
- sensation of blockage in the ear, dizziness, nausea, and vomiting
- obscured or distorted bony landmarks of the tympanic membrane (evident on otoscopy)
- bulging of the tympanic membrane with concomitant erythema
- purulent drainage in the ear canal from tympanic membrane rupture.

Serous symptoms

Many patients with serous otitis media are asymptomatic but end up developing severe conductive hearing loss ranging from 15

to 35 dB, depending on the thickness and amount of fluid in the middle ear cavity. Other signs and symptoms include:
• a sensation of fullness in the ear or hearing an echo when speaking
• popping, crackling, and clicking sounds with swallowing and jaw movement
• experiencing a vague feeling of top-heaviness
• tympanic membrane retraction, which causes the bony landmarks to appear more prominent (seen on otoscopy)
• clear or amber fluid behind the tympanic membrane (seen on otoscopy) with possible presence of an air bubble
• blue-black tympanic membrane (seen on otoscopy) if hemorrhage into the middle ear has occurred.

Long-term liability

Chronic otitis media usually begins in childhood and persists into adulthood. Its effects include:
• decreased or absent tympanic membrane mobility (tympanosclerosis)
• cystlike mass in the middle ear (cholesteatoma)
• erythema and perforation of the eardrum
• painless, purulent discharge (otorrhea)
• conductive hearing loss that varies with the size and type of tympanic membrane perforation and ossicular destruction
• thickening and possible scarring of the tympanic membrane (seen on otoscopy).

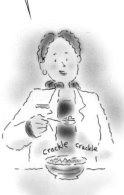

Is that my cereal crackling or a sign of serous otitis media?

crackle crackle

What tests tell you

• Otoscopic examination can determine the need for microscopic examination.
• Computed tomography scanning can reveal effects on structures of the middle ear.
• Culture and sensitivity testing can determine the causative organism.
• Pneumatoscopy can show decreased tympanic membrane mobility. However, this procedure is painful because of the bulging, erythematous tympanic membrane that occurs in acute otitis media.

How it's treated

For acute secretory otitis media, the only treatment required may be inflation of the eustachian tube several times per day using Valsalva's maneuver. Otherwise, nasopharyngeal decongestant therapy may be helpful.

Weighing the evidence

Treatment alternatives for acute otitis media

Because of increasing antibiotic resistance, antibiotics are no longer routinely used to treat uncomplicated cases of otitis media. But how effective are alternative treatments?

To answer that question, researchers looked at treatment alternatives to determine their effectiveness. They compared immediate treatment with antibiotics, treatment with tympanocentesis (drainage of fluid from the middle ear) and antibiotics, and treatment with tympanocentesis and observation. Results showed that none of the three groups showed a significant difference in treatment failure or recurrence of otitis media. The researchers concluded that alternative therapies can reduce the reliance on antibiotics without significantly increasing clinical failure.

Grubb, M.S., & Spaugh, D.C. (2010). Treatment failure, recurrence, and antibiotic prescription rates for different acute otitis media treatment methods. *Clinical Pediatrics, 49*(10), 970–975.

Tube time

If decongestant therapy fails, myringotomy and aspiration of middle ear fluid, followed by insertion of a polyethylene tube into the tympanic membrane, provide immediate and prolonged equalization of pressure. The tube falls out spontaneously after 9 to 12 months.

Broad-spectrum antibiotics may be used to help prevent acute otitis media in high-risk patients. In patients with recurring otitis media, antibiotics must be used sparingly and with discretion to prevent development of resistant strains of bacteria. (See *Treatment alternatives for acute otitis media.*)

Other treatments for acute otitis media include:
• antibiotic therapy with ampicillin (Principen), amoxicillin (Dispermox), or cefaclor (Raniclor) or sulfamethoxazole/trimethoprim (Bactrim) for those who are allergic to penicillin derivatives
• acetaminophen (Tylenol) or ibuprofen (Motrin) to help control pain and fever
• myringotomy for severe, painful bulging of the tympanic membrane.

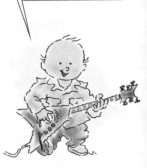

I've got tubes, you don't have to shout. When they're done, they'll just fall out... I got tubes, Babe.

When it goes on and on

For chronic otitis media, therapy includes:
• antibiotics for exacerbations of acute infection
• elimination of eustachian tube obstruction
• myringoplasty (tympanic membrane graft)
• tympanoplasty to reconstruct middle ear structures when thickening and scarring are present, and, possibly, mastoidectomy
• excision of cholesteatoma, if present.

What to do

• After myringotomy, maintain drainage flow. Don't place cotton or plugs deep in the ear canal. Instead, place sterile cotton loosely in the external ear to absorb drainage.
• To prevent infection after the procedure, change the cotton whenever it gets damp and wash your hands before and after providing ear care.
• Watch for and report headache, fever, severe pain, or disorientation.

Tympano treatment

• After tympanoplasty, reinforce dressings, and observe for excessive bleeding from the ear canal. Administer an analgesic, if needed.
• After completing therapy for otitis media, evaluate the patient. Make sure the patient is free from pain and fever, his hearing is completely restored, he understands the importance of completing his antibiotic therapy, and he understands how to prevent recurrence. (See *Otitis media teaching tips.*)

Sinusitis

The prognosis is good for all types of sinusitis. The types include:
• acute, which usually results from the common cold and lingers in subacute form in only about 10% of patients
• chronic, which follows persistent bacterial infection
• allergic, which accompanies allergic rhinitis
• hyperplastic, which is a combination of purulent acute sinusitis and allergic sinusitis or rhinitis
• viral, which follows an upper respiratory tract infection in which the virus penetrates the normal mucous membrane
• fungal, which is generally uncommon but is more common in immunosuppressed or debilitated patients.

What causes it

Sinusitis may result from:
• an upper respiratory tract infection, allergies, or rhinitis
• nasal polyps
• bacterial, viral, or fungal infection (possibly due to swimming in contaminated water or dental manipulation, for example).

Pathophysiology

Ordinarily, bacteria are swept from the sinuses through mucociliary clearance. When the ostia (openings to the sinuses) become

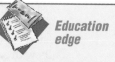

Education edge

Otitis media teaching tips

• Teach the patient the causes, signs and symptoms, and treatment of otitis media.
• Warn the patient against blowing his nose or getting his ears wet when bathing.
• Encourage the patient to complete the prescribed course of antibiotic treatment.
• Instruct the patient or caregiver about medications ordered, correct administration, dosage, and adverse effects.
• Suggest applying warm compresses to the ear to relieve pain.
• Advise the patient with acute otitis media to watch for and immediately report pain and fever, which signal secondary infection.
• To promote eustachian tube patency, instruct the patient to perform Valsalva's maneuver several times daily.
• Urge prompt treatment of otitis media to prevent perforation of the tympanic membrane.

obstructed by inflammation or mucus, however, these bacteria remain in the sinus cavity and multiply. The mucous membrane inside the cavity becomes swollen and inflamed, and the cavity fills with secretions.

What to look for

Signs and symptoms associated with sinusitis include:
• nasal congestion and pressure
• pain over the cheeks and upper teeth (in maxillary sinusitis)
• pain over the eyes (in ethmoid sinusitis)
• pain over the eyebrows (in frontal sinusitis)
• rarely, pain behind the eyes (in sphenoid sinusitis)
• edematous nasal mucosa and edema of the face and periorbital area
• fever (in acute sinusitis)
• nasal discharge (possibly purulent in acute and subacute sinusitis, continuous in chronic sinusitis, and watery in allergic sinusitis)
• nasal stuffiness and possible inflammation and pus on nasal examination.

What tests tell you

• Sinus X-rays may reveal cloudiness in the affected sinus, air-fluid levels, or thickened mucosal lining.
• Antral puncture promotes drainage and removal of purulent material and may provide a specimen for culture and sensitivity identification of the infecting organism (rarely performed).
• Transillumination allows inspection of the sinus cavities by shining a light through them; however, purulent drainage prevents passage of light.

How it's treated

The primary treatment for acute sinusitis is antibiotic therapy. Other appropriate measures include:
• a vasoconstrictor such as phenylephrine (Afrin) to decrease nasal secretions
• an analgesic to help relieve pain
• steam inhalation to promote vasoconstriction and encourage drainage
• local application of heat to relieve pain and congestion
• an antibiotic or antifungal agent (for persistent infection).

Antibiotics, take two

Antibiotic therapy is also the primary treatment for subacute sinusitis. A vasoconstrictor may reduce the amount of nasal secretions.

Allergic sinusitis? Treat rhinitis.

Treatment of allergic sinusitis involves treatment of allergic rhinitis, which includes:
- administration of an antihistamine
- identification of allergens by skin testing and desensitization by immunotherapy
- corticosteroids and epinephrine for severe allergic symptoms.

If all else fails...

For chronic and hyperplastic sinusitis, an antihistamine, an antibiotic, and a steroid nasal spray may relieve pain and congestion. If irrigation fails to relieve symptoms, one or more sinuses may require surgery. Surgeries include:
- sinus tap and irrigation for acute sinusitis
- functional endoscopic sinus surgery
- external ethmoidectomy or sphenoethmoidectomy
- frontal sinusotomy for chronic sinusitis.

What to do

- Enforce bed rest with the head of the bed elevated.
- Encourage the patient to drink plenty of fluids to promote drainage.
- Use a humidifier and nasal saline sprays to decrease dryness.
- Monitor temperature to detect infection. Perform sinus irrigations as ordered.
- To relieve pain and promote drainage, apply warm compresses continuously or four times daily for 2-hour intervals.
- Watch for and report complications, such as vomiting, chills, fever, edema of the forehead or eyelids, blurred or double vision, and personality changes.
- Evaluate the patient. Make sure the patient is free from pain, congestion, headaches, and fever; maintains humidification and drainage of his sinuses; understands the importance of complying with antibiotic therapy; and is able to distinguish common smells. (See *Sinusitis teaching tips*.)

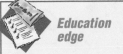

Education edge

Sinusitis teaching tips

- Instruct the patient on how to apply compresses and take his antihistamine.
- Teach him about all prescribed medications, including dosage, frequency, and adverse effects.
- Tell him to finish the prescribed antibiotics, even if his symptoms disappear.
- Encourage the patient to keep all follow-up appointments with the practitioner.

Make sure the patient with sinusitis drinks plenty of fluids to promote drainage. Bottoms up!

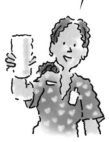

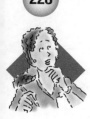

Quick quiz

1. During an otoscopic examination, the nurse should pull the superior posterior auricle of an adult patient's ear:

    A.   up and back.
    B.   up and forward.
    C.   down and back.
    D.   down and forward.

Answer: A. In an adult patient, the superior posterior auricle should be pulled up and back to straighten the ear canal.

2. To assess the frontal sinuses, the nurse should palpate:

    A.   the forehead.
    B.   below the cheekbones.
    C.   over the temporal areas.
    D.   over the preauricular areas.

Answer: A. The frontal sinuses are located in the forehead, the site of palpation for those structures.

3. After a tonsillectomy and adenoidectomy, the nurse should perform all of the following interventions except:

    A.   use a flashlight to check the throat.
    B.   watch for frequent swallowing.
    C.   allow the patient to use a straw and other utensils.
    D.   provide an ice collar for comfort.

Answer: C. Patients shouldn't be allowed to use straws and other utensils because these items might dislodge clots.

4. Pain elicited by palpating the patient's tragus or auricle indicates:

    A.   sinusitis.
    B.   pharyngitis.
    C.   otitis media.
    D.   otitis externa.

Answer: D. If palpating the tragus or auricle causes pain, the problem is otitis externa.

Scoring

☆☆☆   If you answered all four questions correctly, yippee! Your sense of ENT disorders is top-notch.

   ☆☆   If you answered three questions correctly, good for you! You're well on your way to shining a light on the ear, nose, and throat.

     ☆   If you answered fewer than three questions correctly, keep your chin up! Sniff out the difficult areas, and try again!

9

Cardiovascular disorders

Just the facts

In this chapter you'll learn:

◆ anatomy and physiology of the heart and vascular system

◆ history and physical assessment techniques that target cardiac function

◆ appropriate treatments to promote cardiac health

◆ common cardiovascular disorders.

A look at cardiovascular disorders

Although people are living longer than ever before, they're increasingly living with chronic conditions or the effects of acute ones. Of these conditions, cardiovascular disorders head the list. In the United States, over 80 million people suffer from some form of cardiovascular disorder, and many of them suffer from a combination of disorders. Year after year, the number of affected patients continues to rise.

Because of this upward trend, you'll be dealing with cardiovascular patients more often. To provide effective care for these patients, you need a clear understanding of cardiovascular anatomy and physiology, assessment techniques, diagnostic tests, and treatments as well as cardiovascular disorders.

> The number of patients with cardiovascular disease continues to rise.

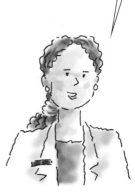

Anatomy and physiology

The cardiovascular system delivers oxygenated blood to tissues and removes waste products. The heart, controlled by the autonomic nervous system, pumps blood to all organs and tissues of the body. Arteries and veins (the vascular system) carry blood throughout the body, keep the heart filled with blood, and maintain blood pressure. Let's look at each part of this critical system.

Heart

The heart is a hollow, muscular organ about the size of a closed fist. Located between the lungs in the mediastinum, it's about 5″ (12.5 cm) long and 3½″ (9 cm) in diameter at its widest point. It weighs between 8.8 and 10 oz (250 to 285 g).

Where's your heart?

The heart spans the area from the second to the fifth intercostal space. The right border of the heart lines up with the right border of the sternum. The left border lines up with the left mid-clavicular line. The exact position of the heart may vary slightly with each patient. Leading into and out of the heart are the great vessels:
- inferior vena cava
- superior vena cava
- aorta
- pulmonary artery
- four pulmonary veins.

> Tell me more about those vessels of yours. I hear they're great!

Slip and slide

A thin sac called the *pericardium* protects the heart. It has an inner, or visceral, layer that forms the epicardium and an outer, or parietal, layer. The space between the two layers contains 10 to 30 ml of serous (pericardial) fluid which prevents friction between the layers as the heart pumps.

Chamber made

The heart has four chambers — two atria and two ventricles — separated by a cardiac septum. The upper atria have thin walls and serve as reservoirs for blood. They also boost the amount of blood moving into the lower ventricles, which fill primarily by gravity. (See *Inside the heart.*)

Blood pathways

Blood moves to and from the heart through specific pathways.

Deoxygenated venous blood returns to the right atrium through three vessels:

superior vena cava — returning blood from the upper body

inferior vena cava — returning blood from the lower body

coronary sinus — returning blood from the heart muscle.

A closer look

Inside the heart

The heart's internal structure consists of the pericardium, 3 layers of the heart wall, 4 chambers, and 4 valves.

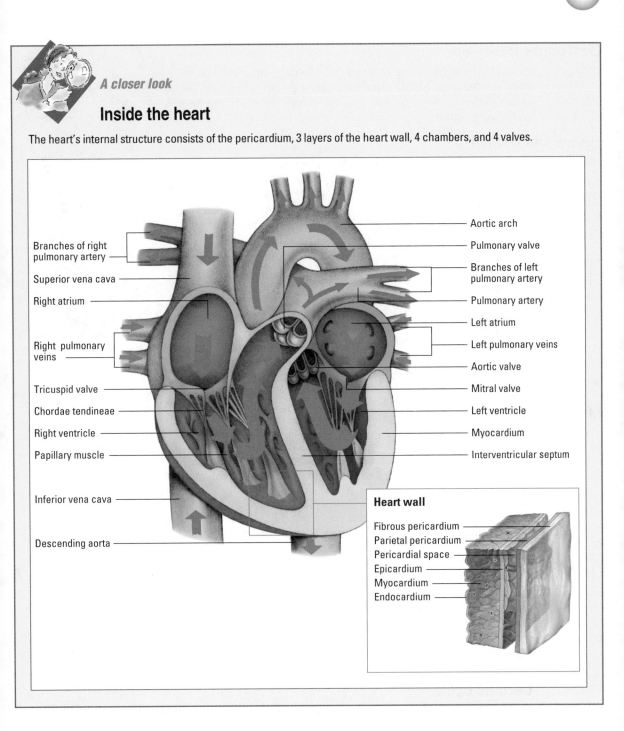

Branches of right pulmonary artery

Superior vena cava

Right atrium

Right pulmonary veins

Tricuspid valve

Chordae tendineae

Right ventricle

Papillary muscle

Inferior vena cava

Descending aorta

Aortic arch

Pulmonary valve

Branches of left pulmonary artery

Pulmonary artery

Left atrium

Left pulmonary veins

Aortic valve

Mitral valve

Left ventricle

Myocardium

Interventricular septum

Heart wall

Fibrous pericardium
Parietal pericardium
Pericardial space
Epicardium
Myocardium
Endocardium

Get some fresh air

Blood in the right atrium empties into the right ventricle and is then ejected through the pulmonic valve into the pulmonary artery when the ventricle contracts. The blood then travels to the lungs to be oxygenated.

Share the wealth

From the lungs, blood travels to the left atrium through the pulmonary veins. The left atrium empties the blood into the left ventricle, which then pumps the blood through the aortic valve into the aorta and throughout the body with each contraction. Because the left ventricle pumps blood against a much higher pressure than the right ventricle, its wall is three times thicker.

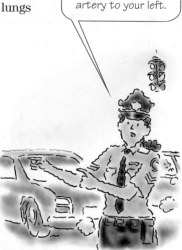

You can't come down this way. Take the first artery to your left.

Valves

Valves in the heart keep blood flowing in only one direction through the heart. Think of the valves as traffic cops at the entrances to one-way streets, preventing blood from traveling the wrong way despite great pressure to do so. Healthy valves open and close as a result of pressure changes within the four heart chambers.

Matching sets

The heart has two sets of valves:

- atrioventricular (between atria and ventricles) — tricuspid valve on the heart's right side and mitral (bicuspid) valve on its left

- semilunar — pulmonary valve (between the right ventricle and pulmonary artery) and aortic valve (between the left ventricle and aorta).

On the cusp

Each valve has cusps (leaflets), which are anchored to the heart wall by cords of fibrous tissue (chordae tendineae). The cusps of the valves act to maintain tight closure. The tricuspid valve has three cusps, the mitral valve has two cusps, and each of the semilunar valves has three cusps.

Cardiac cycle

Contractions of the heart occur in a rhythm — the cardiac cycle — and are regulated by impulses that normally begin at the sinoatrial (SA) node, the heart's pacemaker. The impulses are conducted from there throughout the heart. Impulses from the autonomic nervous system affect the SA node and alter its firing rate to meet the body's needs. The cardiac cycle consists of two phases: diastole and systole.

Just relax... then, kick!

During diastole, the heart relaxes and fills with blood and the heart muscle receives its own supply of blood from the coronary arteries. The mitral and tricuspid valves are open, and the aortic and pulmonic valves are closed. Diastole has three phases:

- isovolumetric relaxation — when ventricular pressure drops below the pressure in the aorta and the pulmonary artery, allowing blood to back up toward the ventricles and causing the aortic and pulmonic valves to snap shut, leading to the second heart sound (S_2) and atrial filling (the beginning of the cardiac cycle)

- ventricular filling (passive) — when 70% of the blood in the atria drains into the ventricles by gravity, which may cause vibrations heard as the third heart sound (S_3)

- atrial contraction (active), also called *atrial kick* — when the remaining 30% of blood is pumped into the ventricles, which may cause the fourth heart sound (S_4).

Outward bound

During systole, ventricular contraction sends blood on its outward journey. Systole has two phases:

- isovolumetric contraction — when pressure within the ventricles rises (because of atrial kick) causing the mitral and tricuspid valves to snap closed, which makes the first heart sound (S_1)

- ventricular ejection — when ventricular pressure rises above the pressure in the aorta and pulmonary artery, causing the aortic and pulmonic valves to open and blood to eject into the pulmonary artery and out to the lungs and into the aorta and out to the rest of the body.

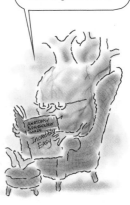

Diastole's such a relaxing time for me. I like to just put my feet up with a good book...

Vascular system

The vascular system consists of a network of arteries, arterioles, capillaries, venules, and veins. This network is constantly filled with about 5 L of blood. The vascular system delivers oxygen, nutrients, and other substances to the body's cells and removes the waste products of cellular metabolism. (See *A close look at the arteries*, page 234, and *A close look at the veins*, page 235.)

(Text continues on page 236.)

A close look at the arteries

This illustration shows the major arteries of the body.

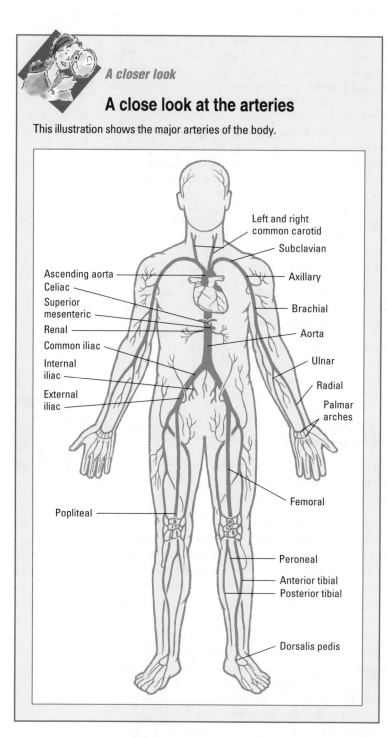

Left and right common carotid

Subclavian

Ascending aorta

Axillary

Celiac

Superior mesenteric

Brachial

Renal

Aorta

Common iliac

Ulnar

Internal iliac

Radial

External iliac

Palmar arches

Femoral

Popliteal

Peroneal

Anterior tibial

Posterior tibial

Dorsalis pedis

A closer look

A close look at the veins

This illustration shows the major veins of the body.

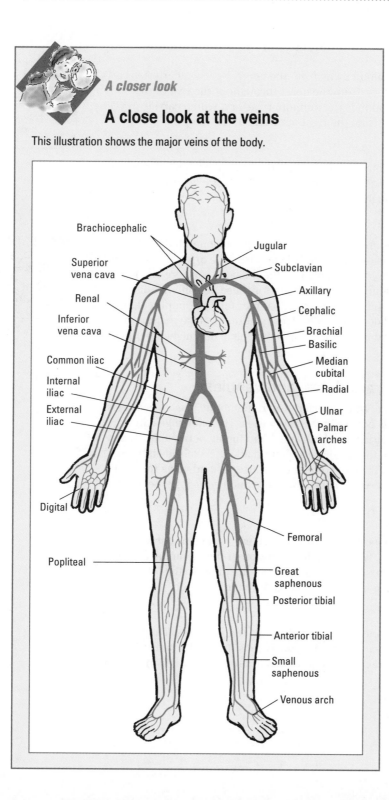

Arteries

Arteries carry blood away from the heart. Nearly all arteries carry oxygen-rich blood from the heart throughout the rest of the body. The only exception is the pulmonary artery, which carries oxygen-depleted blood from the right ventricle to the lungs.

Tough stuff

Arteries have thick walls because they transport blood under high pressure. Arterial walls contain a tough, elastic layer to help propel blood through the arterial system.

Pulse is pressure

Arterial pulses are pressure waves of blood generated by the pumping action of the heart. All vessels in the arterial system have pulsations, but you can only feel the pulsations where an artery lies near the skin. You can palpate for these peripheral pulses: temporal, carotid, brachial, radial, ulnar, femoral, popliteal, posterior tibial, and dorsalis pedis. The location of pulse points varies between individuals. Older adults may have diminished peripheral pulses.

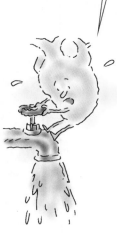

Without the vascular system, I'd be on my own trying to regulate the flow of blood. Talk about pressure!

Capillaries, arterioles, and venules

The exchange of fluid, nutrients, and metabolic wastes between blood and cells occurs in the capillaries. The exchange can occur because capillaries are thin-walled and highly permeable. At any given moment, the capillaries contain about 5% of the circulating blood volume. They're connected to arteries and veins through intermediary vessels called *arterioles* and *venules*, respectively.

Veins

Veins carry blood toward the heart. Nearly all veins carry oxygen-depleted blood, with the sole exception of the pulmonary vein, which carries oxygenated blood from the lungs to the left atrium. Veins serve as a large reservoir for circulating blood.

Feeling flexible

Veins have thinner, more pliable walls than arteries. That pliability allows veins to accommodate variations in blood volume. Veins contain valves at periodic intervals to prevent blood from flowing backward.

Assessment

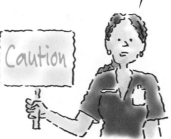

If the patient is in a cardiac crisis, you'll have to rethink assessment priorities.

Baseline information about cardiovascular status that you gather during assessment will help guide your intervention and follow-up care. Note, however, that if your patient is in a cardiac crisis you'll have to rethink your assessment priorities. The patient's condition and the clinical situation will dictate what steps to take.

History

Begin the assessment with a thorough history. You'll find that patients with a cardiovascular problem typically cite specific complaints, including:
• chest, neck, arm, or jaw discomfort or pain
• difficulty breathing or shortness of breath
• a "fluttering" feeling in the chest
• cyanosis, pallor, or other skin changes (such as decreased hair distribution and a thin, shiny appearance to the skin)
• high or low blood pressure, weakness, fatigue, or dizziness
• diaphoresis.

Current health status

Ask the following questions to help the patient elaborate on his current illness:
• How long have you had this problem? When did it begin?
• Where's the pain located? Does the pain radiate to any area of your body? Rate the pain on a scale of 0 to 10.
• Does anything precipitate, exacerbate, or relieve the pain?

Previous health status

Explore all of the patient's previous major illnesses, recurrent minor illnesses, accidents or injuries, surgical procedures, and allergies.

Historic questions

Ask about any history of cardiac-related disorders, such as hypertension, rheumatic fever, scarlet fever, diabetes mellitus, hyperlipidemia, congenital heart defects, and syncope. Ask your patient these questions:
• Have you ever had severe fatigue not caused by exertion?
• Do you consume alcohol, tobacco, or caffeine? How much do you consume?
• Are you taking any prescription, over-the-counter, herbal, or recreational drugs?

- Are you allergic to any drugs, foods, or other products? Can you describe the reaction you experienced?
    If your patient is female, also ask these questions:
- Have you begun menopause?
- Do you use hormonal contraceptives or estrogen?
- Have you experienced any medical problems during pregnancy? Have you ever had gestational hypertension?

Family history

Information about the patient's blood relatives may suggest a specific cardiac problem. Ask him if anyone in his family has ever had hypertension, myocardial infarction (MI), cardiomyopathy, diabetes mellitus, coronary artery disease (CAD), vascular disease, hyperlipidemia, or sudden death. Ask how old the family member was when he or she died.

> Don't forget to ask about hobbies. I find kayaking quite relaxing.

Lifestyle patterns

Always consider the patient's cultural and social background when planning care. Note the patient's education level. What's his occupation and employment status? What kind of support system does he have? Does he live alone or with someone? Does he have any hobbies? How does he view his illness? Assess the patient's self-image as you gather this information.

Physical examination

The first step in the physical examination is to assess the factors that reflect cardiovascular function, including vital signs and physical appearance. After examining these factors, you may assess the patient's cardiovascular system using inspection, palpation, percussion, and auscultation.

Alter to fit

Combine parts of the assessment, as needed, to conserve time and the patient's energy. If the patient is experiencing cardiovascular difficulties, alter the order of your assessment as needed. For example, if he complains of chest pain and dyspnea, quickly check his vital signs and then auscultate the heart. If a female patient feels embarrassed about exposing her chest, explain each assessment step beforehand, use drapes appropriately, and expose only the area being assessed at the moment.

Vital signs

Assessing vital signs includes measuring temperature, blood pressure, pulse rate, and respiration.

Temperature

Temperature change can result from:
- cardiovascular inflammation or infection (higher than normal temperature)
- increased metabolism, which heightens cardiac workload (higher than normal temperature)
- poor perfusion and certain metabolic disorders such as hypothyroidism (lower than normal temperature).

Blood pressure

According to the American Heart Association (AHA), three successive readings of blood pressure above 140/90 mm Hg indicate hypertension. However, emotional stress caused by physical examination may elevate blood pressure. If the patient's blood pressure is high, allow him to relax for several minutes and then measure again to rule out stress.

Take two

When assessing a patient's blood pressure for the first time, take measurements in both arms and use an appropriate-sized cuff. A difference of 10 mm Hg or more between arms may indicate thoracic outlet syndrome or other forms of arterial obstruction.

Pulse rate

If you suspect cardiac disease, auscultate an apical pulse for 1 full minute to detect any arrhythmias. Normally, an adult's pulse ranges from 60 to 100 beats/minute. Its rhythm should feel regular, except for a subtle slowing on expiration, caused by changes in intrathoracic pressure and vagal response. Note whether the pulse feels weak, normal, or bounding.

Respiration

Observe for eupnea — a regular, unlabored, and bilaterally equal breathing pattern. Tachypnea may indicate low cardiac output. Dyspnea, a possible indicator of heart failure, may not be evident at rest. However, the patient may pause after only a few words to take a breath. A Cheyne-Stokes respiratory pattern may accompany severe heart failure, although it's more commonly associated with coma. Shallow breathing may accompany acute pericarditis as the patient attempts to reduce the pain associated with deep respirations.

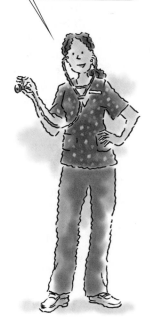

If the patient's blood pressure is high, allow him to relax and then measure again to rule out stress.

Physical appearance

Observe the patient's general appearance, noting:
- weight and muscle composition
- skin turgor, integrity, and color
- energy level
- appearance compared with age
- comfort level or apparent level of anxiety.

Out on a limb

Inspect the hair on the patient's limbs. Hair should be distributed symmetrically and should grow thicker on the anterior surface of the arms and legs. If not, it may indicate diminished arterial blood flow to the arms and legs.

Note whether the length of the arms and legs is proportionate to the length of the trunk. Long, thin arms and legs may indicate Marfan syndrome, a congenital disorder that causes cardiovascular problems, such as aortic dissection, aortic valve incompetence, and cardiomyopathy.

In the pink

Fingernails normally appear pinkish with no markings. A bluish color in the nail beds indicates peripheral cyanosis. To estimate the rate of peripheral blood flow, assess the capillary refill in the fingernails or toenails by applying pressure to the nail for 5 seconds, then assessing the time it takes for color to return. In a patient with a good arterial supply, color should return in less than 3 seconds. Delayed capillary refill suggests reduced circulation to that area, a sign of low cardiac output that may lead to arterial insufficiency.

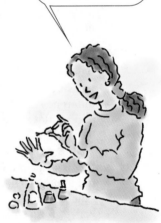

Fingernails normally appear pinkish with no markings. Mine are quite a nice shade of pink!

Inspection

Inspect the patient's chest and thorax. (See *Identifying cardiovascular landmarks.*) Expose the anterior chest and observe its general appearance. Normally, the lateral diameter is twice the size of the anteroposterior diameter. Note any deviations from typical chest shape.

Go for the jugular

When the patient is in a supine position, the jugular veins normally protrude; when the patient stands, the jugular veins normally lie flat. To check for jugular vein distention, place the patient in semi-Fowler's position with his head turned slightly away from the side you're examining. Use tangential lighting (lighting from the side) to cast small shadows along the neck. This will let you see pulse wave movement more easily. If jugular veins appear distended, it

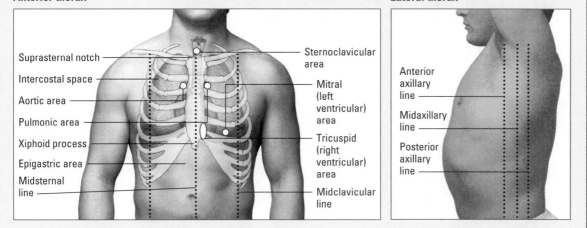

Identifying cardiovascular landmarks

These views show where to find critical landmarks used in cardiovascular assessment.

Anterior thorax

Suprasternal notch
Intercostal space
Aortic area
Pulmonic area
Xiphoid process
Epigastric area
Midsternal line

Sternoclavicular area
Mitral (left ventricular) area
Tricuspid (right ventricular) area
Midclavicular line

Lateral thorax

Anterior axillary line
Midaxillary line
Posterior axillary line

indicates high right atrial pressure and an increase in fluid volume caused by right heart dysfunction. (See *Jugular vein distention,* page 242.)

Precordium pulsations

Using tangential lighting, watch for chest wall movement, visible pulsations, and exaggerated lifts or heaves (strong outward thrusts over the chest during systole) in all areas of the precordium. Ask an obese patient or a patient with large breasts to sit during inspection to bring the heart closer to the anterior chest wall and make pulsations more noticeable.

Impulsive heart

Normally, you'll see pulsations at the point of maximal impulse of the apical impulse (pulsation at the apex of the heart). The apical impulse normally appears in the fifth intercostal space at or just medial to the midclavicular line. This impulse reflects the location and size of the heart, especially of the left ventricle. In thin adults and in children, you may see a slight sternal movement and pulsations over the pulmonary arteries or the aorta as well as visible pulsations in the epigastric area.

Call me impulsive, but I just love a good pulsation in my apex!

Jugular vein distention

Inspecting the jugular veins helps you gather information about blood volume and pressure in the heart's right side. Normally, you won't see a pulsation more than 1½" (4 cm) above the sternal notch. A pulsation higher than this indicates elevated central venous pressure and jugular vein distention. When charting your observations, characterize the distention as mild, moderate, or severe.

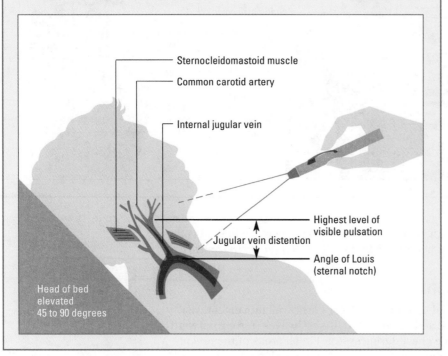

Palpation

Palpate the peripheral pulses and precordium. Make sure the patient is positioned comfortably, draped appropriately, and kept warm. Also, warm your hands and remember to use gentle to moderate pressure.

Feel the flow

You'll already have palpated the radial pulse during your assessment of the patient's vital signs. You'll still need to palpate the other major pulse points to assess blood flow to the tissues. Because the larger central arteries (the carotids) lie closer to the heart, they have slightly higher pressures than the peripheral arteries, allowing you to palpate them more easily. Palpate only one carotid artery at a time; simultaneous palpation can slow the pulse or decrease blood pressure, causing the patient to faint.

After palpating the carotids, continue on to the brachial, radial, femoral, popliteal, dorsalis pedis, and posterior tibial pulses. (See *Assessing arterial pulses*, page 244.) These arteries are close to the body surface and lie over bones, making palpation easier.

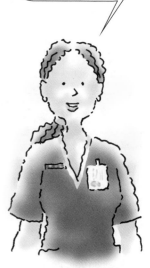

Don't use too much pressure when palpating the pulse, or you may obliterate the pulsation.

A gentle touch

Press gently over these pulse sites; excess pressure can obliterate the pulsation, making the pulse appear absent. Look for the following characteristics:
• pulse rate — varies with age and other factors (usually 60 to 100 beats/minute in adults)
• pulse rhythm — regular
• symmetry — equally strong bilateral pulses
• contour — smooth, wavelike (upstroke and downstroke) pulse flow
• strength — easily palpated pulses (strong finger pressure required to obliterate pulse).

Making the grade

Pulses are graded on a numeric scale:
• 4+ is bounding.
• 3+ is increased.
• 2+ is normal.
• 1+ is weak.
• 0 is absent.

Percussion

As a medical-surgical nurse, you won't routinely percuss the heart. If you note an abnormality in your overall assessment, check the patient's record for a chest X-ray because it provides more accurate information and usually eliminates the need for percussion. Also, lung problems, which commonly accompany cardiovascular disorders, reduce the accuracy of percussion. However, percussion of the abdomen of a patient with right-sided heart failure may reveal dullness that extends several centimeters below the margin of the right ribs, indicating an enlarged liver.

Auscultation

The cardiovascular system requires more auscultation than any other body system.

Assessing arterial pulses

To assess arterial pulses, apply pressure with your index and middle fingers. The following illustrations show where to position your fingers when palpating for various pulses.

Carotid pulse
Lightly place your fingers just medial to the trachea and below the jaw angle. Never palpate both carotid arteries at the same time.

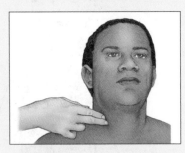

Brachial pulse
Position your fingers medial to the biceps tendon.

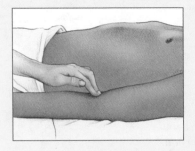

Radial pulse
Apply gentle pressure to the medial and ventral side of the wrist, just below the base of the thumb.

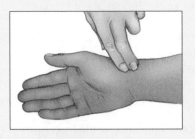

Femoral pulse
Press relatively hard at a point inferior to the inguinal ligament. For an obese patient, palpate in the crease of the groin, halfway between the pubic bone and the hip bone.

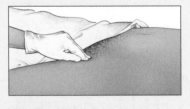

Popliteal pulse
Press firmly in the popliteal fossa at the back of the knee.

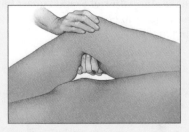

Posterior tibial pulse
Apply pressure behind and slightly below the malleolus of the ankle.

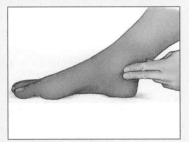

Dorsalis pedis pulse
Place your fingers on the medial dorsum of the foot while the patient points his toes down. The pulse is difficult to palpate here and may seem to be absent in healthy patients.

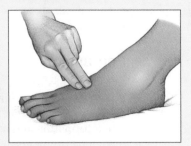

Auscultation aficionado

Heart sounds are auscultated in the precordium. Identifying normal heart sounds, rates, and rhythms isn't routine practice for the medical-surgical nurse, but it's certainly a valuable skill to develop. Even so, expect some difficulty. Even with a stethoscope, the amount of tissue between the source of the sound and the outer chest wall can affect what you hear. Fat, muscle, and air tend to reduce sound transmission. When auscultating an obese patient or a patient with a muscular chest wall or hyperinflated lungs, sounds may seem distant. (See *Positioning the patient for auscultation*.)

See the sites

First, identify cardiac auscultation sites. These include aortic, pulmonic, tricuspid, and mitral areas. Most normal heart sounds

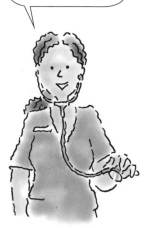

Auscultating heart sounds isn't easy — even if you have fabulous hearing!

Positioning the patient for auscultation

If heart sounds are faint or undetectable, try listening to them with the patient seated and leaning forward or lying on his left side, which brings the heart closer to the surface of the chest. These illustrations show how to position the patient for high- and low-pitched sounds.

Leaning forward

The forward-leaning position is best suited for hearing high-pitched sounds related to semilunar valve problems, such as aortic and pulmonic valve murmurs. To auscultate for these sounds, place the diaphragm of the stethoscope over the aortic and pulmonic areas in the right and left second intercostal spaces, as shown below.

Left lateral recumbent

The left lateral recumbent position is best suited for hearing low-pitched sounds, such as mitral valve murmurs and extra heart sounds. To hear these sounds, place the bell of the stethoscope over the apical area, as shown below.

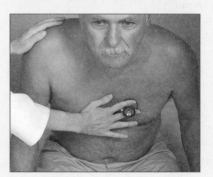

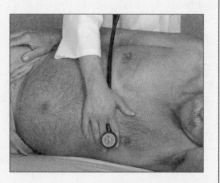

result from vibrations created by the opening and closing of the heart valves. When valves close, they suddenly terminate the motion of blood; when valves open, they accelerate the motion of blood. This sudden deceleration or acceleration produces heart sounds. Auscultation sites don't lie directly over the valves but over the pathways the blood takes as it flows through chambers and valves.

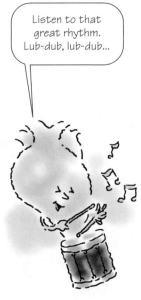

Listen to that great rhythm. Lub-dub, lub-dub...

Sound it out

Next, listen for a few cycles to become accustomed to the rate and rhythm of the sounds. You'll differentiate heart sounds by their pitch (frequency), intensity (loudness), duration, quality (such as musical or harsh), location, and radiation. The timing of heart sounds in relation to the cardiac cycle is particularly important. Two sounds normally occur: S_1 and S_2. They have a relatively high pitch and are separated by a silent period. Normal heart sounds last only a fraction of a second, followed by slightly longer periods of silence. Listen for:

• S_1 — the *lub* of *lub-dub* — which occurs at the beginning of systole when mitral and tricuspid valves close and blood is ejected into the circulation
• S_2 — the *dub* of *lub-dub* — which occurs at the beginning of diastole when aortic and pulmonic valves close (louder in the aortic and pulmonary chest areas), coinciding with the pulse downstroke and followed by a silent period that normally exceeds the pause between S_1 and S_2.

Compare and contrast

At each auscultatory site, use the diaphragm to listen closely to S_1 and S_2 and compare them. Then auscultate again, using the bell of the stethoscope. If you hear any sounds during the diastolic or systolic period or any variations in S_1 or S_2, document the characteristics of the sound. Note the auscultatory site and the part of the cardiac cycle during which it occurred. If you have difficulty identifying normal heart sounds, palpate the patient's carotid artery with your stethoscope over the apex of the heart. The heart sound you hear at the time of the carotid pulse is S_1.

Abnormal findings

Auscultation may also reveal the third and fourth heart sounds as well as a summation gallop, murmur, click, snap, or rub.

Ridin' 3 white horses

Also known as S_3 or *ventricular gallop*, the third heart sound is a low-pitched noise heard best by placing the bell of the stethoscope at the apex of the heart. Its rhythm resembles a horse galloping, and its cadence resembles the word "Ken-tuc-ky" (*lub-dub-by*). Listen for S_3 with the patient in a supine or left-lateral decubitus position.

An S_3 usually occurs during early diastole to mid-diastole, at the end of the passive-filling phase of either ventricle. Listen for this sound immediately after S_2. It may signify that the ventricle isn't compliant enough to accept the filling volume without additional force. You can hear noncompliance in the right ventricle in the tricuspid area, and in the mitral area if the left ventricle is noncompliant. You may also be able to palpate a heave when the sound occurs.

The rhythm of ventricular gallop resembles a horse galloping to the sound of the word Kentucky Giddyap!

Whoa, Nellie

An S_4 is an abnormal heart sound that occurs late in diastole, just before the pulse upstroke. It immediately precedes the S_1 of the next cycle and is associated with acceleration and deceleration of blood entering a chamber that resists additional filling. Known as *atrial gallop* or *presystolic gallop*, it occurs during atrial contraction.

The S_4 shares the same cadence as the word "Ten-nes-see" (*le-lub-dub*). Heard best with the bell of the stethoscope and with the patient in a supine position, S_4 may occur in the tricuspid or mitral area, depending on which ventricle is dysfunctional.

To sum up: A full stable

Occasionally, a patient may have both a third and a fourth heart sound. When this happens, S_3 and S_4 occur so closely together that they appear to be one sound, called *summation gallop*. Auscultation may reveal two separate abnormal heart sounds and two normal sounds. In this case, the patient usually has tachycardia and a shorter diastolic phase.

Murmuring brook

Longer than a heart sound, a murmur occurs as a vibrating, blowing, whistling, or rumbling noise. Just as water in a stream "babbles" as it passes through a narrow point, turbulent blood flow may produce a murmur. If you detect a murmur, identify its loudest location, pinpoint the time it occurs during the cardiac cycle, and describe its pitch, pattern, quality, and intensity. (See *Grading murmurs*, page 248.)

Clicking cusps

Clicks are high-pitched abnormal heart sounds that result from tensing of the chordae tendineae structures and mitral valve cusps. Initially, the mitral valve closes securely, but then a large cusp prolapses into the left atrium, causing the sound. The click usually precedes a late systolic murmur caused by regurgitation of a little blood from the left ventricle into the left atrium. Clicks occur in 5% to 10% of young adults and affect more women than men.

To detect the high-pitched click of mitral valve prolapse, place the stethoscope diaphragm at the heart's apex and listen during midsystole to late systole. To enhance the sound, change the patient's position to sitting or standing, and listen along the lower left sternal border (Erb's point).

Sternal snaps

Place the stethoscope diaphragm medial to the apex along the lower left sternal border to detect a possible opening snap immediately after S_2. This sound results from a stenotic valve (a valve that's constricted or narrowed) attempting to open. The snap resembles the normal S_1 and S_2 in quality, and its high pitch helps differentiate it from an S_3. Because the opening snap may accompany mitral or tricuspid stenosis, it usually precedes a mid-diastolic to late diastolic murmur (classic sign of stenosis).

Rub-a-lub-dub

To detect a pericardial friction rub, use the diaphragm of the stethoscope to auscultate in the third left intercostal space along the lower left sternal border. Listen for a harsh, scratchy, scraping, or squeaking sound that occurs throughout systole, diastole, or both. To enhance the sound, have the patient sit upright and lean forward or exhale. A rub usually indicates pericarditis.

Inaudible arteries

Auscultate the carotid, femoral, and popliteal arteries as well as the abdominal aorta. Over the carotid, femoral, and popliteal arteries, auscultation should reveal no abnormal sounds; over the abdominal aorta, it may detect bowel sounds but no abnormal vascular sounds.

That bruit is brutal

During auscultation of the central and peripheral arteries, you may notice a bruit — a sound caused by turbulent blood flow. A bruit heard over the aorta or the carotid, femoral, popliteal, or brachial arteries can indicate turbulent blood flow caused by tortuous vessels, obstructions, aneurysms (vessels dilated because of weak walls), or dissections (tears in layers of the arterial wall).

Grading murmurs

Use the system outlined below to describe the intensity of a murmur. When recording your findings, use Roman numerals as part of a fraction, always with VI as the denominator. For instance, a grade III murmur would be recorded as "grade III/VI."
- Grade I is a barely audible murmur.
- Grade II is audible but quiet and soft.
- Grade III is moderately loud, without a thrust or thrill.
- Grade IV is loud, with a thrill.
- Grade V is very loud, with a thrust or a thrill.
- Grade VI is loud enough to be heard before the stethoscope comes into contact with the chest.

An opening snap after S_2 makes diagnosing stenosis a, well…a snap!

SNAP

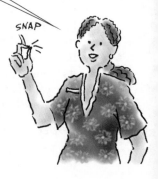

Diagnostic tests

Technological advances have improved the precision of diagnostic tests. Although cardiac marker studies and electrocardiograms (ECGs) are of great value, imaging tests can pinpoint the exact location and extent of cardiac damage within hours of an acute MI, allowing more effective treatment.

Cardiac marker studies

Analysis of cardiac markers (enzymes and proteins) helps diagnose acute MI. After infarction, damaged cardiac tissue releases significant amounts of enzymes into the blood. Serial measurement of enzyme levels reveals the extent of damage and helps monitor healing progress. (See *Release of cardiac enzymes and proteins*, page 250.) These cardiac enzymes include creatine kinase (CK), ischemia-modified albumin (IMA), myoglobin, and troponin I and T. These tests may be used alone or in conjunction with each other. Additional tests that help evaluate the patient's risk of MI include hemoglobin A_{1C} and C-reactive protein.

CK

Heart muscle, skeletal muscle, and brain tissue all contain CK. Its isoenzymes are combinations of the subunits M (muscle) and B (brain). CK-BB appears primarily in brain and nerve tissue; CK-MM, in skeletal muscles; and CK-MB, in the heart muscle. Elevated levels of CK-MB reliably indicate acute MI. Generally, CK-MB levels rise 4 to 8 hours after the onset of acute MI, peak in 12 to 24 hours, and may remain elevated for up to 96 hours.

Nursing considerations
• Explain to the patient that the test will help confirm or rule out MI.
• Tell him he won't need to restrict food or fluids before the test.
• Inform him that blood specimens will be drawn at timed intervals.
• Remember that muscle trauma caused by I.M. injections can raise CK levels.
• Handle the collection tube gently to prevent hemolysis, and send the sample to the laboratory immediately.
• If a hematoma develops at the venipuncture site, apply warm soaks.

Release of cardiac enzymes and proteins

Because they're released by damaged tissue, serum proteins and isoenzymes (catalytic proteins that vary in concentration in specific organs) can help identify the compromised organ and assess the extent of damage. After an acute myocardial infarction, cardiac enzymes and proteins rise and fall in a characteristic pattern, as shown in this graph.

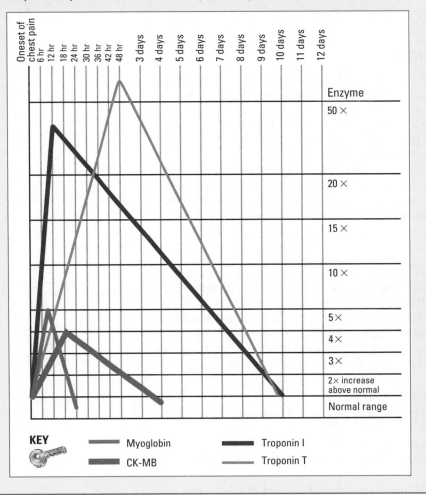

KEY
— Myoglobin
— CK-MB
— Troponin I
— Troponin T

IMA

IMA measures the changes in human serum albumin when it comes in contact with ischemic tissue. Within minutes of the onset of ischemia, IMA reaches detectable levels in the blood because levels rise rapidly when the heart doesn't receive enough oxygen. An increase in IMA occurs significantly sooner than an increase in troponin or CK, but IMA levels don't rise after tissue necrosis. This rapid increase means that IMA levels can be used to detect an MI sooner than possible using other tests. Levels return to normal within 6 hours of the resolution of ischemia.

Nursing considerations
• Handle the collection tube gently to prevent hemolysis, and send the sample to the laboratory immediately.
• IMA is most often performed in conjunction with an ECG and measurement of troponin levels.

Myoglobin

Myoglobin is found in both the myocardium and skeletal muscle. Normally, small amounts of myoglobin are continually released into the bloodstream as a result of the turnover of muscle cells. It's then excreted by the kidneys. During acute MI, myoglobin levels rise as a larger quantity of myoglobin enters the bloodstream. Rising myoglobin levels may be the first marker of cardiac injury after acute MI. Levels may rise within 30 minutes to 4 hours, peak within 6 to 10 hours, and return to baseline by 24 hours. However, because skeletal muscle damage may cause myoglobin levels to rise, it isn't specific to myocardial injury. Myoglobin levels may be available within 30 minutes.

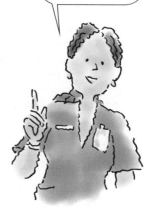

Rising myoglobin levels may be the first marker of cardiac injury after acute MI.

Nursing considerations
• Keep in mind that I.M. injections, recent angina, cardioversion, acute alcohol intoxication, dermatomyositis, hypothermia, muscular dystrophy, polymyositis, severe burns, trauma, severe renal failure, and systemic lupus erythematosus (SLE) can cause elevated myoglobin levels.
• Handle the collection tube gently to prevent hemolysis, and send the sample to the laboratory immediately.
• If a hematoma develops at the venipuncture site, apply warm soaks to help ease discomfort.

Troponin I and troponin T

Troponin is a protein found in skeletal and cardiac muscles. Troponin I and troponin T, two isotypes of troponin, are found in the myocardium. Troponin T may also be found in skeletal muscle.

Troponin I, however, exists in the myocardium — in fact, it's more specific to myocardial damage than CK, CK-MB isoenzymes, and myoglobin. Because troponin T levels can occur in certain muscle disorders or renal failure, it's less specific for myocardial injury than troponin I.

Rise time

Troponin levels rise within 3 to 6 hours after myocardial damage. Troponin I peaks in 12 hours, with a return to baseline in 3 to 10 days, and troponin T peaks in 12 to 48 hours, with a return to baseline in 7 to 10 days. Because troponin levels stay elevated for a prolonged period of time, they can detect an infarction that occurred several days earlier. Rapid troponin T levels can be determined at the bedside in minutes, making them a useful tool for determining treatment in acute MI.

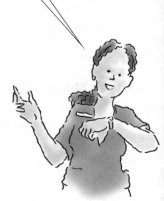

Troponin takes its time. In fact, elevated levels last so long that they can help detect an infarction that occurred several days earlier.

Nursing considerations
• Tell the patient he won't need to restrict food or fluids before the test.
• Tell him that multiple blood samples may be drawn.
• Keep in mind that sustained vigorous exercise, cardiotoxic drugs such as doxorubicin (Adriamycin), renal disease, and certain surgical procedures can cause elevated troponin T levels.
• Handle the collection tube gently to prevent hemolysis, and send the sample to the laboratory immediately.
• If a hematoma develops at the venipuncture site, apply warm soaks to help ease discomfort.

Graphic recording studies

Graphic recording studies to diagnose cardiac disorders include ECG, exercise ECG, and Holter monitoring.

ECG

A valuable diagnostic test that's now a routine part of every cardiovascular evaluation, ECG graphically records electrical current generated by the heart. (See *What the ECG strip shows*.) This test helps identify primary conduction abnormalities, arrhythmias, cardiac hypertrophy, pericarditis, electrolyte imbalance, and MI (site and extent).

Nursing considerations
• Tell the patient that an ECG only takes about 10 minutes and causes no discomfort.
• Explain that he must lie still, relax, breathe normally, and remain quiet.

What the ECG strip shows

On an electrocardiogram (ECG) strip, the horizontal axis correlates the length of each particular electrical event with its duration. Each small block on the horizontal axis represents 0.04 second. Five small blocks form the base of a large block, which in turn represents 0.2 second. The graphic display, or tracing, usually consists of the P wave, the QRS complex, and the T wave.

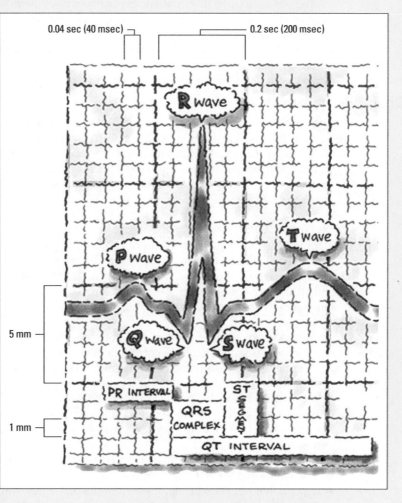

- Keep in mind that evaluation of the recording will guide further treatment.
- Treat chest pain if present (as ordered).

Exercise ECG

Exercise ECG is a noninvasive test that helps the practitioner assess cardiovascular response to an increased workload. Commonly known as a stress test, it provides diagnostic information that can't be obtained from a resting ECG. This test may also assess response to treatment.

The test is stopped if the patient experiences chest pain, fatigue, or other signs and symptoms that reflect exercise intolerance. These may include severe dyspnea, claudication, weakness or dizziness, hypotension, pallor or vasoconstriction, disorientation, ataxia, ischemic ECG changes (with or without pain), rhythm disturbances or heart block, and ventricular conduction abnormalities.

Drugs do it, too

If the patient can't exercise, a stress test can be performed by I.V. injection of a coronary vasodilator, such as dipyridamole or adenosine (Adenocard). Other methods of stressing the heart include dobutamine administration and pacing (in the patient with a pacemaker). During the stress test, nuclear scanning or echocardiography may also be performed.

Nursing considerations
• Inform the patient that he must not eat food, drink caffeinated beverages, or smoke cigarettes for 4 hours before the test.
• Explain that he should wear loose, lightweight clothing and snug-fitting but comfortable shoes, and emphasize that he should immediately report any chest pain, leg discomfort, breathlessness, or fatigue.
• Check the practitioner's orders to determine which cardiac drugs should be administered or withheld before the test. Beta-adrenergic blockers, for example, can limit the patient's ability to raise his heart rate.
• Inform the patient that he may receive an injection of thallium during the test so that the doctor can evaluate coronary blood flow. Reassure him that the injection involves negligible radiation exposure.
• Tell the patient that after the test, his blood pressure and ECG will be monitored for 10 to 15 minutes.
• Explain that he should wait at least 2 hours before showering, and then he should use warm water.

Holter monitoring

Also called *ambulatory ECG*, Holter monitoring allows recording of heart activity as the patient follows his normal routine. Like an exercise ECG, it can provide considerably more diagnostic information than a standard resting ECG. In addition, Holter monitoring can record intermittent arrhythmias.

This test usually lasts about 24 hours (about 100,000 cardiac cycles). The patient wears a small tape recorder connected to bipolar electrodes placed on his chest and keeps a diary of his activities and associated symptoms.

A stress test can also be performed by I.V. injection of a coronary vasodilator.

Nursing considerations

- Urge the patient not to tamper with the monitor or disconnect lead wires or electrodes. Demonstrate how to check the recorder for proper function.
- Tell the patient that he can't bathe or shower while wearing the monitor. He also needs to avoid electrical appliances that can interfere with the monitor's recording.
- Emphasize to the patient the importance of keeping track of his activities, regardless of symptoms.
- Keep in mind that evaluation of the recordings will guide further treatment.

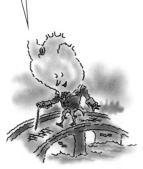

Holter monitoring records heart activity as the patient follows his normal routine.

Imaging studies

Imaging studies used to diagnose cardiovascular disorders include cardiac catheterization and coronary angiography, chest X-ray, echocardiography, magnetic resonance imaging (MRI), multiple-gated acquisition (MUGA) scanning, technetium-99 (^{99m}Tc) pyrophosphate scanning, thallium scanning, transesophageal echocardiography, and ultrafast computed tomography (CT) scan. New methods continue to be developed. (See *Diagnosing CAD: Avoid the invasion.*)

Weighing the evidence

Diagnosing CAD: Avoid the invasion

Over the last decade, computed tomography (CT) technology with ultrafast scanners has advanced significantly. Such advances have helped make CT angiography (CT evaluation of the coronary arteries) a viable noninvasive alternative to conventional invasive coronary angiography.

CT steps up

In certain patient populations and settings, clinicians have found CT angiography can help diagnose coronary artery disease (CAD). For instance, CT angiography can help rule out CAD in some emergency department patients with chest pain. Further research can explore the advantages and limitations of CT angiography compared with invasive testing.

Yerramasu, A., et al. (2010). Evolving role of cardiac CT in the diagnosis of coronary artery disease. *Postgraduate Medical Journal*, August 5, Epub ahead of print.

Cardiac catheterization and coronary angiography

Cardiac catheterization and coronary angiography, two common invasive tests, use a catheter threaded through an artery (for a left-sided catheterization) or vein (for a right-sided catheterization) into the heart to determine the size and location of a coronary lesion, evaluate ventricular function, and measure heart pressures and oxygen saturation.

Nursing considerations

• Make sure the patient understands why he's scheduled for catheterization.
• Check with the practitioner before withholding any medication. Explain to the patient that he won't be able to have anything to eat or drink for 6 to 8 hours before the test.
• Explain that he may receive a mild I.V. or oral sedative before or during the procedure and that a local anesthetic will be used at the insertion site.
• Ask the patient if he's allergic to contrast media or shellfish; document any allergies and report them to the practitioner
• Check the patient's lab values — especially the BUN and creatinine levels — and report abnormal values to the practitioner.

A case of the spins

• Warn the patient that he may feel light-headed, warm, or nauseated for a few moments after the dye injection. He may also receive nitroglycerin during the test to dilate coronary vessels and aid visualization.
• Tell the patient he must cough or breathe deeply as instructed during the test.
• Tell the patient he must lie on his back for several hours after the procedure. Instruct him to notify you if he has any chest pain or feelings of wetness or warmth at the catheter insertion site.
• When the femoral approach is used, tell the patient to keep his leg straight for up to 12 hours or as ordered. Elevate the head of the bed no more than 30 degrees. When the brachial artery is used, tell the patient to keep his arm straight for at least 24 hours or as ordered. To immobilize the leg or arm, place a sandbag over it as ordered.
• Keep in mind that several devices may be used to seal the arterial puncture site, including absorbable collagen protein plugs and a suture tool that's placed inside the puncture site so that the wound can be sutured from below the skin.
• For the first hour after catheterization, monitor the patient's vital signs every 15 minutes and inspect the dressing frequently for signs of bleeding.

Vital checks

- Check the patient's skin color, temperature, and pulses distal to the insertion site. An absent or weak pulse may signify an embolus or other problem requiring immediate attention. Notify the practitioner of any changes in peripheral pulses.
- If the patient's vital signs change or if he has chest pain (possible indications of arrhythmias, angina, or MI), notify the practitioner.
- After the first hour, assess the patient every 30 minutes for 2 hours, then every hour for 4 hours, then once every 4 hours.
- Monitor urine output, especially in cases of impaired renal function.

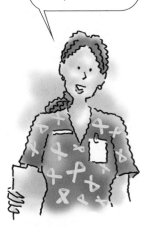

Monitor pulses distal to the insertion site. An absent or weak pulse may signify an occlusion or other problem.

Chest X-ray

A chest X-ray may detect cardiac enlargement, pulmonary congestion, pleural effusion, calcium deposits in or on the heart, pacemaker placement, hemodynamic monitoring lines, and tracheal tube position.

Keep in mind that a chest X-ray alone can't rule out a cardiac problem. Also, clinical signs may reflect the patient's condition 24 to 48 hours before problems appear on an X-ray.

Nursing considerations

- Tell the patient that although this test takes only a few minutes, the practitioner will require extra time to evaluate the quality of the films.
- Inform him that he'll wear a gown without snaps but may keep his pants, socks, and shoes on. Instruct him to remove all jewelry from his neck and chest.
- Tell him that he'll need to take a deep breath and hold it as the technician takes the X-ray.
- Permit the patient to resume activities as ordered.

Echocardiography

Echocardiography, a noninvasive imaging technique, records the reflection of ultra-high frequency sound waves directed at the patient's heart.

A sound image

It allows the practitioner to visualize heart size and shape, myocardial wall thickness and motion, and cardiac valve structure and function. It also helps evaluate overall left ventricular function and detect some MI complications. Plus, it can evaluate prosthetic valve function and help detect mitral valve prolapse; mitral, tricuspid, or pulmonic valve insufficiency; cardiac tamponade; pericardial diseases; cardiac tumors; subvalvular stenosis; ventricular aneurysms; cardiomyopathies; and congenital abnormalities.

Nursing considerations

• Reassure the patient that this 15- to 30-minute test doesn't cause pain or pose any risk.
• Mention that he may undergo other tests, such as ECG and phonocardiography, simultaneously. Tell him that two recordings will be made, one with him on his back, and one with him on his left side.
• Tell him he must sit still while recording takes place because movement may distort results.
• Permit the patient to resume activities as ordered.

MRI

Also known as *nuclear magnetic resonance*, MRI yields high-resolution, tomographic, three-dimensional images of body structures. It takes advantage of certain body nuclei that are magnetically aligned and fall out of alignment after radio frequency transmission. The MRI scanner records the signals the nuclei emit as they realign in a process called *precession* and then translates the signals into detailed pictures of body structures. The resulting images show tissue characteristics without lung or bone interference.

MRI permits visualization of valve leaflets and structures, pericardial abnormalities and processes, ventricular hypertrophy, cardiac neoplasm, infarcted tissue, anatomic malformations, and structural deformities. Applications include monitoring the progression of ischemic heart disease and treatment effectiveness.

Warn your patient he'll hear a loud noise during the MRI — and no, it won't be from my drums!

Nursing considerations

• Instruct the patient that he'll need to lie still during the test.
• Warn him that he'll hear a thumping noise.
• Have him remove all jewelry, his watch, his wallet, and other metallic objects before testing. A patient with an internal surgical clip, scalp vein needle, pacemaker, implanted defibrillator, gold fillings, heart valve prosthesis, or other metal object in his body can't undergo an MRI.

MUGA scanning

MUGA scanning is cardiac blood pool imaging used to evaluate regional and global ventricular performance. During a MUGA scan, the camera records 14 to 64 points of a single cardiac cycle, yielding sequential images that can be studied like a motion picture film to evaluate regional wall motion and determine the ejection fraction and other indices of cardiac function.

Variations on a theme

Many variations of the MUGA scan exist. In the stress MUGA test, the patient undergoes the same test at rest and after exercise to detect changes in ejection fraction and cardiac output. In the nitroglycerin MUGA test, the scintillation camera records points in the cardiac cycle after the sublingual administration of nitroglycerin (Nitrostat) to assess the drug's effect on ventricular function.

> I love being a film star. I'll wave, but no autographs, please.

Nursing considerations
• Keep in mind that an ECG is required to signal the computer and camera to take images for each cardiac cycle.
• Understand that if arrhythmias interfere with a reliable ECG, the test may need to be postponed.

^{99m}Tc pyrophosphate scanning

Also known as *hot spot imaging* or *PYP scanning*, ^{99m}Tc pyrophosphate scanning helps diagnose acute myocardial injury by showing the location and size of newly damaged myocardial tissue. Especially useful for diagnosing transmural infarction, this test works best when performed 12 hours to 6 days after symptom onset. It also helps diagnose right ventricular infarctions; locate true posterior infarctions; assess trauma, ventricular aneurysm, and heart tumors; and detect myocardial damage from a recent electric shock such as defibrillation.

In this test, the patient receives an injection of ^{99m}Tc pyrophosphate, a radioactive material absorbed by injured cells. A scintillation camera scans the heart and displays damaged areas as "hot spots," or bright areas. A spot's size usually corresponds to the injury size.

Nursing considerations
• Tell the patient that the doctor will inject ^{99m}Tc pyrophosphate into an arm vein about 3 hours before the start of this 45-minute test. Reassure him that the injection causes only transient discomfort and that it involves only negligible radiation exposure.
• Instruct the patient to remain still during the test.
• Permit the patient to resume activities as ordered.

Thallium scanning

Also known as *cold spot imaging*, thallium scanning evaluates myocardial blood flow and myocardial cell status. This test helps determine areas of ischemic myocardium and infarcted tissue. It can also help evaluate coronary artery and ventricular function as well as pericardial effusion. (See *Understanding thallium scanning*.) Thallium scanning can also detect an MI in its first few hours.

The test uses thallium-201, a radioactive isotope that emits gamma rays and closely resembles potassium. When injected I.V., the isotope enters healthy myocardial tissue rapidly but enters areas with poor blood flow and damaged cells slowly.

Looking cool

A camera counts the gamma rays and displays an image. Areas with heavy isotope uptake appear light, whereas areas with poor uptake, known as "cold spots," look dark. Cold spots represent areas of reduced myocardial perfusion.

Nursing considerations

• Tell the patient to avoid heavy meals, cigarette smoking, and strenuous activity before the test.
• If the patient is scheduled for an exercise thallium scan, advise him to wear comfortable clothes or pajamas and snug-fitting shoes or slippers.
• Permit the patient to resume activities as ordered.

Transesophageal echocardiography

Transesophageal echocardiography directs high-frequency sound waves at the heart through the esophagus or stomach. This test provides better resolution than echocardiography because the sound waves travel through less tissue. To perform this test, a flexible tube with a transducer at the tip is inserted endoscopically into the esophagus or stomach.

Nursing considerations

• Tell the patient that he must fast for 4 to 6 hours before the test.
• Reassure him that the test only lasts about 15 minutes and that short-acting I.V. sedation is commonly given to reduce anxiety and a topical anesthetic is sprayed in the back of the throat to prevent gagging.
• Inform him that ECG leads will be placed on his chest and his ECG will be continuously monitored.
• Explain that he'll be placed on his left side and will be asked to swallow while the lubricated catheter tip is advanced down his esophagus.

Understanding thallium scanning

In thallium scanning, areas with poor blood flow and ischemic cells fail to take up the isotope (thallium-201 or Cardiolite) and thus appear as cold spots on a scan. Thallium imaging should show normal distribution of the isotope throughout the left ventricle and no defects (cold spots).

To distinguish normal from infarcted myocardial tissue, the practitioner may order an exercise thallium scan followed by a resting perfusion scan. A resting perfusion scan helps differentiate between an ischemic area and an infarcted or scarred area of the myocardium. Ischemic myocardium appears as a reversible defect (the cold spot disappears). Infarcted myocardium shows up as a nonreversible defect (the cold spot remains).

- Warn the patient that he won't be able to have anything to eat or drink after the procedure until his gag reflex has returned, typically in 2 hours.
- Observe the patient for signs and symptoms of esophageal perforation, such as GI bleeding and complaints of pain.

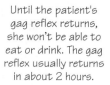

Until the patient's gag reflex returns, she won't be able to eat or drink. The gag reflex usually returns in about 2 hours.

Ultrafast CT scan

Ultrafast CT scan, also called *electron beam CT*, uses a scanner that takes images at fast speeds, resulting in high-resolution pictures. This noninvasive test can identify microcalcifications in the coronary arteries, making it useful for detecting early CAD before symptoms occur, screening symptomatic people at risk for CAD, and evaluating chest pain. This test may also be used to diagnose pulmonary embolus, aortic dissection or aneurysm, congenital heart disease, pericardial disease, and diseases of the great vessels (main vessels that supply organs).

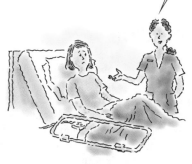

Nursing considerations
- Explain to the patient that he'll need to lie still during scanning.
- If a contrast medium will be used during the test, ask him if he is allergic to contrast media or shellfish.
- If a contrast medium will be used, encourage the patient to increase his fluid intake after the test to promote excretion of the medium. Monitor his blood urea nitrogen (BUN) and creatinine levels before and after the test.

If a contrast medium will be used, encourage your patient to increase his fluid intake after the test to promote excretion of the medium.

Treatments

Ongoing technological advances in the treatment of cardiovascular disorders help patients live longer with a better quality of life than ever before. These treatments include drug therapy, surgery, balloon catheter treatments, and emergency treatment for heart rhythm disturbances.

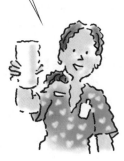

Drug therapy

Drugs are critical to the treatment of many cardiovascular disorders. Drugs that may be used to treat cardiovascular disorders include:
- adrenergics
- antianginals
- antiarrhythmics

- antihypertensives
- antilipemics
- antiplatelet agents
- diuretics
- inotropic agents
- thrombolytics.

Surgery

Despite the drama of successful single- and multiple-organ transplants, improved immunosuppressants, and advanced ventricular assist devices (VADs), far more patients undergo conventional surgeries such as coronary artery bypass grafting (CABG). However, for this and other cardiovascular surgeries, the patient initially recovers in the cardiac intensive care unit (ICU). The role of the medical-surgical nurse is to promote recovery and help smooth the transition from hospital to home using appropriate patient-teaching techniques.

CABG

CABG circumvents an occluded coronary artery with an autogenous graft (usually a segment of the saphenous vein or internal mammary artery), thereby restoring blood flow to the myocardium. CABG techniques vary according to the patient's condition and the number of arteries needing bypass. The most common procedure, aortocoronary bypass, involves suturing one end of the autogenous graft to the ascending aorta and the other end to a coronary artery distal to the occlusion. (See *Bypassing coronary occlusions*.)

CABG caveat

More than 400,000 Americans (most of them male) undergo CABG each year, making it one of the most common cardiac surgeries. Prime candidates include patients with severe angina from atherosclerosis and others with CAD who have a high risk of MI. Successful CABG can relieve anginal pain, improve cardiac function and, possibly, enhance the patient's quality of life.

Even so, although the surgery relieves pain in about 90% of patients, its long-term effectiveness is unclear. Such problems as graft closure and development of atherosclerosis in other coronary arteries may make repeat surgery or other interventions necessary. (See *EECP: Treatment for severe angina*, page 264.) Also, because CABG doesn't resolve the underlying disease associated with arterial blockage, CABG may not reduce the risk of MI recurrence.

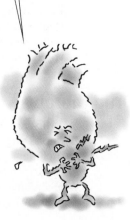

Because CABG doesn't resolve underlying disease, it may not reduce the risk of MI recurrence.

Bypassing coronary occlusions

In this example of coronary artery bypass grafting, the surgeon has used a saphenous vein graft to bypass the right coronary artery and the left internal mammary artery to bypass the left anterior descending artery.

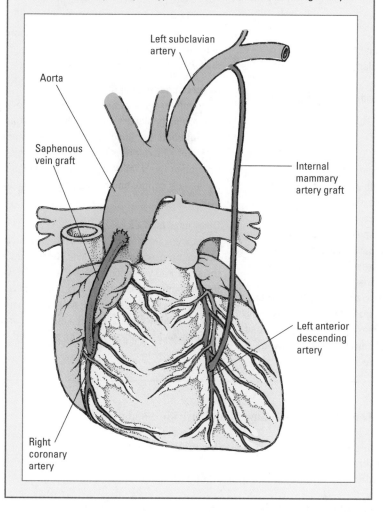

Patient preparation

Take the following steps to help prepare the patient for surgery and support him after surgery:

• Reinforce the surgeon's explanation of the surgery for the patient. Also, explain the complex equipment and procedures used in the ICU or postanesthesia care unit (PACU).

EECP: Treatment for severe angina

For patients with severe angina, enhanced external counterpulsation (EECP) offers an alternative to coronary artery bypass grafting and angioplasty. This procedure can provide pain relief to a patient with recurrent stable angina when standard treatments fail. It can also reduce coronary ischemia, improve exercise tolerance, and stimulate the development of collateral circulation.

Candidates for EECP

A patient may receive EECP if he:
- isn't a candidate for revascularization or if the risk of this procedure is too high
- has recurrent angina even with drug therapy and revascularization
- declines invasive procedures.

Understanding EECP

EECP is usually performed on an outpatient basis over the course of 6 to 7 weeks, with each treatment lasting 1 to 2 hours. For the procedure, the patient has pneumatic cuffs wrapped around his calves, thighs, and lower buttocks and undergoes cardiac monitoring. During diastole, the cuffs sequentially inflate, starting with the calves and moving up the legs. The compression of arteries in the legs promotes retrograde arterial blood flow and coronary perfusion, similar to intra-aortic counterpulsation. At the end of diastole, cuff pressure instantly releases, reducing vascular resistance and decreasing the heart's workload. EECP may also stimulate collateral circulation around stenosed or occluded coronary arteries.

In contrast to intra-aortic counterpulsation, EECP enhances venous return, increasing the filling pressures of the heart and, consequently, cardiac output.

Adverse effects of EECP

Although rare, the patient may experience leg discomfort, bruising, blisters, or skin abrasions from frequent cuff inflation. Because EECP increases venous return, a patient with decreased left ventricular ejection fraction or heart failure requires close monitoring for pulmonary congestion or edema during and after the procedure.

Other uses of EECP

Therapeutic uses of EECP may expand to the treatment of other cardiovascular diseases. Studies are looking at using EECP to treat moderate and severe left ventricular dysfunction and cardiomyopathy. Research is also being conducted on the use of EECP as an interim treatment in acute coronary syndromes and acute myocardial infarction until revascularization can be performed.

- Restrict food and fluids after midnight and provide a sedative, if ordered.
- On the morning of surgery, also provide a sedative, as ordered, to help the patient relax.
- Teach the patient to cough and deep breathe with an incentive spirometer.
- Explain the use of pain medications and nonpharmacologic pain control methods that will be used after surgery.

Monitoring and aftercare

The patient requiring CABG will be monitored in the cardiac ICU after surgery. He'll be transferred to the medical-surgical unit for further postoperative care when his condition is stable. After transfer to the medical-surgical unit:
• Provide analgesia or encourage the use of patient-controlled analgesia (PCA), if appropriate.
• Monitor for postoperative complications, such as stroke, pulmonary embolism, pneumonia, and impaired renal perfusion.
• Gradually allow the patient to increase activities, as ordered.
• Monitor incision sites for signs of infection or drainage.
• Provide support to the patient and his family to help them cope with recovery and lifestyle changes.
• Encourage the patient to do his coughing and deep-breathing exercises.
• Apply compression devices to the patient's lower extremities to help prevent the formation of deep vein thrombosis.

Home care instructions

Instruct the patient to:
• watch for and immediately notify the practitioner of any signs or symptoms of infection (redness, swelling, or drainage from the leg or chest incisions; fever; or sore throat) or possible arterial reocclusion (angina, dizziness, dyspnea, rapid or irregular pulse, or prolonged recovery time from exercise)
• call the practitioner in the case of weight gain greater than 3 lb (1.4 kg) in 1 week
• follow his prescribed diet, especially sodium and cholesterol restrictions
• maintain a balance between activity and rest by trying to sleep at least 8 hours each night, scheduling a short rest period each afternoon, and resting frequently when engaging in tiring physical activity
• follow his exercise program or cardiac rehabilitation if prescribed
• follow lifestyle modifications (no smoking, improved diet, and regular exercise) to reduce atherosclerotic progression
• contact a local chapter of the Mended Hearts Club and the AHA for information and support
• make sure he understands the dose, frequency of administration, and possible adverse effects of prescribed medications
• avoid lifting objects that weigh more than 10 lb (4.5 kg) for the next 4 to 6 weeks

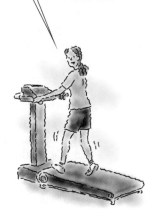

After undergoing CABG, the patient should follow his prescribed exercise program or cardiac rehabilitation.

• perform coughing and deep-beathing exercises, splint the incision with a pillow to reduce pain while doing these exercises, and use an incentive spirometer to prevent pulmonary complications.

MIDCAB

Until recently, cardiac surgery required stopping the heart and using cardiopulmonary bypass to oxygenate and circulate blood. Now, for certain patients, minimally invasive direct coronary artery bypass (MIDCAB) can be performed on a pumping heart through a small thoracotomy incision. The patient may receive only right lung ventilation along with drugs such as beta-adrenergic blockers to slow the heart rate and reduce heart movement during surgery.

It accentuates the positive

Advantages of MIDCAB include shorter hospital stays, use of shorter-acting anesthetic agents, fewer postoperative complications, earlier extubation, reduced cost, smaller incisions, and earlier return to work. Patients eligible for MIDCAB include those with proximal left anterior descending lesions and some lesions of the right coronary and circumflex arteries.

Patient preparation

Before the procedure, take these steps:
• Review the procedure with the patient, and answer his questions. Tell him that he'll be extubated in the operating room or within 2 to 4 hours after surgery.
• Teach the patient to cough and breathe deeply through use of an incentive spirometer.
• Explain the use of pain medications after surgery as well as nonpharmacologic methods to control pain.
• Let the patient know that he should be able to walk with assistance the first postoperative day and be discharged within 48 hours.

Monitoring and aftercare

The patient undergoing MIDCAB may be monitored in a cardiac ICU or step-down unit after surgery. He'll be transferred to the medical-surgical unit for further postoperative care when his condition is stable. After transfer to the medical-surgical unit:
• Provide analgesia or encourage the use of PCA if appropriate.
• Monitor for postoperative complications, such as stroke, pulmonary embolism, pneumonia, and impaired renal perfusion.

> Your patient should be able to walk with assistance the first day after surgery.

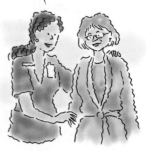

• Gradually allow the patient to increase activities as ordered.
• Monitor the incision site for signs of infection or drainage. Depending on the procedure, the patient will have one to three small chest incisions.
• Provide support to the patient and his family to help them cope with recovery and lifestyle changes.

Home care instructions

Before discharge, instruct the patient to:
• continue with the progressive exercise started in the hospital
• perform coughing and deep-breathing exercises, splint the incision with a pillow to reduce pain while doing these exercises, and use the incentive spirometer to reduce pulmonary complications
• avoid lifting objects that weigh more than 10 lb (4.5 kg) for the next 4 to 6 weeks
• wait 2 to 4 weeks before resuming sexual activity
• check the incision site daily and immediately notify the practitioner of any signs or symptoms of infection (redness, foul-smelling drainage, or swelling) or possible graft occlusion (slow, rapid, or irregular pulse; angina; dizziness; or dyspnea)
• perform any necessary incisional care
• follow lifestyle modifications
• take medications, as prescribed, and report adverse effects to the practitioner
• consider participation in a cardiac rehabilitation program.

Port access cardiac surgery

Port access cardiac surgery is another minimally invasive surgical technique. In this procedure, the surgeon performs coronary bypass grafting through small incisions with the aid of videoscopes. This procedure requires a shorter hospital stay, promoting faster recovery. Also, because the heart can be turned, port access allows the surgeon to perform more bypass grafting.

Picture using ports

This procedure uses a small anterior thoracotomy and several small "port" chest incisions. The surgeon inserts a thorascope through the ports to view the heart. As with traditional cardiac surgery, the surgeon creates a cardiopulmonary bypass. However, the procedure uses the femoral artery and vein cannulation, reducing the risk of atrial fibrillation associated with atrial cannulation. Also, rather than cross-clamping the aorta — increasing the risk of atherosclerotic emboli — port access surgery internally occludes the aorta with an inflated endoaortic balloon, which prevents air and thrombotic emboli during bypass.

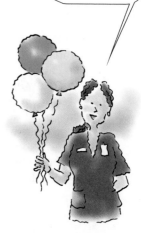

Balloons prevent air and thrombotic emboli during bypass.

Patient preparation

Before the procedure, take these steps:
• Teach the patient to perform coughing and deep-breathing exercises and how to use an incentive spirometer.
• Tell the patient that he'll be assisted to a sitting position and allowed to ambulate as early as the first postoperative evening.

Monitoring and aftercare

The patient undergoing port access cardiac surgery will require nursing care similar to MIDCAB. After transfer to the medical-surgical unit, follow these steps:
• Provide analgesia or encourage the use of PCA, if appropriate.
• Monitor for postoperative complications, such as stroke, femoral artery dissection, and femoral artery or vein occlusion.
• Gradually allow the patient to increase activities, as ordered.
• Monitor the incision site for signs of infection, drainage, or bleeding.
• Provide support to the patient and his family to help them cope with recovery and lifestyle changes.

Home care instructions

Before discharge, instruct the patient to:
• continue with the progressive exercise started in the hospital
• perform coughing and deep-breathing exercises, splint the incision with a pillow to reduce pain while doing these exercises, and use the incentive spirometer to reduce pulmonary complications
• avoid lifting objects that weigh more than 10 lb (4.5 kg) for the next 4 to 6 weeks
• wait 2 to 4 weeks before resuming sexual activity
• check the incision site daily and immediately notify the practitioner of any signs and symptoms of infection (redness, foul-smelling drainage, or swelling) or possible graft occlusion (slow, rapid, or irregular pulse; angina; dizziness; or dyspnea)
• check for bleeding or hematoma at the femoral insertion sites
• follow lifestyle modifications
• take medications as prescribed and report adverse reactions to the practitioner
• comply with the laboratory schedule for monitoring International Normalized Ratio (INR) if the patient is receiving warfarin (Coumadin)
• consider participation in a cardiac rehabilitation program.

Vascular repair

Vascular repair may be used to treat:
- vessels damaged by arteriosclerotic or thromboembolic disorders (such as aortic aneurysm or arterial occlusive disease), trauma, infections, or congenital defects
- vascular obstructions that severely compromise circulation
- vascular disease that doesn't respond to drug therapy or nonsurgical treatments such as balloon catheterization
- life-threatening dissecting or ruptured aortic aneurysms
- limb-threatening acute arterial occlusion.

Vascular repair includes aneurysm resection, endovascular repair, grafting, embolectomy, vena caval filtering, endarterectomy, and vein stripping. The specific surgery used depends on the type, location, and extent of vascular occlusion or damage. (See *Understanding types of vascular repair*, page 270.)

In all vascular surgeries, there's a potential for vessel trauma, emboli, hemorrhage, infection, and other complications. Grafting carries added risks because the graft may occlude, narrow, dilate, or rupture.

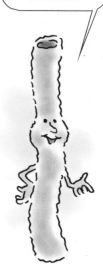

Among other conditions, vascular repair treats vascular obstructions that compromise circulation.

Patient preparation

Vascular surgery may be performed as an emergency procedure or a scheduled event. Take the following steps before surgery:
- Reinforce all explanations about surgery and recovery.
- Perform and document a vascular assessment, focusing on the area that requires treatment.
- If the patient is awaiting surgery for aortic aneurysm repair, be on guard for signs and symptoms of acute dissection or rupture. Note especially sudden severe pain in the chest, abdomen, or lower back; severe weakness; diaphoresis; tachycardia; or a precipitous drop in blood pressure or loss of pulses in the lower extremities. If any of these conditions occur, call the surgeon immediately; he may need to perform life-saving emergency surgery.

Be on the lookout for signs and symptoms of acute dissection or rupture, conditions requiring life-saving emergency treatment.

Monitoring and aftercare

After surgery, the patient will be cared for in the ICU. He'll be transferred to the medical-surgical unit for further postoperative care when his condition is stable. After transfer to the medical-surgical unit, take these steps:
- Frequently assess peripheral pulses, using Doppler ultrasonography if palpation proves difficult.
- Assess extremities bilaterally for muscle strength and movement, color, temperature, and capillary refill time.

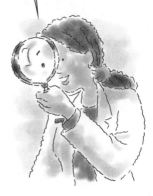

Understanding types of vascular repair

Vascular repair is performed to treat various conditions. Below are five common types of vascular repair.

Aortic aneurysm repair

Aortic aneurysm repair removes an aneurysmal segment of the aorta.

Procedure

The surgeon first makes an incision to expose the aneurysm site. If necessary, he places the patient on a cardiopulmonary bypass machine; then he clamps the aorta. Then the surgeon resects the aneurysm and repairs the damaged portion of the aorta.

Vena caval filter insertion

Vena caval filter insertion traps emboli in the vena cava, preventing them from reaching the pulmonary vessels.

Procedure

A vena caval filter or umbrella (shown at right) is inserted transvenously via a catheter. Once in place in the vena cava, the umbrella or filter traps emboli but allows venous blood flow.

Vein stripping

Vein stripping removes the saphenous vein and its branches to treat varicosities.

Procedure

The surgeon ligates the saphenous vein. He then threads the stripper into the vein, secures it, and pulls it back out, bringing the vein with it.

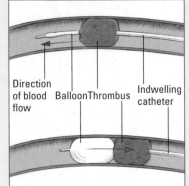

Direction of blood flow   Balloon   Thrombus   Indwelling catheter

Embolectomy

Embolectomy removes an embolism from an artery.

Procedure

The surgeon inserts a balloon-tipped indwelling catheter into the artery and passes it through the thrombus (top). He then inflates the balloon and withdraws the catheter to remove the thrombus (bottom).

Bypass grafting

Bypass grafting bypasses an arterial obstruction resulting from arteriosclerosis.

Procedure

After exposing the affected artery, the surgeon connects a synthetic or autogenous graft to divert blood flow around the occluded arterial segment. The autogenous graft may be a vein harvested from elsewhere in the patient's body. The illustration at right shows a femoropopliteal bypass.

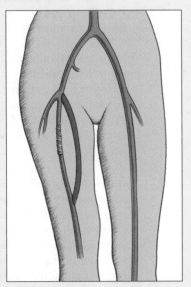

Filter

Direction of blood flow

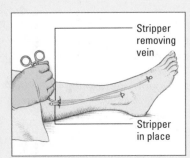

Stripper removing vein

Stripper in place

- Provide analgesia, or encourage the use of PCA, if appropriate.
- Gradually allow the patient to increase activities as ordered.
- Monitor the incision site for signs of infection or drainage.
- Monitor for complications, such as infection, bleeding, and vessel occlusion.
- Provide support to the patient and his family to help them cope with recovery and lifestyle changes.
- Maintain venous compression devices to the patient's lower extremities as appropriate to help prevent deep vein thrombosis.

Home care instructions

Instruct the patient to:
- check his pulse (or have a family member do it) in the affected extremity before rising from bed each morning and to notify the practitioner if he can't palpate his pulse or he develops coldness, pallor, numbness, tingling, pain, or swelling in the extremities
- continue with the progressive exercise started in the hospital
- perform coughing and deep-breathing exercises, splint the incision with a pillow to reduce pain while doing these exercises, and use the incentive spirometer to reduce pulmonary complications
- avoid lifting objects that weigh more than 10 lb (4.5 kg) for the next 4 to 6 weeks
- check the incision site daily and immediately notify the practitioner of any signs and symptoms of infection
- take medications as prescribed and report adverse reactions to the practitioner
- comply with the laboratory schedule for monitoring INR if the patient is receiving warfarin.

Valve surgery

To prevent heart failure, a patient with valvular stenosis or insufficiency accompanied by severe, unmanageable symptoms may require valvuloplasty (valvular repair), commissurotomy (separation of the adherent, thickened leaflets of the mitral valve), or valve replacement (with a mechanical or prosthetic valve).

Because of the high pressure generated by the left ventricle during contraction, stenosis and insufficiency most commonly affect the mitral and aortic valves. Other indications for valve surgery depend on the patient's symptoms and on the affected valve:
- For aortic insufficiency, the patient may need valve replacement after signs and symptoms (palpitations, dizziness, dyspnea on exertion, angina, and murmurs) have developed or the chest X-ray and ECG reveal left ventricular hypertrophy.

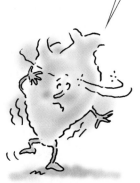

Dizziness is one symptom of aortic insufficiency. I'm not feeling too well...

- For aortic stenosis, valve replacement or balloon valvuloplasty is recommended if cardiac catheterization reveals significant stenosis.
- For mitral stenosis, valvuloplasty or commissurotomy is indicated if the patient develops fatigue, dyspnea, hemoptysis, arrhythmias, pulmonary hypertension, or right ventricular hypertrophy.
- For mitral insufficiency, the patient may undergo valvuloplasty or valve replacement when signs and symptoms (dyspnea, fatigue, and palpitations) interfere with the patient's activities or in acute insufficiency (as in papillary muscle rupture).

It gets complicated

Although valve surgery carries a low risk of mortality, it can cause serious complications. Hemorrhage, for instance, may result from unligated vessels, anticoagulant therapy, or coagulopathy resulting from cardiopulmonary bypass during surgery. Stroke may result from thrombus formation caused by turbulent blood flow through the prosthetic valve or from poor cerebral perfusion during cardiopulmonary bypass. In valve replacement, bacterial endocarditis can develop within days of implantation or months later. Valve dysfunction or failure may occur as the prosthetic device wears out.

Patient preparation

Before surgery, perform these steps:
- As necessary, reinforce and supplement the surgeon's explanation of the procedure.
- Tell the patient that he'll awaken from surgery in an ICU or PACU. Explain that he'll be connected to a cardiac monitor and have I.V. lines, an arterial line and, possibly, a pulmonary artery or left atrial catheter in place.
- Let him know that he'll breathe through an endotracheal tube connected to a mechanical ventilator and that he'll have a chest tube in place.

Monitoring and aftercare

The patient undergoing valve surgery will be cared for in the cardiac ICU after surgery. He'll be transferred to the medical-surgical unit when his condition is stable. After transfer to the medical-surgical unit, take these steps:
- Provide analgesia, or encourage the use of PCA, if appropriate.
- Monitor for postoperative complications, such as stroke, pulmonary embolism, pneumonia, impaired renal perfusion, endocarditis, and hemolytic anemia.
- Gradually allow the patient to increase activities as ordered.

- Monitor the incision site for signs of infection or drainage.
- Provide support to the patient and his family to help them cope with recovery and lifestyle changes.

Home care instructions
Instruct the patient to:
- immediately report chest pain or fever, or redness, swelling, or drainage at the incision site
- immediately notify the practitoner if signs or symptoms of heart failure (weight gain, dyspnea, or edema) develop
- notify the practitioner if signs or symptoms of postpericardiotomy syndrome (fever, muscle and joint pain, weakness, or chest discomfort) develop
- follow the prescribed medication regimen and report adverse reactions
- follow his prescribed diet, especially sodium and fat restrictions
- maintain a balance between activity and rest
- follow exercise or rehabilitation program if prescribed
- inform his dentist and other doctors of his prosthetic valve before undergoing surgery or dental work; he may be ordered to take prophylactic antibiotics before such procedures.

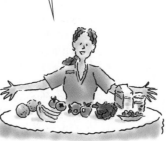

Emphasize the importance of following the prescribed diet, especially sodium and fat restrictions.

Implantable cardioverter-defibrillator
The implantable cardioverter-defibrillator (ICD) has a programmable pulse generator and lead system that monitors the heart's activity, detects ventricular bradyarrhythmias and tachyarrhythmias, and responds with appropriate therapies. Its range of therapies includes antitachycardia and bradycardia pacing, cardioversion, and defibrillation. Some defibrillators also have the ability to pace the atrium and the ventricle, pace both ventricles, or provide therapy for atrial fibrillation.

ICDs are indicated for patients who have experienced sudden cardiac death syndrome or syncope secondary to a ventricular arrhythmia. Those at high risk for ventricular fibrillation or tachycardia—such as those with dilated or hypertropic cardiomyopathy or those with prolonged QT syndrome—may also receive ICDs. The device can be programmed to defibrillate and pace according to the patient's condition. (See *Inserting an ICD*, page 274.)

Patient preparation
Before the procedure, take the following steps:
- Reinforce the cardiologist's instructions to the patient and his family, answering any questions they may have.
- Emphasize the need for the device to the patient, and explain the potential complications and ICD terminology.

Inserting an ICD

To insert an implantable cardioverter-defibrillator (ICD), the cardiologist makes a small incision near the collarbone and accesses the subclavian vein. Then he inserts the lead wires through the subclavian vein, threads them into the heart, and places them in contact with the endocardium.

The leads are connected to the pulse generator, which the cardiologist places under the skin in a specially prepared pocket in the right or left upper chest. (Placement is similar to that used for a pacemaker.) The cardiologist then closes the incision and programs the device.

- Restrict food and fluid for 12 hours before the procedure.
- Provide a sedative on the morning of the procedure as ordered to help the patient relax.

Monitoring and aftercare

The patient undergoing ICD implantation will be monitored on a telemetry or medical-surgical unit. After the procedure, take these steps:
- Monitor for arrhythmias and proper device functioning.
- Gradually allow the patient to increase activities as ordered.
- Monitor the incision site for signs of infection or drainage.
- Provide support to the patient and his family to help them cope with recovery and lifestyle changes.
- Encourage family members to learn cardiopulmonary resuscitation (CPR).

Home care instructions

Before discharge, instruct the patient to:
- avoid placing excessive pressure over the insertion site or moving or jerking the area until the postoperative visit
- check the incision site daily and immediately notify the practitioner of any signs and symptoms of infection
- wear a medical identification band and carry information about his ICD at all times
- take medications as prescribed and report adverse reactions to the practitioner
- keep a log recording discharges and any symptoms.

VAD: Help for the failing heart

A ventricular assist device (VAD), commonly called a "bridge to transplant," is a mechanical pump that relieves the workload of the ventricle as the heart heals or until a donor heart is located. Many types of VAD systems are available. This illustration shows a VAD (from Baxter Novacor) implanted in the left abdominal wall connected to an external controller by a percutaneous lead. This patient also has a reserve power pack. The monitor is a backup power source that can run on electricity.

Typical types

The typical VAD is implanted in the upper abdominal wall. An inflow cannula drains blood from the left ventricle into a pump, which then pushes the blood into the aorta through the outflow cannula. There are two types of VADs:

• continuous flow pump, which fills continuously and returns blood to the aorta at a constant rate

• pulsatile pump, which may fill during systole and pump blood into the aorta during diastole, or pump irrespective of the patient's cardiac cycle.

Complications

The VAD attempts to duplicate the seemingly simple task of the heart; pumping blood throughout the body. Designing a pump is fairly straightforward, but researchers still haven't solved the riddle of how blood swirls through the pulsing chambers of the heart without clotting. Despite the use of anticoagulants and special materials, the VAD usually causes thrombi formation, leading to pulmonary embolism, stroke, and other ominous complications. Thus, a VAD isn't used until other measures have failed. Other possible complications from VAD use include:

• bleeding cardiac tamponade
• right-sided heart failure
• infection
• kidney and liver dysfunction
• hemolysis.

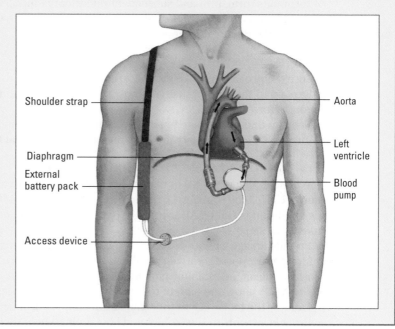

Shoulder strap

Diaphragm

External battery pack

Access device

Aorta

Left ventricle

Blood pump

VAD

A temporary life-sustaining treatment for a failing heart, the VAD diverts systemic blood flow from a diseased ventricle into a pump, which then sends the blood into the aorta. Used most commonly to assist the left ventricle, this device may also assist the right ventricle or both. (See *VAD: Help for the failing heart.*)

Candidates for a VAD include patients with:
- massive MI
- irreversible cardiomyopathy
- acute myocarditis
- inability to wean from cardiopulmonary bypass
- valvular disease
- bacterial endocarditis
- rejection of a heart transplant.

The device may also benefit patients awaiting a heart transplant, enabling them to live for months or years at home with a portable left VAD until a donor heart is located.

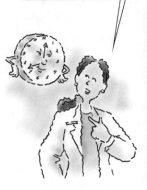

If the patient's ventricular function doesn't improve in 96 hours, the doctor may consider a heart transplant.

The downside

Unfortunately, the VAD carries a high risk of complications. For example, the device damages blood cells, creating the risk of thrombus formation and subsequent pulmonary embolism or stroke. As a result, if ventricular function hasn't improved in 96 hours, the doctor may consider a heart transplant.

Patient preparation

Before the procedure, take the following steps:
- Explain to the patient that you must restrict his food and fluid intake before surgery.
- Tell him that his cardiac function will be continuously monitored using an ECG, a pulmonary artery catheter, and an arterial line.

Monitoring and aftercare

The patient having a VAD implanted will be monitored in the cardiac ICU. He'll be transferred to the medical-surgical unit when his condition is stable. After transfer to the medical-surgical unit, take these steps:
- Provide analgesia, or encourage the use of PCA, if appropriate.
- Monitor for postoperative complications, such as stroke, pulmonary embolism, pneumonia, and impaired renal perfusion.
- Gradually allow the patient to increase activities as ordered.
- Monitor the incision site for signs of infection or drainage.
- Provide support to the patient and his family to help them cope with recovery and lifestyle changes.

Home care instructions

Before discharge, instruct the patient to:
- immediately report redness, swelling, or drainage at the incision site; chest pain; or fever
- immediately notify the practitioner if signs or symptoms of heart failure (weight gain, dyspnea, or edema) develop
- follow the prescribed medication regimen and report adverse reactions

- follow his prescribed diet, especially sodium and fat restrictions
- maintain a balance between activity and rest
- follow exercise or rehabilitation program if prescribed
- comply with the laboratory schedule for monitoring INR if the patient is receiving warfarin.

Balloon catheter treatments

Balloon catheter treatments for cardiovascular disorders include percutaneous balloon valvuloplasty and percutaneous transluminal coronary angioplasty (PTCA).

Percutaneous balloon valvuloplasty

Percutaneous balloon valvuloplasty, which can be performed in the cardiac catheterization laboratory, seeks to improve valvular function. It does so by enlarging the orifice of a stenotic heart valve, which can result from congenital defect, calcification, rheumatic fever, or aging. A small balloon valvuloplasty catheter is introduced through the skin at the femoral vein. Although the treatment of choice for valvular heart disease remains surgery (valvuloplasty, valve replacement, or commissurotomy), percutaneous balloon valvuloplasty offers an alternative for those considered poor candidates for surgery.

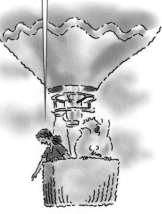

Heart, I know you're nervous, but percutaneous balloon valvuloplasty can help by enlarging the orifice of a stenotic heart valve. And you have to admit the view up here is amazing!

Bursting the balloon

Unfortunately, elderly patients with aortic disease commonly experience restenosis 1 to 2 years after undergoing valvuloplasty. Also, despite the decreased risks associated with more invasive procedures, balloon valvuloplasty can lead to complications, including:
- worsening valvular insufficiency by misshaping the valve so that it doesn't close completely
- pieces breaking off of the calcified valve, which may travel to the brain or lungs and cause embolism (rare)
- severely damaging delicate valve leaflets, requiring immediate surgery to replace the valve (rare)
- bleeding and hematoma at the arterial puncture site
- MI (rare), arrhythmias, myocardial ischemia, and circulatory defects distal to the catheter entry site.

Patient preparation

Before the procedure, take the following steps:
- Reinforce the doctor's explanation of the procedure, including its risks and alternatives.

• Restrict food and fluid intake for at least 6 hours before the procedure or as ordered.

Monitoring and aftercare

The patient undergoing balloon valvuloplasty will be monitored in the cardiac ICU or PACU after the procedure. He'll be transferred to the medical-surgical unit when his condition is stable. After transfer to the medical-surgical unit, take these steps:
• Monitor the effects of I.V. medications such as heparin.
• Assess the cannulation site for bleeding or infection.
• Monitor peripheral pulses distal to the insertion site and the color, temperature, and capillary refill time of the extremity. If pulses are difficult to palpate, use a handheld Doppler instrument.
• Notify the practitioner if pulses are absent.

Home care instructions

Before discharge, instruct the patient to:
• resume normal activity
• notify the practitioner if the patient experiences bleeding or increased bruising at the puncture site or recurrence of symptoms of valvular insufficiency, such as breathlessness or decreased exercise tolerance
• comply with regular follow-up visits.

PTCA

PTCA offers a nonsurgical alternative to coronary artery bypass surgery. The doctor uses a balloon-tipped catheter to dilate a coronary artery that has become narrowed because of atherosclerotic plaque. (See *Understanding angioplasty*.)

Performed in the cardiac catheterization laboratory under local anesthesia, PTCA doesn't involve a thoracotomy, so it's less costly and requires shorter hospitalization. Patients can usually walk the next day and return to work in 2 weeks.

Best working conditions

PTCA works best when lesions are readily accessible, noncalcified, less than 10 mm, concentric, discrete, and smoothly tapered. Patients with a history of less than 1 year of disabling angina make good candidates because their lesions tend to be softer and more compressible. (See *PCI: To intervene or not to intervene*, page 280.) Complications of PTCA are acute vessel closure and late restenosis. To prevent restenosis, the patient may need to undergo such procedures as stenting, atherectomy, and laser angioplasty.

Understanding angioplasty

Percutaneous transluminal coronary angioplasty can open an occluded coronary artery without opening the chest. This procedure is outlined in the steps below.

First, the cardiologist must thread the catheter into the artery. The illustration below shows the entrance of a guide catheter into the coronary artery.

When angiography shows the guide catheter positioned at the occlusion site, the cardiologist carefully inserts a smaller double-lumen balloon catheter through the guide catheter and directs the balloon through the occlusion.

The cardiologist then inflates the balloon, causing arterial stretching and plaque fracture. The balloon may need to be inflated or deflated several times until successful arterial dilation occurs.

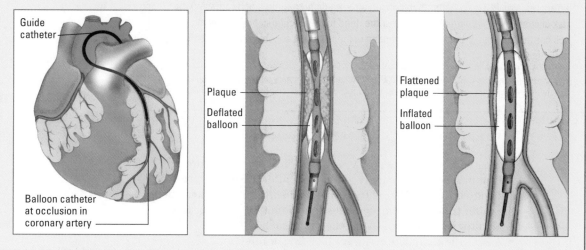

Guide catheter

Balloon catheter at occlusion in coronary artery

Plaque

Deflated balloon

Flattened plaque

Inflated balloon

Patient preparation

Before the procedure, take the following steps:
• Tell the patient that a catheter will be inserted into an artery and a vein in the groin area and that he may feel pressure as the catheter moves along the vessel.
• Advise the patient that the entire procedure lasts from 1 to 4 hours and that he'll have to lie flat on a table during that time.
• Explain to the patient that he'll be awake during the procedure and may have to take deep breaths to allow visualization of the radiopaque balloon catheter and answer questions about how he's feeling during the procedure.
• Tell the patient to notify the cardiologist if he experiences any chest pain or pressure during the procedure.
• Tell the patient he will have to remain on bed rest while the catheter is in place.

Weighing the evidence

PCI: To intervene or not to intervene?

Risk reducer?

Percutaneous coronary intervention (PCI) can improve the symptoms of patients with stable coronary artery disease. But does PCI work better than conservative medical treatment in decreasing the risk of death and myocardial infarction as well as the need for revascularization?

Just symptom reliever

In fact, it doesn't. According to a meta-analysis of patients with chronic stable coronary artery disease, PCI is no better than conservative medical treatment at decreasing the risk of death and myocardial infarction or the need for revascularization. However, it still has the advantage of providing symptom relief, making it a viable option for some patients.

Source: Loannidis, J.P.A., & Katritsis, D.G. (2006). Percutaneous coronary intervention vs. conservative therapy in nonacute coronary artery disease: A meta-analysis. *Circulation, 111*(22):2906–2912.

Monitoring and aftercare

The patient undergoing PTCA may be monitored in the cardiac ICU or interventional care recovery area after the procedure. The patient will be transferred to the medical-surgical unit when stable. After transfer to the medical-surgical unit, take these steps:

- Monitor the effects of I.V. medications such as heparin.
- Assess the cannulation site for bleeding or infection.
- Monitor peripheral pulses distal to the insertion site and the color, temperature, and capillary refill time of the extremity. If pulses are difficult to palpate, use a Doppler stethoscope.
- Notify the practitioner if pulses are absent.

Home care instructions

If the patient doesn't experience complications from the procedure, he may go home in 6 to 12 hours. Instruct the patient to:

- call his practitioner if he experiences any bleeding, bruising, or swelling at the arterial puncture site
- return for a stress thallium imaging test and follow-up angiography, as recommended by his practitioner
- report chest pain to the practitioner because restenosis can occur after PTCA.

Emergency treatment for heart rhythm disturbance

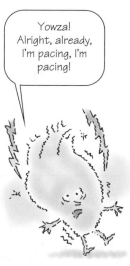

Yowza! Alright, already, I'm pacing, I'm pacing!

Emergency treatment for heart rhythm disturbance may include defibrillation and pacemaker insertion.

Defibrillation

With defibrillation, the heart receives a strong burst of electric current from defibrillator paddles applied to the patient's chest. This brief electric shock completely depolarizes the myocardium, allowing the heart's natural pacemaker to regain control of cardiac rhythm.

First choice

Defibrillation is the treatment of choice for ventricular fibrillation and pulseless ventricular tachycardia. For every minute that defibrillation is delayed, the patient's chance of surviving ventricular fibrillation drops 7% to 10%. If ventricular fibrillation lasts for more than a few minutes, it causes irreparable brain damage. Note that patients with certain arrhythmias such as stable ventricular tachycardia may require a technique similar to defibrillation called *synchronized cardioversion.*

Pacemaker insertion

Pacemakers are battery-operated generators that emit timed electrical signals to trigger contraction of the heart muscle, thus controlling heart rate. Whether temporary or permanent, they're used when the heart's natural pacemaker fails to work properly.

From the temp pool

Temporary pacemakers are used to pace the heart during CPR or open-heart surgery, after cardiac surgery, and when sinus arrest, symptomatic sinus bradycardia, or complete heart block occurs. Temporary pacing may also correct tachyarrhythmias that fail to respond to drug therapy. In emergency situations, the patient may receive a temporary transvenous or transcutaneous pacemaker if time or his condition doesn't permit or require implantation of a permanent pacemaker. The doctor may also use a temporary pacemaker to observe the effects of pacing on cardiac function so he can select an optimal rate before implanting a permanent pacemaker. The method of pacing depends on the device.

Permanent position

Permanent pacemaker implantation is a common procedure; worldwide, about 110,000 people undergo it every year. Permanent pacemakers are inserted when the heart's natural pacemaker becomes irreversibly disrupted. Indications for a permanent pacemaker include:
• acquired atrioventricular (AV) block
• chronic bifascicular and trifascicular block

- AV block associated with acute MI
- sinus node dysfunction
- hypersensitive carotid sinus syndrome
- hypertrophic and dilated cardiomyopathy.

The many types of pacemakers are categorized according to capabilities. Choice of a pacemaker depends on the patient's age and condition, the cardiologist's preference and, increasingly, the cost of the device, which can be several thousand dollars. (See *Reviewing pacemaker codes.*)

Reviewing pacemaker codes

The North American Society of Pacing and Electrophysiology (NASPE) and the British Pacing and Electrophysiology Group (BPEG) developed a five-letter coding system called NASPE/BPEG Generic (NBG) Pacemaker Code to describe pacemaker type and function. Codes may consist of three to five letters. The fourth and fifth letters refer to newer pacemaker functions that aren't used in every pacemaker. Here's a summary of what each of the five letters of the code signifies:

heart chamber being paced — **A** (atrium), **V** (ventricle), **D** (dual, or both chambers), or **O** (none).

heart chamber that the pacemaker senses — **A, V, D,** or **O**.

how the pacemaker responds to the sensed event — **T** (triggered by the event), **I** (inhibited by the event), **D** (dual — triggered and inhibited by the event), or **O** (no response to sensing).

pacemaker's degree of programmability and rate responsiveness — **P** (simple programmable), **M** (multiprogrammable), **C** (communicating functions), **R** (rate responsiveness), or **O** (none).

how the pacemaker reacts to tachycardia — **P** (pacing), **S** (shock), **D** (dual — pacing and shock), or **O** (none).

Common pacing codes

The codes DDD and VVI are the most commonly used pacing codes. A description of each follows, along with its advantages and disadvantages.

DDD
Paces: Atrium and ventricle
Senses: Atrium and ventricle
Response: Inhibited and triggered
Summary: If the atrial rate falls below a preset lower limit, the atrium is paced. If the atrial rate is above this preset lower limit, the atrium isn't paced. However, the ventricle may be paced if the pacemaker doesn't sense a ventricular response within the present atrioventricular (AV) interval.
Advantages: Because both chambers may be paced, AV synchrony is preserved. Used for patients with an intact sinus node but AV block at or below the AV node. May have a rate responsive mode.
Disadvantages: Requires two leads.

VVI
Paces: Ventricle
Senses: Ventricle
Response: Inhibited
Summary: This type of pacemaker paces only when the ventricular rate falls below a preset rate.
Advantages: Requires a single lead and is relatively simple to operate. May be used to treat chronic atrial fibrillation with a slow ventricular response. These patients don't require an atrial lead because a fibrillating atrium can't be paced. May have a rate responsive mode.
Disadvantages: Because only the ventricle is paced, it doesn't preserve AV synchrony.

Nursing diagnoses

When caring for patients with cardiovascular disorders, you'll find that you can use several nursing diagnoses frequently. These commonly used nursing diagnoses appear below, along with appropriate nursing interventions and rationales. See *NANDA-I taxonomy II by domain*, page 936, for the complete list of NANDA diagnoses.

Activity intolerance

Related to an imbalance between oxygen supply and demand, *Activity intolerance* may be associated with such conditions as acute MI, valvular disorders, heart failure, peripheral vascular disorders, and other ailments.

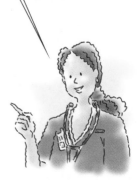

Activity intolerance is related to an imbalance between oxygen supply and demand.

Expected outcomes

• Patient states a desire to increase his activity level.
• Patient identifies controllable factors that cause fatigue.
• Patient demonstrates skill in conserving energy while carrying out activities of daily living (ADLs) to tolerance level.

Nursing interventions and rationales

• Discuss with the patient the need for activity, which will improve physical and psychosocial well-being.
• Identify activities the patient considers desirable and meaningful to enhance their positive impact.
• Encourage the patient to help plan activity progression. Make sure you include activities he considers essential to help compliance.
• Instruct and help the patient to alternate periods of rest and activity to reduce the body's oxygen demand and prevent fatigue.
• Identify and minimize factors that diminish exercise tolerance to help increase activity level.
• Monitor physiologic responses to increased activity (including respirations, heart rate and rhythm, and blood pressure) to ensure they return to normal a few minutes after exercising.
• Teach the patient how to conserve energy while performing ADLs — for example, sitting in a chair while dressing, wearing lightweight clothing that fastens with Velcro or a few large buttons, and wearing slip-on shoes. These measures reduce cellular metabolism and oxygen demand.

Energy boost

- Demonstrate exercises for increasing strength and endurance, which will improve breathing and gradually increase activity level.
- Support and encourage activity to the patient's level of tolerance to help develop his independence.
- Before discharge, formulate a plan with the patient and his caregivers that will enable the patient to continue functioning at maximum activity tolerance or to gradually increase the tolerance. For example, teach the patient and his caregivers how to monitor the patient's pulse during activities; recognize the need for oxygen, if prescribed; and use oxygen equipment properly. Participation in planning encourages patient satisfaction and compliance.

Decreased cardiac output

Related to reduced stroke volume, *Decreased cardiac output* may be associated with such conditions as angina, bacterial endocarditis, heart failure, MI, valvular heart disease, and other ailments.

Expected outcomes

- Patient maintains hemodynamic stability.
- Patient exhibits no arrhythmias.
- Patient maintains adequate cardiac output.

Nursing interventions and rationales

- Monitor and record level of consciousness (LOC), heart rate and rhythm, oxygen saturation (using pulse oximetry), and blood pressure at least every 4 hours, or more often if necessary, to detect cerebral hypoxia possibly resulting from decreased cardiac output.
- Auscultate heart and breath sounds at least every 4 hours. Report abnormal sounds as soon as they develop. Extra heart sounds may indicate early cardiac decompensation. Adventitious breath sounds may indicate pulmonary congestion and decreased cardiac output.
- Measure and record intake and output. Reduced urine output without reduced fluid intake may indicate reduced renal perfusion, possibly from decreased cardiac output.
- Promptly treat life-threatening arrhythmias to avoid the risk of death.
- Weigh the patient daily before breakfast to detect fluid retention.
- Inspect for pedal or sacral edema to detect venous stasis and decreased cardiac output.

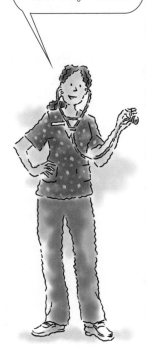

For patients with decreased cardiac output, monitor and record LOC, heart rate and rhythm, oxygen saturation, and blood pressure at least every 4 hours.

Getting a facial

- Provide skin care every 4 hours to enhance skin perfusion and venous flow.
- Gradually increase the patient's activities within limits of the prescribed heart rate to allow the heart to adjust to increased oxygen demand. Monitor pulse rate before and after activity to compare rates and gauge tolerance.
- Plan the patient's activities to avoid fatigue and increased myocardial workload.
- Maintain dietary restrictions as ordered to reduce complications and the risk of cardiac disease.
- Teach the patient stress-reduction techniques to reduce anxiety and provide a sense of control. (See *Biofeedback*.)
- Explain all procedures and tests to enhance understanding and reduce anxiety.

Teaching an old dog new tricks

- Teach the patient about chest pain and other reportable symptoms, prescribed diet, medications (name, dosage, frequency, therapeutic effects, and adverse effects), prescribed activity level, simple methods for lifting and bending, and stress-reduction techniques. These measures involve the patient and his family in care.

Education edge

Biofeedback

Because stress increases the risk of developing hypertension, helping the patient reduce stress will improve his cardiovascular health. Biofeedback is an alternative therapy that teaches people how to exert conscious control over various autonomic functions with the help of electronic monitors. By observing on a monitor the fluctuations of particular body functions (such as breathing, heart rate, and blood pressure), the patient can learn how to bring them under control through mental adjustments. In time, he may be able to regulate conditions, such as high blood pressure, without medication or the use of monitors.

1-2-3, blue light

For example, using monitors initially, a patient with high blood pressure can be taught to recognize and ultimately regulate his body's response to stress. The patient is connected to a skin temperature monitor, which reflects the amount of blood flow beneath the skin. Changes in temperature caused by vasoconstriction or vasodilation trigger lights on the monitor, indicating the stress response. A black light signals if the patient is tense; a blue light shows he's relaxed.

• Carry out the care plan, as ordered. Collaborative practice enhances overall care.
• Administer oxygen as ordered to increase the supply to the myocardium.

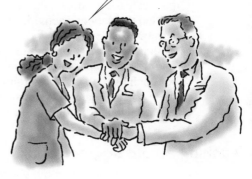

Keep in mind, collaborative practice enhances overall patient care.

Deficient knowledge

Related to heart disease, *Deficient knowledge* can apply to a particular disorder or the risk factors related to cardiovascular disease.

Expected outcomes

• Patient expresses an interest in learning new behaviors.
• Patient sets realistic learning goals.
• Patient practices new health-related behaviors during hospitalization (for example, selects appropriate diet, weighs himself daily, and monitors intake and output).

Nursing interventions and rationales

• Establish an environment of mutual trust and respect to enhance learning. Comfort with growing self-awareness, ability to share this awareness with others, receptiveness to new experiences, and consistency between actions and words form the basis of a trusting relationship.
• Help the patient develop goals for learning. Involving him in planning meaningful goals will encourage follow-through.
• Select teaching strategies (discussion, demonstration, role-playing, or visual materials) appropriate for the patient's individual learning style (specify) to enhance teaching effectiveness.
• Teach skills that the patient must use every day. Have him demonstrate each new skill to help him gain confidence.
• Have the patient incorporate learned skills into his daily routine during hospitalization (specify skills) to allow him to practice new skills and receive feedback.
• Provide the patient with the names and telephone numbers of resource people or organizations to provide continuity of care and follow-up after discharge.

Common cardiovascular disorders

Below are several common cardiovascular disorders, along with their causes, pathophysiology, signs and symptoms, diagnostic test findings, treatments, and nursing interventions.

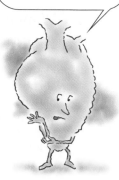

More than half of all patients with untreated abdominal aneurysms 6 cm or larger die within 2 years of diagnosis. Now, that's a scary statistic!

Aneurysm, abdominal aortic

Abdominal aortic aneurysm, an abnormal dilation in the arterial wall, most commonly occurs in the aorta between the renal arteries and iliac branches. More than 50% of patients with untreated abdominal aneurysms 6 cm or larger die within 2 years of diagnosis, primarily from aneurysmal rupture. More than 85% of patients with large aneurysms die within 5 years.

What causes it

Aneurysms commonly result from atherosclerosis, which weakens the aortic wall and gradually distends the lumen. Other causes include:
• fungal infection (mycotic aneurysms) of the aortic arch and descending segments
• congenital disorders, such as coarctation of the aorta, Marfan syndrome, and collagen vascular disorders
• trauma
• syphilis
• hypertension.

Pathophysiology

Degenerative changes in the muscular layer of the aorta (tunica media) create a focal weakness, allowing the inner layer (tunica intima) and outer layer (tunica adventitia) to stretch outward. The resulting outward bulge is called an *aneurysm*. Blood pressure within the aorta progressively weakens the vessel walls and enlarges the aneurysm.

What to look for

Signs and symptoms of an aneurysm include:
• asymptomatic pulsating mass in the periumbilical area
• possible systolic bruit over the aorta on auscultation
• possible abdominal tenderness on deep palpation
• lumbar pain that radiates to the flank and groin (imminent rupture).

Memory jogger

When assessing for signs and symptoms of abdominal aortic aneurysm, remember to jog a few **LAPS:**

Lumbar pain that radiates to the flank and groin (a sign of imminent rupture)

Abdominal tenderness on deep palpation (possible sign)

Pulsating mass in the periumbilical area

Systolic bruit over the aorta (possible sign).

If the aneurysm ruptures, look for:
- severe, tearing abdominal and back pain
- weakness
- sweating
- tachycardia
- hypotension
- circulatory collapse.

What tests tell you

- Serial ultrasonography or computed tomography (CT) angiography determines aneurysm size, shape, and location.
- Anteroposterior and lateral X-rays of the abdomen can detect aortic calcification, which outlines the mass, in at least 75% of patients.
- Aortography shows the condition of vessels proximal and distal to the aneurysm and the extent of the aneurysm. However, this test may underestimate aneurysm diameter because it shows only the flow channel and not the intraluminal clot or dilated walls.

How it's treated

Usually, abdominal aneurysm requires resection of the aneurysm and replacement of the damaged aortic section with a Dacron graft.

Risky business

Large aneurysms or those that produce symptoms involve a significant risk of rupture and require immediate repair.

If the aneurysm appears small and asymptomatic, the practitioner may delay surgery, opting first to treat the patient's hypertension and reduce risk factors. Keep in mind, however, that even small aneurysms may rupture. The patient must undergo regular physical examinations and ultrasound checks to detect enlargement, which may indicate imminent rupture.

Endovascular grafting may also be used to repair an abdominal aortic aneurysm. In this minimally invasive procedure, the surgeon will insert a catheter with an attached graft through the femoral or iliac artery and advance it over a guide wire into the aorta, where he'll position it across the aneurysm. A balloon on the catheter expands, affixing the graft to the vessel wall and excluding the aneurysm.

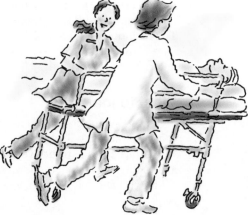

If rupture occurs, there's no time to lose. Get the patient right to surgery.

What to do

• Be alert for signs of rupture, which is life-threatening. Watch closely for any signs of acute blood loss, such as hypotension, increasing pulse and respiratory rate, cool and clammy skin, restlessness, and decreased sensorium.
• If rupture occurs, get the patient to surgery immediately.
• Evaluate the patient. Note whether the patient is free from pain and if he has adequate tissue perfusion with warm, dry skin; adequate pulse and blood pressure; and absence of fatigue. (See *Abdominal aortic aneurysm teaching tips.*)

Aneurysms, femoral and popliteal

Progressive atherosclerotic changes in the medial layer of the femoral and popliteal arteries may lead to aneurysm. Aneurysmal formations may be fusiform (spindle-shaped) or saccular (pouchlike). Fusiform aneurysms are three times more common than saccular aneurysms.

Femoral and popliteal aneurysms may occur as single or multiple segmental lesions, in many cases affecting both legs, and commonly occur with aneurysms in the abdominal aorta or iliac arteries. This condition occurs most commonly in men over age 50. Elective surgery before complications arise greatly improves prognosis.

What causes it

Femoral and popliteal aneurysms can result from:
• atherosclerosis
• congenital weakness in the arterial wall (rare)
• blunt or penetrating trauma
• bacterial infection.

Pathophysiology

An aneurysm is a localized outpouching or dilation of a weakened arterial wall. This weakness can result from either atherosclerotic plaque formation that erodes the vessel wall or the loss of elastin and collagen in the vessel wall.

What to look for

If large enough to compress the medial popliteal nerve and vein, popliteal aneurysms may cause:
• pain in the popliteal space
• edema
• vessel distention and widened pulse

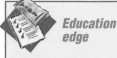

Education edge

Abdominal aortic aneurysm teaching tips

• Provide psychological support for the patient and his family by providing appropriate explanations and answering all questions.
• Explain the postoperative period, and let the patient know that he may be monitored in the intensive care unit.
• Instruct the patient to take all medications as prescribed and to carry a list of current medications in case of an emergency.
• Tell the patient not to push, pull, or lift heavy objects until medically cleared by the surgeon.

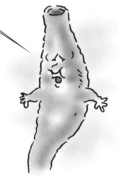

Vessel distention is one sign of aneurysm. And I just thought I was bloated!

- possibly symptoms of severe ischemia (in the leg or foot).
   Signs of a femoral aneurysm include a wide, pulsating mass above or below the inguinal ligament found on palpation.

What tests tell you

- When palpation doesn't provide a positive identification, duplex ultrasonography, CT angiography, or arteriography may help identify femoral and popliteal aneurysms. These tests may also help detect associated aneurysms, especially those in the abdominal aorta and the iliac arteries.
- Ultrasound can also help identify aneurysms and may help to determine the size of the popliteal or femoral artery.

How it's treated

Femoral and popliteal aneurysms require surgical bypass and reconstruction of the artery, usually with an autogenous saphenous vein graft replacement or patch arterioplasty. Arterial occlusion that causes severe ischemia and gangrene may require leg amputation if adequate blood flow can't be restored.

What to do

- Administer prophylactic antibiotics, antihypertensives, or anticoagulants, as ordered.
- Prepare the patient for surgery. (For information on nursing care of patients who undergo vascular surgery, see "Vascular repair," page 269.)
- Evaluate the patient. Document whether the patient shows good color and temperature of extremities and if he no longer has pain. Pulses should be present in his extremities. (See *Femoral or popliteal aneurysm teaching tips*.)

Arterial occlusive disease

A common complication of atherosclerosis, arterial occlusive disease may affect any artery but typically affects the peripheral arteries, such as the carotid (and its branches) and the lower extremity arteries (femoral, popliteal, posterior tibial, anterior tibial, and peroneal). The upper extremity arteries (subclavian, axillary, brachial, radial, and ulnar) are less commonly affected. Arterial occlusions may be acute or chronic. Men suffer from arterial occlusive disease more commonly than women.

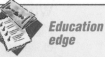

Education edge

Femoral or popliteal aneurysm teaching tips

- Explain what an aneurysm is and how it occurs. Provide emotional support and address concerns.
- Provide preoperative and postoperative teaching. Explain how to care for the incision after surgery and how to recognize complications.
- Teach the patient how to assess daily for a pulse in the affected extremity.
- Tell the patient to report recurrence of symptoms immediately.
- Explain to the patient with popliteal artery resection that swelling may persist. Warn against wearing constrictive clothes.
- If the patient is receiving anticoagulant therapy, suggest measures to prevent excessive bleeding.

What causes it

Risk factors for arterial occlusive disease include smoking, aging, hypertension, hyperlipidemia, diabetes mellitus, and family history of vascular disorders, MI, or stroke. Causes include:
• emboli formation
• infection
• thrombosis
• trauma or fracture
• vasculitis.

Pathophysiology

In arterial occlusive disease, obstruction or narrowing of the lumen of the aorta and its major branches causes an interruption of blood flow, usually to the legs and feet.

Prognosis? It all depends...

Prognosis depends on the location of the occlusion, the development of collateral circulation to counteract reduced blood flow and, in acute disease, the time elapsed between occlusion and its removal.

What to look for

Signs and symptoms depend on the severity and site of the arterial occlusion. Acute arterial occlusion may produce the five classic Ps:

paralysis

pain

paresthesia

pallor

pulselessness.

Other signs and symptoms include:
• unequally cool extremities when compared with each other
• intermittent claudication
• severe pain in the toes or feet (aggravated by elevating the extremity and sometimes relieved by keeping the extremity in a dependent position)
• ulcers or gangrene
• pallor on elevation, followed by redness with dependency
• delayed capillary filling, hair loss, or trophic nail changes
• diminished or absent extremity pulses.

What tests tell you

- Arteriography demonstrates the type (thrombus or embolus), location, and degree of obstruction and helps evaluate the collateral circulation. It's particularly useful for diagnosing chronic forms of the disease and evaluating candidates for reconstructive surgery.
- Duplex Doppler ultrasonography uses ultrasound to visualize vessels and measure the speed, direction, and pattern of blood flow.
- Plethysmography detects arterial pulsations to quantify the blood flow in an extremity.
- Pulse volume recordings can determine the level of ischemia in an extremity.

How it's treated

Treatment for arterial occlusive disease depends on the cause, location, and size of the obstruction.

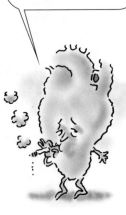

With arterial occlusive disease, treatment consists of such supportive measures as smoking cessation. Time to kick the habit!

Mild disease... moderate measures

For patients with mild chronic disease, it usually consists of risk factor reduction, such as smoking cessation and hypertension control as well as suppportive measures such as walking exercise.

Drug therapy includes dextran and antiplatelet and hemorheologic drugs, such as aspirin, ticlopidine, pentoxifylline (Trental), and cilostazol (Pletal). Thrombolytic therapy may be used to treat an acute arterial thrombosis. Patients with hyperlipidemia may be treated with antilipemic drugs.

Severe disease... surgery

Appropriate surgical procedures may include embolectomy, thromboendarterectomy, patch grafting, and bypass grafting. The patient may require amputation if arterial reconstructive surgery fails or complications develop.

Lower the risk

Invasive endovascular techniques carry less risk than surgery and may include balloon angioplasty, atherectomy, and stenting. Other appropriate therapy includes heparin to prevent emboli (for embolic occlusion) and bowel resection after restoration of blood flow (for mesenteric artery occlusion).

What to do

• For information on nursing care of patients who undergo vascular surgery, see "Vascular repair," page 269.
• Following treatment, evaluate the patient. He should be able to increase exercise tolerance without developing pain and should have normal peripheral pulses. The patient should also maintain good skin color and temperature in his extremities. (See *Arterial occlusive disease teaching tips*.)

Coronary artery disease

Coronary artery disease (CAD) refers to any narrowing or obstruction of arterial lumina that interferes with cardiac perfusion. Deprived of sufficient blood, the myocardium can develop various ischemic diseases, including angina pectoris, MI, heart failure, sudden death, and cardiac arrhythmias.

Not an equal opportunity disease

CAD affects more Whites than Blacks and more men than women. After menopause, however, the risk of CAD in women increases to equal that of men. CAD occurs more commonly in industrial countries than underdeveloped areas and affects affluent people more than poor people.

What causes it

Most commonly, atherosclerosis leads to CAD. Other possible causes include:
• arteritis
• coronary artery spasm
• certain infectious diseases
• congenital abnormalities.
    Patients with certain risk factors appear to face a greater likelihood of developing CAD. These factors include:
• family history of heart disease
• obesity
• smoking
• high-fat, high-carbohydrate diet
• sedentary lifestyle
• menopause
• stress
• diabetes
• hypertension
• hyperlipoproteinemia.

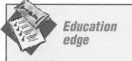

Education edge

Arterial occlusive disease teaching tips

• Teach proper foot care or other appropriate measures, depending on the affected area.
• Instruct the patient about signs and symptoms of recurrence (pain, pallor, numbness, paralysis, absence of pulse) that can result from a recurrent occlusion or occlusion at another site.
• Caution the patient against wearing constrictive clothing or crossing his legs while sitting.
• Advise the patient to stop smoking and refer him to a smoking-cessation program if appropriate.
• Encourage the patient to closely follow his prescribed medication regimen.
• Teach the patient to check his pulses daily.

Pathophysiology

Fatty, fibrous plaques progressively occlude the coronary arteries, reducing the volume of blood that can flow through them, leading to myocardial ischemia.

A precarious balance

As atherosclerosis progresses, luminal narrowing and vascular changes impair the diseased vessel's ability to dilate. This causes a precarious balance between myocardial oxygen supply and demand, threatening the myocardium beyond the lesion.

When the balance tips...

When oxygen demand exceeds what the diseased vessels can supply, localized myocardial ischemia results.

Transient ischemia causes reversible changes at the cellular and tissue levels, depressing myocardial function. Untreated, it can lead to tissue injury or necrosis. Oxygen deprivation forces the myocardium to shift from aerobic to anaerobic metabolism. As a result, lactic acid (the end product of anaerobic metabolism) accumulates and cellular pH decreases.

...things fall apart

The combination of hypoxia, reduced energy availability, and acidosis rapidly impairs left ventricular function. The strength of contractions drops in the affected myocardial region as the fibers shorten inadequately, with less force and velocity. Plus, the ischemic section's wall moves abnormally. This typically results in the heart ejecting less blood with each contraction. If blood flow through the coronary arteries isn't restored, an MI will result. If blood flow is restored, aerobic metabolism and contractility return.

What to look for

Angina, the classic symptom of CAD, occurs as a burning, squeezing, or crushing tightness in the substernal or precordial chest. It may radiate to the left arm, neck, jaw, or shoulder blade. Women, however, may experience atypical chest pain. (See *Atypical chest pain in women.*)

Angina has four major forms:
• stable — pain that's predictable in frequency and duration and relieved with nitrates and rest
• unstable — increased pain that's easily induced
• Prinzmetal's or variant — pain that results from unpredictable coronary artery spasm

---

Atypical chest pain in women

Women with coronary artery disease commonly experience atypical chest pain, vague chest pain, or a lack of chest pain. However, they may also experience classic chest pain, which may occur without any relationship to activity or stress.

Although men tend to complain of crushing pain in the center of the chest, women are more likely to experience arm or shoulder pain; jaw, neck, or throat pain; toothache; back pain; or pain under the breastbone or in the stomach.

Other signs and symptoms women may experience include nausea or dizziness; shortness of breath; unexplained anxiety, weakness, or fatigue; and palpitations, cold sweat, or paleness.

- microvascular — angina-like chest pain in a patient with normal coronary arteries that results from impaired vasodilator reserve.
    Other signs and symptoms of CAD include:
- nausea
- vomiting
- weakness
- diaphoresis
- cool extremities.

What tests tell you

- ECG shows ischemia and, possibly, arrhythmias such as premature ventricular contractions. A pain-free patient may have a normal ECG. Arrhythmias may occur without infarction, secondary to ischemia.
- Exercise ECG may provoke chest pain and signs of myocardial ischemia in response to physical exertion.
- Coronary angiography reveals coronary artery stenosis or obstruction and collateral circulation and shows the condition of the arteries beyond the narrowed area.

Keep on running

- During treadmill exercise, myocardial perfusion imaging with thallium-201 detects ischemic areas of the myocardium, visualized as "cold spots."
- Laboratory evaluation of cardiac markers may be performed to confirm or rule out a diagnosis of MI. The patient may also undergo serum lipid studies to detect and classify hyperlipidemia.
- An elevated Hb A_{1C} level indicates an increased risk for atherosclerosis and adverse cardiac events; an elevated C-reactive protein level points to a higher cadiac risk. Although these two tests alone can't determine if a patient with angina has CAD, they do help detect a higher risk for CAD.

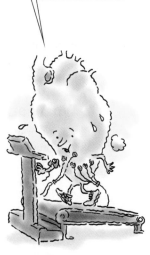

During treadmill exercise, myocardial perfusion imaging detects ischemic areas of the myocardium.

How it's treated

For patients with angina, CAD treatment seeks to reduce myocardial oxygen demand or increase oxygen supply. Nitrates reduce myocardial oxygen consumption. Beta-adrenergic blockers can reduce the workload and oxygen demands of the heart by reducing heart rate and peripheral resistance to blood flow. If angina results from coronary artery spasm, the patient may receive calcium channel blockers. Antiplatelet drugs minimize platelet aggregation and the danger of coronary occlusion. Antilipemic drugs can reduce elevated serum cholesterol or triglyceride levels.

    Obstructive lesions may call for coronary artery bypass surgery or PTCA. Other alternatives include laser angioplasty, minimally invasive surgery, rotational atherectomy, and stent placement.

What to do

- Monitor blood pressure and heart rate during an anginal episode.
- Take an ECG before administering nitroglycerin or other nitrates for angina.
- Record the duration of pain, the amount of medication required to relieve it, and accompanying symptoms. Keep nitroglycerin available for immediate use.
- Evaluate the patient. Note if the patient experiences pain or shortness of breath at rest or with usual activity. Assess whether he can tolerate activity. (See *Coronary artery disease teaching tips*.)

Dilated cardiomyopathy

Dilated cardiomyopathy occurs when myocardial muscle fibers become extensively damaged. This disorder interferes with myocardial metabolism and grossly dilates every heart chamber, giving the heart a globular shape. Dilated cardiomyopathy leads to intractable heart failure, arrhythmias, and emboli. Usually not diagnosed until its advanced stages, this disorder carries a poor prognosis.

What causes it

The primary cause of dilated cardiomyopathy is unknown. Although the relationship remains unclear, it occasionally occurs secondary to:
- viral or bacterial infections
- hypertension
- peripartum syndrome (related to toxemia)
- ischemic heart disease or valvular disease
- drug hypersensitivity or chemotherapy
- cardiotoxic effects of drugs or alcohol.

Pathophysiology

Dilated cardiomyopathy is characterized by a grossly dilated, hypodynamic ventricle that contracts poorly and, to a lesser degree, by myocardial hypertrophy.

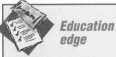

Education edge

Coronary artery disease teaching tips

- Explain all procedures and tests, answer questions appropriately, and provide support.
- Instruct the patient to seek medical attention immediately if he feels symptoms of angina.
- Help the patient determine which activities precipitate episodes of pain. Help him identify and select more effective coping mechanisms to deal with stress.
- Stress the need to follow the prescribed drug regimen.
- Encourage the patient to maintain the prescribed diet.
- Encourage regular moderate exercise. Refer the patient to a local cardiac rehabilitation center if appropriate.
- If the patient smokes, refer him to a smoking-cessation program.
- Refer the patient to the American Heart Association for more information and support.

Pump up the volume

All four chambers enlarge as a result of increased volumes and pressures. Thrombi commonly develop within these chambers from blood pooling and stasis, which may lead to embolization.

If hypertrophy coexists, the heart ejects blood less efficiently. A large volume remains in the left ventricle after systole, causing heart failure from backward blood flow.

What to look for

The patient may develop:
• shortness of breath (orthopnea, exertional dyspnea, or paroxysmal nocturnal dyspnea)
• fatigue
• irritating dry cough at night
• edema
• liver engorgement
• jugular vein distention
• peripheral cyanosis
• sinus tachycardia
• atrial fibrillation
• diffuse apical impulses
• pansystolic murmur (mitral and tricuspid insufficiency secondary to cardiomegaly and weak papillary muscles)
• S_3 and S_4 gallop rhythms.

What tests tell you

• ECG and angiography rule out ischemic heart disease. ECG may also show biventricular hypertrophy, sinus tachycardia, atrial enlargement and, in 20% of patients, atrial fibrillation.
• Chest X-rays may show cardiomegaly (usually affecting all heart chambers), pulmonary congestion, or pleural effusion.
• MUGA scanning and echocardiography show decreased left ventricular function and decreased wall motion.

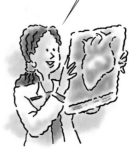

In dilated cardiomyopathy, chest X-rays may show cardiomegaly, pulmonary congestion, or pleural effusion.

How it's treated

Treatment seeks to correct the underlying causes and to improve the heart's pumping ability. Angiotensin-converting enzyme (ACE) inhibitors reduce afterload through vasodilation, thereby reducing heart failure. Diuretics are commonly given with an ACE inhibitor to reduce fluid retention.

When the ACE doesn't fly right

For those without improvement of symptoms on an ACE inhibitor and diuretic, digoxin (Lanoxin) may improve myocardial contractility.

Hydralazine and isosorbide dinitrate in combination produce vasodilation. Antiarrhythmics, cardioversion, and pacemakers may control arrhythmias. Anticoagulants may be prescribed to reduce the risk of emboli. Treatment may also include oxygen, a sodium-restricted diet, and bed rest.

Selective surgery

Surgical interventions in carefully selected patients may include revascularization, such as CABG, if dilated cardiomyopathy results from ischemia. Valvular repair or replacement may help if dilated cardiomyopathy results from valve dysfunction. Cardiomyoplasty — in which the latissimus dorsi muscle is wrapped around the ventricles to help the ventricles pump more efficiently — may work when other medical treatment fails. A cardiomyostimulator delivering bursts of electrical impulses during systole can help the myocardium contract. If the patient doesn't respond to other treatments, he may require a ventricular assist device and eventual heart transplantation.

Living the good life

For all patients with dilated cardiomyopathy, lifestyle changes can help. As applicable, patients should stop smoking and drinking alcohol; adopt a low-fat, low-sodium diet; and maintain appropriate physical activity.

What to do

• Monitor for signs of progressive heart failure (decreased arterial pulses and increased jugular vein distention) and compromised renal perfusion (oliguria, increased blood urea nitrogen [BUN] and serum creatinine levels, and electrolyte imbalances).
• Weigh the patient daily.
• Check blood pressure and heart rate frequently.
• Monitor the patient receiving diuretics for signs of resolving congestion (decreased crackles and dyspnea) or too vigorous diuresis. Check serum potassium level for hypokalemia, especially if therapy includes digoxin.
• Offer support, and encourage the patient to express his feelings.
• Evaluate the patient. Look for adequate tissue perfusion, as evidenced by good color; warm, dry skin; and clear lungs. The patient should maintain his weight and level of activity. He should also have adequate blood pressure and no dizziness or edema. (See *Dilated cardiomyopathy teaching tips*.)

Education edge

Dilated cardiomyopathy teaching tips

• Before discharge, teach the patient about his illness and its treatment.
• Emphasize the need to restrict sodium intake and watch for weight gain.
• Explain the need to take digoxin as prescribed and watch for such adverse reactions as anorexia, nausea, vomiting, and yellow vision.
• Because the patient faces an increased risk of sudden cardiac arrest, encourage family members to learn cardiopulmonary resuscitation.

Endocarditis

Endocarditis — infection of the endocardium, heart valves, or cardiac prosthesis — results from bacterial or fungal invasion. Untreated endocarditis usually proves fatal, but with proper treatment, 70% of patients recover. Prognosis becomes much worse when endocarditis causes severe valvular damage, leading to insufficiency and heart failure, or when it involves a prosthetic valve.

What causes it

Most cases of endocarditis occur in patients who abuse I.V. drugs or those with prosthetic heart valves, mitral valve prolapse, or rheumatic heart disease.

Other predisposing conditions include congenital abnormalities (coarctation of the aorta and tetralogy of Fallot), subaortic and valvular aortic stenosis, ventricular septal defects, pulmonary stenosis, Marfan syndrome, degenerative heart disease, and syphilis.

When bugs attack

Causative organisms may include group A nonhemolytic streptococci, *Pneumococcus*, *Staphylococcus*, *Enterococcus* and, rarely, *Gonococcus*.

Pathophysiology

Infection causes fibrin and platelets to aggregate on the valve tissue and engulf circulating bacteria or fungi. They form friable verrucous (wartlike) vegetative growths on the heart valves, endocardial lining of a heart chamber, or endothelium of a blood vessel. Such vegetations may cover the valve surfaces, causing ulceration and necrosis; they may also extend to the cordae tendineae. Ultimately, they may embolize to the spleen, kidneys, central nervous system, and lungs. (See *Effects of endocarditis*.)

What to look for

Early clinical features are usually nonspecific and include:
- weakness
- fatigue
- weight loss
- anorexia
- arthralgia
- night sweats
- intermittent fever (may recur for weeks)

Effects of endocarditis

This illustration shows vegetative growths on the endocardium produced by fibrin and platelet deposits on infection sites.

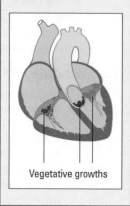

Vegetative growths

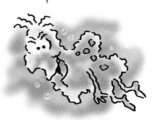

We bacteria like to gather on valve tissue with our fungi friends. Nasty little buggers, aren't we?

• loud, regurgitant murmur that is typical of the underlying rheumatic or congenital heart disease
• murmur that changes or appears suddenly, accompanied by fever.

Lots of spots

Other indications of endocarditis include:
• petechiae on the skin (especially common on the upper anterior trunk); the buccal, pharyngeal, or conjunctival mucosa; and the nails (splinter hemorrhages)
• Osler's nodes (small nodules on the fingers or toes)
• Roth's spots (white spots surrounded by hemorrhage on the retina)
• Janeway lesions (irregular, red lesions on the hands; rare).

When veggies are bad for you

In subacute endocarditis, embolization from vegetating lesions or diseased valve tissue can cause several kinds of problems:
• Splenic infarction causes pain in the left upper quadrant that radiates to the left shoulder as well as abdominal rigidity.
• Renal infarction results in hematuria, pyuria, flank pain, and decreased urine output.
• Cerebral infarction causes hemiparesis, aphasia, and other neurologic deficits.
• Pulmonary infarction — which occurs most commonly in right-sided endocarditis and is common among I.V. drug abusers and after cardiac surgery— can cause cough, pleuritic pain, pleural friction rub, dyspnea, and hemoptysis.
• Peripheral vascular occlusion results in numbness and tingling in an arm, leg, finger, or toe or impending peripheral gangrene.

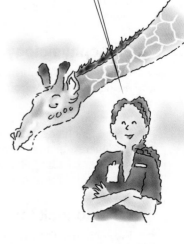

Certain types of spots can indicate endocarditis — but no, I don't think those spots on your neck mean anything!

What tests tell you

• Three or more blood cultures, with samples drawn at least 1 hour apart during a 24-hour period, identify the causative organism in up to 90% of patients. The remaining 10% may have negative blood cultures, possibly suggesting fungal infection.
• Echocardiography, including transesophageal echocardiography, may identify vegetations and valvular damage.
• ECG readings may show atrial fibrillation and other arrhythmias that accompany valvular disease.
• Laboratory abnormalities include elevated white blood cell (WBC) count; abnormal histocytes (macrophages); elevated erythrocyte sedimentation rate (ESR); normocytic, normochromic

anemia (in subacute bacterial endocarditis); and rheumatoid factor (occurs in about half of all patients).

How it's treated

Treatment seeks to eradicate the infecting organism. It should start promptly and continue over several weeks.

Germ warfare

The practitioner bases antibiotic selection on sensitivity studies of the infecting organism — or the probable organism, if blood cultures are negative. I.V. antibiotic therapy usually lasts 4 to 6 weeks and may be followed by oral antibiotics.

Supportive treatment includes bed rest, antipyretics for fever and aches, and sufficient fluid intake. Severe valvular damage, especially aortic insufficiency, or infection of a cardiac prosthesis may require corrective surgery if refractory heart failure develops.

What to do

• Obtain a patient history of allergies.
• Administer antibiotics on time to maintain consistent blood levels. Check dilutions for compatibility with other patient medications, and use a compatible solution (for example, add methicillin to a buffered solution).
• Evaluate the patient. The patient has recovered from endocarditis if he maintains a normal temperature, clear lungs, stable vital signs, and adequate tissue perfusion and is able to tolerate activity for a reasonable period and maintain normal weight.
(See *Endocarditis teaching tips.*)

Heart failure

When the myocardium can't pump effectively enough to meet the body's metabolic needs, heart failure occurs. Pump failure usually occurs in a damaged left ventricle but may also happen in the right ventricle. Usually, left-sided heart failure develops first. Heart failure is classified as:
• acute or chronic
• left-sided or right-sided (see *Understanding left- and right-sided heart failure,* pages 302 and 303)
• systolic or diastolic. (See *Classifying heart failure,* page 305.)

Quality time

Symptoms of heart failure may restrict a person's ability to perform ADLs and severely affect quality of life. Advances in diagnostic and therapeutic techniques have greatly improved outcomes

Education edge

Endocarditis teaching tips

• Teach the patient about the anti-infective medication that he'll continue to take. Stress the importance of taking the medication and restricting activity for as long as recommended.
• Tell the patient to watch for and report signs of embolization and to watch closely for fever, anorexia, and other signs of relapse that could occur about 2 weeks after treatment stops.
• Discuss the importance of completing the full course of antibiotics, even if he's feeling better. Make sure susceptible patients understand the need for prophylactic antibiotics before, during, and after dental work, childbirth, and genitourinary, GI, or gynecologic procedures.

A closer look

Understanding left- and right-sided heart failure

These illustrations show how myocardial damage leads to heart failure.

Left-sided heart failure

Increased workload and end-diastolic volume enlarge the left ventricle (see illustration below). Because of lack of oxygen, the ventricle enlarges with stretched tissue rather than functional tissue. The patient may experience increased heart rate, pale and cool skin, tingling in the extremities, decreased cardiac output, and arrhythmias.

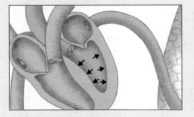

Diminished left ventricular function allows blood to pool in the ventricle and the atrium and eventually back up into the pulmonary veins and capillaries, as shown below. At this stage, the patient may experience dyspnea on exertion, confusion, dizziness, orthostatic hypotension, decreased peripheral pulses and pulse pressure, cyanosis, and an S_3 gallop.

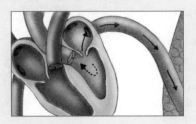

As the pulmonary circulation becomes engorged, rising capillary pressure pushes sodium (Na) and water (H_2O) into the interstitial space (as shown below), causing pulmonary edema. You'll note coughing, subclavian retractions, crackles, tachypnea, elevated pulmonary artery pressure, diminished pulmonary compliance, and increased partial pressure of carbon dioxide.

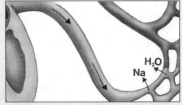

When the patient lies down, fluid in the extremities moves into the systemic circulation. Because the left ventricle can't handle the increased venous return, fluid pools in the pulmonary circulation, worsening pulmonary edema. You may note decreased breath sounds, dullness on percussion, crackles, and orthopnea.

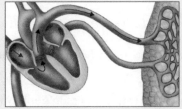

The right ventricle may now become stressed because it's pumping against greater pulmonary vascular resistance and left ventricular pressure (see illustration below). When this occurs, the patient's symptoms worsen.

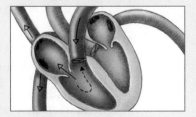

Right-sided heart failure

The stressed right ventricle enlarges with the formation of stretched tissue (see illustration below). Increasing conduction time and deviation of the heart from its normal axis can cause arrhythmias. If the patient doesn't already have left-sided heart failure, he may experience increased heart rate, cool skin, cyanosis, decreased cardiac output, palpitations, and dyspnea.

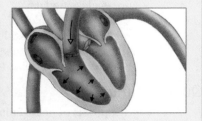

Understanding left- and right-sided heart failure (continued)

Blood pools in the right ventricle and right atrium. The backed-up blood causes pressure and congestion in the vena cava and systemic circulation (see illustration below). The patient will have elevated central venous pressure, jugular vein distention, and hepatojugular reflux.

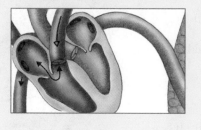

Backed-up blood also distends the visceral veins, especially the hepatic vein. As the liver and spleen become engorged (see illustration below), their function is impaired. The patient may develop anorexia, nausea, abdominal pain, palpable liver and spleen, weakness, and dyspnea secondary to abdominal distention.

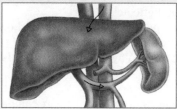

Rising capillary pressure forces excess fluid from the capillaries into the interstitial space (see illustration below). This causes tissue edema, especially in the lower extremities and abdomen. The patient may experience weight gain, pitting edema, and nocturia.

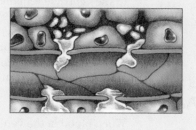

for these patients. However, prognosis still depends on the underlying cause and its response to treatment.

What causes it

Cardiovascular disorders that lead to heart failure include:
- atherosclerotic heart disease
- MI
- hypertension
- rheumatic heart disease
- congenital heart disease
- ischemic heart disease
- cardiomyopathy
- valvular diseases
- arrhythmias.
    Noncardiovascular causes of heart failure include:
- pregnancy and childbirth
- increased environmental temperature or humidity
- severe physical or mental stress
- thyrotoxicosis

- acute blood loss
- pulmonary embolism
- severe infection
- chronic obstructive pulmonary disease.

Pathophysiology

The patient's underlying condition determines whether heart failure is acute or chronic. Heart failure is commonly associated with systolic or diastolic overloading and myocardial weakness. As stress on the heart muscle reaches a critical level, the muscle's contractility is reduced and cardiac output declines. Venous input to the ventricle remains the same, however.

The body's responses to decreased cardiac output include:
- reflex increase in sympathetic activity
- release of renin from the juxtaglomerular cells of the kidney
- anaerobic metabolism by affected cells
- increased extraction of oxygen by the peripheral cells.

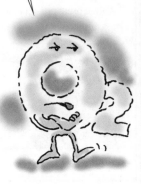

The body responds to decreased cardiac output by increasing oxygen extraction by the peripheral cells. You'd think I'd at least get overtime...

Adept at adaptation

When blood in the ventricles increases, the heart compensates, or adapts. Compensation may occur for long periods before signs and symptoms develop. Adaptations may be short- or long-term. In short-term adaptations, the end-diastolic fiber length increases, causing the ventricular muscle to respond by dilating and increasing the force of contractions. (This is called the *Frank-Starling curve*.) In long-term adaptations, ventricular hypertrophy increases the heart muscle's ability to contract and push its volume of blood into the circulation.

What to look for

Clinical signs of left-sided heart failure include:
- dyspnea, initially upon exertion
- paroxysmal nocturnal dyspnea
- Cheyne-Stokes respirations
- cough
- orthopnea
- tachycardia
- fatigue
- muscle weakness
- edema and weight gain
- irritability
- restlessness

Classifying heart failure

Heart failure is classified according to its pathophysiology. It may be left- or right-sided, systolic or diastolic, and acute or chronic.

Left-sided or right-sided

Left-sided heart failure stems from ineffective left ventricular contraction, which may in turn lead to pulmonary congestion or pulmonary edema and decreased cardiac output. Common causes of left-sided heart failure include left ventricular myocardial infarction, hypertension, and aortic and mitral valve stenosis or regurgitation. As the decreased pumping ability of the left ventricle persists, fluid accumulates, backing up into the left atrium and then into the lungs. If this worsens, pulmonary edema and right-sided heart failure may also result.

Right-sided heart failure is the result of ineffective right ventricular contraction. It may be caused by an acute right ventricular infarction or pulmonary embolus. However, the most common cause is profound backward flow due to left-sided heart failure.

Systolic or diastolic

In systolic heart failure, the left ventricle can't pump enough blood out to the systemic circulation during systole and the ejection fraction falls. Consequently, blood backs up into the pulmonary circulation, pressure rises in the pulmonary venous system, and cardiac output falls.

In diastolic heart failure, the left ventricle can't relax and fill properly during diastole and the stroke volume falls. This results in the need for larger ventricular volumes to maintain cardiac output.

Acute or chronic

Acute refers to the timing of the onset of symptoms and whether compensatory mechanisms kick in. Typically, fluid status is normal or low, and sodium and water retention don't occur.

In chronic heart failure, the patient has had signs and symptoms for some time, compensatory mechanisms have taken effect, and fluid volume overload persists. Drugs, diet changes, and activity restrictions usually control signs and symptoms. Chronic failure is irreversible.

- shortened attention span
- ventricular gallop (heard over the apex)
- bibasilar crackles
- frothy, blood-tinged sputum.
    The patient with right-sided heart failure may develop:
- edema, initially dependent
- jugular vein distention
- hepatomegaly.

What tests tell you

- Blood tests may show elevated BUN and creatinine levels, elevated serum norepinephrine levels, and elevated transaminase and bilirubin levels if hepatic function is impaired.
- Elevated blood levels of B-type natriuretic peptide (BNP) may correctly identify heart failure in as many as 83% of patients. (See *BNP: A potent predictor*, page 306.)

Weighing the evidence

BNP: A potent predictor

It's already been shown that elevated levels of B-type natriuretic peptide (BNP) can predict sudden death in patients with heart failure. But is it the best mortality predictor?

To determine that, researchers compared BNP levels with four other established mortality predictors: peak oxygen consumption, blood urea nitrogen levels, systolic blood pressure, and pulmonary capillary wedge pressure. Analyzing the data from 1,215 congestive heart failure patients, they determined that BNP was the most robust predictor of mortality. They concluded that analyzing BNP levels could help determine the urgency and timing of cardiac transplantation.

Sachdeva, A., et al. (2010). Comparison of usefulness of each of five predictors of mortality and urgent transplantation in patients with advanced heart failure. *American Journal of Cardiology, 106*(6), 830–835.

- ECG reflects heart strain or ventricular enlargement (ischemia). It may also reveal atrial enlargement, tachycardia, and extrasystoles, suggesting heart failure.
- Chest X-ray shows increased pulmonary vascular markings, interstitial edema, or pleural effusion and cardiomegaly.
- MUGA scan shows a decreased ejection fraction in left-sided heart failure.
- Cardiac catheterization may show ventricular dilation, coronary artery occlusion, and valvular disorders (such as aortic stenosis) in both left- and right-sided heart failure.
- Echocardiography may show ventricular hypertrophy, decreased contractility, and valvular disorders in both left- and right-sided heart failure. Serial echocardiograms may help assess the patient's response to therapy.
- Cardiopulmonary exercise testing to evaluate the patient's ventricular performance during exercise may show decreased oxygen uptake.

How it's treated

Treatment for heart failure can be planned by using the New York Heart Association classification system and the patient's BNP level to determine his degree of heart failure. (See *Correlating the degree of heart failure with BNP level.*)

Correlating the degree of heart failure with BNP level

The higher a patient's level of B-type natriuretic peptide (BNP), the greater the degree of heart failure. In turn, the greater the degree of heart failure, the more the patient's ability to perform activities of daily living will be impaired. Use this chart to plan your nursing care.

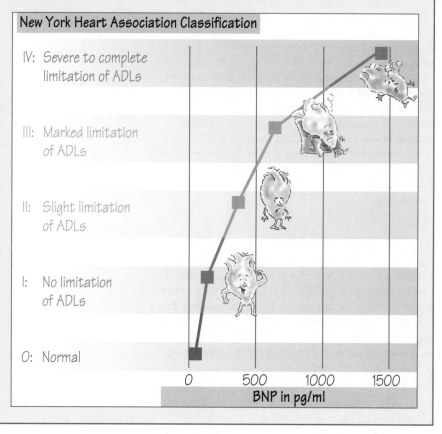

New York Heart Association Classification

IV: Severe to complete limitation of ADLs

III: Marked limitation of ADLs

II: Slight limitation of ADLs

I: No limitation of ADLs

0: Normal

0   500   1000   1500

BNP in pg/ml

Treatments include diuretics that reduce preload by decreasing total blood volume and circulatory congestion. ACE inhibitors dilate blood vessels and decrease systemic vascular resistance, reducing the heart's workload. The patient who can't tolerate ACE inhibitors can instead receive vasodilators. These increase cardiac output by reducing impedance to ventricular outflow, which decreases afterload.

Strengthening medicine

- Digoxin may help strengthen myocardial contractility. Beta-adrenergic blockers may prevent cardiac remodeling (left ventricular dilation and hypertrophy). Nesiritide (Natrecor), a human BNP, can augment diuresis and decrease afterload. Positive inotropic agents, such as I.V. dopamine or dobutamine, are reserved for those with end-stage heart failure or those awaiting heart transplantion.

Stop and go

The patient must alternate periods of rest with periods of activity and follow a sodium-restricted diet with smaller, more frequent meals. He may have to wear antiembolism stockings to prevent venostasis and possible thromboembolism formation. The practitioner may also order oxygen therapy.

Although controversial, surgery may be performed if the patient's heart failure doesn't improve after therapy and lifestyle modifications. If the patient with valve dysfunction has recurrent acute heart failure, he may undergo surgical valve replacement. A patient with heart failure caused by ischemia may undergo CABG, PTCA, or stenting.

Remodeling show

The Dor procedure, also called *partial left ventriculectomy* or *ventricular remodeling*, involves the removal of nonviable heart muscle to reduce the size of the hypertrophied ventricle, thereby allowing the heart to pump more efficiently. Patients with severe heart failure may benefit from a mechanical VAD or cardiac transplantation. A patient with life-threatening arrhythmias may have an internal cardioverter-defibrillator implanted. Insertion of a biventricular pacemaker can control ventricular dyssynchrony.

What to do

- Frequently monitor BUN, serum creatinine, potassium, sodium, chloride, and magnesium levels.
- Reinforce the importance of adhering to the prescribed diet. If fluid restrictions have been ordered, arrange a mutually acceptable schedule for allowable fluids.
- Weigh the patient daily to assess for fluid overload.
- To prevent deep vein thrombosis from vascular congestion, assist the patient with range-of-motion (ROM) exercises. Enforce bed rest, and apply antiembolism stockings. Watch for calf pain and tenderness and unilateral edema. Organize activities to provide periods of rest.

Education edge

Heart failure teaching tips

• Teach the patient about lifestyle changes. Advise him to avoid foods high in sodium to help curb fluid overload. Explain that he'll need to take the prescribed potassium supplement and eat high-potassium foods to replace the potassium lost through diuretic therapy. Stress the need for regular checkups and the benefits of balancing activity and rest.
• Stress the importance of taking cardiac glycosides exactly as prescribed. Tell him to watch for and report signs of toxicity.
• Tell him to notify the practitioner if his pulse is unusually irregular or less than 60 beats/minute; if he experiences signs and symptoms such as dizziness, blurred vision, shortness of breath, paroxysmal nocturnal dyspnea, swollen ankles, or decreased urine output; or if he gains 3 to 5 lb (1.5 to 2.5 kg) in 1 week.

• Evaluate the patient. Successful recovery should reveal clear lungs, normal heart sounds, adequate blood pressure, and absence of dyspnea or edema. The patient should be able to perform ADLs and maintain his normal weight. (See *Heart failure teaching tips.*)

Hypertension

Hypertension refers to an intermittent or sustained elevation in diastolic or systolic blood pressure. Essential (idiopathic) hypertension is the most common form. Secondary hypertension results from a number of disorders. Malignant hypertension is a severe, fulminant form of hypertension common to both types.

Hypertension represents a major cause of stroke, cardiac disease, and renal failure. Detecting and treating it before complications develop greatly improves the patient's prognosis. Severely elevated blood pressure may become fatal.

What causes it

Scientists haven't been able to identify a single cause for essential hypertension. The disorder probably reflects an interaction of multiple homeostatic forces, including changes in renal regulation of sodium and extracellular fluids, in aldosterone secretion and metabolism, and in norepinephrine secretion and metabolism.

Secondary hypertension may be caused by renal vascular disease, pheochromocytoma, primary hyperaldosteronism,

Cushing's syndrome, or dysfunction of the thyroid, pituitary, or parathyroid glands. It may also result from coarctation of the aorta, pregnancy, and neurologic disorders.

Certain risk factors appear to increase the likelihood of hypertension. These include:

- family history of hypertension
- race (more common in blacks)
- gender (more common in men)
- diabetes mellitus
- stress
- obesity
- high dietary intake of saturated fats or sodium
- tobacco use
- hormonal contraceptive use
- sedentary lifestyle
- aging.

> Men are at greater risk for hypertension than women.

Pathophysiology

Essential hypertension usually begins insidiously as a benign disease, slowly progressing to a malignant state. If left untreated, even mild cases can cause major complications and death.

Why? Why? Why?

Several theories help to explain the development of hypertension. It's thought to arise from:

- changes in the arteriolar bed that cause increased resistance
- abnormally increased tone in the sensory nervous system that originates in the vasomotor system centers, causing increased peripheral vascular resistance
- increased blood volume resulting from renal or hormonal dysfunction
- increased arteriolar thickening caused by genetic factors, leading to increased peripheral vascular resistance
- abnormal renin release, resulting in the formation of angiotensin II, which constricts the arterioles and increases blood volume. (See *Blood vessel damage*.)

The domino effect

The pathophysiology of secondary hypertension is related to the underlying disease. The most common cause is chronic renal disease. Insult to the kidney from chronic glomerulonephritis or renal artery stenosis can interfere with sodium excretion, the renin-angiotensin-aldosterone system, or renal perfusion. This in turn causes blood pressure to rise.

Other diseases can also underlie secondary hypertension. In Cushing's syndrome, increased cortisol levels raise blood pressure by increasing renal sodium retention, angiotensin II levels, and

> The most common cause of secondary hypertension is chronic renal disease. I don't feel so well...

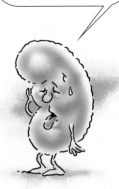

Blood vessel damage

Sustained hypertension damages blood vessels. Vascular injury begins with alternating areas of dilation and constriction in the arterioles. The illustrations below show how damage occurs.

Increased intra-arterial pressure damages the endothelium.

Angiotensin induces endothelial wall contraction, allowing plasma to leak through interendothelial spaces.

Plasma constituents deposited in the vessel wall cause medial necrosis.

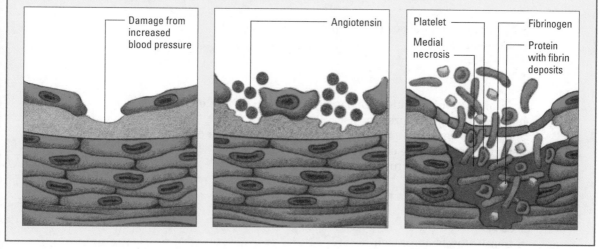

Damage from increased blood pressure

Angiotensin

Platelet

Fibrinogen

Medial necrosis

Protein with fibrin deposits

vascular response to norepinephrine. In primary aldosteronism, increased intravascular volume, altered sodium concentrations in vessel walls, or very high aldosterone levels cause vasoconstriction (increased resistance).

Pheochromocytoma is a secreting tumor of chromaffin cells, usually of the adrenal medulla. It causes hypertension by increasing epinephrine and norepinephrine secretion. Epinephrine functions mainly to increase cardiac contractility and rate; norepinephrine, mainly to increase peripheral vascular resistance.

What to look for

Signs and symptoms may include:
• blood pressure measurements of more than 140/90 mm Hg on two or more readings taken at two or more visits after an initial screening (see *Blood pressure classifications*, page 312.)

Blood pressure classifications

The degree of elevation of the readings determines blood pressure (BP) classifications. This table classifies BP according to systolic blood pressure (SBP) and diastolic blood pressure (DBP).

BP classification	Normal	Prehypertensive	Stage 1	Stage 2
SBP (mm Hg)	< 120	120 to 139	140 to 159	≥ 160
	and	or	or	or
DBP (mm Hg)	< 80	80 to 89	90 to 99	≥ 100

- throbbing occipital headaches upon waking
- drowsiness
- confusion
- vision problems
- nausea.

Expect a patient with secondary hypertension to have clinical manifestations of the primary disease. Other clinical effects don't appear until complications develop as a result of vascular changes in target organs. These effects include:
- left ventricular hypertrophy
- angina
- MI
- heart failure
- stroke
- transient ischemic attack
- nephropathy
- peripheral arterial disease
- retinopathy.

What tests tell you

- In urinalysis, protein, red blood cell (RBC), and WBC levels may indicate glomerulonephritis.
- Elevated blood glucose levels may indicate diabetes.
- Complete blood count may reveal anemia (causes a high output state resulting in hypertension) or polycythemia (increases the risk of hypertension and stroke).
- Lipid profile reveals elevated total cholesterol and low-density lipoprotein levels.
- Excretory urography shows renal atrophy, indicating chronic renal disease; one kidney more than 5/8" (1.5 cm) shorter than the other suggests unilateral renal disease.

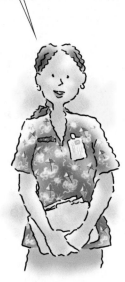

Elevated blood glucose levels may indicate diabetes, a condition that predisposes the patient to vascular changes and hypertension.

- Serum potassium levels are less than 3.5 mEq/L, indicating adrenal dysfunction (primary hyperaldosteronism).
- BUN level is greater than 20 mg/dl and creatinine level is greater than 1.5 mg/dl, suggesting renal disease.

Other tests help detect cardiovascular damage and other complications:

- ECG may show left ventricular hypertrophy or ischemia.
- Echocardiography may show left ventricular hypertrophy.
- Chest X-ray may show cardiomegaly.

How it's treated

Treatment of secondary hypertension includes correcting the underlying cause and controlling hypertensive effects. Although essential hypertension has no cure, lifestyle modifications along with drug therapy can control it. Lifestyle modifications for all patients may include changing diet (including restricting sodium and saturated fat intake), learning relaxation techniques, exercising regularly, quitting smoking, and limiting alcohol use.

Drugs can drop the pressure

The need for drug therapy is determined by blood pressure and the presence of target organ damage or risk factors. Drug therapy for uncomplicated hypertension usually begins with a thiazide diuretic, an ACE inhibitor, or a beta-adrenergic blocker. Other antihypertensive drugs include angiotensin II receptor blockers, alpha-receptor blockers, direct arteriole dilators, and calcium channel blockers.

What to do

- If a patient enters the hospital with hypertension, find out if he was taking his prescribed medication. If not, help the patient to identify reasons for noncompliance. If the patient can't afford the medication, refer him to an appropriate social service agency. If he suffered severe adverse effects, he may need different medication.
- Routinely screen all patients for hypertension, especially those at high risk.
- Evaluate the patient. After successful treatment for hypertension, the patient will have a blood pressure under 140/90 mm Hg at rest, the ability to tolerate activity, and the absence of enlargement of the left ventricle (as revealed by ECG or chest X-ray). (See *Hypertension teaching tips*.)

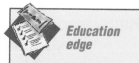

Education edge

Hypertension teaching tips

- Teach the patient to use a self-monitoring blood pressure cuff and to record readings at the same time of the day at least twice weekly to review with his primary health care provider.
- Warn the patient that uncontrolled hypertension may cause a stroke or myocardial infarction.
- To encourage compliance with antihypertensive therapy, suggest that the patient establish a daily routine for taking medication. Tell him to report drug adverse effects and to keep a record of the effectiveness of drugs. Advise him to avoid high-sodium antacids and over-the-counter cold and sinus medications, which contain harmful vasoconstrictors.
- Help the patient examine and modify his lifestyle, and encourage necessary diet changes.
- If the patient smokes, encourage quitting and refer him to a smoking-cessation program.

Hypertrophic cardiomyopathy

Hypertrophic cardiomyopathy is a primary disease of the cardiac muscle characterized by disproportionate, asymmetrical thickening of the interventricular septum, particularly in the anterior-superior part. It affects both diastolic and systolic function. As the septum hypertrophies, blood flow through the aortic valve becomes obstructed. Mitral insufficiency develops as the papillary muscles become affected. The course of illness varies; some patients demonstrate progressive deterioration. Others remain stable for several years. Sudden cardiac death may also occur.

What causes it

Almost all patients inherit hypertrophic cardiomyopathy as a non–sex-linked autosomal dominant trait.

Pathophysiology

In hypertrophic cardiomyopathy, hypertrophy of the left ventricle and interventricular septum obstruct left ventricular outflow. The heart compensates for the resulting decreased cardiac output by increasing the rate and force of contractions. The hypertrophied ventricle becomes stiff and unable to relax and fill during diastole. As left ventricular volume diminishes and filling pressure rises, pulmonary venous pressure also rises, leading to venous congestion and dyspnea.

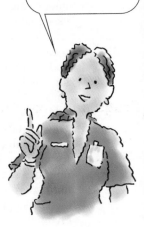

Hypertrophic cardiomyopathy is almost always a genetically inherited disorder.

What to look for

Clinical features of hypertrophic cardiomyopathy include:
- angina pectoris
- arrhythmias
- dyspnea
- syncope
- heart failure
- systolic ejection murmur (of medium pitch, heard along the left sternal border and at the apex)
- pulsus bisferiens
- irregular pulse (with atrial fibrillation).

What tests tell you

- Echocardiography shows increased thickness of the interventricular septum and abnormal motion of the anterior mitral leaflet during systole.
- Cardiac catheterization reveals elevated left ventricular end-diastolic pressure and possibly mitral insufficiency.

- ECG may demonstrate left ventricular hypertrophy, ST-segment and T-wave abnormalities, deep waves (from hypertrophy, not infarction), left anterior hemiblock, ventricular arrhythmias and, possibly, atrial fibrillation.
- Phonocardiography confirms an early systolic murmur.

How it's treated

Treatment seeks to relax the ventricle and to relieve outflow tract obstruction. Propranolol (Inderal), a beta-adrenergic blocker, slows heart rate and increases ventricular filling by relaxing the obstructing muscle, thereby reducing angina, syncope, dyspnea, and arrhythmias. However, propranolol may aggravate symptoms of cardiac decompensation. Calcium channel blockers may be prescribed to relax the heart muscle and improve ventricular filling. Antiarrhythmic drugs may be prescribed to treat arrhythmias. Atrial fibrillation calls for cardioversion to treat the arrhythmia and, because of the high risk of systemic embolism, anticoagulant therapy until fibrillation subsides.

When drugs don't do it

If drug therapy fails, the patient may undergo surgery. Septal myectomy (resection of the hypertrophied septum) alone or combined with mitral valve replacement may ease outflow tract obstruction and relieve symptoms. However, this is an experimental procedure and can cause complications, such as complete heart block and ventricular septal defect. Dual-chamber pacing can prevent progression of hypertrophy and obstruction. Implantable defibrillators may be used in patients with ventricular arrhythmias.

What to do

- Administer medication as ordered. Warn the patient not to stop taking propranolol abruptly because doing so may cause rebound effects, resulting in MI or sudden death. Before surgery, administer prophylaxis for subacute bacterial endocarditis; tell the patient he'll also need prophylactic antibiotics before dental work.
- Provide psychological support. Refer the patient for psychosocial counseling to help him and his family accept his restricted lifestyle and cope with his poor prognosis. Urge parents of a school-age child to arrange for continuation of studies in the hospital.
- Evaluate the patient. If treatment proves successful, the patient will show adequate tissue perfusion, clear lungs, and absence of edema and syncopal episodes. He'll be able to maintain his weight, tolerate activity, and maintain adequate blood pressure. (See *Hypertrophic cardiomyopathy teaching tips.*)

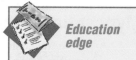

Education edge

Hypertrophic cardiomyopathy teaching tips

- Instruct the patient to take his medication as ordered.
- Warn the patient against strenuous physical activity such as running. Syncope or sudden death may follow well-tolerated exercise. Advise him to avoid Valsalva's maneuver or sudden position changes; both may worsen obstruction.
- Inform the patient that before dental work or surgery he needs a prophylactic antibiotic to prevent bacterial endocarditis.
- Because the patient is at risk for sudden cardiac arrest, urge his family to learn cardiopulmonary resuscitation.

Myocardial infarction

An occlusion of a coronary artery, MI leads to oxygen deprivation, myocardial ischemia, and eventual necrosis. It's one component of acute coronary syndrome. (See *Understanding MI*, pages 317 and 318.)

The extent of functional impairment and the patient's prognosis depend on the size and location of the infarct, the condition of the uninvolved myocardium, the potential for collateral circulation, and the effectiveness of compensatory mechanisms. In the United States, MI is the leading cause of death in adults.

What causes it

MI can arise from any condition in which the myocardial oxygen supply can't keep pace with demand, including:
- CAD
- coronary artery emboli
- thrombus
- coronary artery spasm
- severe hematologic and coagulation disorders
- myocardial contusion
- congenital coronary artery anomalies.

Certain risk factors increase a patient's vulnerability to MI. These factors include family history of MI, gender (men are more susceptible), hypertension, smoking, diabetes mellitus, obesity, sedentary lifestyle, aging, stress, menopause, elevated serum triglyceride, cholesterol, and low-density lipoprotein (LDL) levels.

Pathophysiology

MI results from prolonged ischemia to the myocardium with irreversible cell damage and muscle death. Functionally, MI causes:
- reduced contractility with abnormal wall motion
- altered left ventricular compliance
- reduced stroke volume
- reduced ejection fraction
- elevated left ventricular end-diastolic pressure.

What to look for

The patient experiences severe, persistent chest pain that's unrelieved by rest or nitroglycerin. He may describe the pain as crushing or squeezing. Usually substernal, pain may radiate to the left arm, jaw, neck, or shoulder blades. Other signs and symptoms include a feeling of impending doom, fatigue, nausea and vomiting, shortness of breath, cool extremities, perspiration, anxiety, hypotension or hypertension, palpable precordial pulse and, possibly, muffled heart sounds.

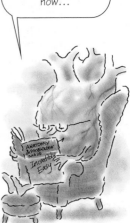

Says here that a sedentary lifestyle is one of the risk factors for MI. Maybe I should get up now...

A closer look

Understanding MI

In myocardial infarction (MI), blood supply to the myocardium is interrupted. Here's what happens.

Injury to the endothelial lining of the coronary arteries causes platelets, white blood cells, fibrin, and lipids to gather at the injured site, as shown below. Foam cells, or resident macrophages, gather beneath the damaged lining and absorb oxidized cholesterol, forming a fatty streak that narrows the arterial lumen.

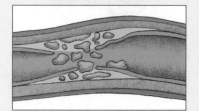

As the arterial lumen narrows gradually, collateral circulation develops, which helps to maintain myocardial perfusion distal to the obstructed vessel lumen. The illustration below shows collateral circulation.

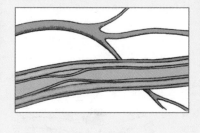

When myocardial demand for oxygen is more than the collateral circulation can supply, myocardial metabolism shifts from aerobic to anaerobic, producing lactic acid (A), which stimulates nerve endings, as shown below.

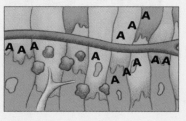

Lacking oxygen, the myocardial cells die. This decreases contractility, stroke volume, and blood pressure.

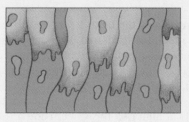

Hypotension stimulates baroreceptors, which in turn stimulate the adrenal glands to release epinephrine and norepinephrine. This cycle is shown below. These catecholamines increase heart rate and cause peripheral vasoconstriction, further increasing myocardial oxygen demand.

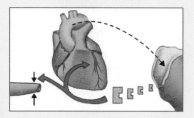

Damaged cell membranes in the infarcted area allow intracellular contents into the vascular circulation, as shown below. Ventricular arrhythmias then develop with elevated serum levels of potassium, creatine kinase (CK), CK-MB, aspartate aminotransferase, and lactate dehydrogenase.

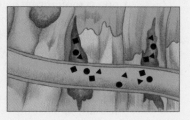

(continued)

Understanding MI (continued)

 All myocardial cells are capable of spontaneous depolarization and repolarization, so the electrical conduction system may be affected by infarct, injury, or ischemia. The illustration below shows an injury site.

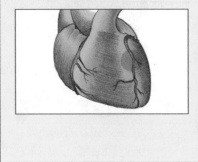

Extensive damage to the left ventricle may impair its ability to pump, allowing blood to back up into the left atrium and, eventually, into the pulmonary veins and capillaries, as shown in the illustration below. Crackles may be heard in the lungs on auscultation. Pulmonary artery wedge pressure is increased.

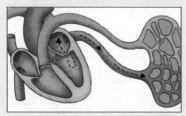

As back pressure rises, fluid crosses the alveolar-capillary membrane, impeding diffusion of oxygen (O_2) and carbon dioxide (CO_2). Arterial blood gas measurements may show decreased partial pressure of arterial oxygen and arterial pH and increased partial pressure of arterial carbon dioxide.

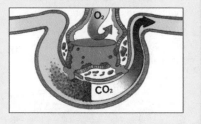

What tests tell you

• Serial 12-lead ECG may show no abnormalities or may prove inconclusive during the first few hours after MI. When present, characteristic abnormalities on the ECG can help pinpoint the location of the MI.
• ST-segment monitoring tracks the heart's response to MI. Continuous monitoring can immediately detect ischemic episodes. During an MI, monitoring can help differentiate between an ST-segment elevated MI (STEMI) and a non ST-segment elevated MI (NSTEMI); differentiating between a STEMI and NSTEMI helps the practitioner better guide treatment. ST-segment monitoring can also identify patients at high risk for reocclusion after PTCA or MI and permits prompt intervention if reocclusion occurs. After MI, monitoring may reduce or eliminate the need for angiography in patients receiving thrombolytic drugs by gauging the efficacy of the drugs.
• Serial serum cardiac marker measurements show elevated CK, especially the CK-MB isoenzyme (the cardiac muscle fraction of CK), troponin I and T, and myoglobin.
• Echocardiography shows ventricular wall dyskinesia (with transmural MI).

Characteristic abnormalities on the ECG can help pinpoint the location of an MI.

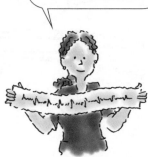

Thrombolytic drug precautions

Although you'll rarely see thrombolytic drugs given on a medical-surgical unit, you should still know and understand their contraindications and precautions.

Contraindications

Thrombolytic drugs are contraindicated in patients:
- with active internal bleeding
- with intracranial neoplasm
- with arteriovenous malformation
- with aneurysm
- with severe uncontrolled hypertension
- with a history of recent stroke (within the past 2 months)
- with subarachnoid hemorrhage
- with known bleeding diathesis
- who have experienced intraspinal or intracranial trauma
- who have undergone surgery within the past 2 months
- who are pregnant.

Precautions

Thrombolytic drugs should be used cautiously in patients who:
- have undergone major surgery within the past 10 days
- have undergone organ biopsy
- have experienced traumatic injury (including cardiopulmonary resuscitation)
- have GI or genitourinary bleeding
- have cerebrovascular disease
- are hypertensive
- have mitral stenosis, atrial fibrillation, or another condition that may lead to left-sided heart thrombus
- have acute pericarditis or subacute bacterial endocarditis
- have septic thrombophlebitis
- have diabetic hemorrhagic retinopathy
- are receiving anticoagulants
- are 10 days or fewer postpartum
- are lactating.

How it's treated

Primary treatment for MI seeks to relieve pain, stabilize heart rhythm, revascularize the coronary artery, preserve myocardial tissue, and reduce cardiac workload. These treatments include thrombolytic therapy and PTCA.

Thrombolytic thrill

To preserve myocardial tissue, thrombolytic therapy should start within 3 hours of the onset of symptoms. This therapy involves administrating medications such as alteplase (Activase) or reteplase (Retavase). However, because of the nature of thrombolytic drugs, they carry many precautions and contraindications. (See *Thrombolytic drug precautions*.)

PTCA, please!

PTCA is another option for opening blocked or narrowed arteries. If PTCA is performed soon after the onset of symptoms, the thrombolytic agent can be administered directly into the coronary artery.

Other options

Other treatments include:
- delivering oxygen to increase oxygenation of the blood
- administering sublingual or I.V. nitroglycerin to relieve chest pain, unless systolic blood pressure is less than 90 mm Hg or heart rate is less than 50 or greater than 100 beats/minute
- administering morphine for analgesia (because pain stimulates the sympathetic nervous system, leading to an increase in heart rate and vasoconstriction)
- administering aspirin to inhibit platelet aggregation
- administering I.V. heparin for patients who have received tissue plasminogen activator to increase the chances of patency in the affected coronary artery
- limiting physical activity for the first 12 hours to reduce cardiac workload, which should limit the area of necrosis
- administering atropine or lidocaine as appropriate
- administering I.V. nitroglycerin for 24 to 48 hours in patients without hypotension, bradycardia, or excessive tachycardia to reduce afterload and preload and relieve chest pain
- administering glycoprotein IIb/IIIa inhibitors to patients with continued unstable angina, acute chest pain, or following invasive cardiac procedures, to reduce platelet aggregation
- providing an early I.V. beta-adrenergic blocker to patients with evolving acute MI, followed by oral therapy (if no contraindications exist) to reduce heart rate and myocardial contractile force, which should reduce myocardial oxygen requirements
- administering an ACE inhibitor to those with evolving MI with ST-segment elevation or left bundle-branch block but without hypotension or other contraindications to reduce afterload and preload and prevent remodeling
- performing laser angioplasty, atherectomy, stent placement, or transmyocardial revascularization
- administering lipid-lowering drugs to patients with elevated LDL and cholesterol levels
- transcutaneous or transvenous pacing
- emergency interventions for cardiac arrest.

What to do

- When caring for the post-MI patient, direct your efforts toward detecting complications, preventing further myocardial damage, and promoting comfort, rest, and emotional well-being. Many patients with MI receive treatment in the ICU, under constant observation for complications.

• Monitor and record ECG readings, blood pressure, temperature, and heart and breath sounds.

• Assess pain and administer analgesics, as ordered. Always record the severity and duration of pain. Don't give I.M. injections because absorption from the muscle is unpredictable. Also, muscle damage increases CK, myoglobin, and LD levels, making diagnosis of MI more difficult.

• Check the patient's blood pressure after giving nitroglycerin, especially the first dose.

• Frequently monitor the ECG to detect rate changes or arrhythmias.

• During episodes of chest pain, obtain ECG, blood pressure, and pulmonary artery catheter measurements to determine changes.

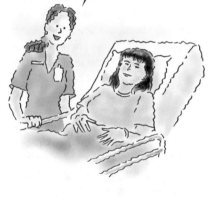

Promoting comfort, rest, and emotional well-being is an important nursing objective when caring for MI patients.

• Watch for signs and symptoms of fluid retention (crackles, cough, tachypnea, and edema), which may indicate impending heart failure. Carefully monitor daily weight, intake and output, respirations, serum enzyme levels, and blood pressure. Auscultate for adventitious breath sounds periodically (patients on bed rest commonly have atelectatic crackles) and for S_3 or S_4 gallops.

Do not disturb

• Organize patient care and activities to maximize periods of uninterrupted rest.

• Ask the dietary department to provide a clear liquid diet until nausea subsides. A low-cholesterol, low-sodium diet may be ordered.

• Provide a stool softener to prevent straining, which causes vagal stimulation and may slow heart rate. Allow the patient to use a bedside commode, and provide as much privacy as possible.

• Administer a histamine$_2$ receptor blocker to help prevent stress ulcers from forming.

• Assist with ROM exercises and ambulation as allowed. If the patient is completely immobilized by a severe MI, turn him often. Antiembolism stockings help prevent venostasis and thrombophlebitis in patients on prolonged bed rest.

• Provide emotional support, and help reduce stress and anxiety; administer tranquilizers, as needed. Involve his family as much as possible in his care.

• Evaluate the patient. When assessing treatment outcomes, look for clear breath sounds; normal heart sounds and blood pressure; absence of arrhythmias, chest pain, shortness of breath, fatigue, and edema; and evidence of ability to tolerate exercise. The patient

Education edge

MI teaching tips

- Explain procedures and answer questions.
- Carefully prepare the patient with a myocardial infarction (MI) for discharge. To promote compliance with the prescribed medication regimen and other treatment measures, thoroughly explain dosages and therapy. Warn about drug adverse effects, and advise the patient to watch for and report signs of toxicity. If the patient has a Holter monitor in place, explain its purpose and use.
- Counsel the patient about lifestyle changes. Review dietary restrictions. If the patient must follow a low-sodium or low-fat and low-cholesterol diet, provide a list of undesirable foods. Ask the dietitian to speak to the patient and his family.
- Advise the patient to resume sexual activity progressively, usually after 2 to 4 weeks.

- If appropriate, stress the need to stop smoking and refer the patient to a smoking-cessation program.
- Advise the patient to control hypertension, strive for ideal body weight and, if necessary, manage blood glucose levels.
- Help the patient learn about support groups and community resources. Refer him to the American Heart Association for further information and support.
- Recommend his participation in a cardiac rehabilitation program for exercise, education, symptom management, and support with risk modification.
- Instruct the patient to report chest pain. Postinfarction syndrome may develop, producing chest pain that must be differentiated from recurrent MI, pulmonary infarct, or heart failure.

should also have adequate cardiac output, as shown by a normal LOC; warm, dry skin; and no dizziness. (See *MI teaching tips*.)

Myocarditis

Myocarditis, a focal or diffuse inflammation of the cardiac muscle (myocardium), may be acute or chronic and can strike at any age. In many cases, myocarditis fails to produce specific cardiovascular symptoms or ECG abnormalities. The patient will commonly experience spontaneous recovery without residual effects. Occasionally, myocarditis is complicated by heart failure and, rarely, leads to cardiomyopathy.

> The myocarditis patient commonly experiences spontaneous recovery without residual effects.

> That's such good news! It makes me feel like dancing.

What causes it

Potential causes of myocarditis include:
• viral infections (most common cause in the United States), such as coxsackievirus A and B strains and, possibly, poliomyelitis, influenza, rubeola, rubella, adenoviruses, and echoviruses
• bacterial infections, such as diphtheria, tuberculosis, typhoid fever, tetanus, and staphylococcal, pneumococcal, and gonococcal infections
• hypersensitivity reactions, such as acute rheumatic fever and postcardiotomy syndrome
• radiation therapy to the chest in treating lung or breast cancer
• chronic alcoholism
• parasitic infections, such as toxoplasmosis and, especially, South American trypanosomiasis (Chagas' disease) in infants and immunosuppressed adults
• helminthic infections such as trichinosis.

Pathophysiology

Damage to the myocardium occurs when an infectious organism triggers an autoimmune, cellular, or humoral reaction; toxic inflammation can also result from a noninfectious cause. In either case, inflammation may lead to hypertrophy, fibrosis, and inflammatory changes of the myocardium and conduction system.

Feeling flabby

The heart muscle weakens and contractility is reduced. The heart muscle becomes flabby and dilated and pinpoint hemorrhages may develop.

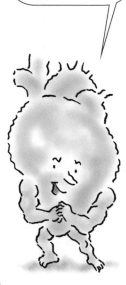

Who are you calling flabby?! I may have let myself go a little, but I'm still in pretty good shape.

What to look for

Signs and symptoms of myocarditis may include:
• fatigue
• dyspnea
• palpitations
• fever
• mild, continuous pressure or soreness in the chest
• signs and symptoms of heart failure (with advanced disease).

What tests tell you

• Laboratory tests may reveal elevated cardiac enzymes, such as CK and CK-MB, an increased WBC count and ESR, and elevated antibody titers (such as antistreptolysin-O titer in rheumatic fever).

- ECG changes provide the most reliable diagnostic aid. Typically, the ECG shows diffuse ST-segment and T-wave abnormalities, such as those that occur with pericarditis, conduction defects (prolonged PR interval), and other supraventricular ectopic arrhythmias.
- Stool and throat cultures may identify bacteria.
- Endomyocardial biopsy provides a definitive diagnosis.

How it's treated

Treatment includes antibiotics for bacterial infection, modified bed rest to decrease heart workload, and careful management of complications. Thromboembolism requires anticoagulant therapy. Inotropic drugs, such as dobutamine or dopamine, may be necessary. Some patients may require nitroprusside and nitroglycerin for afterload reduction. Treatment with immunosuppressive drugs is controversial but may help after the acute inflammation has passed. Patients with low cardiac output may benefit from intra-aortic balloon pulsation and left VADs. Patients will only receive heart transplantation as a last resort.

What to do

- Assess cardiovascular status frequently, watching for signs of heart failure, such as dyspnea, hypotension, and tachycardia.
- Assist the patient with bathing as necessary. Provide a bedside commode because this stresses the heart less than using a bedpan.
- Evaluate the patient. After successful treatment, the patient should have adequate cardiac output as evidenced by normal blood pressure, warm and dry skin, normal LOC, and no dizziness. He should be able to tolerate a normal level of activity. His temperature should be normal, and he shouldn't be dyspneic. (See *Myocarditis teaching tips*.)

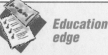

Pericarditis

Pericarditis is an acute or chronic inflammation that affects the pericardium, the fibroserous sac that envelops, supports, and protects the heart. Acute pericarditis can be fibrinous or effusive, with purulent serous or hemorrhagic exudate. Chronic constrictive pericarditis characteristically leads to dense fibrous pericardial thickening. Because pericarditis commonly coexists with other conditions, diagnosis of acute pericarditis depends on typical clinical features and the elimination of other possible causes. Prognosis depends on the underlying cause. Most patients recover from acute pericarditis, unless constriction occurs.

What causes it

Pericarditis may result from:
- bacterial, fungal, or viral infection (infectious pericarditis)
- neoplasms (primary or metastatic from lungs, breasts, or other organs)
- high-dose radiation to the chest
- uremia

Don't be so sensitive!

- hypersensitivity or autoimmune diseases, such as rheumatic fever (the most common cause of pericarditis in children), systemic lupus erythematosus, and rheumatoid arthritis
- postcardiac injury, such as MI (which later causes an autoimmune reaction [Dressler's syndrome] in the pericardium), trauma, and surgery that leaves the pericardium intact but causes blood to leak into the pericardial cavity
- neoplastic disease
- idiopathic factors (most common in acute pericarditis)
- less commonly, aortic aneurysm with pericardial leakage, and myxedema with cholesterol deposits in the pericardium.

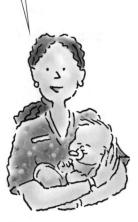

Rheumatic fever is the most common cause of pericarditis in children.

Pathophysiology

As the pericardium becomes inflamed, it may become thickened and fibrotic. If it doesn't heal completely after an acute episode, it may calcify over a long period and form a firm scar around the heart. This scarring interferes with diastolic filling of the ventricles.

What to look for

Pericarditis causes a sharp, sudden pain that usually starts over the sternum and radiates to the neck, shoulders, back, and arms. Unlike the pain of MI, pericardial pain is usually pleuritic, increasing with deep inspiration and decreasing when the patient sits up and leans forward.

One of the classics

A classic sign, pericardial friction rub is a grating sound that occurs as the heart moves. You will usually hear the friction rub best during forced expiration while the patient leans forward or is on his hands and knees in bed. Occasionally, you'll hear the friction rub only briefly or not at all. Pericarditis also causes signs similar to those of chronic right-sided heart failure, such as fluid retention, ascites, and hepatomegaly (with chronic constrictive pericarditis).

What tests tell you

• Laboratory results don't establish a diagnosis. Instead,they indicate the presence of inflammation and may help identify its cause. They may include normal or elevated WBC count (especially in infectious pericarditis), an elevated ESR, and slightly elevated cardiac enzymes (with associated myocarditis).
• A culture of pericardial fluid obtained by open surgical drainage or cardiocentesis sometimes identifies a causative organism in bacterial or fungal pericarditis.
• Echocardiography may establish the diagnosis of pericardial effusion by revealing an echo-free space between the ventricular wall and the pericardium.
• Chest X-ray may show an enlarged cardiac silhouette (with large effusion).

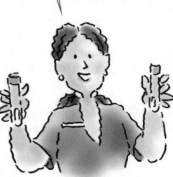

Although lab results don't establish a diagnosis of pericarditis, they can indicate inflammation and help identify a cause.

Get the rhythm

ECG changes in acute pericarditis may include:
• elevated ST segments in the standard limb leads and most precordial leads without the significant changes in QRS morphology that occur with MI
• atrial ectopic rhythms such as atrial fibrillation
• diminished QRS voltage (in pericardial effusion).

How it's treated

Treatment for pericarditis seeks to relieve symptoms and manage underlying systemic disease. In acute idiopathic pericarditis, post-MI pericarditis, and postthoracotomy pericarditis, treatment consists of bed rest as long as fever and pain persist and nonsteroidal anti-inflammatory drugs, such as aspirin and indomethacin (Indocin), to relieve pain and reduce inflammation. If these drugs fail to relieve symptoms, expect to administer corticosteroids.

Infectious pericarditis that results from disease of the left pleural space, mediastinal abscesses, or septicemia requires antibiotics, surgical drainage, or both. If cardiac tamponade develops, the doctor may perform emergency pericardiocentesis. Signs of cardiac tamponade include pulsus paradoxus, jugular vein distention, dyspnea, and shock.

Open a window

Recurrent pericarditis may necessitate partial pericardiectomy, which creates a "window" that allows fluid to drain into the pleural space. In constrictive pericarditis, the surgeon may need to perform total pericardiectomy to permit adequate filling and contraction of the heart. Treatment must also include management of rheumatic fever, uremia, tuberculosis, and other underlying disorders.

What to do

- Encourage complete bed rest.
- Assess pain in relation to respiration and body position to distinguish pericardial pain from myocardial ischemic pain.
- Place the patient in an upright position to relieve dyspnea and chest pain.
- Provide analgesics and oxygen, as ordered.
- Reassure the patient with acute pericarditis that his condition is temporary and treatable.
- Monitor for signs of cardiac compression or cardiac tamponade, both possible complications of pericardial effusion. Signs include decreased blood pressure, increased central venous pressure, jugular vein distention, and pulsus paradoxus. Because cardiac tamponade requires immediate treatment, keep a pericardiocentesis set at bedside whenever pericardial effusion is suspected.
- Evaluate the patient. Evidence of successful treatment includes normal temperature, absence of pain and shortness of breath, adequate blood pressure, and warm, dry skin. (See *Pericarditis teaching tips*.)

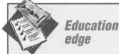

Education edge

Pericarditis teaching tips

- Explain tests and treatments to the patient.
- Instruct him to resume his daily activities slowly and to schedule rest periods into his daily routine.
- Show him how to position himself to relieve pain.

Raynaud's phenomenon

Primary Raynaud's phenomenon is one of several arteriospastic diseases characterized by episodic vasospasm in the small peripheral arteries and arterioles. It occurs bilaterally and usually affects the hands or, less commonly, the feet. Upon exposure to cold or stress, the patient experiences skin color changes (blanching, cyanosis, and rubor). He may develop pain, numbness, and throbbing after an attack, but his arterial pulses remain normal. Primary Raynaud's phenomenon is usually relatively mild and rarely leads to the development of other diseases.

What causes it

The cause of primary Raynaud's phenomenon is unknown. However, secondary Raynaud's phenomenon is a condition commonly associated with several connective tissue disorders, such as systemic sclerosis, SLE, and polymyositis, and has a progressive course, leading to ischemia, gangrene, and amputation. Distinction between the two disorders is difficult; some patients who experience mild symptoms of secondary Raynaud's phenomenon for several years may later develop overt connective tissue disease, such as systemic lupus erythematosus or scleroderma.

Pathophysiology

Raynaud's phenomenon is a syndrome of episodic constriction of the arterioles and arteries of the extremities, resulting in pallor and cyanosis of the fingers and toes. Several mechanisms may account for the reduced digital blood flow, including:
• intrinsic vascular wall hyperactivity to cold
• increased vasomotor tone due to sympathetic stimulation
• antigen-antibody immune response (most likely because abnormal immunologic test results accompany secondary Raynaud's phenomenon).

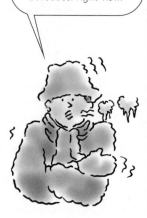

In Raynaud's phenomenon, exposure to cold or stress triggers skin blanching on the fingertips. I'm feeling both cold and stressed right now!

What to look for

After exposure to cold or stress, the patient will typically experience:
• blanching of the skin on the fingertips, which then becomes cyanotic before changing to red and from cold to normal temperature
• numbness and tingling of fingers
• sclerodactyly, ulcerations, or chronic paronychia (in long-standing disease).

What tests tell you

• Diagnosis requires that clinical symptoms last at least 2 years, after which the patient may undergo tests to rule out secondary disease processes, such as chronic arterial occlusive or connective tissue disease.
• Antinuclear antibody (ANA) titer may identify autoimmune disease as an underlying cause of Raynaud's phenomenon; more specific tests must be performed if ANA titer is positive.
• Erythrocyte sedimentation rate measures inflammation. It will be elevated in secondary Raynaud's phenomenon but not in the primary form.
• Doppler ultrasonography may show reduced blood flow if the patient also has an associated arterial occlusive disease.

How it's treated

Initially, the patient must avoid cold, safeguard against mechanical or chemical injury, and quit smoking. Drug therapy is usually reserved for patients with unusually severe symptoms.

Calcium channel blockers, such as nifedipine (Procardia), diltiazem (Cardizem), and nicardipine (Cardene), may be prescribed to produce vasodilation and prevent vasospasm. Adrenergic blockers, such as phenoxybenzamine or reserpine, may improve blood flow to fingers or toes.

What to do

• For a patient with a less advanced form of illness, provide reassurance that symptoms are benign. As the disorder progresses, try to allay the patient's fears about disfigurement.
• Evaluate the patient. The patient who responds well to treatment will have warm hands and feet. The skin of his hands and feet will retain its normal color. (See *Raynaud's phenomenon teaching tips.*)

Restrictive cardiomyopathy

Characterized by restricted ventricular filling and failure to contract completely during systole, restrictive cardiomyopathy is a rare disorder of the myocardial musculature that results in low cardiac output, and eventually endocardial fibrosis and thickening. If severe, it's irreversible.

What causes it

The cause of primary restrictive cardiomyopathy remains unknown. In amyloidosis, infiltration of amyloid into the intracellular spaces in the myocardium, endocardium, and subendocardium may lead to restrictive cardiomyopathy syndrome.

Pathophysiology

In restrictive cardiomyopathy, left ventricular hypertrophy and endocardial fibrosis limit myocardial contraction and emptying during systole as well as ventricular relaxation and filling during diastole. As a result, cardiac output falls.

What to look for

Restrictive cardiomyopathy produces:
• fatigue
• dyspnea
• orthopnea
• chest pain
• generalized edema
• liver engorgement
• peripheral cyanosis
• pallor
• S_3 or S_4 gallop rhythms.

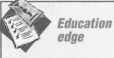

Education edge

Raynaud's phenomenon teaching tips

• Warn against exposure to the cold. Tell the patient to wear mittens or gloves in cold weather or when handling cold items.
• Advise the patient to avoid stressful situations and to stop smoking. Refer him to a smoking-cessation program, if needed.
• Encourage the patient to avoid decongestants and caffeine to reduce vasoconstriction.
• Instruct the patient to inspect his skin frequently and to seek immediate care for signs of skin breakdown or infection.
• Teach the patient about prescribed drugs, inlcuding their use and their adverse effects.

What tests tell you

• ECG may show low-voltage complexes, hypertrophy, or AV conduction defects. Arterial pulsation reveals blunt carotid upstroke with small volume.
• Chest X-ray shows massive cardiomegaly, affecting all four chambers of the heart (in advanced stages).
• Echocardiography rules out constrictive pericarditis as the cause of restricted filling by detecting increased left ventricular muscle mass and differences in end-diastolic pressures between the ventricles.
• Cardiac catheterization demonstrates increased left ventricular end-diastolic pressure and also rules out constrictive pericarditis as the cause of restricted filling.
• Endomyocardial biopsy may reveal amyloidosis.

How it's treated

Although no therapy currently exists for restricted ventricular filling, digoxin, diuretics, and a sodium-restricted diet can ease symptoms. Anticoagulant therapy may prevent thrombophlebitis in the patient on prolonged bed rest.

What to do

• In the acute phase, monitor heart rate and rhythm, blood pressure, and urine output.
• Be supportive and understanding, and encourage the patient to express his fears.
• Provide appropriate diversionary activities for the patient restricted to prolonged bed rest.
• If the patient needs additional help in coping with his restricted lifestyle, refer him for psychosocial counseling.
• Evaluate the patient. When assessing his response to therapy, look for adequate tissue perfusion, demonstrated by good color; warm, dry skin; and clear lungs. The patient should maintain his weight and level of activity. He should have adequate blood pressure and no dizziness or edema. (See *Restrictive cardiomyopathy teaching tips.*)

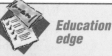

> *Education edge*
>
> ## Restrictive cardiomyopathy teaching tips
>
> • Teach the patient to watch for and report signs and symptoms of digoxin (Lanoxin) toxicity (anorexia, nausea, vomiting, yellow vision).
> • Advise the patient to record his weight daily and report weight gain of 2 lb (0.9 kg) in 1 day or 5 lb (2.3 kg) in 1 week.
> • If the patient must restrict sodium intake, tell him to avoid canned foods, pickles, smoked meats, and excessive use of table salt.

Thrombophlebitis

An acute condition characterized by inflammation and thrombus formation, thrombophlebitis may occur in deep (intermuscular or intramuscular) or superficial (subcutaneous) veins.

That's deep

Deep vein thrombophlebitis commonly begins in the small veins, such as the soleal venous sinuses or calf veins. Clots can also form or extend into the large veins, such as the vena cava and the femoral, iliac, and subclavian veins. Usually progressive, this disorder may lead to pulmonary embolism, a potentially fatal condition.

So superficial

Superficial thrombophlebitis is usually self-limiting and rarely leads to pulmonary embolism.

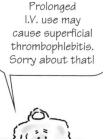

Prolonged I.V. use may cause superficial thrombophlebitis. Sorry about that!

What causes it

Although deep vein thrombophlebitis may be idiopathic, it usually results from endothelial damage, accelerated blood clotting, or reduced blood flow. Superficial thrombophlebitis may follow:
- trauma
- infection
- I.V. drug abuse
- chemical irritation caused by prolonged I.V. use
- coagulation problems.

Risk on the rise

Certain risk factors appear to increase the risk of developing deep vein or superficial thrombophlebitis. These include:
- immobility
- trauma
- childbirth
- use of hormonal contraceptives
- major abdominal surgery
- joint replacement.

Pathophysiology

Alteration in the epithelial lining causes platelet aggregation and fibrin entrapment of RBCs, WBCs, and additional platelets. The thrombus initiates a chemical inflammatory process in the vessel epithelium that leads to fibrosis, which may either occlude the vessel lumen or embolize.

What to look for

Clinical features vary with the site and length of the affected vein. Deep vein thrombophlebitis may produce:
- severe pain
- fever
- chills
- malaise

- nonpitting edema greater than 1" (2.5 cm) of the affected arm or leg
- possible warmth to the touch in the affected area
- positive Homans' sign (pain on dorsiflexion of the foot); false-positives are common.

Signs and symptoms of superficial thrombophlebitis occur along the length of the affected vein. They include:
- heat
- pain
- swelling
- redness
- tenderness
- induration
- lymphadenitis (with extensive vein involvement)
- palpable cord.

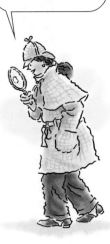

Thrombophlebitis causes filling defects and diverted blood flow that can be detected with phlebography...

What tests tell you

- Doppler ultrasonography identifies reduced blood flow to a specific area and any obstruction to venous flow, particularly in iliofemoral deep vein thrombophlebitis.
- CT angiography can help visualize the thrombus.
- Phlebography (also called venography), which is performed infrequently, shows filling defects and diverted blood flow.

How it's treated

Treatment aims to control thrombus development, prevent complications, relieve pain, and prevent recurrence of the disorder. Symptomatic measures include bed rest, with elevation of the affected arm or leg; warm, moist soaks to the affected area; and analgesics, as ordered. After an acute episode of deep vein thrombophlebitis subsides, the patient may begin to walk while wearing antiembolism stockings (applied before getting out of bed).

You can never be too thin...

Treatment for thrombophlebitis may also include anticoagulants (initially, unfractionated or low-molecular-weight heparin [Lovenox]; later, warfarin) to prolong clotting time. Before any surgical procedure, discontinue the full anticoagulant dose as ordered to reduce the risk of hemorrhage. After some types of surgery, especially major abdominal or pelvic operations and joint replacements, prophylactic doses of anticoagulants may reduce the risk of deep vein thrombophlebitis and pulmonary embolism.

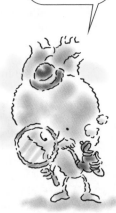

...which usually confirms the diagnosis.

Acute, but not so cute

For lysis of acute, extensive deep vein thrombosis, treatment may include thrombolytics such as alteplase. In rare cases, deep vein thrombophlebitis may cause complete venous occlusion, and embolectomy may need to be performed.

Superficial treatment

Therapy for severe superficial thrombophlebitis may include an anti-inflammatory drug, such as indomethacin, along with antiembolism stockings, warm soaks, and elevation of the patient's leg. A patient with a high risk for deep vein thrombophlebitis and pulmonary embolus combined with contraindications to anticoagulant therapy or with a high risk for bleeding complications might undergo insertion of a vena caval umbrella or filter.

What to do

• To prevent thrombophlebitis in high-risk patients, perform ROM exercises while the patient is on bed rest. Use an intermittent external venous compression device during lengthy surgical or diagnostic procedures. Apply antiembolism stockings postoperatively, and encourage early ambulation.
• Remain alert for signs of pulmonary emboli, such as sudden sharp chest pain that's worse on inspiration, crackles, dyspnea, hemoptysis, sudden changes in mental status, restlessness, and hypotension.
• Closely monitor anticoagulant therapy to prevent serious complications such as internal hemorrhage. Watch for signs of bleeding, such as dark, tarry stools; coffee-ground vomitus; and ecchymoses. Encourage the patient to use an electric razor and to avoid medications that contain aspirin.

Keep it flowing

To prevent venostasis in patients with thrombophlebitis, take the following steps:
• Enforce bed rest, as ordered, and elevate the patient's affected arm or leg. If you plan to use pillows for elevating the leg, place them to support the entire length of the affected extremity and to avoid compressing the popliteal space.
• Apply warm soaks to improve circulation to the affected area and to relieve pain and inflammation. Give analgesics to relieve pain as ordered.
• Measure and record the circumference of the affected arm or leg daily. Compare this with the circumference of the other arm or leg. To ensure accuracy and consistency of serial measurements, mark the skin over the area and measure at the same spot daily.
• Administer heparin I.V. or S.C. as ordered. Use an infusion monitor or pump to control the flow rate of I.V. infusions.
• Evaluate the patient. After successful therapy, the patient shouldn't feel pain in the affected area or have a fever. He should also have normal skin temperature and pulses in the affected arm or leg. (See *Deep vein thrombophlebitis teaching tips*.)

Education edge

Deep vein thrombophlebitis teaching tips

• To prepare the patient with deep vein thrombophlebitis for discharge, emphasize the importance of follow-up blood studies to monitor anticoagulant therapy. If the practitioner has ordered postdischarge heparin therapy, teach the patient or a family member how to give subcutaneous injections. If he requires further help, arrange for a visiting nurse.
• Tell the patient to avoid prolonged sitting or standing to help prevent recurrence.
• Teach him how to apply and use antiembolism stockings properly.
• Tell the patient to immediately report signs of increasing edema or pain in the affected extremity.

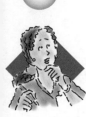

Quick quiz

1. The test that's most specific for myocardial damage is:
    A. CK.
    B. CK-MB.
    C. troponin I.
    D. myoglobin.

Answer: C. Troponin is a protein found in skeletal and cardiac muscles. However, troponin I is found only in the myocardium; it's more specific to myocardial damage than the other choices.

2. Modifiable risk factors associated with CAD include:
    A. age, weight, and cholesterol level.
    B. smoking, diet, and blood pressure.
    C. family history, weight, and blood pressure.
    D. blood glucose level, activity level, and family history.

Answer: B. Smoking, diet, and blood pressure are modifiable risk factors; age and family history aren't.

3. A primary goal in the treatment of MI is to:
    A. prevent blood loss.
    B. decrease blood pressure.
    C. relieve pain.
    D. administer I.V. fluids.

Answer: C. The primary goals in the treatment of MI are to relieve pain, stabilize heart rhythm, revascularize the coronary artery, preserve myocardial tissue, and reduce cardiac workload.

4. One sign of arterial occlusive disease is:
    A. a bounding pulse.
    B. abdominal pain.
    C. high blood pressure.
    D. intermittent claudication.

Answer: D. Intermittent claudication is a sign of arterial occlusive disease.

Scoring

⭐⭐⭐ If you answered all four questions correctly, yahoo! You got to the heart of cardiovascular disorders.

⭐⭐ If you answered three questions correctly, terrific! You are pumping cardiovascular information very efficiently.

⭐ If you answered fewer than three questions correctly, don't get tachycardic! Review the chapter, take deep breaths, and try again.

Respiratory disorders

Just the facts

In this chapter, you'll learn:

♦ structures and functions of the respiratory system

♦ techniques for assessing the respiratory system

♦ nursing diagnoses appropriate for respiratory disorders

♦ common respiratory disorders and treatments.

A look at respiratory disorders

The respiratory system functions primarily to maintain the exchange of oxygen and carbon dioxide in the lungs and tissues and to regulate acid-base balance. Any change in this system affects every other body system. Conversely, changes in other body systems may reduce the lungs' ability to provide oxygen and eliminate carbon dioxide.

The respiratory system delivers oxygen to the bloodstream and removes excess carbon dioxide from the body. Good job!

Anatomy and physiology

The respiratory system consists of the airways, lungs, bony thorax, and respiratory muscles and functions in conjunction with the central nervous system (CNS). (See *Understanding the respiratory system*, page 336.) These structures work together to deliver oxygen to the bloodstream and remove excess carbon dioxide from the body.

A closer look

Understanding the respiratory system

This illustration shows the major structures of the upper and lower airways. The inset shows the alveoli in detail.

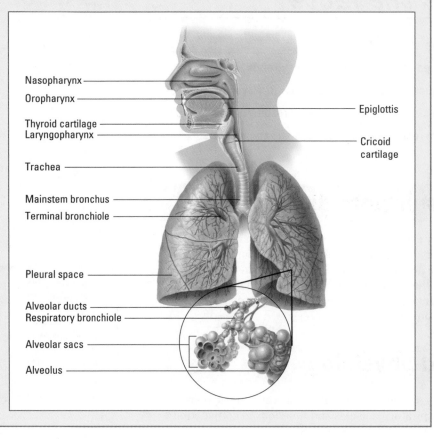

Nasopharynx

Oropharynx

Thyroid cartilage

Laryngopharynx

Trachea

Mainstem bronchus

Terminal bronchiole

Pleural space

Alveolar ducts

Respiratory bronchiole

Alveolar sacs

Alveolus

Epiglottis

Cricoid cartilage

Airways

The airways are divided into the upper and lower airways. The upper airways include the nasopharynx (nose), oropharynx (mouth), laryngopharynx, and larynx. Their purpose is to warm, filter, and humidify inhaled air. They also help make sound and send air to the lower airways.

The top tier

The epiglottis is a flap of tissue that closes over the top of the larynx when the patient swallows. It protects the patient from aspirating food or fluid into the lower airways.

The larynx is located at the top of the trachea and houses the vocal cords. It's the transition point between the upper and lower airways.

Lowdown on the lower airways

The lower airways begin with the trachea, which then divides into the right and left mainstem bronchial tubes. The mainstem bronchi divide into the lobar bronchi, which are lined with mucus-producing ciliated epithelium, one of the lungs' major defense systems.

The lobar bronchi then divide into secondary bronchi, tertiary bronchi, terminal bronchioles, respiratory bronchioles, alveolar ducts and, finally, into the alveoli, the gas-exchange units of the lungs. The lungs in a typical adult contain about 300 million alveoli.

Lungs

Each lung is wrapped in a lining called the visceral pleura. The larger of the two lungs, the right lung has three lobes: upper, middle, and lower. The smaller left lung has only an upper and a lower lobe.

Smooth sliding

The lungs share space in the thoracic cavity with the heart, great vessels, trachea, esophagus, and bronchi. All areas of the thoracic cavity that come in contact with the lungs are lined with parietal pleura.

A small amount of fluid fills the area between the two layers of the pleura. This pleural fluid allows the layers of the pleura to slide smoothly over one another as the chest expands and contracts. The parietal pleurae also contain nerve endings that transmit pain signals when inflammation occurs.

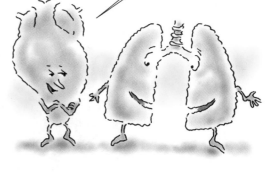

The lungs share space in the thoracic cavity with the great vessels, trachea, esophagus, bronchi—and me!

Thorax

The bony thorax includes the clavicles, sternum, scapula, 12 sets of ribs, and 12 thoracic vertebrae. You can use specific parts of the thorax, along with some imaginary vertical lines drawn on the

Respiratory assessment landmarks

The illustrations below show common landmarks used in respiratory assessment.

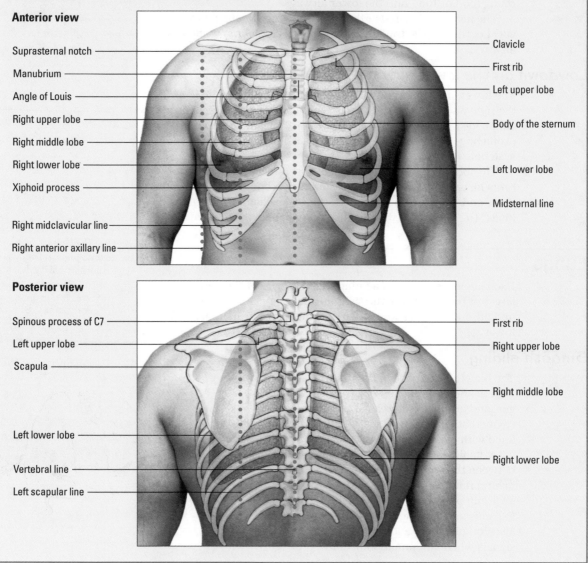

Anterior view

- Suprasternal notch
- Manubrium
- Angle of Louis
- Right upper lobe
- Right middle lobe
- Right lower lobe
- Xiphoid process
- Right midclavicular line
- Right anterior axillary line

- Clavicle
- First rib
- Left upper lobe
- Body of the sternum
- Left lower lobe
- Midsternal line

Posterior view

- Spinous process of C7
- Left upper lobe
- Scapula
- Left lower lobe
- Vertebral line
- Left scapular line

- First rib
- Right upper lobe
- Right middle lobe
- Right lower lobe

chest, to help describe the locations of your findings. (See *Respiratory assessment landmarks.*)

A closer look

A close look at breathing

These illustrations show how mechanical forces, such as the movement of the diaphragm and intercostal muscles, produce a breath. A plus sign (+) indicates positive pressure, and a minus sign (−) indicates negative pressure.

At rest
- Inspiratory muscles relax.
- Atmospheric pressure is maintained in the tracheobronchial tree.
- No air movement occurs.

Inhalation
- Inspiratory muscles contract.
- The diaphragm descends.
- Negative alveolar pressure is maintained.
- Air moves into the lungs.

Exhalation
- Inspiratory muscles relax, causing the lungs to recoil to their resting size and position.
- The diaphragm ascends.
- Positive alveolar pressure is maintained.
- Air moves out of the lungs.

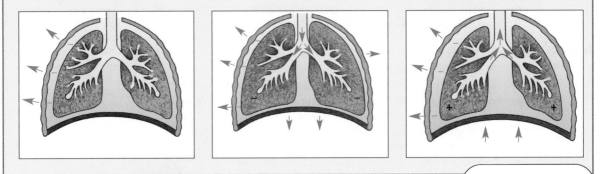

Ribs are made of bone and cartilage and allow the chest to expand and contract during each breath. All ribs attach to the vertebrae. The first seven ribs also attach directly to the sternum. The 8th, 9th, and 10th ribs attach to the costal cartilage of the ribs above. The 11th and 12th ribs are called floating ribs because they don't attach to anything in the front.

The medulla initiates each breath by sending messages to primary respiratory muscles.

Hey, thanks for that!

My pleasure!

Respiratory muscles

The diaphragm and the external intercostal muscles are the primary muscles used in breathing. They contract when the patient inhales and relax when the patient exhales. The respiratory center in the medulla initiates each breath by sending messages to the primary respiratory muscles over the phrenic nerve. Impulses from the phrenic nerve adjust the rate and depth of breathing, depending on the carbon dioxide and pH levels in the cerebrospinal fluid (CSF). (See *A close look at breathing*.)

Accessory to breathing

Accessory inspiratory muscles also assist in breathing. They include the trapezius, sternocleidomastoid, and scalenes, which work together to elevate the scapula, clavicle, sternum, and upper ribs. That elevation expands the front-to-back diameter of the chest when use of the diaphragm and intercostal muscles isn't effective. If the patient has an airway obstruction, he may also use the abdominal and internal intercostal muscles to exhale.

Pulmonary circulation

Oxygen-depleted blood enters the lungs from the pulmonary artery off the right ventricle, then flows through the main pulmonary vessels into the pleural cavities and the main bronchi, where it continues to flow through progressively smaller vessels until it reaches the single-celled endothelial capillaries serving the alveoli. Here, oxygen and carbon dioxide diffusion takes place.

> Here's the plan. We enter the lungs from the pulmonary artery and make our way to the endothelial capillaries serving the alveoli. Then we grab the oxygen we need. Got it?

Movin' and diffusin'

In diffusion, molecules of oxygen and carbon dioxide move in opposite directions between the alveoli and the capillaries. Partial pressure — the pressure exerted by one gas in a mixture of gases — dictates the direction of movement, which is always from an area of greater concentration to one of lesser concentration. During diffusion, oxygen moves across the alveolar and capillary membranes into the bloodstream, where it's taken up by the hemoglobin (Hb) in the red blood cells (RBCs). This oxygen movement displaces the carbon dioxide in those RBCs, which then moves back through the alveoli.

Where do we go from here?

After passing through the pulmonary capillaries, the oxygenated blood flows through progressively larger vessels, enters the main pulmonary vein, and flows into the left atrium for distribution throughout the body. (See *Understanding pulmonary circulation.*)

Acid-base balance

The lungs help maintain acid-base balance in the body by maintaining external respiration (gas exchange in the lungs) and internal respiration (gas exchange in the tissues). Oxygen collected in the lungs is transported to the tissues by the circulatory system, which exchanges it for the carbon dioxide produced by cellular

Understanding pulmonary circulation

The right and left pulmonary arteries carry deoxygenated blood from the right side of the heart to the lungs. These arteries divide into distal branches, called arterioles, which eventually terminate as a concentrated capillary network in the alveoli and alveolar sacs, where gas exchange occurs. The end branches of the pulmonary veins, called venules, collect the oxygenated blood from the capillaries and transport it to larger vessels, which lead to the pulmonary veins. The pulmonary veins enter the left side of the heart and deliver the oxygenated blood for distribution throughout the body.

During the gas exchange process, oxygen and carbon dioxide continuously diffuse across a very thin pulmonary membrane. To understand the direction of movement, remember that gases travel from areas of greater to lesser concentration. Carbon dioxide diffuses from the venous end of the capillary into the alveolus, and oxygen diffuses from the alveolus into the capillary.

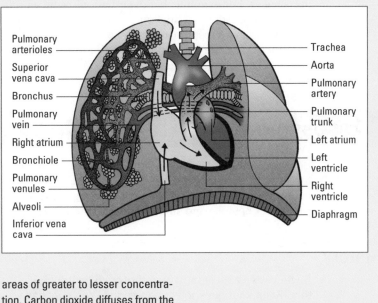

Pulmonary arterioles — Superior vena cava — Bronchus — Pulmonary vein — Right atrium — Bronchiole — Pulmonary venules — Alveoli — Inferior vena cava

Trachea — Aorta — Pulmonary artery — Pulmonary trunk — Left atrium — Left ventricle — Right ventricle — Diaphragm

metabolism. Because carbon dioxide is 20 times more soluble than oxygen, it dissolves in the blood, where most of it forms bicarbonate (base) and smaller amounts form carbonic acid (acid).

Balancing act

The lungs control hydrogen ion concentration and bicarbonate levels by controlling the amount of carbon dioxide eliminated. In response to signals from the medulla, the lungs can change the rate and depth of ventilation. Such changes maintain acid-base balance by adjusting the amount of carbon dioxide that's lost. For example, in metabolic alkalosis, which results from excess bicarbonate retention, the rate and depth of ventilation decrease so that carbon dioxide is retained. This increases carbonic acid levels. In metabolic acidosis (a condition resulting from excess acid retention or excess bicarbonate loss), the lungs increase the rate and depth of ventilation to exhale excess carbon dioxide, thereby reducing carbonic acid levels.

When the balance tips

Inadequately functioning lungs, however, can produce acid-base imbalances. For example, hypoventilation (reduced rate and depth of ventilation) of the lungs, which results in carbon dioxide retention, causes respiratory acidosis. Conversely, hyperventilation (increased rate and depth of ventilation) of the lungs leads to increased exhalation of carbon dioxide and results in respiratory alkalosis.

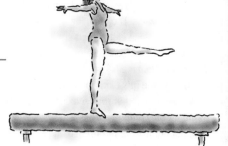

The lungs work hard to keep acids and bases in balance. It's not as easy as it looks!

Assessment

Because the body depends on the respiratory system for survival, respiratory assessment is a critical nursing responsibility. By performing it thoroughly, you can detect obvious and subtle respiratory changes.

History

Begin your assessment with a thorough health history. Keep your questions open-ended. You may have to conduct the interview in several short sessions, depending on the severity of your patient's condition.

Current health status

Ask your patient to tell you about his reason for seeking care. Because many respiratory disorders are chronic, ask him how the latest episode compared with the previous episode and what relief measures helped or didn't help. A patient with a respiratory disorder may complain of shortness of breath, cough, sputum production, wheezing, chest pain, and ankle and leg edema.

Gain a history of the patient's shortness of breath by determining its severity. (See *Grading dyspnea.*) Ask the patient these questions:
• What do you do to relieve the shortness of breath?
• How well does it work?

Three-pillow pileup

A patient with orthopnea (shortness of breath when lying down) tends to sleep with his upper body elevated. Ask this patient how many pillows he uses. The answer describes the severity of orthopnea. For instance, a patient who uses three pillows can be said to have "three-pillow orthopnea."

Cough it up

Ask the patient with a cough these questions:
• When did the cough start?
• Is the cough productive?
• If the cough is chronic, has it changed recently? If so, how?
• What makes the cough better?
• What makes it worse?
• What medications are you taking? (Angiotensin-converting enzyme inhibitors can cause a cough in some patients.) (See *Chronic cough algorithm*, pages 344 and 345.)

Spit it out

When a patient produces sputum, ask him to estimate the amount produced in teaspoons or some other common measurement. Also ask him these questions:
• At what time of day do you cough most often?
• What's the color and consistency of the sputum?
• If sputum is a chronic problem, has it changed recently? If so, how?

Tell me about the wheeze, please

If a patient wheezes, ask these questions:
• At what time of day does wheezing occur?
• What makes you wheeze?
• Do you wheeze loudly enough for others to hear it?
• What helps stop your wheezing?

A pain in the chest

Chest pain that occurs from a respiratory problem usually results from pleural inflammation, inflammation of the costochondral junctions, soreness of chest muscles because of coughing, or indigestion. Less common causes of pain include rib or vertebral fractures caused by coughing or by osteoporosis. If the patient has chest pain, ask him these questions:
• Where is the pain exactly?
• What does it feel like? Is it sharp, stabbing, burning, or aching?
• Does it move to another area?
• How long does it last?
• What causes it to occur or makes it better?
• Do you have associated symptoms, such as shortness of breath or nausea and vomiting?

Previous health status

Focus your questions on identifying previous respiratory problems, such as asthma or emphysema. A history of these conditions provides instant clues to the patient's current condition. Ask

---

Grading dyspnea

To assess dyspnea as objectively as possible, ask your patient to briefly describe how various activities affect his breathing. Then document his response using the grading system below.
Grade 0: Not troubled by breathlessness except with strenuous exercise
Grade 1: Troubled by shortness of breath when hurrying on a level path or walking up a slight hill
Grade 2: Walks more slowly on a level path because of breathlessness than people of the same age, or has to stop to breathe when walking on a level path at his own pace
Grade 3: Stops to breathe after walking about 100 yards (91.4 m) on a level path
Grade 4: Too breathless to leave the house or breathless when dressing or undressing

Weighing the evidence

Chronic cough algorithm

The American Academy of Chest Physicians recommends this algorithm for guiding treatment of a chronic cough.

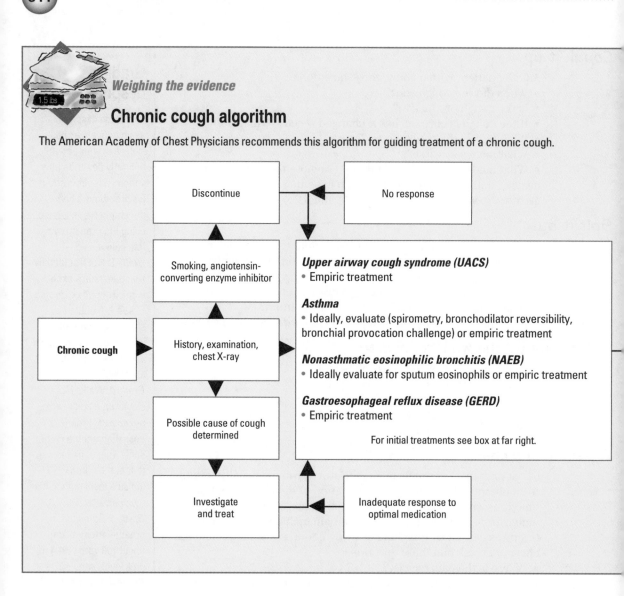

about his smoking history. Then ask about childhood illnesses. Infantile eczema, atopic dermatitis, or allergic rhinitis, for example, may precipitate current respiratory problems such as asthma.

Family history

Ask the patient if anyone in his family has had cancer, diabetes, sickle cell anemia, heart disease, or a chronic illness, such as asthma or emphysema. Be sure to determine whether the patient lives with anyone who has an infectious disease, such as influenza or tuberculosis (TB).

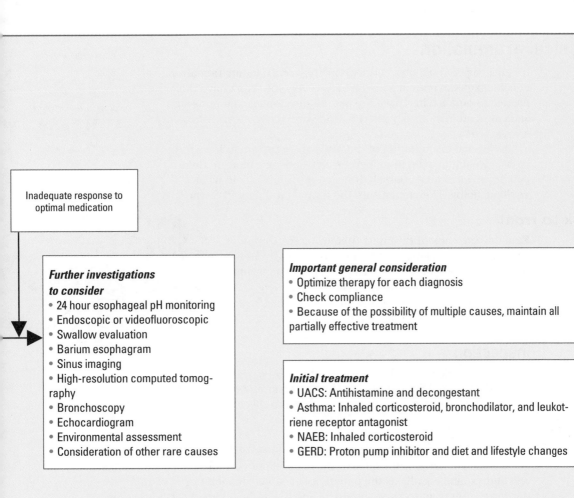

Inadequate response to optimal medication

Further investigations to consider
• 24 hour esophageal pH monitoring
• Endoscopic or videofluoroscopic
• Swallow evaluation
• Barium esophagram
• Sinus imaging
• High-resolution computed tomography
• Bronchoscopy
• Echocardiogram
• Environmental assessment
• Consideration of other rare causes

Important general consideration
• Optimize therapy for each diagnosis
• Check compliance
• Because of the possibility of multiple causes, maintain all partially effective treatment

Initial treatment
• UACS: Antihistamine and decongestant
• Asthma: Inhaled corticosteroid, bronchodilator, and leukotriene receptor antagonist
• NAEB: Inhaled corticosteroid
• GERD: Proton pump inhibitor and diet and lifestyle changes

Source: Baumann, M.H. et al. (2006). Diagnosis and management of cough executive summary: ACCP evidence-based clinical practice guideline. *Chest, 129*(1 Suppl), 1S–23S.

Lifestyle patterns

The patient's history should also include information about lifestyle, community, and other environmental factors that might affect his respiratory status or how he deals with respiratory problems. Most importantly, ask the patient if he smokes; if he does, ask when he started and how many cigarettes he smokes per day.

Also ask about interpersonal relationships, mental status, stress management, and coping style. Keep in mind that a patient's sex habits or drug use may be connected with acquired immunodeficiency syndrome-related respiratory disorders.

Physical examination

In most cases, you'll proceed with the physical examination after you've taken the patient's history. However, you won't have the chance to obtain a history if the patient develops an ominous sign such as acute respiratory distress. (See *Emergency respiratory assessment*.)

A physical examination of the respiratory system follows four steps: inspection, palpation, percussion, and auscultation. Before you begin, introduce yourself, if necessary, and explain what you'll be doing. Then make sure the room is well lit and warm.

> When performing a physical examination of the chest, make sure the room is well lit and warm. Well, maybe it doesn't have to be quite this warm, though.

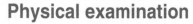

Back to front

Examine the back of the chest first, using inspection, palpation, percussion, and auscultation. Always compare one side with the other. Then examine the front of the chest using the same sequence. The patient can lie back when you examine the front of the chest if that's more comfortable for him.

Inspection

First, inspect the chest. Help the patient into an upright position. The patient should be undressed from the waist up or clothed in an examination gown that allows easy access to his chest.

Beauty in symmetry

Note masses or scars that indicate trauma or surgery. Look for chest wall symmetry. Both sides of the chest should be equal at rest and expand equally as the patient inhales. The diameter of the chest from front to back should be about half the width of the chest.

A new angle

Also, look at the angle between the ribs and the sternum at the point immediately above the xiphoid process. This angle — the costal angle — should be less than 90 degrees in an adult. The angle will be larger if the chest wall is chronically expanded because of an enlargement of the intercostal muscles, as can happen with chronic obstructive pulmonary disease (COPD).

Breathing rate and pattern

To find the patient's respiratory rate, count his respirations for a full minute — longer if you note abnormalities. Don't tell him what you're doing, or he might alter his natural breathing pattern.

What do I do?

Emergency respiratory assessment

When your patient is in acute respiratory distress, immediately assess his airway, breathing, and circulation (ABCs). If they're compromised, call for help and start cardiopulmonary resuscitation as necessary. If his airway is patent and he's breathing and has a pulse, proceed with the following rapid assessment.

Crisis questions

Quickly check for these signs of impending crisis:
• Is the patient having trouble breathing?
• What's his respiratory rate? Is he breathing faster or slower than normal?
• Is he using accessory muscles to breathe? If chest excursion is less than the normal $1^1/8''$ to $2^3/8''$ (3 to 6 cm), he'll use accessory muscles when he breathes. Look for shoulder elevation, intercostal muscle retraction, and the use of scalene and sternocleidomastoid muscles.
• Has his level of consciousness diminished?
• Is he confused, anxious, or agitated?
• Does he change his body position to ease breathing?

• Does his skin look pale or cyanotic?
• Is he diaphoretic?

Setting priorities

When your patient is in respiratory distress, establish priorities for your nursing assessment. Don't assume the obvious. Note positive and negative factors, starting with the most critical (the ABCs) and progressing to less critical factors.

Although you won't have time to go through each step of the nursing process, make sure you gather enough data to clarify the problem. Remember, a single sign or symptom has many possible meanings. Rely on a group of findings for problem solving and appropriate intervention.

Adults normally breathe at a rate of 12 to 20 breaths/minute. The respiratory pattern should be even, coordinated, and regular, with occasional sighs. The inspiratory-expiratory ratio (length of inspiration to length of expiration) is about 1:2.

Muscles in motion

When the patient inhales, his diaphragm should descend and the intercostal muscles should contract. This dual motion causes the abdomen to push out and the lower ribs to expand laterally.

When the patient exhales, his abdomen and ribs return to their resting position. The upper chest shouldn't move much. Accessory muscles may hypertrophy with frequent use. Frequent use of accessory muscles may be normal in some athletes, but for other patients it indicates a respiratory problem, particularly when the patient purses his lips and flares his nostrils when breathing.

Inspecting related structures

Inspection of the skin, tongue, mouth, fingers, and nail beds may also provide information about respiratory status.

> Count respirations for more than 1 minute if you notice abnormalities.

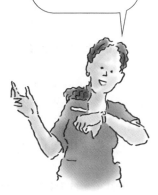

Gettin' the blues

Skin color varies considerably among patients, but in all cases, a patient with a bluish tint to his skin and mucous membranes is considered cyanotic. Cyanosis, which occurs when oxygenation to the tissues is poor, is a late sign of hypoxemia.

The most reliable place to check for cyanosis is the tongue and mucous membranes of the mouth. Cyanotic nail beds, nose, or ears can sometimes occur when the patient is cold, indicating low blood flow to those areas but not necessarily to major organs.

Clubbing clues

When you check the fingers, look for clubbing, a possible sign of long-term hypoxia. A fingernail normally enters the skin at an angle of less than 180 degrees. When clubbing occurs, the angle is greater than or equal to 180 degrees.

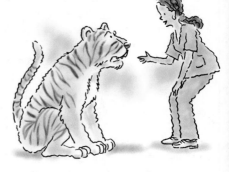

The most reliable place to check for cyanosis is the tongue and mucous membranes of the mouth. Now, open wide!

Palpation

Palpation of the chest provides important information about the respiratory system and the processes involved in breathing. Here's what to look for when palpating the chest.

No extra air

The chest wall should feel smooth, warm, and dry. Crepitus indicates subcutaneous air in the chest, an abnormal condition. Crepitus feels like puffed-rice cereal crackling under the skin and indicates that air is leaking from the airways or lungs.

If a patient has a chest tube, you may find a small amount of subcutaneous air around the insertion site. If the patient has no chest tube or the area of crepitus is getting larger, alert the practitioner immediately.

Ouch! That hurts...

Gentle palpation shouldn't cause the patient pain. If the patient complains of chest pain, check for painful areas on the chest wall. Painful costochondral joints are typically located at the midclavicular line or next to the sternum. Rib or vertebral fractures will be quite painful over the fracture, although pain may radiate around the chest as well. Pain may also stem from sore muscles from protracted coughing or a collapsed lung.

Good — and bad — vibrations

Palpate for tactile fremitus, palpable vibrations caused by the transmission of air through the bronchopulmonary system. Fremitus is decreased over areas where pleural fluid collects, at times

Checking for tactile fremitus

When you check the back of the thorax for tactile fremitus, ask the patient to fold his arms across his chest. This movement shifts the scapulae out of the way.

What to do
Check for tactile fremitus by lightly placing your open palms on both sides of the patient's back, as shown, without touching his back with your fingers. Ask the patient to repeat the phrase "ninety-nine" loudly enough to produce palpable vibrations. Then palpate the front of the chest using the same hand positions.

What the results mean
Vibrations that feel more intense on one side than the other indicate tissue consolidation on that side. Less intense vibrations may indicate emphysema, pneumothorax, or pleural effusion. Faint or no vibrations in the upper posterior thorax may indicate bronchial obstruction or a fluid-filled space.

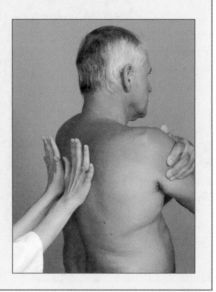

when the patient speaks softly, and within pneumothorax, pleural effusion, and emphysema. Fremitus is increased normally over the large bronchial tubes and abnormally over areas in which alveoli are filled with fluid or exudate, as happens in pneumonia. (See *Checking for tactile fremitus.*)

Measure up

To evaluate the patient's chest wall symmetry and expansion, place your hands on the front of the chest wall, with your thumbs touching each other at the second intercostal space. As the patient inhales deeply, watch your thumbs. They should separate simultaneously and equally, to a distance several centimeters away from the sternum. Repeat the measurement at the fifth intercostal space. You can make the same measurement on the back of the chest near the tenth rib.

Percussion

Percuss the chest to find the boundaries of the lungs; determine whether the lungs are filled with air, fluid, or solid material; and evaluate the distance the diaphragm travels between the patient's inhalation and exhalation. (See *Percussing the chest*, page 350.)

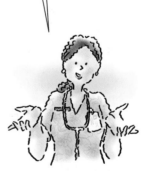

To evaluate chest wall symmetry and expansion, watch your thumbs!

Percussing the chest

To percuss the chest, hyperextend the middle finger of your left hand if you're right-handed or the middle finger of your right hand if you're left-handed. Place your hand firmly on the patient's chest. Use the tip of the middle finger of your dominant hand — your right hand if you're right-handed, left hand if you're left-handed — to tap on the middle finger of your other hand just below the distal joint (as shown).

The movement should come from the wrist of your dominant hand, not your elbow or upper arm. Keep the fingernail you use for tapping short so you won't hurt yourself. Follow the standard percussion sequence over the front and back chest walls.

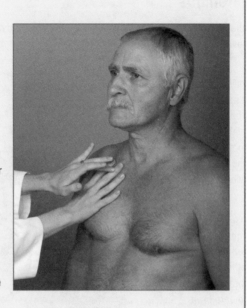

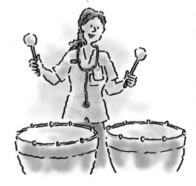

Normally, my percussion isn't dull — except over the heart, of course!

Different sites, different sounds

Percussion allows you to assess structures as deep as 3″ (7.6 cm). You'll hear different percussion sounds in different areas of the chest. (See *Percussion sounds.*)

You also may hear different sounds after certain treatments. For instance, if your patient has atelectasis and you percuss his chest before chest physiotherapy, you'll hear a high-pitched, dull, soft sound. After physiotherapy, you should hear a low-pitched, hollow sound.

Ringing with resonance

You'll hear resonant sounds over normal lung tissue, which you should find over most of the chest. In the left front chest, from the third or fourth intercostal space at the sternum to the third or fourth intercostal space at the midclavicular line, you should hear a dull sound. Percussion is dull here because that's the space occupied by the heart. Resonance resumes at the sixth intercostal space.

Descending diaphragm

Percussion also allows you to assess how much the diaphragm moves during inspiration and expiration. The normal diaphragm descends $1^{1}/8$″ to 2″ (3 to 5 cm) when the patient inhales. The

Percussion sounds

Use the chart below to become more comfortable with percussion and interpret percussion sounds quickly. Learn the different percussion sounds by practicing on yourself, your patients, and any other person willing to help.

Sound	Description	Clinical significance
Flat	Short, soft, high-pitched, extremely dull, found over the thigh	Consolidation, as in atelectasis and extensive pleural effusion
Dull	Medium in intensity and pitch, moderate length, thudlike, found over the liver	Solid area as in pleural effusion
Resonant	Long, loud, low-pitched, hollow	Normal lung tissue
Hyperresonant	Very loud, lower-pitched, found over the stomach	Hyperinflated lung, as in emphysema or pneumothorax
Tympanic	Loud, high-pitched, moderate length, musical, drumlike, found over a puffed-out cheek	Air collection, as in a gastric air bubble or air in the intestines

diaphragm doesn't move as far in patients with emphysema, respiratory depression, diaphragm paralysis, atelectasis, obesity, or ascites. (See *Measuring diaphragm movement*, page 352.)

Auscultation

Auscultation helps you determine the condition of the alveoli and surrounding pleura. As air moves through the bronchial tubes, it creates sound waves that travel to the chest wall. The sounds produced by breathing change as air moves from larger airways to smaller airways. Sounds also change if they pass through fluid, mucus, or narrowed airways.

Preparing to auscultate
Auscultation sites are the same as percussion sites. Listen to a full inspiration and a full expiration at each site, using the diaphragm of the stethoscope. Ask the patient to breathe through his mouth; nose breathing alters the pitch of breath sounds.

Be firm

To auscultate for breath sounds, press the stethoscope firmly against the skin. If the patient has abundant chest hair, press the diaphragm of the stethoscope down even more firmly so the hair doesn't make a sound that might be mistaken for crackles.

You'll use the same sites for auscultation that you used for percussion. That makes life simple!

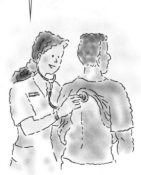

Measuring diaphragm movement

You can measure how much the diaphragm moves by asking the patient to exhale. Percuss the back on one side to locate the upper edge of the diaphragm, the point at which normal lung resonance changes to dullness. Use a pen to mark the spot where the diaphragm is at full expiration on that side of the back.

Then ask the patient to inhale as deeply as possible. Percuss the back when the patient has breathed in fully until you locate the diaphragm. Use the pen to mark this spot as well. Repeat on the opposite side of the back.

Measure

Use a ruler or tape measure to determine the distance between the marks. The distance, normally $1^1/_8''$ to 2" (3 to 5 cm), should be equal on the right and left sides.

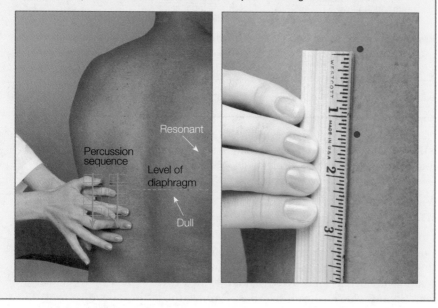

Percussion sequence

Resonant

Level of diaphragm

Dull

Remember that if you listen through clothing or chest hair, you may hear unusual, deceptive sounds.

Normal breath sounds

You'll hear four types of breath sounds over normal lungs. The type of sound you hear depends on where you listen:
• Tracheal breath sounds, heard over the trachea, are harsh, high-pitched, discontinuous sounds. They occur when a patient inhales or exhales.
• Bronchial breath sounds, usually heard next to the trachea, are loud, high-pitched, and discontinuous. They're loudest when the patient exhales.

Qualities of normal breath sounds

Breath sound	Quality	Inspiration-expiration (I:E) ratio	Location
Tracheal	Harsh, high-pitched, discontinuous	I = E	Above the supraclavicular notch, over the trachea
Bronchial	Loud, high-pitched, discontinuous	I < E	Just above the clavicles on each side of the sternum, over the manubrium
Bronchovesicular	Medium in loudness and pitch, continuous	I = E	Next to the sternum, between the scapulae
Vesicular	Soft, low-pitched	I > E	Remainder of the lungs

• Bronchovesicular sounds, heard when the patient inhales or exhales, are medium-pitched and continuous. They're heard next to the sternum, between the scapulae.
• Vesicular sounds, heard over the rest of the lungs, are soft and low-pitched. They're prolonged during inhalation and shortened during exhalation.

What's that sound?

Classify each sound according to its intensity, location, pitch, duration, and characteristic. Note whether the sound occurs when the patient inhales, exhales, or both. If you hear a sound in an area other than where you would expect to hear it, consider the sound abnormal. (See *Qualities of normal breath sounds.*)

For instance, bronchial or bronchovesicular breath sounds found in an area where you would normally hear vesicular breath sounds indicates that the alveoli and small bronchioles in that area might be filled with fluid or exudate, as occurs in pneumonia and atelectasis. In such a situation, you won't hear vesicular sounds in those areas because no air is moving through the small airways.

Testing, testing

A patient with abnormal findings during a respiratory assessment may need further evaluation with such diagnostic tests as arterial blood gas (ABG) analysis or pulmonary function tests.

Vocal fremitus

Vocal fremitus is the sound produced by chest vibrations as the patient speaks. Abnormal transmission of voice sounds may occur

> If you hear a sound in an area where you wouldn't expect to hear it, consider it abnormal.

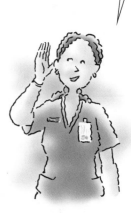

over consolidated areas. The most common abnormal voice sounds are called *bronchophony, egophony,* and *whispered pectoriloquy.* Here's what they sound like:
• Ask the patient to say "ninety-nine" or "blue moon." Over normal lung tissue, the words sound muffled. In bronchophony, the words sound unusually loud over consolidated areas.
• Ask the patient to say "E." Over normal lung tissue, the sound is muffled. In egophony, it will sound like the letter *a* over consolidated lung tissue.
• Ask the patient to whisper "1, 2, 3." Over normal lung tissue, the numbers will be almost indistinguishable. In whispered pectoriloquy, the numbers will be loud and clear over consolidated lung tissue.

Diagnostic tests

If the history and physical examination reveal evidence of respiratory dysfunction, diagnostic tests will help identify and evaluate the dysfunction. These tests include blood and sputum studies and endoscopic and imaging tests as well as other diagnostic tests, such as pulse oximetry, thoracentesis, and pulmonary function tests.

Blood and sputum studies

Blood and sputum studies include ABG analysis and sputum analysis.

ABG analysis

A practitioner will typically order an ABG analysis as one of the first tests to assess respiratory status because it helps evaluate gas exchange in the lungs. ABG analysis includes several measures:
• An indication of hydrogen ion concentration in the blood, *pH* shows the blood's acidity or alkalinity.
• Known as the respiratory parameter, *partial pressure of arterial carbon dioxide* ($Paco_2$), reflects the adequacy of the lungs' ventilation and carbon dioxide elimination.
• *Partial pressure of arterial oxygen* (Pao_2) reflects the body's ability to pick up oxygen from the lungs.
• Known as the metabolic parameter, the *bicarbonate* (HCO_3^-) *level* reflects the kidneys' ability to retain and excrete bicarbonate.

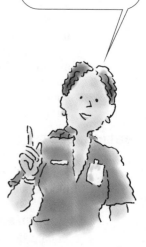

ABG analysis is one of the first tests used to assess respiratory status because it evaluates gas exchange in the lungs.

Teamwork

The respiratory and metabolic systems work together to keep the body's acid-base balance within normal limits. If respiratory acidosis develops, for example, the kidneys attempt to compensate by conserving bicarbonate. Therefore, if respiratory acidosis is present, expect to see the bicarbonate value rise above normal. Similarly, if metabolic acidosis develops, the lungs try to compensate by increasing the respiratory rate and depth to eliminate carbon dioxide. Therefore, expect to see the $Paco_2$ level fall below normal. (See *Understanding acid-base disorders*, page 356.)

Nursing considerations

• Blood for an ABG analysis should be drawn from an arterial line if the patient has one. If a percutaneous puncture is necessary, the site must be chosen carefully. The brachial, radial, or femoral arteries can be used.
• After the sample is obtained, apply pressure to the puncture site for 5 minutes and tape a gauze pad firmly in place. (Don't apply tape around the arm; it could restrict circulation.) Regularly monitor the site for bleeding, and check the arm for signs of complications, such as swelling, discoloration, pain, numbness, and tingling.
• Make sure you note on the slip whether the patient is breathing room air or oxygen. If oxygen, document the number of liters. If the patient is receiving mechanical ventilation, document the fraction of inspired oxygen. Also include the patient's temperature on the slip; results may be corrected if the patient has a fever or hypothermia.
• Keep in mind that certain conditions may interfere with test results — for example, failing to properly heparinize the syringe before drawing a blood sample or exposing the sample to air. Venous blood in the sample may lower Pao_2 levels and elevate $Paco_2$ levels.

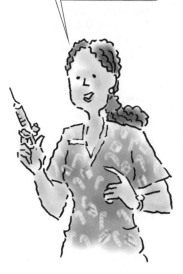

When drawing blood for an ABG analysis, keep in mind that certain conditions may interfere with test results — such as not properly heparinizing the syringe before drawing the sample.

Sputum analysis

Analysis of a sputum specimen (the material expectorated from a patient's lungs and bronchi during deep coughing) helps diagnose respiratory disease, determine the cause of respiratory infection (including viral and bacterial causes), identify abnormal lung cells, and manage lung disease.

Understanding acid-base disorders

Disorder and ABG findings	Possible causes	Signs and symptoms
Respiratory acidosis (excess carbon dioxide retention) pH <7.35 HCO_3^- >26 mEq/L (if compensating) $Paco_2$ >45 mm Hg	• Central nervous system depression due to drugs, injury, or disease • Asphyxia • Hypoventilation due to pulmonary, cardiac, musculoskeletal, or neuromuscular disease	Diaphoresis, headache, tachycardia, confusion, restlessness, apprehension, flushed face
Respiratory alkalosis (excess carbon dioxide excretion) pH >7.45 HCO_3^- <22 mEq/L (if compensating) $Paco_2$ <35 mm Hg	• Hyperventilation due to anxiety, pain, or improper ventilator settings • Respiratory stimulation due to drugs, disease, hypoxia, fever, or high room temperature • Gram-negative bacteremia	Rapid, deep respirations; paresthesia; light-headedness; twitching; anxiety; fear
Metabolic acidosis (HCO_3^- loss, acid retention) pH <7.35 HCO_3^- <22 mEq/L $Paco_2$ <35 mm Hg (if compensating)	• HCO_3^- depletion due to diarrhea • Excessive production of organic acids due to hepatic disease, endocrine disorders, shock, or drug intoxication • Inadequate excretion of acids due to renal disease	Rapid, deep breathing; fruity breath; fatigue; headache; lethargy; drowsiness; nausea; vomiting; abdominal pain; coma (if severe)
Metabolic alkalosis (HCO_3^- retention, acid loss) pH >7.45 HCO_3^- >26 mEq/L $Paco_2$ >45 mm Hg (if compensating)	• Loss of hydrochloric acid due to prolonged vomiting or gastric suctioning • Loss of potassium due to increased renal excretion (as in diuretic therapy) or steroids • Excessive alkali ingestion	Slow, shallow breathing; hypertonic muscles; restlessness; twitching; confusion; irritability; apathy; tetany; seizures; coma (if severe)

Under the microscope

A sputum specimen is stained and examined under a microscope and, depending on the patient's condition, sometimes cultured. Culture and sensitivity testing identifies a specific microorganism and its antibiotic sensitivities. A negative culture may suggest a viral infection.

Nursing considerations
• Encourage the patient to increase his fluid intake the night before sputum collection to aid expectoration.
• To prevent foreign particles from contaminating the specimen, instruct the patient not to eat, brush his teeth, or use a mouthwash before expectorating. He may rinse his mouth with water.
• When the patient is ready to expectorate, instruct him to take three deep breaths and force a deep cough.

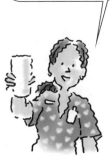

Encourage the patient to drink fluids the night before sputum collection. Bottoms up!

• Before sending the specimen to the laboratory, make sure it's sputum, not saliva. Saliva has a thinner consistency and more bubbles (froth) than sputum.

Endoscopic and imaging tests

Endoscopic and imaging tests include bronchoscopy, chest X-ray, magnetic resonance imaging (MRI), pulmonary angiography, thoracic computed tomography (CT) scan, and ventilation-perfusion ($\dot{V}/\dot{Q}$) scan.

Bronchoscopy

Bronchoscopy is direct inspection of the trachea and bronchi through a flexible fiber-optic or rigid bronchoscope. It allows the doctor to determine the location and extent of pathologic processes, assess resectability of a tumor, diagnose bleeding sites, collect tissue or sputum specimens, and remove foreign bodies, mucus plugs, or excessive secretions.

Nursing considerations
• Tell the patient that he'll receive a sedative, such as diazepam (Valium), midazolam, or meperidine (Demerol).
• Explain that the doctor will introduce the bronchoscope tube through the patient's nose or mouth into the airway. Then he'll flush small amounts of anesthetic through the tube to suppress coughing and gagging.
• Explain to the patient that he'll be asked to lie on his side or sit with his head elevated at least 30 degrees until his gag reflex returns; food, fluid, and oral drugs will be withheld as well until this time. Explain that hoarseness or a sore throat is temporary, and when his gag reflex returns, he can have throat lozenges or a gargle.
• Report bloody mucus, dyspnea, wheezing, or chest pain to the practitioner immediately. A chest X-ray will be taken after the procedure and the patient may receive an aerosolized bronchodilator treatment.
• Monitor for subcutaneous crepitus around the patient's face and neck, which may indicate tracheal or bronchial perforation.
• Watch for breathing problems from laryngeal edema or laryngospasm; call the practitioner immediately if you note labored breathing.

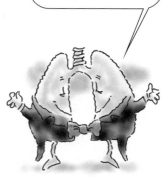

Bronchoscopy inspects the trachea and lungs through a bronchoscope. How do I look? Am I ready for my close-up?

- Observe the patient for signs of hypoxia, pneumothorax, bronchospasm, or bleeding.
- Keep resuscitative equipment and a tracheostomy tray available during the procedure and for 24 hours afterward.

Chest X-ray

Because normal pulmonary tissue is radiolucent, foreign bodies, infiltrates, fluids, tumors, and other abnormalities appear as densities (white areas) on a chest X-ray. It's most useful when compared with the patient's previous films, which allows the radiologist to detect changes.

By itself, a chest X-ray film may not provide information for a definitive diagnosis. For example, it may not reveal mild to moderate obstructive pulmonary disease. Even so, it can show the location and size of lesions and identify structural abnormalities that influence ventilation and diffusion. Examples of abnormalities visible on X-ray include pneumothorax, fibrosis, atelectasis, and infiltrates.

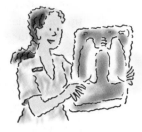

A chest X-ray alone may not confirm a diagnosis, but it can show structural abnormalities and lesion location and size.

Nursing considerations

- Tell the patient that he must wear a gown without snaps and must remove all jewelry from his neck and chest but need not remove his pants, socks, and shoes.
- If the test is performed in the radiology department, tell the patient that he'll stand or sit in front of a machine. If it's performed at the bedside, someone will help him to a sitting position and a cold, hard film plate will be placed behind his back. He'll be asked to take a deep breath and to hold it for a few seconds while the X-ray is taken. He should remain still for those few seconds.
- Reassure the patient that the amount of radiation exposure is minimal. Explain that facility personnel will leave the area when the technician takes the X-ray because they're potentially exposed to radiation many times each day.

MRI

MRI is a noninvasive test that employs a powerful magnet, radio waves, and a computer to help diagnose respiratory disorders. It provides high-resolution, cross-sectional images of lung structures and traces blood flow. MRI's greatest advantage is its ability to "see through" bone and to delineate fluid-filled soft tissue in great detail, without using ionizing radiation or contrast media.

Nursing considerations

• Tell the patient that he must remove all jewelry and take everything out of his pockets. Explain that no metal can be in the test room; the powerful magnet may demagnetize the magnetic strip on a credit card or stop a watch from ticking. If he has any metal inside his body, such as a pacemaker, orthopedic pins or disks, and bullets or shrapnel fragments, tell him he must notify the practitioner.
• Explain to the patient that he'll be asked to lie on a table that slides into an 8′ (2.4 m) tunnel inside the magnet.
• Tell him to breathe normally but not talk or move during the test to avoid distorting the results; the test usually takes 15 to 30 minutes but may take up to 45 minutes.
• Warn the patient that the machinery will be noisy, with sounds ranging from a constant ping to a loud bang. Tell him ear protection will be provided. He may feel claustrophobic or bored. Suggest that he try to relax and concentrate on breathing or a favorite image.

Pulmonary angiography

Also called pulmonary arteriography, pulmonary angiography allows radiographic examination of the pulmonary circulation.

Dyeing to find out

After injecting a radioactive contrast dye through a catheter inserted into the pulmonary artery or one of its branches, a series of X-rays is taken to detect blood flow abnormalities, possibly caused by emboli or pulmonary infarction. This test provides more reliable results than a $\dot{V}/\dot{Q}$ scan but carries higher risks, including cardiac arrhythmias.

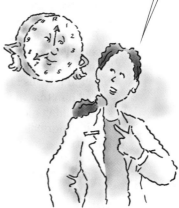

Tell the patient he'll need to fast for 6 hours before pulmonary angiography or as ordered.

Nursing considerations

• Tell the patient who will perform the test and where and when it will take place. Explain that the test takes about 1 hour and allows confirmation of pulmonary emboli.
• Tell the patient he must fast for 6 hours before the test or as ordered. He may continue his prescribed drug regimen unless the practitioner orders otherwise.
• Ask the patient if he has ever had an allergic reaction to contrast media, shellfish, or iodine. If he has, notify the doctor before starting the procedure.
• Explain that he'll be given a sedative, such as diazepam, as ordered. He may also be given diphenhydramine (Benadryl) to reduce the risk of a reaction to the dye.
• Explain the procedure to the patient. The doctor will make a percutaneous needle puncture in an antecubital, femoral, jugular, or subclavian vein. The patient may feel pressure at the site. The doctor will then insert and advance a catheter.

• After catheter insertion, check the pressure dressing for bleeding and assess for arterial occlusion by checking the patient's temperature, sensation, color, and peripheral pulse distal to the insertion site.
• After the test, monitor the patient for hypersensitivity to the contrast medium or to the local anesthetic. Keep emergency equipment nearby and watch for dyspnea.

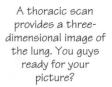

A thoracic scan provides a three-dimensional image of the lung. You guys ready for your picture?

Thoracic CT scan

A thoracic CT scan provides cross-sectional views of the chest by passing an X-ray beam from a computerized scanner through the body at different angles and depths. The CT scan provides a three-dimensional image of the lung, allowing the doctor to assess abnormalities in the configuration of the trachea or major bronchi and evaluate masses or lesions, such as tumors and abscesses, and abnormal lung shadows. (See *Diagnosing pulmonary embolism: Testing the tests.*) A contrast agent is sometimes used to highlight blood vessels and to allow greater visual discrimination.

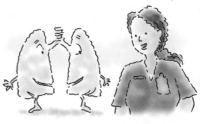

Nursing considerations

• Ask the patient if he has ever had an allergic reaction to contrast media, shellfish, or iodine. If he has, notify the practitioner before the procedure.
• Tell the patient that, if a contrast dye will be used, he should fast for 4 hours before the test.
• Explain that he'll lie on a large, noisy, tunnel-shaped machine. If a contrast dye will be used, tell him that he may experience transient nausea, flushing, warmth, and a salty taste when the dye is injected into his arm vein.
• Tell him that the equipment may make him feel claustrophobic. He shouldn't move during the test but should try to relax and breathe normally. Movement may invalidate the results and require repeat testing.
• Reassure the patient that he'll receive only minimal radiation exposure during the test.

V̇/Q̇ scan

Although less reliable than pulmonary angiography, a V̇/Q̇ scan carries fewer risks. This test indicates lung perfusion and ventilation. It's used to evaluate V̇/Q̇ mismatch, to detect pulmonary emboli, and to evaluate pulmonary function, particularly in preoperative patients with marginal lung reserves.

Weighing the evidence

Diagnosing pulmonary embolism: Testing the tests

Which tests work best?

Each year, emergency departments see a steady stream of patients with respiratory difficulties. Many of these patients are suspected of having pulmonary embolism—but what combination of tests would allow health care workers to identify those patients? One study set out to determine the effectiveness of combining D-dimer testing and computed tomography (CT) scanning.

Two-test combo

To test the effectiveness of these two tests, researchers studied 3,306 patients suspected of having pulmonary embolism. They concluded that CT scanning and D-dimer (fibrin degradation fragment) testing work effectively together. Along with the overall clinical picture, these two tests helped health care workers identify patients with pulmonary embolism.

Source: van Belle, A., et al. (2006). Effectiveness of managing suspected pulmonary embolism using an algorithm combining clinical probability, D-dimer testing, and computed tomography. *Journal of the American Medical Association, 295*(2), 172–179.

Nursing considerations

- Tell the patient that a V̇/Q̇ scan requires injection of a radioactive contrast dye. Explain that he'll lie in a supine position on a table as a radioactive protein substance is injected into an arm vein.
- While he remains in a supine position, a large camera will take pictures, continuing as he lies on his side, lies prone, and sits up. When he's prone, more dye will be injected.
- Reassure the patient that the amount of radioactivity in the dye is minimal. However, he may experience some discomfort from the venipuncture and from lying on a cold, hard table. He may also feel claustrophobic when surrounded by the camera equipment.

Other diagnostic tests

Other diagnostic tests include pulse oximetry, thoracentesis, and pulmonary function tests (PFTs).

Pulse oximetry

Pulse oximetry is a continuous noninvasive study of arterial blood oxygen saturation using a clip or probe attached to a sensor site (usually an earlobe or a fingertip). The percentage expressed is the ratio of oxygen to Hb. (See *Pulse oximetry levels.*)

Nursing considerations
• Place the probe or clip over the finger or other intended sensor site so that the light beams and sensors are opposite each other.
• Protect the transducer from exposure to strong light. Check the transducer site frequently to make sure the device is in place, and examine the skin for abrasion and circulatory impairment.
• Rotate the transducer at least every 4 hours to avoid skin irritation.
• If oximetry has been performed properly, the saturation readings are usually within 2% of ABG values when saturations range between 84% and 98%.

Thoracentesis
Also known as pleural fluid aspiration, thoracentesis is used to obtain a sample of pleural fluid for analysis, relieve lung compression and, occasionally, obtain a lung tissue biopsy specimen.

Nursing considerations
• Tell the patient that his vital signs will be taken and then the area around the needle insertion site will be shaved.
• Explain that the doctor will clean the needle insertion site with a cold antiseptic solution, then inject a local anesthetic. Tell the patient that he may feel a burning sensation as the doctor injects the anesthetic.

Settle into stillness
• Explain to him that after his skin is numb, the doctor will insert the needle. He'll feel pressure during needle insertion and withdrawal. He'll need to remain still during the test to avoid the risk of lung injury. He should try to relax and breathe normally during the test and shouldn't cough, breathe deeply, or move.
• Emphasize that he should tell the doctor if he experiences dyspnea, palpitations, wheezing, dizziness, weakness, or diaphoresis; these symptoms may indicate respiratory distress. After withdrawing the needle, the doctor will apply slight pressure to the site and then an adhesive bandage.
• Tell the patient to report fluid or blood leakage from the needle insertion site as well as signs and symptoms of respiratory distress.

Pulse oximetry levels

Pulse oximetry, which may be intermittent or continuous, monitors arterial oxygen saturation. Normal oxygen saturation levels are 95% to 100% for adults and 94% to 100% for full-term neonates. Lower levels may indicate hypoxemia and warrant intervention.

Interfering factors
Certain factors can interfere with accuracy. For example, an elevated bilirubin level may falsely lower oxygen saturation readings, whereas elevated carboxyhemoglobin or methemoglobin levels can falsely elevate oxygen saturation readings. Certain intravascular substances, such as lipid emulsions and dyes, can also affect readings. Other interfering factors include excessive light (such as from phototherapy or direct sunlight), excessive patient movement, excessive ear pigment, severe peripheral vascular disease, hypothermia, hypotension, and vasoconstriction.

PFTs

PFTs can measure either volume or capacity. These tests aid diagnosis in patients with suspected respiratory dysfunction. The practitioner orders these tests to:
• evaluate ventilatory function through spirometric measurements
• determine the cause of dyspnea
• assess the effectiveness of medications, such as bronchodilators and steroids
• determine whether a respiratory abnormality stems from an obstructive or restrictive disease process
• evaluate the extent of dysfunction.

Verifying volume

Direct spirography measures tidal volume and expiratory reserve volume, two of the five pulmonary function tests. Minute volume, inspiratory reserve volume, and residual volume are calculated from the results of other PFTs.

Calculating capacity

Of the pulmonary capacity tests, functional residual capacity, total lung capacity, and maximal midexpiratory flow must be calculated. Either direct measurement or calculation provides vital capacity and inspiratory capacity. Direct spirographic measurements include forced vital capacity, forced expiratory volume, and maximal voluntary ventilation. The amount of carbon monoxide exhaled permits calculation of the diffusing capacity for carbon monoxide. (See *Interpreting pulmonary function test results*, page 364.)

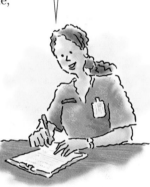

Some pulmonary capacity tests must be calculated. Good thing my math skills are in top form!

Nursing considerations

• For some tests, the patient will sit upright and wear a noseclip.
• Explain that he may receive an aerosolized bronchodilator. He may need to receive the bronchodilator more than once to evaluate the drug's effectiveness.
• Emphasize that the test will proceed quickly if the patient follows directions, tries hard, and keeps a tight seal around the mouthpiece or tube to ensure accurate results.
• Instruct the patient to loosen tight clothing so he can breathe freely. Tell him he must not smoke or eat a large meal for 4 hours before the test.

Interpreting pulmonary function test results

You may need to interpret pulmonary test results in your assessment of a patient's respiratory status. Use the chart below as a guide to common pulmonary function tests.

Restrictive and obstructive
The chart mentions restrictive and obstructive defects. A restrictive defect is one in which a person can't inhale a normal amount of air. It may occur with chest-wall deformities, neuromuscular diseases, or acute respiratory tract infections.

An obstructive defect is one in which something obstructs the flow of air into or out of the lungs. It may occur with such disorders as asthma, chronic bronchitis, emphysema, and cystic fibrosis.

Test	Implications
Tidal volume (V_T): amount of air inhaled or exhaled during normal breathing	Decreased V_T may indicate restrictive disease and necessitate further tests, such as full pulmonary function studies and chest X-rays.
Minute volume (MV): amount of air breathed per minute	Normal MV can occur in emphysema. Decreased MV may indicate other diseases such as pulmonary edema.
Inspiratory reserve volume (IRV): amount of air inhaled after normal inspiration	Abnormal IRV alone doesn't indicate respiratory dysfunction. IRV decreases during normal exercise.
Expiratory reserve volume (ERV): amount of air that can be exhaled after normal expiration	ERV varies, even in healthy people.
Vital capacity (VC): amount of air that can be exhaled after maximum inspiration	Normal or increased VC with decreased flow rates may indicate a reduction in functional pulmonary tissue. Decreased VC with normal or increased flow rates may indicate respiratory effort, decreased thoracic expansion, or limited movement of the diaphragm.
Inspiratory capacity (IC): amount of air that can be inhaled after normal expiration	Decreased IC indicates restrictive disease.
Forced vital capacity (FVC): amount of air that can be exhaled after maximum inspiration	Decreased FVC indicates flow resistance in the respiratory system from obstructive disorders, such as chronic bronchitis, emphysema, and asthma.
Forced expiratory volume (FEV): volume of air exhaled in the first (FEV_1), second (FEV_2), or third (FEV_3) FVC maneuver	Decreased FEV_1 and increased FEV_2 and FEV_3 may indicate obstructive disease. Decreased or normal FEV_1 may indicate restrictive disease.

• Keep in mind that anxiety can affect test accuracy. Also remember that medications, such as analgesics and bronchodilators, may produce misleading results. You may be asked to withhold bronchodilators and other respiratory treatments before the test. If the patient receives a bronchodilator during the test, don't give another dose for 4 hours.

Treatments

Respiratory disorders interfere with airway clearance, breathing patterns, and gas exchange. If not corrected, they can adversely affect many other body systems and can be life-threatening. Treatments for respiratory disorders include drug therapy, surgery, inhalation therapy, and chest physiotherapy.

Drug therapy

Drugs are used for airway management in such disorders as bronchial asthma and chronic bronchitis and may include:
• xanthines (theophylline and derivatives) and adrenergics to dilate bronchial passages and reduce airway resistance, making it easier for the patient to breathe and allowing sufficient ventilation
• corticosteroids to reduce inflammation and make the airways more responsive to bronchodilators
• antihistamines, antitussives, and expectorants to help suppress coughing and mobilize secretions
• antimicrobials to reduce or eliminate infective organisms
• leukotrine receptor modifiers to help block the bronchoconstrictive effect of leukotrines
• antihistamines to block or reverse inflammation caused by sensitivity to allergens.

Surgery

If drugs or other therapeutic approaches fail to maintain airway patency and protect healthy tissues from disease, the patient may need surgical intervention. Respiratory surgeries include tracheotomy, chest tube insertion, and thoracotomy. Lung resection, lung reduction, pneumonectomy, or lung transplant surgery may also be indicated.

Tracheotomy

A tracheotomy provides an airway for an intubated patient who needs prolonged mechanical ventilation and helps remove lower tracheobronchial secretions in a patient who can't clear them. It's also performed in emergencies when endotracheal (ET) intubation isn't possible, to prevent an unconscious or paralyzed patient from aspirating food or secretions, and to bypass upper airway obstruction due to trauma, burns, epiglottiditis, or a tumor.

A tracheotomy helps remove lower tracheobronchial secretions in a patient who can't clear them. A little help here!

After the doctor creates the surgical opening, he inserts a tracheostomy tube to permit access to the airway. He may select from several tube styles, depending on the patient's condition. (See *Comparing tracheostomy tubes*.)

Patient preparation

Before a tracheotomy, take these steps:
• For an emergency tracheotomy, briefly explain the procedure to the patient as time permits and quickly obtain supplies or a tracheotomy tray.
• For a scheduled tracheotomy, explain the procedure and the need for general anesthesia to the patient and his family. If possible, mention whether the tracheostomy will be temporary or permanent.
• Set up a communication system with the patient (letter board or flash cards), and practice it with him to ensure he'll be able to communicate comfortably while his speech is limited.

A friend in need

• Introduce a patient requiring a long-term or permanent tracheostomy to someone who has experienced the procedure and has adjusted well to tracheostomy care.
• Ensure that samples for ABG analysis and other diagnostic tests have been collected and that the patient or a responsible family member has signed a consent form.

Monitoring and aftercare

After a tracheotomy, take these steps:
• Auscultate breath sounds every 2 hours after the procedure. Note crackles, rhonchi, or diminished breath sounds.
• Observe for abnormal bleeding at the tracheostomy site. A small amount of bloody drainage is normal for the first 24 hours.
• Turn the patient every 2 hours to avoid pooling tracheal secretions. As ordered, provide chest physiotherapy to help mobilize secretions, and note their quantity, consistency, color, and odor.
• Replace humidity lost in bypassing the nose, mouth, and upper airway mucosa to reduce the drying effects of oxygen on mucous membranes. Humidification will also help to thin secretions. Oxygen administered through a T-piece or tracheostomy mask should be connected to a nebulizer or heated cascade humidifier.
• Monitor ABG results and compare them with baseline values to check adequacy of oxygenation and carbon dioxide removal. Also monitor the patient's oximetry values as ordered.
• Suction the tracheostomy using sterile technique to remove excess secretions only when necessary. Avoid suctioning a

Avoid suctioning the patient for longer than 10 seconds at a time, and stop if the patient develops respiratory distress.

Comparing tracheostomy tubes

Tracheostomy tubes are made of plastic or metal and come in uncuffed, cuffed, or fenestrated varieties. Tube selection depends on the patient's condition and the doctor's preference. Make sure you're familiar with the advantages and disadvantages of these commonly used tracheostomy tubes.

Uncuffed

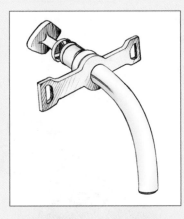

Advantages
• Free flow of air around tube and through larynx
• Reduced risk of tracheal damage
• Mechanical ventilation possible in patient with neuromuscular disease

Disadvantages
• Increased risk of aspiration in adults due to lack of cuff
• Adapter possibly needed for ventilation

Plastic cuffed
(low pressure and high volume)

Advantages
• Disposable
• Cuff bonded to tube (won't detach accidentally inside trachea)
• Low cuff pressure that's evenly distributed against tracheal wall (no need to deflate periodically to lower pressure)
• Reduced risk of tracheal damage

Disadvantages
• Possibly more expensive than other tubes

Fenestrated

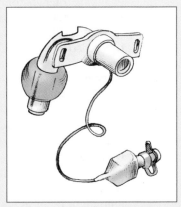

Advantages
• Speech possible through upper airway when external opening is capped and cuff is deflated
• Breathing by mechanical ventilation possible with inner cannula in place and cuff inflated
• Easy removal of inner cannula for cleaning

Disadvantages
• Possible occlusion of fenestration
• Possible dislodgment of inner cannula
• Cap removal necessary before inflating cuff

patient for longer than 10 seconds at a time, and discontinue the procedure if the patient develops respiratory distress.

A secure feeling

• Make sure the tracheostomy ties are secure but not too tight. To prevent accidental tube dislodgment or expulsion, avoid changing

the ties until the stoma track is stable. Report any tube pulsation to the practitioner; this may indicate the tube is close to the innominate artery, which predisposes the patient to hemorrhage.
• Change the tracheostomy dressing when soiled or once per shift using sterile technique, and check the color, odor, amount, and type of drainage. Also check for swelling, crepitus, erythema, and bleeding at the site and report excessive bleeding or unusual drainage immediately. Wear goggles, gloves, and a mask when changing tracheostomy tubes.
• Keep a sterile tracheostomy tube (with obturator) at the patient's bedside and be prepared to replace an expelled or contaminated tube. Also keep available a sterile tracheostomy tube (with obturator) that's one size smaller than the tube currently being used. You may need the smaller tube if the trachea begins to close after tube expulsion, making insertion of the same size tube difficult.

Home care instructions
Take these steps to help the patient and his family prepare for returning home:
• Tell the patient or his family to notify the practitioner of breathing problems, chest or stoma pain, or a change in the amount or color of his secretions.
• Make sure that the patient or his family can care for the stoma and tracheostomy tube effectively.
• Tell the patient to place a foam filter over his stoma in winter to warm the inspired air and to wear a bib over the filter.
• Teach the patient to bend at the waist during coughing to help expel secretions. Tell him to keep a tissue handy to catch expelled secretions.
• Instruct the patient and his family to keep an extra sterile tracheostomy tube available; make sure all family members know where it's located.

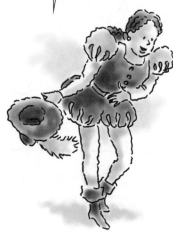

Tell the patient to bend at the waist during coughing to help expel secretions.

Chest tube insertion
A chest tube may be required to help treat pneumothorax, hemothorax, empyema, pleural effusion, or chylothorax. Inserted into the pleural space, the tube allows blood, fluid, pus, or air to drain and allows the lungs to reinflate.

Water tight
In pneumothorax, the tube restores negative pressure to the pleural space through an underwater-seal drainage system. The water in the system prevents air from being sucked back into the pleural space during inspiration. If a leak occurs through the bronchi and can't be sealed, suction applied to the underwater-seal system removes air from the pleural space faster than it can collect.

Patient preparation

Before the procedure, take these steps:
• If time permits, the doctor will obtain a signed consent form after explaining the procedure. Reassure the patient that chest tube insertion will help him breathe more easily.
• Obtain baseline vital signs and administer a sedative as ordered.
• If the patient requires an underwater-seal drainage system, collect necessary equipment, including a thoracotomy tray and an underwater-seal drainage system. Prepare lidocaine (Xylocaine) for local anesthesia as directed. The doctor will clean the insertion site with antimicrobial solution. Set up the drainage system according to the manufacturer's instructions and place it at the bedside, below the patient's chest level. Stabilize the unit to avoid knocking it over. (See *Closed chest drainage system*.)

Closed chest drainage system

One-piece, disposable plastic drainage systems, such as the Pleur-evac, contain three chambers. The drainage chamber is on the right and has three calibrated columns that display the amount of drainage collected. When the first column fills, drainage carries over into the second and, when that fills, into the third. The water-seal chamber is located in the center. The suction-control chamber on the left is filled with water to achieve various suction levels. Rubber diaphragms are provided at the rear of the device to change the water level or remove samples of drainage. A positive-pressure relief valve at the top of the water-seal chamber vents excess pressure into the atmosphere, preventing pressure buildup.

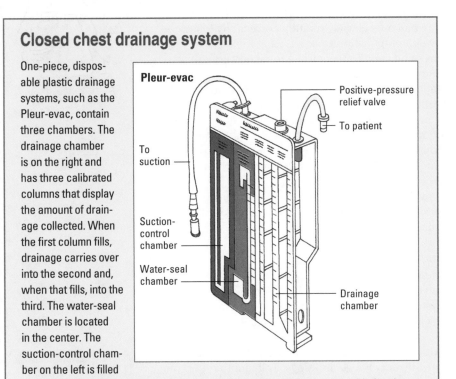

Pleur-evac

Positive-pressure relief valve

To patient

To suction

Suction-control chamber

Water-seal chamber

Drainage chamber

Monitoring and aftercare

After tube insertion, take these steps:
• When the patient's chest tube is stabilized, instruct him to take several deep breaths to inflate his lungs fully and help push pleural air out through the tube.
• Obtain vital signs immediately after tube insertion and every 15 minutes thereafter, according to facility policy (usually for 1 hour).
• Routinely assess chest tube function. Describe and record the amount of drainage on the intake and output sheet.
• Monitor the suction chamber to make sure it has a consistent water level. You may need to add water if any is lost through evaporation.
• After most of the air has been removed, the drainage system should bubble only during forced expiration unless the patient has a bronchopleural fistula. Constant bubbling in the system may indicate that a connection is loose or that the tube has advanced slightly out of the patient's chest. Promptly correct any loose connections to prevent complications.
• Change the dressing daily (or according to facility policy) to clean the site and remove drainage.
• If the chest tube becomes dislodged, cover the opening immediately with petroleum gauze and apply pressure to prevent negative inspiratory pressure from sucking air into the chest. Call the practitioner and have an assistant collect equipment for tube reinsertion while you keep the opening closed. Reassure the patient, and monitor him closely for signs of tension pneumothorax. (See *Combating tension pneumothorax.*)
• The practitioner will remove the patient's chest tube after the lung has fully reexpanded. As soon as the tube is removed, apply an airtight, sterile petroleum dressing.

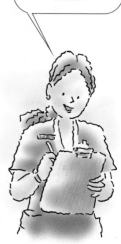

Describe and record the amount of chest tube drainage on the intake and output sheet.

Home care instructions

Typically, a patient is discharged with a chest tube only if it's used to drain a loculated empyema, which doesn't require an underwater-seal drainage system. Teach this patient how to care for his tube, perform wound care and dressing changes, and dispose of soiled dressings.

Teach the patient with a recently removed chest tube how to clean the wound site and change dressings. Tell him to report any signs of infection.

Thoracotomy

A thoracotomy is the surgical removal of all or part of a lung; it aims to spare healthy lung tissue from disease. Lung excision may

What do I do?

Combating tension pneumothorax

Tension pneumothorax, the entrapment of air within the pleural space, can be fatal without prompt treatment.

What causes it?

An obstructed or dislodged chest tube is a common cause of tension pneumothorax. Other causes include blunt chest trauma or high-pressure mechanical ventilation. In such cases, increased positive pressure within the patient's chest cavity compresses the affected lung and the mediastinum, shifting them toward the opposite lung. This impairs venous return and cardiac output and may cause the lung to collapse.

Telltale signs

Suspect tension pneumothorax if the patient develops dyspnea, chest pain, an irritating cough, vertigo, syncope,

or anxiety after a blunt chest trauma or if the patient has a chest tube in place. Is his skin cold, pale, and clammy? Are his respiratory and pulse rates unusually rapid? Does the patient have unequal bilateral chest expansion?

If you note these signs and symptoms, palpate the patient's neck, face, and chest wall for subcutaneous emphysema and palpate his trachea for deviation from midline. Auscultate the lungs for decreased or absent breath sounds on one side. Then percuss them for hyper-resonance. If you suspect tension pneumotorax, notify the practitioner at once and help identify the cause.

---

involve a pneumonectomy, lobectomy, segmental resection, or wedge resection.

The whole shebang

A pneumonectomy is the excision of an entire lung; it's usually performed to treat bronchogenic carcinoma but may also be used to treat TB, bronchiectasis, or a lung abscess. It's used only when a less radical approach can't remove all diseased tissue. Chest cavity pressures stabilize after a pneumonectomy and, over time, fluid enters the cavity where lung tissue was removed, preventing significant mediastinal shift.

One out, four remaining

A lobectomy is the removal of one of the five lung lobes; it's used to treat bronchogenic carcinoma, TB, a lung abscess, emphysematous blebs or bullae, benign tumors, and localized fungal infections. After this surgery, the remaining lobes expand to fill the entire pleural cavity.

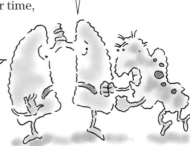

A lobectomy can be used to remove a lobe that has a localized fungal infection. Yikes! Get away!

Bits and pieces

A segmental resection is the removal of one or more lung segments; it preserves more functional tissue than lobectomy and is commonly used to treat bronchiectasis. A wedge resection is the removal of a small portion of the lung without regard to segments;

it preserves the most functional tissue of all the surgeries but can treat only a small, well-circumscribed lesion. Remaining lung tissue must be reexpanded after both types of resection.

Patient preparation

Take these steps to help prepare the patient:
• Explain the anticipated surgery to the patient and inform him that he'll receive a general anesthetic.
• Tell the patient that postoperatively he may have chest tubes in place and may receive oxygen.
• Teach him deep-breathing techniques, and explain that he'll perform these after surgery to promote lung reexpansion. Also teach him to use an incentive spirometer; record the volumes he achieves to provide a baseline.

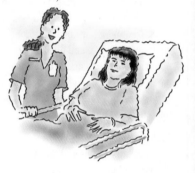

Explain to the patient that she may have chest tubes in place and may receive oxygen after surgery.

Monitoring and aftercare

After surgery, take these steps:
• After a pneumonectomy, make sure the patient lies only on the operative side or on his back until stabilized. This prevents fluid from draining into the unaffected lung if the sutured bronchus opens.
• Make sure the chest tube is functioning, if present, and observe for signs of tension pneumothorax.
• Provide analgesics as ordered.
• Have the patient begin coughing and deep-breathing exercises as soon as his condition is stable. Auscultate his lungs, place him in semi-Fowler's position, and have him splint his incision to promote coughing and deep breathing.
• Perform passive range-of-motion (ROM) exercises the evening of surgery and two or three times daily thereafter. Progress to active ROM exercises.

Home care instructions

Before discharge, teach the patient to:
• continue his coughing and deep-breathing exercises to prevent complications and report changes in sputum characteristics to his practitioner
• continue performing ROM exercises to maintain mobility of his shoulder and chest wall
• avoid contact with people who have an upper respiratory tract infection
• refrain from smoking
• care for his wound and change the dressing as necessary.

Inhalation therapy

Inhalation therapy uses carefully controlled ventilation techniques to help the patient maintain optimal ventilation in the event of respiratory failure. Techniques include mechanical ventilation, continuous positive airway pressure (CPAP), and oxygen therapy.

Mechanical ventilation

> Mechanical ventilation corrects profoundly impaired ventilation. I could really use that right now!

Mechanical ventilation corrects profoundly impaired ventilation, evidenced by hypercapnia, hypoxia, and signs of respiratory distress (such as nostril flaring, intercostal retractions, decreased blood pressure, and diaphoresis). Typically requiring an ET or tracheostomy tube, it delivers up to 100% room air under positive pressure or oxygen-enriched air in concentrations up to 100%.

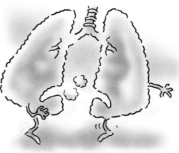

Pressure's on

Major types of mechanical ventilation systems include positive-pressure, negative-pressure, and high-frequency ventilation (HFV). Positive-pressure systems, the most commonly used, can be volume-cycled or pressure-cycled. During a cycled breath, inspiration ceases when a preset pressure or volume is met.

Pressure's off

Negative-pressure systems provide ventilation for patients who can't generate adequate inspiratory pressures. HFV systems provide high ventilation rates with low peak airway pressures, synchronized to the patient's own inspiratory efforts.

Who's in control

Mechanical ventilators can be programmed to assist, control, or assist-control. In assist mode, the patient initiates inspiration and receives a preset tidal volume from the machine, which augments his ventilatory effort while letting him determine his own rate. In control mode, a ventilator delivers a set tidal volume at a prescribed rate, using predetermined inspiratory and expiratory times. This mode can fully regulate ventilation in a patient with paralysis or respiratory arrest. In assist-control mode, the patient initiates breathing and a backup control delivers a preset number of breaths at a set volume.

Synchronicity

In synchronized intermittent mandatory ventilation (SIMV), the ventilator delivers a set number of specific-volume breaths. The patient may breathe spontaneously between the SIMV breaths at volumes that differ from those on the machine, however. Commonly used as a weaning tool, SIMV may also be used for ventilation and helps to condition respiratory muscles.

Patient preparation

Before mechanical ventilation begins, take these steps:
• Describe to the patient what mechanical ventilation system will be used, including its benefits and what he may experience.
• If he's not already intubated or doesn't have a tracheostomy tube in place, describe the intubation process.
• Set up a communication system with the patient (such as a letter board), and reassure him that a nurse will always be nearby. Keep in mind that an apprehensive patient may fight the machine, defeating its purpose.
• If possible, place the patient in semi-Fowler's position to promote lung expansion. Obtain baseline vital signs and ABG readings.

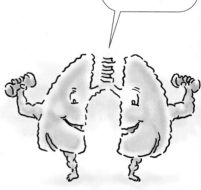

SIMV helps condition respiratory muscles.

Monitoring and aftercare

The patient must be intubated to establish an artificial airway. A bite block is commonly used with an oral ET tube to prevent the patient from biting the tube. After the patient is intubated, arrange for a chest X-ray to evaluate tube placement. Secure the tube to the patient's face and mark the proximal end to identify position. Make sure he has a communication device and a call bell within reach, and continuously monitor his pulse oximetry level.

For all patients, check ABG levels as ordered. Overventilation may cause respiratory alkalosis from decreased carbon dioxide levels. Inadequate alveolar ventilation or atelectasis from an inappropriate tidal volume may cause respiratory acidosis.

Perform the following steps every 1 to 2 hours and as needed:
• Check all connections between the ventilator and the patient. Make sure critical alarms are turned on, such as the low-pressure alarm that indicates a disconnection in the system and is set at not less than 3 cm H_2O and the high-pressure alarm that prevents excessive airway pressures. The high-pressure alarm should be set 20 to 30 cm H_2O greater than the patient's peak airway pressure. Volume alarms should also be used if available. Make sure the patient can reach his call bell.
• Verify that ventilator settings are correct and that the ventilator is operating at those settings; compare the patient's respiratory rate with the setting and, for a volume-cycled machine, watch that

Check ABG levels as ordered to detect respiratory alkalosis or acidosis. I like to keep things in balance!

the spirometer reaches the correct volume. For a pressure-cycled machine, use a respirometer to check exhaled tidal volume.

Water, water, everywhere

• Check the humidifier and refill it if necessary. Check the corrugated tubing for condensation; drain collected water into a container and discard. Don't drain condensation — which may be contaminated with bacteria — into the humidifier, and be careful not to drain condensation into the patient's airway.
• If ordered, give the patient several deep breaths (usually two or three) each hour by setting the sigh mechanism on the ventilator or by using a handheld resuscitation bag.
• Check oxygen concentration every 8 hours and ABG values whenever ventilator settings are changed. Assess respiratory status at least every 2 hours in the acute patient and every 4 hours in the stable chronic patient to detect the need for suctioning and to evaluate the response to treatment. Suction the patient as necessary, noting the amount, color, odor, and consistency of secretions. Auscultate for decreased breath sounds on the left side — an indication of tube slippage into the right mainstem bronchus.
   Also perform the following:
• Monitor the patient's fluid intake and output and his electrolyte balance. Weigh him as ordered.
• Using sterile technique, change the humidifier, nebulizer, and ventilator tubing according to facility protocol.
• Reposition the patient frequently, and perform chest physiotherapy as necessary.

No more heartburn

• Provide emotional support to reduce stress, and give antacids and other medications as ordered to reduce gastric acid production and to help prevent GI complications.
• Monitor for decreased bowel sounds and abdominal distention, which may indicate paralytic ileus.
• Check nasogastric (NG) aspirate and stools for blood; stress ulcers are a common complication of mechanical ventilation.
• If the patient is receiving high-pressure ventilation, assess for signs and symptoms of a pneumothorax (absent or diminished breath sounds on the affected side, acute chest pain and, possibly, tracheal deviation or subcutaneous or mediastinal emphysema).
• If the patient is receiving a high oxygen concentration, watch for signs and symptoms of toxicity (substernal chest pain, increased coughing, tachypnea, decreased lung compliance and vital capacity, and decreased $Paco_2$ without a change in oxygen concentration).

To detect tube slippage in a patient receiving mechanical ventilation, auscultate for decreased breath sounds on the left side of the chest.

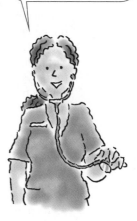

- If the patient resists mechanical ventilation and ineffective ventilation results, give him a sedative, an antianxiety agent, a neuromuscular blocking agent, or a short-acting anesthetic, as ordered, and observe him closely.

Home care instructions

If the patient requires a ventilator at home, teach him and a family member:
- how to check the device and its settings for accuracy and the nebulizer and oxygen equipment for proper functioning at least once per day
- to refill his humidifier as necessary
- that his ABG levels will be measured periodically to evaluate his therapy
- how to count his pulse rate and to report changes in rate or rhythm as well as chest pain, fever, dyspnea, or swollen extremities
- to call his practitioner or respiratory therapist if he has questions or problems.

CPAP

As its name suggests, CPAP ventilation maintains positive pressure in the airways throughout the patient's respiratory cycle. Originally delivered only with a ventilator, CPAP may now be delivered to intubated or nonintubated patients through an artificial airway, a mask, or nasal prongs by means of a ventilator or a separate high-flow generating system. (See *Using CPAP.*)

Goes with the flows

CPAP is available as a continuous-flow system and a demand system. In the continuous-flow system, an air-oxygen blend flows through a humidifier and a reservoir bag into a T-piece. In the demand system, a valve opens in response to the patient's inspiratory flow.

Other talents

CPAP not only treats respiratory distress syndrome, it has also successfully treated pulmonary edema, pulmonary emboli, bronchiolitis, fat emboli, pneumonitis, viral pneumonia, postoperative atelectasis, and sleep apnea. In mild to moderate cases of these disorders, CPAP provides an alternative to intubation and mechanical ventilation. It increases the

> CPAP has successfully treated several disorders, including respiratory distress syndrome, pulmonary edema and emboli, bronchiolitis, and sleep apnea.

Using CPAP

Continuous positive airway pressure (CPAP) devices apply positive pressure to the airway to prevent obstruction during inspiration in patients with sleep apnea. Two types of CPAP devices are shown below. Patient and practitioner preference typically determines which device is used.

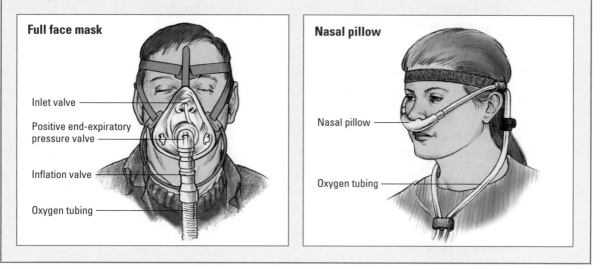

Full face mask

Inlet valve

Positive end-expiratory pressure valve

Inflation valve

Oxygen tubing

Nasal pillow

Nasal pillow

Oxygen tubing

functional residual capacity by distending collapsed alveoli, which improves PaO_2 and decreases intrapulmonary shunting and oxygen consumption. It also reduces the work of breathing. CPAP can also be used to wean a patient from mechanical ventilation.

Through the nose

Nasal CPAP has proved successful as a long-term treatment for obstructive sleep apnea. In this type of CPAP, high-flow compressed air is directed into a mask that covers only the patient's nose. The pressure supplied through the mask serves as a back-pressure splint, preventing the unstable upper airway from collapsing during inspiration. It also helps reduce other risks from sleep apnea. (See *CPAP and the heart*, page 378.)

Not so positive

CPAP may cause gastric distress if the patient swallows air during the treatment (most common when CPAP is delivered without intubation). The patient may feel claustrophobic. Because mask CPAP can also cause nausea and vomiting, it shouldn't be used in patients who are unresponsive or at risk for vomiting and aspiration. Rarely, CPAP causes barotrauma or lowers cardiac output.

Weighing the evidence

CPAP and the heart

Obstructive sleep apnea (OSA) can certainly disrupt sleep, but it's also associated with such cardiovascular disorders as coronary artery disease, congestive heart failure, hypertension, cardiac arrhythmias, and stroke. Researchers believe that endothelial dysfunction, coagulopathies, inflammatory processes, and neurovascular mechanisms are likely responsible for the development of cardiac disease with OSA. The good news is that multiple studies have shown that using CPAP improves cardiac status and slows cardiac disease progression in OSA patients. Researchers now recommend that patients with OSA be screened for cardiac disease and vice versa.

Butt, M., et al. (2010). Obstructive sleep apnea and cardiovascular disease. *International Journal of Cardiology, 139*(1), 7–16.

Patient preparation

If the patient is intubated or has a tracheostomy, you can accomplish CPAP with a mechanical ventilator by adjusting the settings. Assess vital signs and breath sounds during CPAP.

If CPAP is to be delivered through a mask, a respiratory therapist usually sets up the system and fits the mask. The mask should be transparent and lightweight, with a soft, pliable seal. A tight seal isn't required as long as pressure can be maintained. Obtain ABG results and bedside pulmonary function studies to establish a baseline.

Monitoring and aftercare

After CPAP has begun, take these steps:
• Check for decreased cardiac output, which may result from increased intrathoracic pressure associated with CPAP.
• Watch closely for changes in respiratory rate and pattern. Uncoordinated breathing patterns may indicate severe respiratory muscle fatigue that CPAP can't help. Report this to the practitioner; the patient may need mechanical ventilation.
• Check the CPAP system for pressure fluctuations.

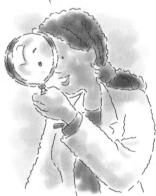

Watch closely for uncoordinated breathing patterns that may indicate severe respiratory muscle fatigue that CPAP can't help.

- Keep in mind that high airway pressures increase the risk of pneumothorax, so monitor for chest pain and decreased breath sounds.
- Use oximetry, if possible, to monitor oxygen saturation, especially when you remove the CPAP mask to provide routine care.
- If the patient is stable, remove his mask briefly every 2 to 4 hours to provide mouth and skin care along with fluids. Don't apply oils or lotions under the mask — they may react with the mask seal material. Increase the length of time the mask is off as the patient's ability to maintain oxygenation without CPAP improves.
- Check closely for air leaks around the mask near the eyes (an area difficult to seal); escaping air can dry the eyes, causing conjunctivitis or other problems.
- If the patient is using a nasal CPAP device for sleep apnea, observe for decreased snoring and mouth breathing while he sleeps. If these signs don't subside, notify the practitioner; either the system is leaking or the pressure is inadequate.

Home care instructions

CPAP for sleep apnea is the only treatment requiring instructions for home care.
- Have the patient demonstrate his ability to maintain the prescribed pressures without excess leakage in the system. Teach him how to clean the mask and change the air filter.
- Explain to the patient that he must use nasal CPAP every night, even when feeling better after initial treatments; apneic episodes will recur if CPAP isn't used as directed. He should call his practitioner if symptoms recur despite consistent use.
- If the patient is obese, explain that CPAP treatments might be decreased or eliminated with weight loss.

Oxygen therapy

In oxygen therapy, oxygen is delivered by mask, nasal prongs, nasal catheter, or transtracheal catheter to prevent or reverse hypoxemia and reduce the work of breathing. Possible causes of hypoxemia include emphysema, pneumonia, Guillain-Barré syndrome, heart failure, and myocardial infarction (MI).

Fully equipped

The equipment depends on the patient's condition and the required fraction of inspired oxygen (FIO_2). High-flow systems, such as a Venturi mask and ventilators, deliver a precisely controlled air-oxygen mixture. Low-flow systems, such as nasal prongs, a nasal catheter, a simple mask, a partial rebreather

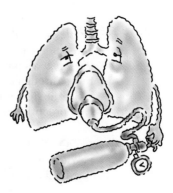

Oxygen therapy prevents or reverses hypoxemia and reduces the work of breathing. Thank you!

mask, and a nonrebreather mask, allow variation in the oxygen percentage delivered, based on the patient's respiratory pattern.

Compare and contrast

Nasal prongs deliver oxygen at flow rates from 0.5 to 6 L/minute. Inexpensive and easy to use, the prongs permit talking, eating, and suctioning — interfering less with the patient's activities than other devices. Even so, the prongs may cause nasal drying and can't deliver high oxygen concentrations. In contrast, a nasal catheter can deliver low-flow oxygen at somewhat higher concentrations, but it isn't commonly used because of discomfort and drying of the mucous membranes. Masks deliver up to 100% oxygen concentrations but can't be used to deliver controlled oxygen concentrations. Also, they may fit poorly, causing discomfort, and must be removed to eat. Transtracheal oxygen catheters, used for patients requiring chronic oxygen therapy, permit highly efficient oxygen delivery and increased mobility with portable oxygen systems and avoid the adverse effects of nasal delivery systems. Even so, they may become a source of infection and require close monitoring and follow-up after insertion as well as daily maintenance care.

Patient preparation

Before oxygen therapy begins, take these steps:
• Instruct the patient, his roommates, and visitors not to use improperly grounded radios, televisions, electric razors, or other equipment. Place an OXYGEN PRECAUTIONS sign on the outside of the patient's door.
• Perform a cardiopulmonary assessment, and check that baseline ABG or oximetry values have been obtained.
• Check the patency of the patient's nostrils (he may need a mask if they're blocked). Consult the practitioner if the patient requires a change in administration route.

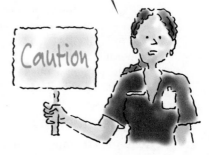

Make sure there's an OXYGEN THERAPY sign on the outside of the patient's door.

Some assembly required

• Assemble the equipment, check the connections, and turn on the oxygen source. Make sure the humidifier bubbles and oxygen flows through the prongs, catheter, or mask.
• Set the flow rate as ordered. If necessary, have the respiratory care practitioner check the flowmeter for accuracy.

Procedure

• When applying a nasal cannula, direct the curved prongs inward, following the nostrils' natural curvature. Hook the tubing

behind the patient's ears and under his chin. Set the flow rate as ordered.
• If you're inserting a nasal catheter, determine the length to insert by stretching one end of the catheter from the tip of the patient's nose to his earlobe. Mark this spot. Then lubricate the catheter with sterile water or water-soluble lubricant and gently insert the catheter through the nostril into the nasopharynx to the premeasured length. Use a flashlight and a tongue blade to check that the catheter is positioned correctly: It should be directly behind the uvula but not beyond it (misdirected airflow may cause gastric distention). If the catheter causes the patient to gag or choke, withdraw it slightly. Secure the catheter by taping it at the nose and cheek, and set the flow rate as ordered.
• When applying a mask, make sure the flow rate is at least 5 L/minute. Lower flow rates won't flush carbon dioxide from the mask. Place the mask over the patient's nose, mouth, and chin and press the flexible metal strip so it fits the bridge of the patient's nose. Use gauze padding to ensure comfort and proper fit.

To rebreathe or not to rebreathe?

• The partial rebreather mask has an attached reservoir bag that conserves the first portion of the patient's exhalation and fills with 100% oxygen before the next breath. The mask delivers oxygen concentrations ranging from 40% at a flow rate of 8 L/minute to 60% at a flow rate of 15 L/minute and depends on the patient's breathing pattern and rate. The nonrebreather mask also has a reservoir bag and can deliver oxygen concentrations ranging from 60% at a flow rate of 8 L/minute to 90% at a flow rate of 15 L/minute. Set flow rates for these masks as ordered, but keep in mind that the reservoir bag should deflate only slightly during inspiration. If it deflates markedly or completely, increase the flow rate until only slight deflation occurs.
• The Venturi mask, another alternative, delivers the most precise oxygen concentrations (to within 1% of the setting). When using this mask, make sure its air entrainment ports don't become blocked or the patient's FIO_2 level could rise dangerously. Venturi masks are available with adapters that allow various oxygen concentrations ranging from 24% to 60%. Adjust oxygen flow to the rate indicated on the adapter.
• If a transtracheal oxygen catheter will be used to deliver oxygen, the doctor will give the patient a local anesthetic before inserting this device into the patient's trachea.

Monitoring and aftercare

After the oxygen delivery system is in place, take these steps:

• Periodically perform a cardiopulmonary assessment on the patient receiving any form of oxygen therapy.

Bed restless

• If the patient is on bed rest, change his position frequently to ensure adequate ventilation and circulation.

• Provide good skin care to prevent irritation and breakdown caused by the tubing, prongs, or mask.

• Humidify oxygen flow exceeding 3 L/minute to help prevent drying of mucous membranes. However, keep in mind that humidity isn't added with Venturi masks because water can block the Venturi jets.

• Assess for signs of hypoxia, including decreased level of consciousness (LOC), tachycardia, arrhythmias, diaphoresis, restlessness, altered blood pressure or respiratory rate, clammy skin, and cyanosis. If these occur, notify the practitioner, obtain a pulse oximetry reading, and check the oxygen delivery equipment to see if it's malfunctioning. Be especially alert for changes in respiratory status when you change or discontinue oxygen therapy.

• If your patient has COPD, monitor him closely. High oxygen levels may decrease respiratory drive in such patients, causing high carbon dioxide levels and respiratory depression.

• If your patient is using a nonrebreather mask, periodically check the valves to see if they're functioning properly. If the valves stick closed, the patient will reinhale carbon dioxide and not receive adequate oxygen. Replace the mask if necessary.

Oxygen high

• If the patient receives high oxygen concentrations (exceeding 50%) for more than 24 hours, ask about signs and symptoms of oxygen toxicity, such as dyspnea, dry cough, and burning, substernal chest pain. Atelectasis and pulmonary edema may also occur. Encourage coughing and deep breathing to help prevent atelectasis. Monitor ABG levels frequently and reduce oxygen concentrations as soon as ABG results indicate this is feasible.

• Use a low flow rate if your patient has chronic pulmonary disease. However, don't use a simple face mask because low flow rates won't flush carbon dioxide from the mask, and the patient will rebreathe carbon dioxide. Watch for alterations in LOC, heart rate, and respiratory rate, which may signal carbon dioxide narcosis or worsening hypoxemia.

> If the patient receives high oxygen concentrations for more than 24 hours, ask about dyspnea, dry cough, and burning, substernal chest pain — signs of oxygen toxicity.

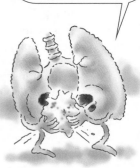

Home care instructions

If the patient needs oxygen at home, the practitioner will order the flow rate, the number of hours per day to be used, and the conditions of use. Several types of delivery systems are available, including a tank, concentrator, and liquid oxygen system. Choose the system based on the patient's needs and the system's availability and cost. Make sure the patient can use the prescribed system safely and effectively. He'll need regular follow-up care to evaluate his response to therapy.

Chest physiotherapy

Chest physiotherapy is usually performed with other treatments, such as suctioning, incentive spirometry, and administration of such medications as small-volume nebulizer aerosol treatments and expectorants. (See *Types of chest physiotherapy.*) Recent studies indicate that percussional vibration isn't an effective treatment for most diseases; exceptions include cystic fibrosis and bronchiectasis. Improved breath sounds, increased PaO_2, sputum production, and improved airflow suggest successful treatment.

Patient preparation

Before chest physiotherapy begins, take these steps:
• Administer pain medication before the treatment as ordered, and teach the patient to splint his incision.
• Auscultate the lungs to determine baseline status, and check the doctor's order to determine which lung areas require treatment.
• Obtain pillows and a tilt board if necessary.
• Don't schedule therapy immediately after a meal; wait 2 to 3 hours to reduce the risk of nausea and vomiting.
• Make sure the patient is adequately hydrated to promote secretion removal.
• If ordered, administer bronchodilator and mist therapies before the treatment.
• Provide tissues, an emesis basin, and a cup for sputum.
• Set up suction equipment if the patient doesn't have an adequate cough to clear secretions.
• If he needs oxygen therapy or is borderline hypoxemic without it, provide adequate flow rates of oxygen during therapy. (See *Performing chest physiotherapy,* page 384.)

Types of chest physiotherapy

Especially important for the bedridden patient, chest physiotherapy improves secretion clearance and ventilation and helps prevent or treat atelectasis and pneumonia. Procedures include:
• postural drainage, which uses gravity to promote drainage of secretions from the lungs and bronchi into the trachea
• percussion, which involves cupping the hands and fingers together and clapping them alternately over the patient's lung fields to loosen secretions (also achieved with the gentler technique of vibration)
• vibration, which can be used with percussion or as an alternative to it in a patient who's frail, in pain, or recovering from thoracic surgery or trauma
• deep-breathing exercises, which help loosen secretions and promote more effective coughing
• coughing, which helps clear the lungs, bronchi, and trachea of secretions and prevents aspiration.

Performing chest physiotherapy

Chest physiotherapy includes postural drainage, percussion, and vibration. Outlined below are the procedures for each method.

Postural drainage

• Position the patient as ordered. (The practitioner usually determines a position sequence after auscultation and chest X-ray review.) Make sure you position the patient so drainage is always oriented toward larger, more central airways.
• If the patient has a localized condition, such as pneumonia in a specific lobe, expect to start with that area first to avoid infecting uninvolved areas. If the patient has a diffuse disorder, such as bronchiectasis, expect to start with the lower lobes and work toward the upper ones.

Percussion

• Place your cupped hands against the patient's chest wall and rapidly flex and extend your wrists, generating a rhythmic, popping sound (a hollow sound helps verify correct performance of the technique).
• Percuss each segment for a minimum of 3 minutes. The vibrations you generate pass through the chest wall and help loosen secretions from the airways.
• Perform percussion throughout inspiration and expiration, and encourage the patient to take slow, deep breaths.
• Don't percuss over the spine, sternum, liver, kidneys, or the female patient's breasts because you may cause trauma, especially in elderly patients.
• Percussion is painless when done properly; the cushion of air formed in the cupped palm diminishes the impact. This technique requires practice.

Vibration

• Ask the patient to inhale deeply and then exhale slowly through pursed lips.
• During exhalation, firmly press your fingers and the palms of your hands against the chest wall. Tense the muscles of your arms and shoulders in an isometric contraction to send fine vibrations through the chest wall.
• Repeat vibration for five exhalations over each chest segment.
• When the patient says "ah" on exhalation, you should hear a tremble in his voice.

Be aware that postural drainage positions can cause nausea, dizziness, dyspnea, and hypoxemia. Ooh, the room keeps spinning!

Monitoring and aftercare

After therapy, take these steps:
• Evaluate the patient's tolerance for therapy and make adjustments as needed. Watch for fatigue and remember that the patient's ability to cough and breathe deeply diminishes as he tires.
• Assess for difficulty expectorating secretions. Use suction if the patient has an ineffective cough or a diminished gag reflex.
• Provide oral hygiene after therapy; secretions may taste foul or have an unpleasant odor.
• Be aware that postural drainage positions can cause nausea, dizziness, dyspnea, and hypoxemia.

Home care instructions

The patient with chronic bronchitis, bronchiectasis, or cystic fibrosis may need chest physiotherapy at home. Teach him and his family the appropriate techniques and positions. Arrange for the patient to get a mechanical percussion and vibration device if necessary.

Nursing diagnoses

After completing your assessment, you're ready to analyze the findings and select nursing diagnoses. Below you'll find nursing diagnoses commonly used in patients with respiratory problems. For each diagnosis, you'll also find nursing interventions along with rationales. See *NANDA-I taxonomy II by domain*, page 936, for the complete list of NANDA diagnoses.

Ineffective breathing pattern

Related to decreased energy or increased fatigue, *Ineffective breathing pattern* is commonly associated with such conditions as COPD and pulmonary embolus.

Expected outcomes

- Patient reports feeling comfortable when breathing.
- Patient achieves maximum lung expansion with adequate ventilation.
- Patient's respiratory rate remains within 5 breaths/minute of baseline.
- Patient's oxygen level remains within acceptable limits.

Nursing interventions and rationales

- Auscultate breath sounds at least every 4 hours to detect decreased or adventitious breath sounds.
- Assess adequacy of ventilation to detect early signs of respiratory compromise.
- Teach breathing techniques to help the patient improve ventilation.
- Teach relaxation techniques to help reduce the patient's anxiety and enhance his feeling of self-control.
- Administer bronchodilators to help relieve bronchospasm and wheezing.
- Administer oxygen as ordered to help relieve hypoxemia and respiratory distress.

Ineffective airway clearance

Related to the presence of tracheobronchial secretions or obstruction, *Ineffective airway clearance* commonly accompanies such conditions as asthma, COPD, interstitial lung disease, cystic fibrosis, and pneumonia.

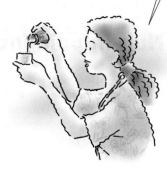

Give expectorants and mucolytics as ordered to enhance airway clearance.

Expected outcomes

- Patient coughs effectively.
- Patient's airway remains patent.
- Adventitious breath sounds are absent.

Nursing interventions and rationales

- Teach coughing techniques to promote chest expansion and ventilation, enhance clearance of secretions from airways, and involve the patient in his own care.
- Perform postural drainage, percussion, and vibration to promote secretion movement.
- Encourage fluids to ensure adequate hydration and liquefy secretions.
- Give expectorants and mucolytics as ordered to enhance airway clearance.
- Provide an artificial airway as needed to maintain airway patency.

Impaired gas exchange

Related to altered oxygen supply or oxygen-carrying capacity of the blood, *Impaired gas exchange* can occur with acute respiratory failure (ARF), COPD, pneumonia, pulmonary embolism, and other respiratory problems.

Expected outcomes

- Patient's respiratory rate remains within 5 breaths/minute of baseline.
- Patient has normal breath sounds.
- Patient's ABG levels return to baseline.

Nursing interventions and rationales

- Give antibiotics as ordered, and monitor their effectiveness in treating infection and improving alveolar expansion.
- Teach deep breathing and incentive spirometry to enhance lung expansion and ventilation.

- Monitor ABG values and notify the practitioner immediately if Pao_2 drops or $Paco_2$ rises. If needed, start mechanical ventilation to improve ventilation.
- Provide CPAP or positive end-expiratory pressure (PEEP) as needed to improve the driving pressure of oxygen across the alveolocapillary membrane, enhance arterial blood oxygenation, and increase lung compliance.

Common respiratory disorders

Below are several common respiratory disorders, along with their causes, pathophysiology, signs and symptoms, diagnostic test findings, treatments, and nursing interventions.

Acute respiratory distress syndrome

A form of pulmonary edema that leads to ARF, acute respiratory distress syndrome (ARDS) results from increased permeability of the alveolocapillary membrane. Although severe ARDS may be fatal, recovering patients may have little or no permanent lung damage.

What causes it

ARDS may result from:
- aspiration of gastric contents
- sepsis (primarily gram-negative)
- trauma (such as lung contusion, head injury, and long-bone fracture with fat emboli)
- oxygen toxicity
- viral, bacterial, or fungal pneumonia
- microemboli (fat or air emboli or disseminated intravascular coagulation)
- drug overdose (such as barbiturates and opioids)
- blood transfusion
- smoke or chemical inhalation (such as nitrous oxide, chlorine, ammonia, and organophosphate)
- hydrocarbon or paraquat ingestion
- pancreatitis, uremia, or miliary TB (rare)
- near drowning.

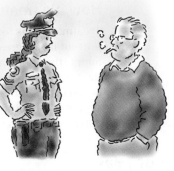

Smoke or chemical inhalation can cause ARDS. Put out that cigarette!

Pathophysiology

In ARDS, fluid accumulates in the lung interstitium, alveolar spaces, and small airways, causing the lung to stiffen. This impairs ventilation and reduces oxygenation of pulmonary capillary blood. (See *What happens in ARDS.*)

What to look for

Assess your patient for the following signs and symptoms:
- rapid, shallow breathing; dyspnea; and hypoxemia
- tachycardia
- intercostal and suprasternal retractions, crackles, and rhonchi
- restlessness, apprehension, mental sluggishness, and motor dysfunction.

What tests tell you

- ABG values on room air show decreased PaO_2 (less than 60 mm Hg) and $PaCO_2$ (less than 35 mm Hg). As ARDS becomes more severe, ABG values show respiratory acidosis, with $PaCO_2$ values elevated above 45 mm Hg. The patient's PaO_2 decreases despite oxygen therapy.
- Noninvasive cardiac output monitoring can help determine the patient's fluid volume status and heart function.
- Pulmonary artery catheterization helps identify the cause of pulmonary edema by evaluating pulmonary artery wedge pressure and allows collection of pulmonary artery blood, which shows decreased oxygen saturation, a sign of tissue hypoxia. It also measures pulmonary artery pressureas well as cardiac output by thermodilution techniques.
- Serial chest X-rays initially show bilateral infiltrates. In later stages, the X-rays have a ground-glass appearance and, as hypoxemia becomes irreversible, shows "whiteouts" in both lung fields.
- Other tests may be done to detect infections, drug ingestion, or pancreatitis.

How it's treated

Treatment aims to correct the underlying cause of ARDS to prevent its progression toward potentially fatal complications. Supportive medical care includes humidified oxygen through a tight-fitting mask, allowing the use of CPAP. When hypoxemia doesn't respond to these measures, patients require ventilatory support with intubation, volume ventilation, and PEEP. Other supportive measures include fluid restriction, diuretics, and correction of electrolyte and acid-base abnormalities.

Just relax...

Patients who receive mechanical ventilation commonly require sedatives and narcotics or neuromuscular blocking agents, such as vecuronium and pancuronium, to minimize anxiety. Decreasing anxiety enhances ventilation by reducing oxygen consumption and carbon dioxide production. If given early, a short course of high-dose steroids

A closer look

What happens in ARDS

The illustrations below show the development of acute respiratory distress syndrome (ARDS).

 Injury reduces normal blood flow to the lungs, allowing platelets to aggregate. These platelets release substances, such as serotonin (S), bradykinin (B), and histamine (H), that inflame and damage the alveolar membrane and later increase capillary permeability.

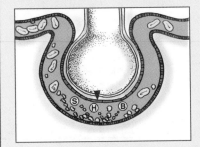

 Histamines (H) and other inflammatory substances increase capillary permeability. Fluids shift into the interstitial space.

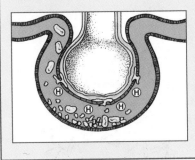

 As capillary permeability increases, proteins and more fluid leak out, causing pulmonary edema.

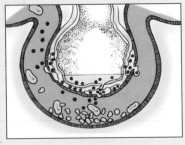

 Fluid in the alveoli and decreased blood flow damage surfactant in the alveoli. This reduces the alveolar cells' ability to produce more surfactant. Without surfactant, alveoli collapse, impairing gas exchange.

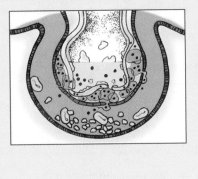

 The patient breathes faster, but sufficient oxygen (O_2) can't cross the alveolar capillary membrane. Carbon dioxide (CO_2), however, crosses more easily and is lost with every exhalation. Both O_2 and CO_2 levels in the blood decrease.

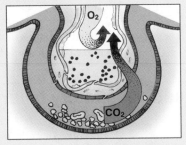

 Pulmonary edema worsens. Meanwhile, inflammation leads to fibrosis, which further impedes gas exchange. The resulting hypoxemia leads to respiratory acidosis.

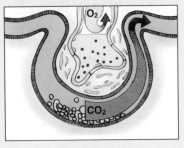

may help patients with ARDS that results from fat emboli or chemical injury to the lungs. Fluids and vasopressors maintain the patient's blood pressure. Nonviral infections require antimicrobial drugs.

What to do

• Carefully monitor your patient and provide supportive care to prepare him for transfer to an intensive care unit (ICU).
• Frequently assess his respiratory status. Watch for retractions on inspiration. Note the rate, rhythm, and depth of respirations, and watch for dyspnea and the use of accessory muscles of respiration. On auscultation, listen for adventitious or diminished breath sounds. Check for pink, frothy sputum, which may indicate pulmonary edema.
• Observe and document the hypoxemic patient's neurologic status. Assess his LOC and observe for mental sluggishness.
• Maintain a patent airway by suctioning the patient as needed.
• Closely monitor heart rate and rhythm and blood pressure.
• Reposition the patient often and observe for hypotension, increased secretions, or elevated body temperature — all signs of deterioration.
• Evaluate the patient. After successful treatment, he should have normal ABG values; a normal respiratory rate, depth, and pattern; and clear breath sounds. (See *ARDS teaching tips.*)

Acute respiratory failure

When the lungs no longer meet the body's metabolic needs, ARF results. In patients with essentially normal lung tissue, ARF usually means $Paco_2$ above 50 mm Hg and Pao_2 below 50 mm Hg. These limits, however, don't apply to patients with COPD, who commonly have a consistently high $Paco_2$ and low Pao_2. In patients with COPD, only acute deterioration in ABG values, with corresponding clinical deterioration, indicates ARF.

What causes it

ARF may develop from any condition that increases the work of breathing and decreases the respiratory drive. Respiratory tract infections, such as bronchitis and pneumonia, are the most common precipitating factors but bronchospasm or accumulated secretions due to cough suppression can also lead to ARF. Other causes of ARF include:
• CNS depression — head trauma or injudicious use of sedatives, narcotics, tranquilizers, or oxygen
• cardiovascular disorders — MI, heart failure, or pulmonary emboli
• airway irritants — smoke or fumes

Education edge

ARDS teaching tips

• Provide emotional support. Advise the patient with acute respiratory distress syndrome (ARDS) that recovery will take some time, with a gradual return to strength.
• If the patient requires mechanical ventilation, provide him with an alternate means of communication.
• Explain medications that are administered and any necessary fluid restrictions.

Cardiovascular disorders can lead to ARF. I didn't mean to cause trouble!

• endocrine and metabolic disorders — myxedema or metabolic alkalosis
• thoracic abnormalities — chest trauma, pneumothorax, or thoracic or abdominal surgery.

Pathophysiology

Respiratory failure results from impaired gas exchange, when the lungs don't oxygenate the blood adequately and fail to prevent carbon dioxide retention. Any condition associated with hypoventilation (a reduction in the volume of air moving into and out of the lung), $\dot{V}/\dot{Q}$ mismatch (too little ventilation with normal blood flow or too little blood flow with normal ventilation), or intrapulmonary shunting (right-to-left shunting in which blood passes from the heart's right side to its left without being oxygenated) can cause ARF if left untreated.

What to look for

Patients with ARF experience hypoxemia and acidemia affecting all body organs, especially the central nervous, respiratory, and cardiovascular systems. Although specific symptoms vary with the underlying cause, you should always assess for:
• altered respirations (increased, decreased, or normal rate; shallow, deep, or alternating shallow and deep respirations; possible cyanosis; crackles, rhonchi, wheezes, or diminished breath sounds on chest auscultation)
• altered mentation (restlessness, confusion, loss of concentration, irritability, tremulousness, diminished tendon reflexes, or papilledema)
• cardiac arrhythmias (from myocardial hypoxia)
• tachycardia (occurs early in response to low PaO_2)
• pulmonary hypertension (increased pressures on the right side of the heart, elevated jugular veins, enlarged liver, and peripheral edema).

What tests tell you

• Progressive deterioration in ABG levels and pH, when compared with the patient's baseline values, strongly suggests ARF. (In patients with essentially normal lung tissue, a pH value below 7.35 usually indicates ARF. However, COPD patients display an even greater deviation in pH values, along with deviations in $PaCO_2$ and PaO_2.)
• Arterial blood gas levels show a pH value of 7.35 or less, PaO_2 of 50 mm Hg or less, and PCO_2 of 50 mm Hg or greater.
• Hematocrit and Hb levels are abnormally low, possibly from blood loss, indicating decreased oxygen-carrying capacity.

• The white blood cell (WBC) count is elevated if ARF results from bacterial infection (Gram stain and sputum culture identify pathogens).

Get the picture

• A chest X-ray shows pulmonary abnormalities, such as emphysema, atelectasis, lesions, pneumothorax, infiltrates, and effusions.
• An electrocardiogram (ECG) shows arrhythmias, which commonly suggest cor pulmonale and myocardial hypoxia.

How it's treated

ARF is an emergency requiring immediate action to correct the underlying cause and restore adequate pulmonary gas exchange. If significant respiratory acidosis persists, the patient may require mechanical ventilation through an ET or a tracheostomy tube. If he doesn't respond to conventional mechanical ventilation, the practitioner may try HFV; prone positioning may also help. Treatment routinely includes antibiotics for infection, bronchodilators and possibly steroids.

What to do

• Closely monitor airway patency and oxygen supply.
• To reverse hypoxemia, administer oxygen at appropriate concentrations to maintain Pao_2 at a minimum of 50 mm Hg. Patients with COPD usually require only small amounts of supplemental oxygen. Watch for a positive response, such as improvement in ABG results and the patient's breathing and color.
• Maintain a patent airway. If the patient is intubated and lethargic, turn him every 1 to 2 hours. Use postural drainage and chest physiotherapy to help clear secretions.
• In an intubated patient, suction the airways as required, after hyperoxygenation. Observe for changes in quantity, consistency, and color of sputum. To prevent aspiration and reduce the risk of ventilator-associated pneumonia, always suction the oropharynx and the area above the cuff of the ET tube before deflating the cuff. Provide humidity to liquefy secretions.
• Observe the patient closely for respiratory arrest. Auscultate for breath sounds. Monitor ABG levels and report any changes immediately.

Fluid situation

• Monitor serum electrolyte levels and correct imbalances; monitor fluid balance by recording fluid intake and output and daily weight.
• Check the cardiac monitor for arrhythmias.
• If the patient requires mechanical ventilation and is unstable, he'll probably be transferred to an ICU. Arrange for his safe transfer.
• Evaluate the patient. Make sure that ABG values are returning to normal, with a PaO_2 greater than 50 mm Hg, and that the patient can make a normal respiratory effort. (See *ARF teaching tips*.)

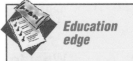

Education edge

ARF teaching tips

• If the patient isn't on mechanical ventilation and is retaining carbon dioxide, encourage him to cough and breathe deeply with pursed lips.
• If the patient is alert, teach and encourage him to use an incentive spirometer.

Atelectasis

Atelectasis (collapsed or airless condition of all or part of the lung) may be chronic or acute and commonly occurs to some degree in patients undergoing abdominal or thoracic surgery. The prognosis depends on prompt removal of airway obstruction, relief of hypoxia, and reexpansion of the collapsed lobules or lung.

What causes it

Atelectasis may result from:
• bronchial occlusion by mucus plugs (a common problem in heavy smokers or people with COPD, bronchiectasis, or cystic fibrosis)
• occlusion by foreign bodies
• bronchogenic carcinoma
• inflammatory lung disease
• oxygen toxicity
• pulmonary edema
• any condition that inhibits full lung expansion or makes deep breathing painful, such as abdominal surgical incisions, rib fractures, tight dressings, obesity, and neuromuscular disorders
• prolonged immobility
• mechanical ventilation using constant small tidal volumes without intermittent deep breaths
• CNS depression (as in drug overdose), which eliminates periodic sighing.

Atelectasis is a collapsed or airless condition in all or part of the lung. I'm feeling a bit flat...

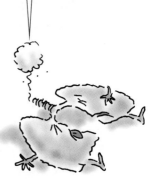

Pathophysiology

In atelectasis, incomplete expansion of lobules (clusters of alveoli) or lung segments leads to partial or complete lung collapse. Because parts of the lung are unavailable for gas exchange, unoxygenated blood passes through these areas unchanged, resulting in hypoxemia.

What to look for

Your assessment findings will vary with the cause and degree of hypoxia and may include:
• dyspnea, possibly mild and subsiding without treatment if atelectasis involves only a small area of the lung; severe if massive collapse has occurred
• cyanosis
• anxiety, diaphoresis
• dull sound on percussion if a large portion of the lung has collapsed
• hypoxemia, tachycardia
• substernal or intercostal retraction
• compensatory hyperinflation of unaffected areas of the lung
• mediastinal shift to the affected side
• decreased or absent breath sounds.

A chest X-ray shows characteristic horizontal lines in the lower lung zones.

What tests tell you

• A chest X-ray shows characteristic horizontal lines in the lower lung zones. Dense shadows accompany segmental or lobar collapse and are commonly associated with hyperinflation of neighboring lung zones during widespread atelectasis. However, extensive areas of "micro-atelectasis" may exist without showing abnormalities on the patient's chest X-ray.
• When the cause of atelectasis is unknown, bronchoscopy may rule out an obstructing neoplasm or a foreign body.

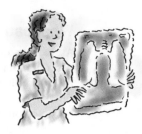

How it's treated

Atelectasis is treated with incentive spirometry, chest percussion, postural drainage, and frequent coughing and deep-breathing exercises. If these measures fail, bronchoscopy may help remove secretions. Humidity and bronchodilators can improve mucociliary clearance and dilate airways and are sometimes used with a nebulizer. Atelectasis secondary to an obstructing neoplasm may require surgery or radiation therapy.

What to do

• Take appropriate steps to keep the patient's airways clear and relieve hypoxia.
• To prevent atelectasis, encourage the patient to cough, turn, and breathe deeply every 1 to 2 hours as ordered. Teach the patient to splint his incision when coughing. Gently reposition a postoperative

patient often and help him walk as soon as possible. Administer adequate analgesics to control pain.
• During mechanical ventilation, make sure tidal volume is maintained at 10 to 15 ml/kg of the patient's body weight to ensure adequate lung expansion. Use the sigh mechanism on the ventilator, if appropriate, to intermittently increase tidal volume at the rate of three to four sighs per hour.
• Humidify inspired air and encourage adequate fluid intake to mobilize secretions. Loosen and clear secretions with postural drainage and chest percussion.
• Assess breath sounds and ventilatory status frequently and report any changes.
• Evaluate the patient. Secretions should be clear and the patient should show no signs of hypoxia. (See *Atelectasis teaching tips*.)

Bronchiectasis

An irreversible condition marked by chronic abnormal dilation of bronchi and destruction of bronchial walls, bronchiectasis can occur throughout the tracheobronchial tree or can be confined to one segment or lobe. However, it's usually bilateral, involving the basilar segments of the lower lobes. It affects people of both sexes and all ages.

What causes it

Bronchiectasis may be caused by such conditions as:
• cystic fibrosis
• immunologic disorders
• recurrent, inadequately treated bacterial respiratory tract infections such as TB
• measles, pneumonia, pertussis, or influenza
• obstruction by a foreign body, tumor, or stenosis associated with recurrent infection
• inhalation of corrosive gas or repeated aspiration of gastric content into the lungs.

Pathophysiology

Bronchiectasis results from repeated damage of bronchial walls and abnormal mucociliary clearance that causes breakdown of supportive tissue adjacent to the airways. This disease has three forms: cylindrical (fusiform), varicose, and saccular (cystic). (See *Forms of bronchiectasis*, page 396.)

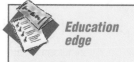

Education edge

Atelectasis teaching tips

• Provide reassurance and emotional support because the patient may be frightened by his limited breathing capacity.
• Teach the patient how to use an incentive spirometer. Encourage him to use it for 10 to 20 breaths every hour while he's awake.
• Teach him about respiratory care, including postural drainage, coughing, and deep breathing.
• Encourage the patient to stop smoking and lose weight as needed. Refer him to appropriate support groups for help.

Forms of bronchiectasis

The different forms of bronchiectasis may occur separately
or simultaneously. In cylindrical
bronchiectasis, the bronchi expand unevenly, with little change
in diameter, and end suddenly in
a squared-off fashion. In varicose
bronchiectasis, abnormal, irregular dilation and narrowing of
the bronchi give the appearance
of varicose veins. In saccular
bronchiectasis, many large dila-
tions end in sacs. These sacs

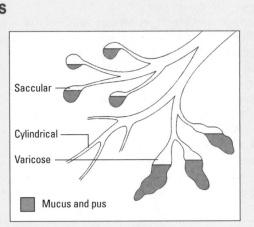

balloon into pus-filled cavities as they approach the periphery and are then called sac-
cules.

What to look for

Initially, bronchiectasis may not produce symptoms. Assess your
patient for a chronic cough that produces copious, foul-smelling,
mucopurulent secretions, possibly totaling several cupfuls daily
(classic symptom). Other characteristic findings include:
• coarse crackles during inspiration over involved lobes or segments
• occasional wheezes
• dyspnea
• weight loss, malaise
• clubbing
• recurrent fever, chills, and other signs of infection.

What tests tell you

• The most reliable diagnostic test, bronchography reveals the
location and extent of disease.
• Chest X-rays show peribronchial thickening, areas of atelecta-
sis, and scattered cystic changes.
• Bronchoscopy helps identify the source of secretions or the site
of bleeding in hemoptysis.
• Sputum culture and Gram stain identify predominant organisms.
• Complete blood count and WBC differential identify anemia and
leukocytosis.
• PFTs detect decreased vital capacity and decreased expiratory
flow.
• ABG analysis shows hypoxemia.

How it's treated

Treatment for bronchiectasis includes:
• antibiotics given by mouth or I.V. for 7 to 10 days or until sputum production decreases
• bronchodilators, with postural drainage and chest percussion, to help remove secretions if the patient has bronchospasm and thick, tenacious sputum
• bronchoscopy used occasionally to aid removal of secretions
• oxygen therapy for hypoxemia
• lobectomy or segmental resection for severe hemoptysis.

What to do

• Provide a warm, quiet, comfortable environment, and urge the patient to rest as much as possible.
• Administer antibiotics as ordered.
• Perform chest physiotherapy several times per day (early morning and bedtime are best); include postural drainage and chest percussion for involved lobes. Have the patient maintain each position for 10 minutes; then perform percussion and tell him to cough.
• Encourage balanced, high-protein meals to promote good health and tissue healing and plenty of fluids to aid expectoration.
• Provide frequent mouth care to remove foul-smelling sputum.
• Evaluate the patient. His secretions should be thin and clear or white. (See *Bronchiectasis teaching tips*.)

Chronic obstructive pulmonary disease

COPD is an umbrella term that could refer to emphysema and chronic bronchitis and, more commonly, a combination of these conditions. Asthma was once classified as a type of COPD and shares some of the same characteristics but it's now considered a distinct chronic inflammatory disorder. The most common chronic lung disease, COPD affects an estimated 30 million Americans, and its incidence is rising. It now ranks fourth among the major causes of death in the United States.

Equal opportunity disease?

The disorder affects more men than women, probably because until recently men were more likely to smoke heavily. However, the rate of COPD among women is increasing. Early COPD may not produce symptoms and may cause only minimal disability in many patients, but it tends to worsen with time.

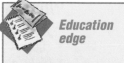

Education edge

Bronchiectasis teaching tips

• Explain all diagnostic tests.
• Show family members how to perform postural drainage and percussion. Also, teach the patient coughing and deep-breathing techniques to promote good ventilation and the removal of secretions.
• Advise the patient to stop smoking, which stimulates secretions and irritates the airways. Refer the patient to a local self-help group.
• Teach the patient to dispose of secretions properly.
• Tell the patient to avoid air pollutants and people with upper respiratory tract infections. Instruct him to take medications (especially antibiotics) exactly as ordered.
• To help prevent this disease, vigorously treat bacterial pneumonia and stress the need for immunization to prevent childhood diseases.

What causes it

COPD may result from:
- cigarette smoking
- recurrent or chronic respiratory tract infection
- allergies
- familial and hereditary factors such as alpha$_1$-antitrypsin deficiency.

Pathophysiology

Smoking, one of the major causes of COPD, impairs ciliary action and macrophage function and causes inflammation in the airways, increased mucus production, destruction of alveolar septa, and peribronchiolar fibrosis. Early inflammatory changes may reverse if the patient stops smoking before lung disease becomes extensive.

The mucus plugs and narrowed airways trap air, as occurs in chronic bronchitis and emphysema, and the alveoli hyperinflate on expiration. On inspiration, airways enlarge, allowing air to pass beyond the obstruction, but they narrow on expiration, preventing gas flow. Air trapping (also called ball valving) occurs commonly in asthma and chronic bronchitis.

What to look for

The typical COPD patient is asymptomatic until middle age, when the following signs and symptoms may occur:
- reduced ability to exercise or do strenuous work
- productive cough
- dyspnea with minimal exertion.

What tests tell you

For specific diagnostic tests used to determine COPD, see *Types of COPD*, pages 400 and 401.

How it's treated

Treatment for COPD aims to relieve symptoms and prevent complications. Most patients receive beta-agonist bronchodilators (albuterol [Proventil HFA] or salmeterol), anticholinergic bronchodilators (ipratropium [Atrovent]), and corticosteroids (beclomethasone [Beconase AQ]). These drugs are usually given by metered dose inhaler.

What to do
• Administer antibiotics as ordered to treat respiratory tract infections.
• Administer low concentrations of oxygen as ordered.
• Check ABG levels regularly to determine oxygen need and to avoid carbon dioxide narcosis.
• Evaluate the patient. The patient's chest X-rays, respiratory rate and rhythm, ABG values, and pH should be approaching normal. He should have a PaO_2 level above 60 mm Hg. He should also have normal body weight and urine output. (See *COPD teaching tips*.)

Pleural effusion

Pleural effusion is an excess of fluid in the pleural space. Normally this space contains a small amount of extracellular fluid that lubricates the pleural surfaces. Increased production or inadequate removal of this fluid results in transudative or exudative pleural effusion. Empyema is the accumulation of pus and necrotic tissue in the pleural space.

What causes it
Transudative pleural effusion can stem from:
• heart failure
• hepatic disease with ascites
• peritoneal dialysis
• hypoalbuminemia
• disorders resulting in overexpanded intravascular volume.
 Exudative pleural effusion can stem from:
• TB
• subphrenic abscess
• esophageal rupture
• pancreatitis
• bacterial or fungal pneumonitis or empyema
• cancer
• pulmonary embolism with or without infarction
• collagen disorders (such as lupus erythematosus and rheumatoid arthritis)
• myxedema
• chest trauma.

Pathophysiology
In transudative pleural effusion, excessive hydrostatic pressure or decreased osmotic pressure allows excessive fluid to pass across intact capillaries, resulting in an ultrafiltrate of plasma containing
(Text continues on page 402.)

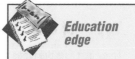

Education edge

COPD teaching tips

• Urge the patient to stop smoking and to avoid other respiratory irritants. Suggest that an air conditioner with an air filter may prove helpful.
• Explain that bronchodilators alleviate bronchospasm and enhance mucociliary clearance of secretions. Familiarize the patient with prescribed bronchodilators. Teach or reinforce the correct method of using an inhaler.
• To strengthen the muscles of respiration, teach the patient to take slow, deep breaths and exhale through pursed lips.
• Teach the patient how to cough effectively to help mobilize secretions. If secretions are thick, urge the patient to maintain adequate hydration.
• If the patient will continue oxygen therapy at home, teach him how to use the equipment correctly.

Types of COPD

This chart lists the types of chronic obstructive pulmonary disease (COPD) along with their causes, pathophysiology, clinical features, confirming diagnostic measures, and management.

Disease	Causes and pathophysiology	Clinical features
Emphysema • Abnormal, irreversible enlargement of air spaces distal to terminal bronchioles due to destruction of alveolar walls, resulting in decreased elastic recoil properties of lungs • Most common cause of death from respiratory disease in the United States	• Cigarette smoking and congenital deficiency of alpha$_1$-antitrypsin • Recurrent inflammation associated with release of proteolytic enzymes from cells in lungs that causes bronchiolar and alveolar wall damage and, ultimately, destruction; decreased elastic recoil and airway collapse on expiration due to loss of lung supporting structure; decreased surface area for gas exchange due to alveolar wall destruction	• Insidious onset, with dyspnea the predominant symptom • *Other signs and symptoms of long-term disease:* anorexia, weight loss, malaise, barrel chest, use of accessory muscles of respiration, prolonged expiratory period with grunting, pursed-lip breathing, and tachypnea • *Complications:* recurrent respiratory tract infections, cor pulmonale, respiratory failure
Chronic bronchitis • Excessive mucus production with productive cough for at least 3 months per year for 2 successive years • Development of significant airway obstruction in only a minority of patients with clinical syndrome of chronic bronchitis	• Severity of disease related to amount and duration of smoking; symptoms exacerbated by respiratory infection • Hypertrophy and hyperplasia of bronchial mucous glands, increased goblet cells, damage to cilia, squamous metaplasia of columnar epithelium, and chronic leukocytic and lymphocytic infiltration of bronchial walls; resistance in small airways and severe ventilation-perfusion imbalance due to widespread inflammation, distortion, narrowing of airways, and mucus within airways	• Insidious onset, with productive cough and exertional dyspnea predominant symptoms • *Other signs and symptoms:* colds associated with increased sputum production and worsening dyspnea, which take progressively longer to resolve; copious sputum (gray, white, or yellow); weight gain due to edema; cyanosis; tachypnea; wheezing; prolonged expiratory time; use of accessory muscles of respiration

Confirming diagnostic measures	Management
• *Physical examination:* hyperresonance on percussion, decreased breath sounds, expiratory prolongation, and quiet heart sounds • *Chest X-ray:* in advanced disease, flattened diaphragm, reduced vascular markings at lung periphery, hyperinflation of lungs, vertical heart, enlarged anteroposterior chest diameter, large retrosternal air space • *Pulmonary function tests:* increased residual volume, total lung capacity, and compliance; decreased vital capacity, diffusing capacity, and expiratory volumes • *Arterial blood gas* (ABG) *analysis:* reduced partial pressure of arterial oxygen (Pao_2) with normal partial pressure of arterial carbon dioxide ($Paco_2$) until late in disease • *Electrocardiogram* (ECG): tall, symmetrical P waves in leads II, III, and aV_F; vertical QRS axis; signs of right ventricular hypertrophy late in disease • *Red blood cell count:* increased hemoglobin level late in disease when persistent severe hypoxia is present	• Oxygen at low-flow settings for hypoxia • Avoidance of smoking and air pollutants • Breathing techniques to control dyspnea • Lung volume reduction surgery for selected patients
• *Physical examination:* rhonchi and wheezes on auscultation, prolonged expiration, jugular vein distention, and pedal edema • *Chest X-ray:* possibly hyperinflation and increased bronchovascular markings • *Pulmonary function tests:* increased residual volume, decreased vital capacity and forced expiratory volumes, normal static compliance and diffusing capacity • *ABG analysis:* decreased Pao_2, normal or increased $Paco_2$ • *ECG:* may show atrial arrhythmias; peaked P waves in leads II, III, and aV_F; and, occasionally, right ventricular hypertrophy	• Antibiotics for infections • Avoidance of smoking and air pollutants • Bronchodilators to relieve bronchospasm and promote mucociliary clearance • Adequate fluid intake and chest physiotherapy to mobilize secretions • Ultrasonic or mechanical nebulizer treatments to loosen and help mobilize secretions • Occasionally, corticosteroids • Diuretics for edema • Oxygen for hypoxemia

low concentrations of protein. In exudative pleural effusion, capillaries exhibit increased permeability, with or without changes in hydrostatic and colloid osmotic pressures, allowing protein-rich fluid to leak into the pleural space. Empyema is usually associated with infection in the pleural space.

What to look for

Assess your patient for the following signs and symptoms:
- dyspnea, dry cough
- pleural friction rub
- possible pleuritic pain that worsens with coughing or deep breathing
- dullness on percussion
- tachycardia, tachypnea
- decreased chest motion and breath sounds.

What tests tell you

- In transudative effusions, pleural fluid (obtained by thoracentesis) has a specific gravity that's usually less than 1.015 and protein less than 3 g/dl.
- In exudative effusions, pleural fluid has a specific gravity that's greater than 1.02, and the ratio of protein in pleural fluid to serum is equal to or greater than 0.5. Pleural fluid lactate dehydrogenase (LD) is equal to or greater than 200 IU, and the ratio of LD in pleural fluid to LD in serum is equal to or greater than 0.6.
- If a pleural effusion results from esophageal rupture or pancreatitis, amylase levels in aspirated fluid are usually higher than serum levels.
- In empyema, cell analysis shows leukocytosis.
- Aspirated fluid may also be tested for lupus erythematosus cells, antinuclear antibodies, and neoplastic cells. It may be analyzed for color and consistency; acid-fast bacillus, fungal, and bacterial cultures; and triglycerides (in chylothorax).
- Chest X-ray shows radiopaque fluid in dependent regions.
- Pleural biopsy may be particularly useful for confirming TB or cancer.

How it's treated

Depending on the amount of fluid present, symptomatic effusion requires either thoracentesis to remove fluid or careful monitoring of the patient's own fluid reabsorption. Hemothorax requires drainage to prevent fibrothorax formation. Associated hypoxia requires supplemental oxygen.

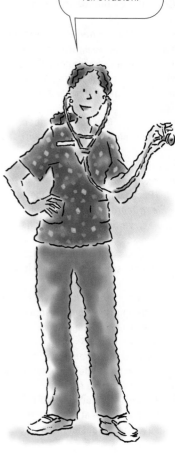

Assess your patient for decreased breath sounds, a sign of pleural effusion.

What to do

- Administer oxygen as ordered.
- Provide meticulous chest tube care and use sterile technique for changing dressings around the tube insertion site in empyema. Record the amount, color, and consistency of tube drainage.
- If the patient has open drainage through a rib resection or an intercostal tube, use hand hygiene and contact precautions. Because weeks of such drainage are usually necessary to obliterate the space, make visiting nurse referrals for patients who will be discharged with the tube in place.
- If pleural effusion was a complication of pneumonia or influenza, advise prompt medical attention for chest colds.
- Evaluate the patient. He should have minimal chest discomfort, be afebrile, and have a normal respiratory pattern. (See *Pleural effusion teaching tips.*)

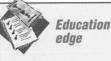

Education edge

Pleural effusion teaching tips

- Explain thoracentesis to the patient.
- Reassure him during the procedure and observe for complications during and after the procedure.
- Encourage the patient to do deep-breathing exercises to promote lung expansion and use an incentive spirometer to promote deep breathing.

Pneumonia

Pneumonia is an acute infection of the lung parenchyma that commonly impairs gas exchange. The prognosis is usually good for people who have normal lungs and adequate host defenses before the onset of pneumonia; however, bacterial pneumonia is the fifth leading cause of death in debilitated patients. The disorder occurs in primary and secondary forms.

What causes it

Pneumonia is caused by an infecting pathogen (bacterial or viral) or by a chemical or other irritant (such as aspirated material). Certain predisposing factors increase the risk of pneumonia. For bacterial and viral pneumonia, these include:

- chronic illness and debilitation
- cancer (particularly lung cancer)
- abdominal and thoracic surgery
- atelectasis, aspiration
- colds or other viral respiratory infections
- chronic respiratory disease, such as COPD, asthma, bronchiectasis, and cystic fibrosis
- smoking, alcoholism
- malnutrition
- sickle cell disease
- tracheostomy
- exposure to noxious gases
- immunosuppressive therapy
- immobility or decreased activity level.

Aspiration pneumonia is more likely to occur in elderly patients.

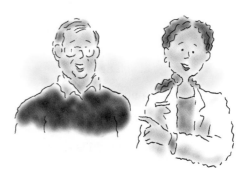

Aspiration pneumonia is more likely to occur in elderly or debilitated patients, those receiving NG tube feedings, and those with an impaired gag reflex, poor oral hygiene, or a decreased LOC.

Pathophysiology

In general, the lower respiratory tract can be exposed to pathogens by inhalation, aspiration, vascular dissemination, or direct contact with contaminated equipment such as suction catheters. After pathogens are inside, they begin to colonize and infection develops.

Stasis report

In bacterial pneumonia, which can occur in any part of the lungs, an infection initially triggers alveolar inflammation and edema. This produces an area of low ventilation with normal perfusion. Capillaries become engorged with blood, causing stasis. As the alveolar capillary membrane breaks down, alveoli fill with blood and exudate, resulting in atelectasis. In severe bacterial infections, the lungs look heavy and liverlike — similar to ARDS.

Virus attack!

In viral pneumonia, the virus first attacks bronchiolar epithelial cells. This causes interstitial inflammation and desquamation. The virus also invades bronchial mucous glands and goblet cells. It then spreads to the alveoli, which fill with blood and fluid.

Subtracting surfactant

In aspiration pneumonia, inhalation of gastric juices or hydrocarbons triggers inflammatory changes and inactivates surfactant over a large area. Decreased surfactant leads to alveolar collapse. Acidic gastric juices may damage the airways and alveoli. Particles containing aspirated gastric juices may obstruct the airways and reduce airflow, leading to secondary bacterial pneumonia.

There are five cardinal signs and symptoms of bacterial pneumonia.

What to look for

The five cardinal signs and symptoms of early bacterial pneumonia are:

- coughing
- sputum production
- pleuritic chest pain
- shaking chills
- fever.

Other signs vary widely, ranging from diffuse, fine crackles to signs of localized or extensive consolidation and pleural effusion.

What tests tell you

• Chest X-rays showing infiltrates and a sputum smear demonstrating acute inflammatory cells support the diagnosis.
• Positive blood cultures in patients with pulmonary infiltrates strongly suggest pneumonia produced by the organisms isolated from the blood cultures.
• Occasionally, a transtracheal aspirate of tracheobronchial secretions or bronchoscopy with brushings may be done to obtain material for smear and culture.

How it's treated

Antimicrobial therapy varies with the infecting agent. Therapy should be reevaluated early in the course of treatment. Supportive measures include:
• humidified oxygen therapy for hypoxemia
• mechanical ventilation for respiratory failure
• a high-calorie diet and adequate fluid intake
• bed rest
• an analgesic to relieve pleuritic chest pain.

What to do

• Maintain a patent airway and adequate oxygenation. Measure ABG levels, especially in hypoxic patients. Administer supplemental oxygen as ordered. If the patient has underlying COPD, give oxygen cautiously.
• Administer antibiotics as ordered and pain medication as needed. Fever and dehydration may require I.V. fluids and electrolyte replacement.

Mangi, mangi!

• Maintain adequate nutrition to offset extra calories burned during infection. Ask the dietary department to provide a high-calorie, high-protein diet consisting of soft, easy-to-eat foods. Encourage the patient to eat and to drink fluids. Monitor fluid intake and output.
• To control the spread of infection, dispose of secretions properly. Teach the patient respiratory hygiene/cough etiquette, and tell him to sneeze and cough into a disposable tissue; tape a waxed bag to the side of the bed for used tissues.
• To prevent aspiration during NG tube feedings, elevate the patient's head, check the position of the tube, and administer feedings slowly. Don't give large volumes at one time because this

could cause vomiting. If the patient has a tracheostomy or an ET tube, inflate the tube cuff. Keep his head elevated for at least 30 minutes after feeding.

• Be aware that antimicrobial agents used to treat cytomegalovirus, PCP, and respiratory syncytial virus pneumonia may be hazardous to fetal development. Pregnant health care workers or those attempting conception should minimize exposure to these agents (such as acyclovir [Zovirax], ribavirin [Virazole], and pentamidine [Pentam 300]).

• Evaluate the patient. His chest X-rays should be normal and his ABG levels should show PaO_2 of 50 to 60 mm Hg. (See *Pneumonia teaching tips.*)

Pneumonia teaching tips

• Teach the patient how to cough and perform deep-breathing exercises to clear secretions.

• Urge all postoperative and bedridden patients to perform deep-breathing exercises frequently. Position patients properly to promote full ventilation and drainage of secretions.

• Encourage annual influenza and pneumococcal vaccination for high-risk patients, such as those with COPD, chronic heart disease, or sickle cell disease.

• To prevent pneumonia, advise the patient to avoid using antibiotics indiscriminately during minor viral infections because this may result in upper airway colonization with antibiotic-resistant bacteria. If the patient then develops pneumonia, the infecting organisms may require treatment with more toxic antibiotics.

Pneumothorax

In pneumothorax, air or gas accumulates between the parietal and visceral pleurae, causing the lungs to collapse. The amount of air or gas trapped determines the degree of lung collapse. In some cases, venous return to the heart is impeded, causing a life-threatening condition called tension pneumothorax.

When spontaneity is a bad thing

Pneumothorax is classified as either traumatic or spontaneous. Traumatic pneumothorax may be further classified as open (sucking chest wound) or closed (blunt or penetrating trauma). An open (penetrating) wound may in turn cause closed pneumothorax if communication between the atmosphere and the pleural space seals itself off. Spontaneous pneumothorax — also considered closed — can be further classified as primary (idiopathic) or secondary (related to a specific disease).

What causes it

Spontaneous pneumothorax can result from:
• ruptured congenital blebs
• ruptured emphysematous bullae
• tubercular or malignant lesions that erode into the pleural space
• interstitial lung disease such as eosinophilic granuloma.
    Traumatic pneumothorax can result from:
• insertion of a central venous access device
• thoracic surgery
• thoracentesis or closed access device
• penetrating chest injury
• transbronchial biopsy.

Understanding tension pneumothorax

In tension pneumothorax, air accumulates intrapleurally and can't escape. Intrapleural pressure rises, collapsing the ipsilateral lung.

On inspiration, the mediastinum shifts toward the unaffected lung, impairing ventilation.

On expiration, the mediastinal shift distorts the vena cava and reduces venous return.

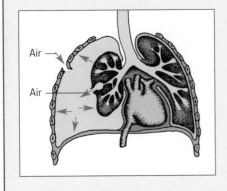

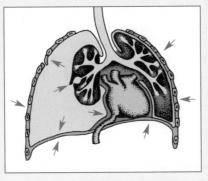

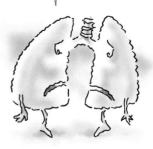

It gets worse! Spontaneous and traumatic pneumothorax can further develop into tension pneumothorax. I'm feeling tense just thinking about it!

Tension pneumothorax can develop from either spontaneous or traumatic pneumothorax. (See *Understanding tension pneumothorax.*)

Pathophysiology

The pathophysiology of pneumothorax varies according to classification.

A change in atmosphere

Open pneumothorax results when atmospheric air (positive pressure) flows directly into the pleural cavity (negative pressure). As the air pressure in the pleural cavity becomes positive, the lung collapses on the affected side. Lung collapse leads to decreased total lung capacity. The patient then develops $\dot{V}/\dot{Q}$ imbalance, leading to hypoxia.

Leaking lung

Closed pneumothorax occurs when air enters the pleural space from within the lung, causing increased pleural pressure and preventing lung expansion during inspiration. It may be called traumatic pneumothorax when blunt chest trauma causes lung tissue to rupture, resulting in air leakage.

The domino effect

Spontaneous pneumothorax is a type of closed pneumothorax. The usual cause is rupture of a subpleural bleb (a small cystic space) at the surface of the lung. This rupture causes air leakage into the pleural spaces; then the lung collapses, causing decreased total lung capacity, vital capacity, and lung compliance — leading, in turn, to hypoxia.

What to look for

Spontaneous pneumothorax may not produce symptoms in mild cases, but profound respiratory distress occurs in moderate to severe cases. Weak and rapid pulse, pallor, jugular vein distention, and anxiety indicate tension pneumothorax. In most cases, look for these symptoms:
- sudden, sharp, pleuritic pain
- asymmetrical chest wall movement
- shortness of breath
- cyanosis
- decreased or absent breath sounds over the collapsed lung
- hyperresonance on the affected side
- crackling beneath the skin on palpation (subcutaneous emphysema).

What tests tell you

- Chest X-rays show air in the pleural space and may reveal mediastinal shift.
- If pneumothorax is significant, ABG findings include pH less than 7.35, PaO_2 less than 80 mm Hg, and $PaCO_2$ above 45 mm Hg.

How it's treated

Treatment is conservative for spontaneous pneumothorax in cases where no signs of increased pleural pressure appear, lung collapse is less than 30%, and the patient shows no signs of dyspnea or other indications of physiologic compromise. Such treatment consists of:
- bed rest or activity as tolerated by the patient
- careful monitoring of blood pressure, pulse rate, and respirations
- oxygen administration
- in some cases, needle aspiration of air with a large-bore needle attached to a syringe.

Conservative treatment for spontaneous pneumothorax includes bed rest. I'm just going to take a nap now...

Also, keep in mind these treatment pointers:
• When more than 30% of the lung has collapsed, reexpansion of the lung is performed by placing a thoracotomy tube in the second or third intercostal space at the midclavicular line. This procedure is done to allow air to rise to the top of the intrapleural space. The tube is connected to an underwater seal with suction at low pressures.
• Recurring spontaneous pneumothorax requires thoracotomy and pleurectomy. These procedures prevent recurrence by causing the lung to adhere to the parietal pleura.
• Traumatic or tension pneumothorax requires chest tube drainage.
• Traumatic pneumothorax may also require surgical repair.

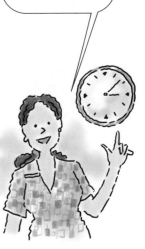

In the patient with pneumothorax, carefully monitor vital signs at least every hour.

What to do
• Watch for pallor, gasping respirations, and sudden chest pain.
• Carefully monitor vital signs at least every hour for indications of shock, increasing respiratory distress, or mediastinal shift. Listen for breath sounds over both lungs. Falling blood pressure with rising pulse and respiratory rates may indicate tension pneumothorax, which can be fatal if not promptly treated.
• Make the patient as comfortable as possible — a patient with pneumothorax is usually most comfortable sitting upright.
• Urge the patient to control coughing and gasping during thoracotomy.

Take a deep breath
• After the chest tube is in place, encourage the patient to cough and breathe deeply at least once per hour to promote lung expansion.
• In the patient undergoing chest tube drainage, watch for continuing air leakage (bubbling) in the water-seal chamber. This indicates the lung defect has failed to close and may require surgery. Also observe for increasing subcutaneous emphysema by checking around the neck or at the tube insertion site for crackling beneath the skin. If the patient is on a ventilator, be alert for any difficulty in breathing in time with the ventilator as you monitor its gauges for pressure increases.
• Change dressings around the chest tube insertion site as needed and as per your facility's policy. Don't reposition or dislodge the tube; if the tube does dislodge, immediately place a petroleum gauze dressing over the opening to prevent rapid lung collapse.
• Observe the chest tube site for leakage, and note the amount and color of drainage. Walk the patient as ordered (usually on the

first postoperative day) to promote deep inspiration and lung expansion.
• Reassure the patient by explaining what occurs with pneumothorax, its causes, and all accompanying diagnostic tests and procedures.
• Evaluate the patient. He should have normal chest X-rays, respiratory rate and depth, and vital signs. (See *Pneumothorax teaching tips*.)

Pulmonary embolism and infarction

Pulmonary embolism is an obstruction of the pulmonary arterial bed by a dislodged thrombus or foreign substance. Pulmonary infarction, or lung tissue death from a pulmonary embolus, is sometimes mild and may not produce symptoms. However, when a massive embolism occurs involving more than 50% obstruction of pulmonary arterial circulation, it can be rapidly fatal.

What causes it

Pulmonary embolism usually results from dislodged thrombi that originate in the leg veins. Other less common sources of thrombi are the pelvic, renal, hepatic, and arm veins and the right side of the heart.

Pathophysiology

Trauma, clot dissolution, sudden muscle spasm, intravascular pressure changes, or a change in peripheral blood flow can cause the thrombus to loosen or fragmentize. Then the thrombus — now called an embolus — floats to the heart's right side and enters the lung through the pulmonary artery. There, the embolus may dissolve, continue to fragmentize, or grow.

Death threat

If the embolus occludes the pulmonary artery, alveoli collapse and atelectasis develops. If the embolus enlarges, it may clog most or all of the pulmonary vessels and cause death.

A rare find

Rarely, the emboli contain air, fat, amniotic fluid, or tumor cells. They may also contain talc from drugs intended for oral administration that I.V. drug addicts have injected. Pulmonary embolism may lead to pulmonary infarction, especially in patients with chronic heart or pulmonary disease.

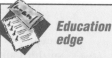

Education edge

Pneumothorax teaching tips

• Encourage the patient to perform hourly deep-breathing exercises when awake.
• Discuss the potential for recurrent spontaneous pneumothorax, and review its signs and symptoms. Emphasize the need for immediate medical intervention if these occur.

What to look for

Total occlusion of the main pulmonary artery is rapidly fatal; smaller or fragmented emboli produce symptoms that vary with the size, number, and location of the emboli. Dyspnea is usually the first symptom of pulmonary embolism and may be accompanied by anginal or sharp pleuritic chest pain that worsens with inspiration. Other clinical features include tachycardia, productive cough (sputum may be blood-tinged), and low-grade fever.

Less common signs include massive hemoptysis, splinting of the chest, and leg edema. A large embolus may produce right-sided heart failure with cyanosis, syncope, and distended jugular veins. Signs of shock (such as weak, rapid pulse and hypotension) and hypoxia (such as restlessness) may also occur. Cardiac auscultation occasionally reveals a right ventricular third heart sound audible at the lower sternum and increased intensity of a pulmonary component of the second heart sound. Crackles and a pleural friction rub may be heard at the infarction site.

What tests tell you

• Chest X-rays show a characteristic wedge-shaped infiltrate that suggests pulmonary embolism. X-ray studies may also rule out other pulmonary diseases and reveal areas of atelectasis, an elevated diaphragm, pleural effusion, and a prominent pulmonary artery.
• Lung scan shows perfusion defects in areas beyond occluded vessels; a normal lung scan rules out pulmonary embolism.
• Spiral CT angiography can help visualize the embolus and lungs.

Risky business

• Pulmonary angiography is the most definitive test but poses some risk to the patient (such as allergic reaction to the dye, infection at the catheter site, and kidney failure related to difficulty excreting dye). Its use depends on the uncertainty of the diagnosis and the need to avoid unnecessary anti-coagulant therapy (treatment of pulmonary embolism) in high-risk patients.
• ECG is inconclusive but helps distinguish pulmonary embolism from MI. In extensive embolism, the ECG may show right axis deviation; right bundle-branch block; tall, peaked P waves; depressed ST segments and T-wave inversions (indicating right heart strain); and supraventricular tachyarrhythmias.

Memory jogger

When you assess a patient with a possible pulmonary embolism who has a productive cough—especially if the sputum is tinged with blood—assess for these signs, and think **FAST**:

Fever (low grade)

Anginal or pleuritic chest pain (possible)

Shortness of breath (dyspnea)

Tachycardia.

An ECG can help distinguish pulmonary embolism from MI.

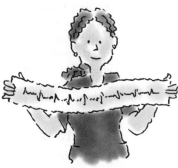

- ABG measurements showing decreased Pao_2 and $Paco_2$ are characteristic but don't always occur.
- An elevated D-dimer level indicates the presence of a blood clot in the body and strongly suggests a pulmonary embolism.

How it's treated

Treatment aims to maintain adequate cardiovascular and pulmonary function as the obstruction resolves and to prevent recurrence. Because most emboli resolve within 10 days, treatment consists of oxygen therapy as needed and anticoagulation with heparin to inhibit new thrombus formation.

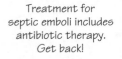

Treatment for septic emboli includes antibiotic therapy. Get back!

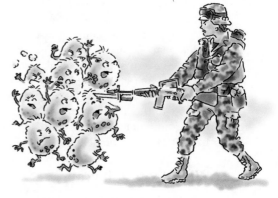

Massive means more

Patients with massive pulmonary embolism and shock may require thrombolytic therapy with a tissue plasminogen activator such as (Alteplase) to enhance fibrinolysis of the pulmonary emboli and remaining thrombi. Hypotension related to pulmonary emboli may be treated with vasopressors.

Seek the septic source

Treatment for septic emboli requires antibiotic therapy as well as evaluation of the source of infection, particularly in cases of endocarditis. Anticoagulants aren't used to treat septic emboli.

Surgery saved for last

Surgery to interrupt the inferior vena cava is reserved for patients for whom anticoagulants are contraindicated (for example, because of age, recent surgery, or blood dyscrasia) or who have recurrent emboli during anticoagulant therapy. It should only be performed when pulmonary embolism is confirmed by angiography. Surgery may consist of vena caval ligation, plication, or insertion of an umbrella filter for blood returning to the heart and lungs. The patient may receive a combination of low-dose heparin or low-molecular-weight heparin (enoxaparin [Lovenox]) to prevent postoperative venous thromboembolism.

What to do

- Give oxygen by nasal cannula or mask.
- Check ABG levels if fresh emboli develop or dyspnea worsens.

• Be prepared to provide equipment for ET intubation and assisted ventilation if breathing is severely compromised. If necessary, prepare to transfer the patient to an ICU according to facility policy.
• Administer heparin as ordered through continuous drip.
• Monitor coagulation studies daily and after changes in heparin dosage. Maintain adequate hydration to avoid the risk of hypercoagulability.

Walking the walk

• After the patient is stable, encourage him to move about often and assist with isometric and ROM exercises. Check his temperature and the color of his feet to detect venostasis. Never vigorously massage the patient's legs. Walk the patient as soon as possible after surgery to prevent venostasis.
• Report frequent pleuritic chest pain so that analgesics can be prescribed.
• Evaluate the patient. His vital signs should be within normal limits, and he should show no signs of bleeding after anticoagulant therapy. (See *Pulmonary embolism and infarction teaching tips.*)

Education edge

Pulmonary embolism and infarction teaching tips

• Teach the patient how to use an incentive spirometer to assist in deep breathing.
• Encourage activity as tolerated to reduce venous stasis and prevent thrombus formation. Warn the patient not to cross his legs; this promotes thrombus formation.
• Encourage family participation in care. Most patients need treatment with an oral anticoagulant (such as warfarin [Coumadin]) for 4 to 6 months (sometimes longer) after a pulmonary embolism.
• Advise the patient to watch for signs of bleeding from anticoagulants, to take the prescribed medication exactly as ordered, and to avoid taking any additional medication (even for headaches or colds) or changing medication dosages without consulting his doctor.
• Stress the importance of follow-up laboratory tests to monitor anticoagulant therapy.

Tuberculosis

TB is an acute or chronic infection characterized by pulmonary infiltrates and formation of granulomas with caseation, fibrosis, and cavitation. The American Lung Association estimates that active TB afflicts nearly 5 out of every 100,000 people. The prognosis is excellent with correct treatment.

What causes it

Mycobacterium tuberculosis is the major cause of TB. Other strains of mycobacteria may also be involved. Several factors increase the risk of infection, including:
- gastrectomy
- uncontrolled diabetes mellitus
- Hodgkin's disease
- leukemia
- treatment with corticosteroid therapy or immunosuppressant therapy
- silicosis
- human immunodeficiency virus infection.

Pathophysiology

TB spreads by inhalation of droplet nuclei when infected persons cough or sneeze. Here's what happens:

On the move

- *Transmission* — An infected person coughs or sneezes, spreading infected droplets. When someone without immunity inhales these droplets, the bacilli are deposited in the lungs.

Rallying the troops

- *Immune response* — The immune system responds by sending leukocytes, and inflammation results. After a few days, macrophages replace the leukocytes. The macrophages then ingest the bacilli, and the lymphatics carry the bacilli off to the lymph nodes.

We have you surrounded...

- *Tubercle formation* — Macrophages that ingest the bacilli fuse to form epithelioid cell tubercles (tiny nodules surrounded by lymphocytes). Within the lesion, caseous necrosis develops and scar

The first step in TB infection is inhalation of infected droplets. Then the battle begins!

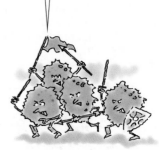

tissue encapsulates the tubercle. The organism may be killed in the process.

...come out with your hands up!

• *Dissemination* — If the tubercles and inflamed nodes rupture, the infection contaminates the surrounding tissue and may spread through the blood and lymphatic circulation to distant sites. This process is called *hematogenous dissemination.*

What to look for

In primary infection, the disease usually doesn't produce symptoms. However, it may produce nonspecific signs and symptoms such as:
• fatigue
• cough
• anorexia
• weight loss
• night sweats
• low-grade fever.

In reinfection, the patient may experience cough, productive mucopurulent sputum, and chest pain.

What tests tell you

• Chest X-rays show nodular lesions, patchy infiltrates (many in upper lobes), cavity formation, scar tissue, and calcium deposits. However, they may not distinguish active from inactive TB.
• Tuberculin skin tests detect exposure to TB but don't distinguish the disease from uncomplicated infection. Patients from non–North American countries may test positive for TB by skin test because of the positive antibody titer produced by the bacille Calmette-Guérin live vaccine they received as children.
• Stains and cultures of sputum, CSF, urine, drainage from abscesses, or pleural fluid show heat-sensitive, nonmotile, aerobic, acid-fast bacilli and confirm the diagnosis.

How it's treated

Antitubercular therapy with daily oral doses of isoniazid, rifampin (Rifadin), and pyrazinamide (and sometimes with ethambutol [Myambutol] or streptomycin) for at least 6 months usually cures TB. After 2 to 4 weeks, the disease is typically no longer infectious, and the patient can resume his normal lifestyle while continuing to take medication. The patient with atypical myco- bacterial disease or drug-resistant TB may require second-line drugs, such as capreomycin (Capastat), streptomycin, cycloserine (Seromycin), amikacin, and quinolones.

What to do

• Isolate the infectious patient in a negative-pressure room until he's no longer contagious.
• Watch for adverse effects of medications. Pyridoxine (vitamin B_6) is sometimes recommended to prevent peripheral neuropathy caused by large doses of isoniazid. If the patient receives etham- butol, watch for optic neuritis; if it develops, discontinue the drug. Observe for hepatitis and purpura in patients receiving rifampin.
• Evaluate the patient. His sputum culture should be negative and secretions should be thin and clear. (See *Tuberculosis teaching tips*.)

Education edge

Tuberculosis teaching tips

• Teach the isolated patient to cough and sneeze into tissues and to dispose of secretions properly.
• Instruct the patient to wear a mask when he leaves his room. Visitors and personnel should wear high-efficiency particulate air respirator masks when in his room.
• Remind the patient to get plenty of rest.
• Stress the importance of eating balanced meals. Record weight weekly.
• Teach him the signs of adverse medication effects; warn him to report them immediately.
• Emphasize the importance of regular follow-up examinations to watch for recurring tuberculosis.
• Advise persons who have been exposed to infected patients to re- ceive appropriate tests.

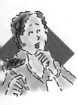

Quick quiz

1. Which type of breath sound is medium-pitched and continuous, occurs over the upper third of the sternum in the interscapular area, and is equally audible during inspiration and expiration?
    A. Vesicular
    B. Bronchial
    C. Bronchovesicular
    D. Tracheal

Answer: C. Bronchovesicular breath sounds demonstrate these characteristics.

2. Your patient's ABG analysis shows a pH less than 7.35, bicarbonate greater than 26 mEq/L, and a $Paco_2$ greater than 45 mm Hg. He's diaphoretic, has tachycardia, and is restless. Which condition does he probably have?
    A. Respiratory alkalosis
    B. Respiratory acidosis
    C. Metabolic alkalosis
    D. Metabolic acidosis

Answer: B. The patient with respiratory acidosis can display all of these signs and symptoms and can also have headache, confusion, apprehension, and a flushed face.

3. When suctioning a patient, you should:
    A. apply suction intermittently as the catheter is inserted.
    B. suction the patient for longer than 10 seconds each time.
    C. oxygenate the patient's lungs before and after suctioning.
    D. apply suction continuously while inserting the catheter.

Answer: C. The patient should be oxygenated before and after suctioning to reduce the risk of hypoxemia. Avoid suctioning for longer than 10 seconds and apply suction intermittently as you withdraw — not insert — the catheter.

4. TB is transmitted through:
    A. inhalation of infected droplets.
    B. contact with blood.
    C. the fecal-oral route.
    D. skin-to-skin contact.

Answer: A. TB spreads by inhalation of droplet nuclei when an infected person coughs or sneezes.

Scoring

★★★ If you answered all four questions correctly, way to go! You can breathe easy about your knowledge of respiratory disorders.

★★ If you answered three questions correctly, great! Your understanding of respiratory disorders is circulating well!

★ If you answered fewer than three questions correctly, no worries! Take a deep breath, oxygenate those tissues, and review the chapter.

Gastrointestinal disorders

Just the facts

In this chapter, you'll learn:

◆ anatomy and physiology of the GI system

◆ important questions and discussion topics for the health history

◆ techniques for assessing the GI system and interpreting abnormal findings

◆ relevant nursing diagnoses for GI disorders

◆ nursing care for common GI disorders.

A look at gastrointestinal disorders

As the site of the body's digestive processes, the GI system has the critical task of supplying essential nutrients to fuel the brain, heart, and lungs. GI function also profoundly affects the quality of life through its impact on overall health.

Anatomy and physiology

The GI system's major functions include ingestion and digestion of food and elimination of waste products. When these processes are interrupted, the patient can experience problems ranging from loss of appetite to acid-base imbalances.

The GI system consists of two major divisions: the GI tract and the accessory organs. (See *GI system structures*, page 420.)

> The GI system has the critical task of supplying essential nutrients to fuel the brain, heart, and lungs. Okay, everyone, time for some dinner!

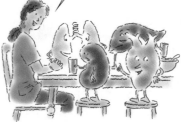

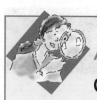

A closer look

GI system structures

This illustration shows the GI system's major anatomic structures. Knowing these structures will help you conduct an accurate physical assessment.

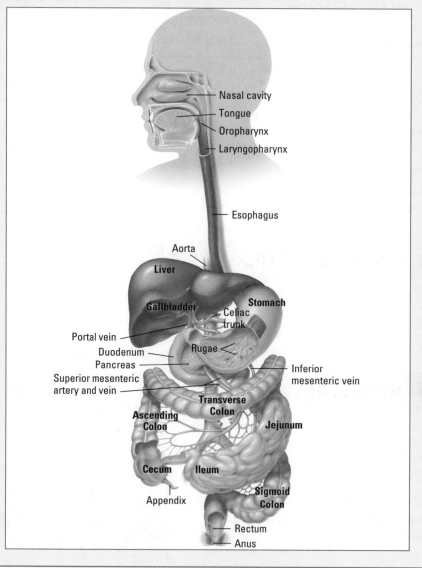

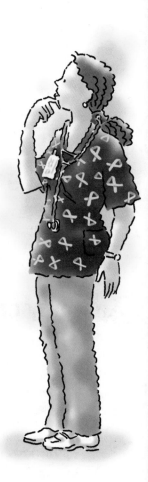

GI tract

The GI tract is a hollow tube that begins at the mouth and ends at the anus. About 25′ (7.5 m) long, it consists of smooth muscle alternating with blood vessels and nerve tissue. Specialized circular and longitudinal fibers contract, causing peristalsis, which helps propel food through the GI tract. The GI tract includes the pharynx, esophagus, stomach, small intestine, and large intestine.

Move into the mouth

Digestive processes begin in the mouth with chewing, salivating, and swallowing. The tongue provides the sense of taste. Saliva is produced by three pairs of glands: the parotid, submandibular, and sublingual.

Proceed to the pharynx

The pharynx, or throat, allows the passage of food from the mouth to the esophagus. The pharynx assists in the swallowing process and secretes mucus that aids in digestion. The epiglottis — a thin, leaf-shaped structure made of fibrocartilage — lies directly behind the root of the tongue. When food is swallowed, the epiglottis closes over the larynx, and the soft palate lifts to block the nasal cavity. These actions keep food and fluid from being aspirated into the airway.

Enter the esophagus

The esophagus is a muscular, hollow tube about 10″ (25.5 cm) long that moves food from the pharynx to the stomach. When food is swallowed, the upper esophageal sphincter relaxes, and the food moves into the esophagus. Peristalsis then propels the food toward the stomach. The gastroesophageal sphincter at the lower end of the esophagus normally remains closed to prevent reflux of gastric contents. The sphincter opens during swallowing, belching, and vomiting.

Slide into the stomach

The stomach, a reservoir for food, is a dilated, saclike structure that lies obliquely in the left upper quadrant below the esophagus and diaphragm, to the right of the spleen, and partly under the liver. The stomach contains two important sphincters: the cardiac sphincter, which protects the entrance to the stomach, and the pyloric sphincter, which guards the exit.

The stomach has three major functions. It:

stores food

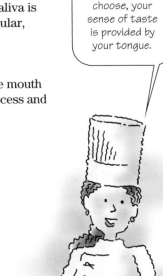

No matter what you choose, your sense of taste is provided by your tongue.

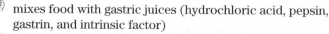 mixes food with gastric juices (hydrochloric acid, pepsin, gastrin, and intrinsic factor)

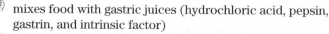 passes chyme — a watery mixture of partly digested food and digestive juices — into the small intestine for further digestion and absorption.

An average meal can remain in the stomach for 3 to 4 hours. Accordion-like folds in the stomach lining called *rugae* allow the stomach to expand when large amounts of food and fluid are ingested.

I can hold on to an average meal for 3 to 4 hours. Thanks to my rugae, I can expand for those larger-than-average meals, too!

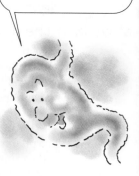

Slip through the small intestine

The small intestine is about 20′ (6 m) long and is named for its diameter, not its length. It has three sections: the duodenum, the jejunum, and the ileum. As food passes into the small intestine, the end products of digestion are absorbed through its thin mucous membrane lining into the bloodstream.

Carbohydrates, fats, and proteins are broken down in the small intestine. Enzymes from the pancreas, bile from the liver, and hormones from glands of the small intestine all aid digestion. These secretions mix with the food as it moves through the intestines by peristalsis.

Last stop, the large intestine

The large intestine, or colon, is about 5′ (1.5 m) long and is responsible for:
• absorbing excess water and electrolytes
• storing food residue
• eliminating waste products in the form of feces.

The large intestine includes the cecum; the ascending, transverse, descending, and sigmoid colons; the rectum; and the anus — in that order. The appendix, a fingerlike projection, is attached to the cecum. Bacteria in the colon produce gas or flatus.

Accessory organs

Accessory GI organs include the liver, pancreas, gallbladder, and bile ducts. The abdominal aorta and the gastric and splenic veins also aid the GI system.

Look at the liver

The liver is located in the right upper quadrant under the diaphragm. It has two major lobes, divided by the falciform ligament. The liver is the heaviest organ in the body, weighing about 3 lb (1.5 kg) in an adult.

The liver's functions include:
• metabolizing carbohydrates, fats, and proteins

- detoxifying blood
- converting ammonia to urea for excretion
- synthesizing plasma proteins, nonessential amino acids, vitamin A, and essential nutrients, such as iron and vitamins D, K, and B_{12}.

The liver also secretes bile, a greenish fluid that helps digest fats and absorb fatty acids, cholesterol, and other lipids. Bile also gives stool its color.

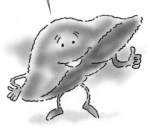

I'm a metabolizing, detoxifying, synthesizing wonder!

Gaze at the gallbladder

The gallbladder is a small, pear-shaped organ about 4″ (10 cm) long that lies halfway under the right lobe of the liver. Its main function is to store bile from the liver until the bile is emptied into the duodenum. This process occurs when the small intestine initiates chemical impulses that cause the gallbladder to contract.

Presenting the pancreas

The pancreas, which measures 6″ to 8″ (15 to 20 cm) in length, lies horizontally in the abdomen behind the stomach. It consists of a head, tail, and body. The body of the pancreas lies in the right upper quadrant, and the tail is in the left upper quadrant, attached to the duodenum. The tail of the pancreas touches the spleen. The pancreas releases insulin and glycogen into the bloodstream and releases pancreatic enzymes into the duodenum for digestion.

Behold the bile ducts

The bile ducts provide a passageway for bile to travel from the liver to the intestines. Two hepatic ducts drain the liver, and the cystic duct drains the gallbladder. These ducts converge into the common bile duct, which then empties into the duodenum.

View the vasculature

The abdominal aorta supplies blood to the GI tract. It enters the abdomen and then splits into many branches that supply blood to the length of the GI tract.

The gastric and splenic veins drain absorbed nutrients into the portal vein of the liver. After entering the liver, the venous blood circulates and then exits the liver through the hepatic vein, emptying into the inferior vena cava.

Assessment

GI disorders can have many baffling signs and symptoms. To help sort out significant symptoms, you'll need to take a thorough patient history. Then you'll probe further by conducting a thorough physical examination, using inspection, auscultation, palpation, and percussion.

History

To help track the development of relevant signs and symptoms over time, you'll need to develop a detailed patient history.

Current health status

Ask the patient about changes in appetite, difficulty chewing or swallowing, indigestion, nausea, vomiting, diarrhea, constipation, and abdominal pain. Has he noticed a change in bowel movements? Has he ever seen blood in his stool?

Drug difficulties

Ask the patient if he's taking any medications. Some drugs — including aspirin, sulfonamides, nonsteroidal anti-inflammatory drugs (NSAIDs), and some antihypertensives — can cause GI signs and symptoms.

Don't forget to ask about laxative use; habitual use may cause constipation. Also ask the patient if he's allergic to medications or foods. Such allergies commonly cause GI symptoms.

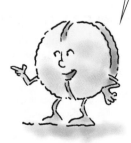

Ask your patient about medications he's taking. Some drugs — including aspirin — can cause GI symptoms.

Previous health status

To determine if your patient's problem is new or recurring, ask about past GI illnesses, such as ulcers, gallbladder disease, inflammatory bowel disease, gastroesophageal reflux, or GI bleeding. Also ask if he has had abdominal surgery or trauma.

Family history

Because some GI disorders are hereditary, ask the patient whether anyone in his family has had a GI disorder. Disorders with a familial link include:
• ulcerative colitis
• GI cancer
• stomach ulcers
• diabetes
• alcoholism
• Crohn's disease.

Lifestyle patterns

Inquire about your patient's occupation, home life, financial situation, stress level, and recent life changes. Be sure to ask about alcohol, caffeine, and tobacco use as well as food consumption, meal frequency, exercise habits, and oral hygiene. Also ask about sleep patterns. How many hours of sleep does he feel he needs? How many does he get?

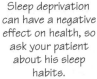

Sleep deprivation can have a negative effect on health, so ask your patient about his sleep habits.

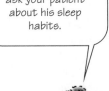

Physical examination

Physical assessment of the GI system includes evaluation of the mouth, abdomen, liver, and rectum. To perform an abdominal assessment, use this sequence: inspection, auscultation, percussion, and palpation. Palpating or percussing the abdomen before you auscultate it can change the character of the patient's bowel sounds and lead to an inaccurate assessment.

Mouth

Use inspection and palpation to assess the mouth.

Open wide

First, inspect the patient's mouth and jaw for asymmetry and swelling. Check his bite, noting malocclusion from an overbite or underbite. Inspect the inner and outer lips, teeth, and gums with a penlight. Note bleeding, gum ulcerations, and missing, displaced, or broken teeth. Palpate the gums for tenderness and the inner lips and cheeks for lesions.

Now, stick out your tongue

Assess the tongue, checking for coating, tremors, swelling, and ulcerations. Note unusual breath odors. Finally, examine the pharynx, looking for uvular deviation, tonsillar abnormalities, lesions, plaques, and exudate.

Abdomen

Have the patient lie in the supine position, with knees slightly flexed. Use inspection, auscultation, percussion, and palpation to examine the abdomen. Assess painful areas last to help prevent the patient from experiencing increased discomfort and tension.

Inspection

Begin by mentally dividing the abdomen into four quadrants and then imagining the organs in each quadrant. (See *Abdominal quadrants*, page 426.)

Abdominal quadrants

To perform a systematic GI assessment, you can visualize abdominal structures by dividing the abdomen into four quadrants, as shown here.

Right upper quadrant
- Right lobe of liver
- Gallbladder
- Pylorus
- Duodenum
- Head of the pancreas
- Hepatic flexure of the colon
- Portions of the ascending and transverse colon

Left upper quadrant
- Left lobe of liver
- Stomach
- Body of the pancreas
- Splenic flexure of the colon
- Portions of the transverse and descending colon

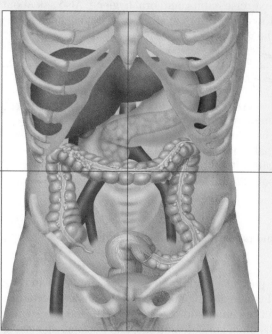

Right lower quadrant
- Cecum and appendix
- Portion of the ascending colon

Left lower quadrant
- Sigmoid colon
- Portion of the descending colon

Learn the lingo

You can more accurately pinpoint your physical findings at the midline by knowing these three terms:

epigastric — above the umbilicus and between the costal margins

umbilical — around the navel

suprapubic — above the symphysis pubis.

The shape of things

Observe the abdomen for symmetry, checking for bumps, bulges, or masses. Also note the patient's abdominal shape and contour.

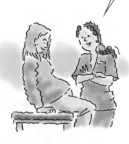

Observe the patient's abdomen for symmetry, checking for bumps, bulges, and masses. Now, *that's* a bulge that should be gone very soon!

Assess the umbilicus, which should be located midline in the abdomen and inverted. If his umbilicus protrudes, the patient may have an umbilical hernia.

Scanning the skin

The skin of the abdomen should be smooth and uniform in color. Note stretch marks, or *striae*, and dilated veins. Record the length of any surgical scars on the abdomen.

Riding the peristaltic wave

Note abdominal movements and pulsations. Usually, waves of peristalsis can't be seen; if they're visible, they look like slight, wavelike motions. If you observe visible rippling waves, report them immediately; they may indicate bowel obstruction. In thin patients, pulsation of the aorta is visible in the epigastric area. Marked pulsations may occur with hypertension, aortic aneurysm, and other conditions causing widening pulse pressure.

Auscultation

Lightly place the stethoscope diaphragm in the right lower quadrant, slightly below and to the right of the umbilicus. Auscultate in a clockwise fashion in each of the four quadrants, spending at least 2 minutes in each area. Note the character and quality of bowel sounds in each quadrant. In some cases, you may need to auscultate for 5 minutes before you hear sounds. Be sure to allow enough time for listening in each quadrant before you decide that bowel sounds are absent.

Before auscultating the abdomen of a patient with a gastric or an abdominal tube connected to suction, such as a nasogastric (NG) tube, briefly clamp the tube or turn off the suction. Suction noises can obscure or mimic actual bowel sounds.

Pardon my borborygmus

In a normal bowel, you'll hear high-pitched, gurgling noises caused by air mixing with fluid during peristalsis. The noises vary in frequency, pitch, and intensity and occur irregularly from 5 to 34 times per minute. They're loudest before mealtimes. Borborygmus, or stomach growling, is the loud, gurgling, splashing bowel sound heard over the large intestine as gas passes through it.

Bowel sounds are classified as normal, hypoactive, or hyperactive.

Humming along

Auscultate for vascular sounds with the bell of the stethoscope. (See *Vascular sounds.*) Using firm pressure, listen over the aorta and renal, iliac, and femoral arteries for bruits. Check for venous hums over the portal vein, inferior vein cava, and common iliac veins.

Vascular sounds

Use the bell of your stethoscope to auscultate for vascular sounds at the sites shown in this illustration.

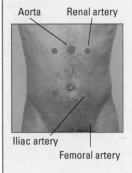

Aorta   Renal artery

Iliac artery

Femoral artery

Percussion

Direct or indirect percussion is used to determine the size and location of abdominal organs and to detect air or fluid in the abdomen, stomach, or bowel. In direct percussion, strike your hand or finger directly against the patient's abdomen. In indirect percussion, use the middle finger of your dominant hand or a percussion hammer to strike a finger resting on the patient's abdomen. Begin percussion in the right lower quadrant and proceed clockwise, covering all four quadrants. Don't percuss the abdomen of a patient with an abdominal aortic aneurysm because doing so can precipitate a rupture.

Tympany: Never a dull moment

Normally, you'll hear two sounds during percussion of the abdomen: tympany and dullness. When you percuss over hollow organs, such as an empty stomach or bowel, you'll hear a clear, hollow sound like a drum beating. This sound, tympany, predominates because the stomach and bowel normally contain air. The degree of tympany depends on the amount of air and gastric dilation.

When you percuss over solid organs — such as the liver, kidney, or feces-filled intestines — the sound changes to dullness. Note where percussed sounds change from tympany to dullness.

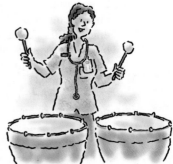

I've always loved the percussion section — especially the tympany. You won't hear any dull playing here!

Sounding out the liver

Percussion of the liver can help you estimate its size. (See *Percussing and measuring the liver.*) Hepatomegaly is commonly associated with hepatitis and other liver diseases. Liver borders may be obscured and difficult to assess.

Dull, yes — but never boring!

The spleen is located at about the level of the 10th rib, in the left midaxillary line. Percussion may produce a small area of dullness, generally 7″ (18 cm) or less in adults. However, the spleen usually can't be percussed because tympany from the colon masks the dullness of the spleen.

To assess a patient for splenic enlargement, ask him to breathe deeply. Then percuss along the 9th to 11th intercostal spaces on the left, listening for a change from tympany to dullness. Measure the area of dullness.

Palpation

Palpate all four quadrants, leaving painful and tender areas for last.

Percussing and measuring the liver

To percuss and measure the liver, follow these steps:
• Identify the upper border of liver dullness. Start in the right midclavicular line in an area of lung resonance, and percuss downward toward the liver. Use a pen to mark the spot where the sound changes to dullness.
• Start in the right midclavicular line at a level below the umbilicus, and lightly percuss upward toward the liver. Mark the spot where the sound changes from tympany to dullness.
• Use a ruler to measure the vertical span between the two marked spots, as shown. In an adult, a normal liver span ranges from 2^1/$_2$" to 4^3/$_4$" (6.5 to 12 cm).

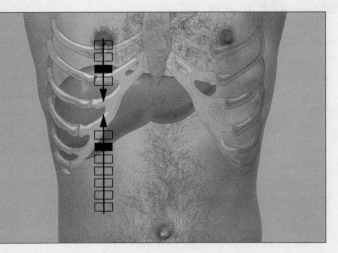

Light touch

Light palpation helps identify muscle resistance and tenderness as well as the location of some superficial organs. To palpate, put the fingers of one hand close together, depress the skin about ^{1}/$_2$" (1.3 cm) with your fingertips, and make gentle, rotating movements. Avoid short, quick jabs.

The abdomen should be soft and nontender. As you palpate the four quadrants, note organs, masses, and areas of tenderness or increased resistance.

In deep

To perform deep palpation, push the abdomen down about 2" to 3" (5 to 7.5 cm). In an obese patient, put one hand on top of the other and push. Palpate the entire abdomen in a clockwise direction, checking for tenderness, pulsations, organ enlargement, and masses.

If the patient's abdomen is rigid, don't palpate it. He could have peritoneal inflammation, and palpation could cause pain or could rupture an inflamed organ. (See *Emergency signals*, page 430.)

Palpate the patient's liver to check for enlargement and tenderness. (See *Palpating the liver*, page 431.) Unless the spleen is enlarged, it isn't palpable. To attempt to palpate the spleen, stand at the patient's right side. Use your left hand to support his back left lower rib cage, and ask him to take a deep breath. Then, with your right hand on his abdomen,

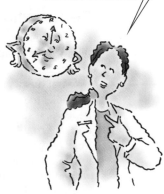

When you palpate the entire abdomen, move in a clockwise direction.

What do I do?

Emergency signals

When assessing a patient with a GI problem, stay alert for the signs and symptoms described here because they may signal an emergency. If you note any of these signs or symptoms, notify the practitioner and assess the patient for deterioration such as signs of shock. Intervene, as necessary, by providing oxygen therapy and I.V. fluids as ordered. Place the patient on a cardiac monitor if appropriate. Provide emotional support.

Abdominal pain
- Progressive, severe, or colicky pain for more than 6 hours without improvement
- Acute pain associated with hypertension
- Acute pain in an elderly patient (Such a patient may have minimal tenderness, even with a ruptured abdominal organ or appendicitis.)
- Severe pain with guarding and a history of recent abdominal surgery
- Pain accompanied by X-ray evidence of free intraperitoneal air (gas) or mediastinal gas
- Disproportionately severe pain under benign conditions (soft abdomen with normal physical findings)

Vomitus and stools
- Vomitus containing fresh blood
- Prolonged vomiting or heaving, with or without obstipation (intractable constipation)
- Bloody or black, tarry stools

Abdominal tenderness
- Abdominal tenderness and rigidity, even when the patient is distracted
- Rebound tenderness

Other signs
- Fever
- Tachycardia
- Hypotension
- Dehydration

press up and in toward the spleen. If you do feel the spleen, stop palpating immediately because compression can cause rupture.

Rectum and anus

If the patient is age 40 or older, perform a rectal examination as part of your GI assessment. Explain the procedure to him before you begin.

First, inspect the perianal area. Put on gloves and spread the buttocks to expose the anus and surrounding tissue, checking for fissures, lesions, scars, inflammation, discharge, rectal prolapse, and external hemorrhoids. Ask the patient to strain as if he's having a bowel movement; this may reveal internal hemorrhoids, polyps, or fissures. The skin in the perianal area is normally somewhat darker than that of the surrounding area.

Next, palpate the rectum. Apply a water-soluble lubricant to your gloved index finger. Tell the patient to relax, and warn him

Palpating the liver

These illustrations show the correct hand positions for two ways of palpating the liver.

Simple palpation

• Place the patient in the supine position. Standing at his right side, place your left hand under his back at the approximate location of the liver.
• Place your right hand slightly below the mark you made at the liver's upper border during percussion and measurement. Point the fingers of your right hand toward the patient's head just under the right costal margin.
• As the patient inhales deeply, gently press in and up on the abdomen until the liver brushes under your right hand. The edge should be smooth, firm, and somewhat round. Note any tenderness.

Hooking

• Hooking is an alternate way of palpating the liver. To hook the liver, stand next to the patient's right shoulder, facing his feet. Place your hands side-by-side, and hook your fingertips over the right costal margin, below the lower mark of dullness.
• Ask the patient to take a deep breath as you push your fingertips in and up. If the liver is palpable, you may feel its edge as it slides down in the abdomen as he breathes in.

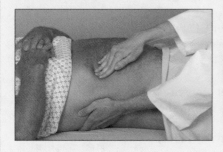
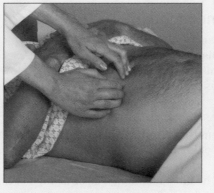

that he'll feel some pressure. Then insert your finger into the rectum, toward the umbilicus. To palpate as much of the rectal wall as possible, rotate your finger clockwise and then counterclockwise. The rectal walls should feel soft and smooth, without masses, fecal impaction, or tenderness.

Inspect and test

Remove your finger from the rectum, and inspect the glove for stool, blood, and mucus. Test fecal matter adhering to the glove for occult blood using a guaiac test.

Diagnostic tests

Many tests provide information that will help direct your care of the patient with a GI problem. Even if you don't participate in testing, you'll need to know why the practitioner ordered each test, what the results mean, and what responsibilities you'll need to carry out before, during, and after the test.

Endoscopy

Using a fiber-optic endoscope, the doctor can directly view hollow visceral linings to diagnose inflammatory, ulcerative, and infectious diseases; benign and malignant neoplasms; and other esophageal, gastric, and intestinal mucosal lesions. Endoscopy can also be used for therapeutic interventions or to obtain biopsy specimens.

Lower GI endoscopy

Lower GI endoscopy, also called *colonoscopy* or *proctosigmoidoscopy*, helps diagnose inflammatory and ulcerative bowel disease, pinpoints lower GI bleeding, and detects lower GI abnormalities, such as tumors, polyps, hemorrhoids, and abscesses.

Nursing considerations
• Tell the patient that he will need to undergo a bowel preparation consisting of laxatives and enemas for 1 or 2 days before the procedure.
• Tell him that he must maintain a clear liquid diet the day before the procedure and then fast the morning of the test.
• Explain that he should review the medications he should take before the procedure with his practitioner.

Try to relax
• If the patient will undergo a sigmoidoscopy, explain that he most likely won't be sedated; if he will undergo a colonoscopy, tell him he'll be under I.V. sedation.
• Inform the patient that the doctor will insert a flexible tube into his rectum.
• Tell him that he may feel some lower abdominal discomfort and the urge to move his bowels as the tube is advanced. To control the urge to defecate and ease the discomfort, instruct him to breathe deeply and slowly through his mouth.

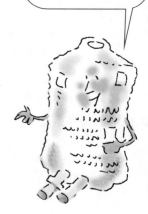

If the patient will undergo a colonoscopy, he'll be under I.V. sedation.

• Explain that air may be introduced into the bowel through the tube. If he feels the urge to expel some air, tell him not to try to control it.
• Tell him that he may hear and feel a suction machine removing any liquid that may obscure the doctor's view, but it won't cause any discomfort.
• Let him know he can eat after recovering from the sedative, usually about 1 hour after the test.
• If air was introduced into the bowel, the patient may pass large amounts of flatus. Explain that this is normal and helps prevent abdominal cramping.
• Tell him to report any blood in his stool.

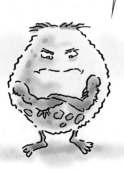

H. pylori is my name and infecting the alimentary canal is my game.

Upper GI endoscopy

Upper GI endoscopy, also called *esophagogastro-duodenoscopy*, identifies abnormalities of the esophagus, stomach, and small intestine, such as esophagitis, inflammatory bowel disease, Mallory-Weiss syndrome, lesions, tumors, gastritis, and polyps. During endoscopy, biopsies may be taken to detect the presence of *Helicobacter pylori* or to rule out gastric carcinoma.

Nursing considerations
• Tell the patient that he must restrict food and fluids for at least 6 hours before the test.
• If the test is an emergency procedure, inform the patient that he'll have his stomach contents suctioned to permit better visualization.
• Explain that he'll be given I.V. sedation to help keep him comfortable.

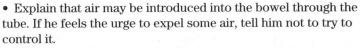

I can't feel my lipths...

• Before insertion of the tube, the patient's throat will be sprayed with a local anesthetic. Explain that the spray will taste unpleasant and will make his mouth feel swollen and numb, causing difficulty swallowing.
• Reassure the patient that he'll have a mouthguard to protect his teeth from the tube.
• Before the test, ask the patient to remove dentures and dental appliances, as applicable.
• Tell the patient that he can expect to feel some pressure in the abdomen and some fullness or bloating as the tube is inserted and advanced and as air is introduced to inflate the stomach.
• The patient can resume eating when his gag reflex returns — usually in about 1 hour.

Laboratory tests

Common laboratory tests used to diagnose GI disorders include studies of stool, urine, and esophageal, gastric, and peritoneal contents as well as percutaneous liver biopsy.

24-hour pH testing

The lower esophageal sphincter (LES) normally prevents gastric reflux. However, if this sphincter is incompetent, the recurrent backflow of acidic juices (and of bile salts, if the pyloric sphincter is also incompetent) into the esophagus inflames the esophageal mucosa. This inflammation (esophagitis) causes burning epigastric or retrosternal pain that radiates to the back or arms. To distinguish such pain from angina pectoris, patients who also complain of chest pain would have received cardiac testing to eliminate that possibility.

Performed on an outpatient basis, 24-hour pH testing provides 24 hours of continuous acidity data.

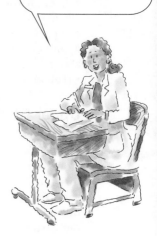

The patient will need to keep a diary of activities during 24-hour pH testing. But I'm afraid this diary can't be secret!

Dear Diary...

At the same time, the patient keeps a diary of activities — such as walking, sitting, lying down, and eating — and signs and symptoms — such as burping, vomiting, and chest pain. Then the diary and the data from the 24-hour pH study are entered into a computer, which compares the patient's symptoms and activities with acid levels to determine the severity of the reflux disease.

Although 24-hour pH monitoring provides accurate results, it's an uncomfortable procedure. A shorter monitoring period may provide the same results, with less discomfort to the patient. (See *Detecting reflux: The long and short of it.*)

Nursing considerations

• Document medications the patient takes for reflux, including the date and time of the last dose.
• Tell the patient not to use any antacids, chewing gum, lozenges, or hard candy during the study.
• Encourage him to follow his usual routine so that the study can accurately demonstrate the correlations between activities and reflux disease.
• To help relieve throat discomfort, tell the patient to suck ice chips or use dyclonine hydrochloride (Cepacol) spray.
• To help prevent reflux, tell the patient to avoid large meals, caffeine, alcohol, and lying in a supine position after meals.

Weighing the evidence

Detecting reflux: The long and short of it

24 works well...

Patients typically undergo 24-hour gastric pH monitoring to diagnose acid reflux, but such monitoring is invasive and uncomfortable. Researchers set out to determine if monitoring for a shorter period—and decreasing the time patients would have to undergo the procedure—would still help accurately diagnose gastroesophageal reflux. To find out, they studied a group of about 200 patients undergoing 24-hour gastric pH monitoring, comparing the results for a 3-hour period during and after mealtimes with the 24-hour results.

... but 3 does the job

They found that the 3-hour results just as accurately detected acid reflux as the 24-hour results. The long and short of it? The decreased monitoring period can not only decrease patient discomfort, but it might even enhance patient compliance.

Source: Guijian, F., et al. (2010). Comparing 3-hour pH monitoring in esophagus with 24-hour pH monitoring to diagnose GERD. *Hepatogastroenterology, 57*(97), 86–89.

Fecal studies

Normal stool appears brown and formed but soft. Narrow, ribbonlike stool signals spastic or irritable bowel, or partial bowel or rectal obstruction. Diet and medication can cause constipation. Diarrhea may indicate spastic bowel or viral infection. Soft stool mixed with blood and mucus can signal bacterial infection; mixed with blood and pus, colitis.

Yellow or green stool suggests severe, prolonged diarrhea; black stool suggests GI bleeding or intake of iron supplements or raw-to-rare meat. Tan or white stool shows hepatic-duct or gallbladder-duct blockage, hepatitis, or cancer. Red stool may signal colon or rectal bleeding, but some drugs and foods can also cause this coloration.

Most stool contains 10% to 20% fat. However, higher fat content can turn stool pasty or greasy — a possible sign of intestinal malabsorption or pancreatic disease. (See *Fecal and urine tests,* page 436.)

Nursing considerations

- Collect the stool specimen in a clean, dry container.
- Don't use stool that has been in contact with toilet-bowl water or urine.

Fecal and urine tests

This table lists fecal and urine tests, their normal values and purpose, and the implications of abnormal results.

Test and normal values	Purpose	Implications of abnormal results
Bilirubin None	Detects bile pigments in urine	• Presence: biliary obstruction
Clostridium difficile *toxin assay* Negative	Detects pseudomembranous entero-colitis	• Indicates presence of *C. difficile* • False-negative result possible
Fecal lipid Less than 7 g/24 hours	Tests 72-hour stool collection for increased fat content if malabsorption is suspected	• Elevated: possible malabsorption caused by insufficient pancreatic enzyme excretion
Fecal occult blood test Less than 2.5 ml/day	Measures occult (concealed) blood in stool samples	• Positive: GI bleeding or colorectal cancer, anal outlet bleeding
Fecal urobilinogen Males: 0.3 to 2.1 Ehrlich units/2 hours Females: 0.1 to 1.1 Ehrlich units/2 hours	Detects impaired liver function	• Elevated: impaired liver function • Lowered: total biliary obstruction
Stool culture No pathogens	Detects pathogens causing GI disease	• Presence of pathogens: bacterial, viral, or fungal GI infection
Stool examination for ova and parasites No parasites or ova in stool	Confirms or rules out intestinal parasitic infestation and disease	• Presence of parasites or ova: parasitic infestation and possible infection

• Send the specimen to the laboratory immediately for accurate results.

• Keep in mind that serial stool specimens are usually collected once per day with the first morning stool.

• Instruct the patient being tested for fecal occult blood to avoid eating red meat, poultry, fish, turnips, or horseradish or taking iron preparations, ascorbic acid (vitamin C), or anti-inflammatory agents for 48 to 72 hours before the specimens are collected.

• Use commercial Hemoccult slides as a simple method of testing for blood in stool. Follow the package directions.

Percutaneous liver biopsy

A percutaneous liver biopsy involves the needle aspiration of a core of liver tissue for histologic analysis. It's done under local or general anesthesia. This biopsy can detect hepatic disorders and can confirm cancer if ultrasonography, computed tomography (CT) scans, and radionuclide studies have proved inconclusive.

What's your profile?

Because many patients with hepatic disorders have clotting defects, a clotting profile (prothrombin time [PT], partial thromboplastin time [PTT]) along with type and crossmatching should precede liver biopsy.

In a liver biopsy, a Menghini needle attached to a 5-ml syringe containing normal saline solution is introduced through the chest wall and intercostal space. Negative pressure is created in the syringe. The needle is then pushed rapidly into the liver and pulled out of the body entirely to obtain a tissue specimen.

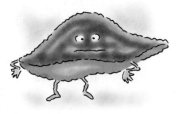

Percutaneous liver biopsy can detect hepatic disorders and cancer. Okay, I'm officially worried.

Nursing considerations

• Tell the patient to restrict food and fluids for at least 4 hours before the test.
• Explain the testing procedure to the patient:
– He will be awake during the test and, although the test is uncomfortable, medication is available to help him relax.
– The doctor will drape and clean an area on his abdomen. Then he'll receive a local anesthetic, which may sting and cause brief discomfort.
– He'll be instructed how and when to hold his breath and to lie still as the doctor inserts the biopsy needle into the liver.
– The needle may cause a sensation of pressure and some discomfort in the right upper back but will remain in his liver for only a few seconds.

When it's all over

After the procedure:
• The patient must remain in bed on his right side for at least 2 hours and maintain bed rest for 24 hours.
• The patient may experience discomfort for several hours and may take ibuprofen (Motrin) but not aspirin.
• Let the patient know that he may resume his normal diet.
• Watch for bleeding and symptoms of bile peritonitis — tenderness and rigidity around the biopsy site.
• Be alert for signs and symptoms of a pneumothorax, such as rising respiratory rate, depressed breath sounds, dyspnea, persistent shoulder pain, and pleuritic chest pain. Report these complications promptly.
• Apply a gauze dressing to the puncture site. Check the dressing frequently, whenever you check vital signs. Reinforce or apply a pressure dressing if needed.

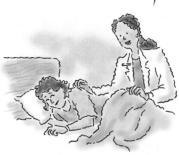

After the procedure, the patient should remain in bed on her right side for 2 hours.

- Maintain the patient in a right side-lying position for at least 2 hours because the pressure will enhance coagulation at the site.
- Monitor urine output for at least 24 hours and watch for hematuria, which may indicate bladder trauma.

Peritoneal fluid analysis

The peritoneal fluid analysis series includes examination of gross appearance, erythrocyte and leukocyte counts, cytologic studies, microbiological studies for bacteria and fungi, and determinations of protein, glucose, amylase, ammonia, and alkaline phosphatase levels. A sample of peritoneal fluid is obtained by paracentesis, which involves inserting a trocar and cannula through the abdominal wall while the patient is under a local anesthetic. If the sample of fluid is being removed for therapeutic purposes, the cannula can be connected to a drainage system.

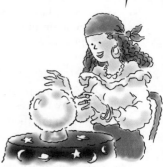

You don't need a crystal ball to know that increasing pain and abdominal tenderness after paracentesis could be serious.

Nursing considerations
- Before the procedure, have the patient empty his bladder.
- Observe the patient for dizziness, pallor, perspiration, and increased anxiety.
- Check the site for peritoneal fluid leakage.

Shocking signs
- Watch for signs of hemorrhage, shock, and increasing pain and abdominal tenderness. These signs may indicate a perforated intestine or, depending on the site of the paracentesis, puncture of the inferior epigastric artery, hematoma of the anterior cecal wall, or rupture of the iliac vein or bladder.

Urine tests

Urinalysis provides valuable information about hepatic and biliary function. Urinary bilirubin and urobilinogen tests are commonly used to evaluate liver function.

The name's Rubin, Billy Rubin
Bilirubin results from the breakdown of the heme fraction of hemoglobin. In the liver, free bilirubin conjugates with glucuronic acid, which allows the glomeruli to filter bilirubin (unconjugated bilirubin isn't filtered). Bilirubin is normally excreted in bile as its principal pigment, but it also occurs abnormally in urine. Conjugated bilirubin appears in urine when serum bilirubin levels rise — as in biliary tract obstruction or hepatocellular damage — and is accompanied by jaundice.

Formed in the intestine by bacterial action on conjugated bilirubin, urobilinogen is primarily excreted in stool, producing its characteristic brown color. A small amount is reabsorbed by the portal system and is mainly reexcreted in bile, although the kidneys also excrete some. As a result, elevated urine urobilinogen levels may be an early indication of hepatic damage. In biliary obstruction, urine urobilinogen levels decline.

Nursing considerations
• Collect a freshly voided random urine specimen in the container provided.

No time to lose
• You can analyze bilirubin at the patient's bedside using dip strips. Wait 20 seconds before interpreting the color change on the dip strip. Bilirubin must be tested within 30 minutes, before it disintegrates. If it's to be tested in the laboratory, send it immediately and record the collection time on the patient's chart.
• For urobilinogen, obtain a random specimen and send it to the laboratory immediately; it, too, must be tested within 30 minutes, before the sample deteriorates.

Nuclear imaging and ultrasonography

Nuclear imaging methods, which include liver-spleen scanning and magnetic resonance imaging (MRI), analyze concentrations of injected or ingested radiopaque substances to enhance visual evaluation of possible disease processes. Nuclear imaging methods can study the liver, spleen, and other abdominal organs.

Ultrasonography creates images of internal organs, such as the gallbladder and liver. Gas-filled structures, such as the intestines, can't be seen with this technique.

Liver-spleen scan

In a liver-spleen scan, a scanner or gamma camera records the distribution of radioactivity within the liver and spleen after I.V. injection of a radioactive colloid. Most of this colloid is taken up by Kupffer's cells in the liver, while smaller amounts lodge in the spleen and bone marrow. By registering the extent of this absorption, the imaging device detects such abnormalities as tumors, cysts, and abscesses. Because the test demonstrates disease nonspecifically (as an area that fails to take up the colloid, or a *cold spot*), test results usually require confirmation by ultrasonography, CT scan, gallium scan, or biopsy.

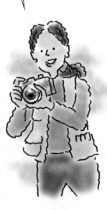

A liver-spleen scan uses a scanner or gamma camera to obtain its results. Somehow, I don't think this camera is up to the job.

Nursing considerations

• Explain the testing procedure to the patient:

– This test examines the liver and spleen through pictures taken with a special scanner or camera.

– The patient will receive an injection of a radioactive substance (technetium-99m) through an I.V. line in his hand or arm to allow better visualization of the liver and spleen. The injection contains only trace amounts of radioactivity, and he won't be radioactive after the test.

– He should immediately report any adverse reactions, such as flushing, fever, light-headedness, or difficulty breathing.

– If the test uses a rectilinear scanner, he'll hear a soft, irregular clicking noise as the scanner moves across his abdomen.

– If the test uses a gamma camera, the patient will feel the camera lightly touch his abdomen. He should lie still, relax, and breathe normally. He may be asked to hold his breath briefly to ensure good-quality pictures.

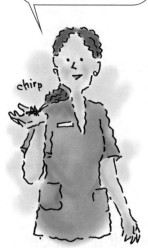

Tell the patient undergoing a rectilinear scan that he'll hear a soft, irregular clicking noise. No, Cricket, it's not you!

MRI

Used in imaging the liver and abdominal organs, MRI generates an image by energizing protons into a strong magnetic field. Radio waves emitted as protons return to their former equilibrium state and are recorded. MRI transmits no ionizing radiation during the scan. One disadvantage of the process is the closed, tubelike space that's required for the scan, although newer MRI centers offer a less confining "open-MRI" scan. Patients with metal or implanted devices such as pacemakers can't undergo this test because of the strong magnetic field it generates. MRI is useful in evaluating liver disease to help characterize tumors, masses, or cysts found on previous studies.

Nursing considerations

• Explain the testing procedure to the patient:

– He must lie still during the procedure, which may last from 30 to 90 minutes.

– He must remove any metal, such as jewelry, before the procedure.

– If he becomes claustrophobic during the test, he may be given mild sedation.

Ultrasonography

Ultrasonography uses a focused beam of high-frequency sound waves to create echoes, which then appear as images on a monitor. Echoes vary with tissue density. The test helps differentiate between obstructive and nonobstructive jaundice and diagnoses cholelithiasis, cholecystitis, and certain metastases and hematomas.

Spotlight on cold spots

When used with liver-spleen scanning, it can clarify the nature of cold spots, such as tumors, abscesses, and cysts. The technique also helps diagnose pancreatitis, pseudocysts, pancreatic cancer, ascites, and splenomegaly.

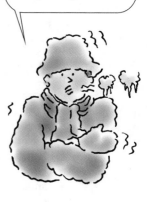

Ultrasonography can help clarify the nature of cold spots, such as tumors. I'm in a bit of a cold spot myself right now!

Nursing considerations

• If the patient is undergoing pelvic ultrasonography, he'll need a full bladder; therefore, he must drink three or four glasses of water before the test and must avoid urinating until after the test.
• For gallbladder evaluation, tell the patient that he shouldn't eat solid food for 12 hours before the test.
• For pancreas, liver, or spleen evaluation, tell the patient that he should fast for 8 hours before the test.
• If the patient is undergoing a barium enema or an upper GI series, make sure it occurs after abdominal ultrasonography because sound waves can't penetrate barium.

Radiographic tests

Radiographic tests include abdominal X-rays, CT scans, various contrast medium studies, and virtual colonoscopy.

Abdominal X-rays

An abdominal X-ray, also called *flat plate of the abdomen* or *kidney-ureter-bladder radiography*, helps detect and evaluate tumors, kidney stones, abnormal gas collection, and other abdominal disorders. The test consists of two plates: one taken with the patient supine and the other taken while he stands. On X-ray, air appears black, adipose tissue appears gray, and bone appears white.

Compare and contrast

Although a routine X-ray won't reveal most abdominal organs, it will show the contrast between air and fluid. For example, intestinal blockage traps large amounts of detectable fluids and air inside organs. When an intestinal wall tears, air leaks into the abdomen and becomes visible on X-ray.

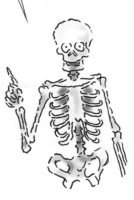

On X-ray, I'm white, air is black, and adipose tissue is gray. Of course, I look fabulous in any color, but white is my signature color.

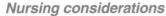
Nursing considerations

• Radiography requires no special pretest or posttest care. Explain the procedure to the patient.
• X-ray interpretation involves locating normal anatomic structures, discerning any abnormal images, and correlating findings with assessment data.

CT scan

In CT scanning, a computer translates the action of multiple X-ray beams into three-dimensional oscilloscope images of the biliary tract, liver, and pancreas. The test can be done with or without a contrast medium, but contrast is preferred (unless the patient is allergic to contrast medium). This test:
• helps distinguish between obstructive and nonobstructive jaundice
• identifies abscesses, cysts, hematomas, tumors, and pseudocysts
• can help evaluate the cause of weight loss
• detects occult malignancy
• can help diagnose and evaluate pancreatitis.

Nursing considerations

• Tell the patient to restrict food and fluids after midnight before the test but to continue any drug regimen, as ordered.
• Explain that the patient should lie still, relax, breathe normally, and remain quiet during the test because movement blurs the X-ray picture and prolongs the test.
• If the practitioner orders an I.V. contrast medium, the patient may experience discomfort from the needle puncture and a localized feeling of warmth on injection.
• If the patient has a seafood or dye allergy, a pretest preparation kit containing prednisone, cimetidine, and diphenhydramine may be given to him. He should immediately report any adverse reactions, such as nausea, vomiting, dizziness, headache, and urticaria (hives). Assure him that reactions are rare.
• Explain that the patient may resume his normal diet after the test.

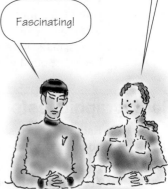

Contrast radiography

Some X-ray tests require contrast media to more accurately assess the GI system because the media accentuate differences among densities of air, fat, soft tissue, and bone. These tests include barium enema, barium swallow test, cholangiography, endoscopic retrograde cholangiopancreatography (ERCP), small-bowel series and enema, and upper GI series.

Barium below, barium above

The barium enema is most commonly used to evaluate suspected lower intestinal disorders. It helps diagnose inflammatory disorders, colorectal cancer, polyps, diverticula, and large-intestine structural changes such as intussusception.

The barium swallow test allows examination of the pharynx and esophagus to detect strictures, ulcers, tumors, polyps, diverticula, hiatal hernia, esophageal webs, gastroesophageal reflux disease (GERD), motility disorders and, sometimes, achalasia.

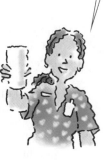

A barium swallow allows examination of the pharynx and esophagus. Bottoms up!

Cholangiography clues

In cholangiography (percutaneous and postoperative), a contrast agent is injected into the biliary tree through a flexible needle. In percutaneous transhepatic cholangiography (PTHC), a radiopaque dye is injected directly into the liver through the eighth or ninth midaxillary intercostal space. If done postoperatively, the dye is injected by way of a T tube. In an oral cholangiogram, the patient is given the contrast medium by mouth. These tests are used to determine the cause of upper abdominal pain that persists after cholecystectomy, to evaluate jaundice, and to determine the location, extent and, usually, the cause of mechanical obstructions.

Down endoscope

In ERCP, the doctor passes an endoscope into the duodenum and injects dye through a cannula inserted into the ampulla of Vater. This test helps to determine the cause of jaundice; evaluate tumors and inflammation of the pancreas, gallbladder, or liver; and locate obstructions in the pancreatic duct and hepatobiliary tree.

Shorter series or better distender?

Results of a small-bowel series or enema, which follow the contrast agent through the small intestine, may suggest sprue, obstruction, motility disorders, malabsorption syndrome, Hodgkin's disease, lymphosarcoma, ischemia, bleeding, inflammation, or Crohn's disease of the small intestine. Although longer and more uncomfortable than the small-bowel series, the enema study better distends the bowel, making lesion identification easier.

I spy with an upper GI

In an upper GI series, the practitioner follows the barium's passage from the esophagus to the stomach. Usually combined with a small-bowel series, the upper GI series helps diagnose gastritis, cancer, hiatal hernia, diverticula, strictures, and (most commonly) gastric and duodenal ulcers. It may also suggest motility disorders.

Nursing considerations

- Tell the patient where and when the test will take place.
- Explain that the test will take only 30 to 40 minutes for a barium swallow or enema but can take up to 6 hours for an upper GI or small-bowel series.
- Instruct the patient to maintain a low-residue diet for 2 to 3 days and restrict food, fluids, and smoking after midnight before the test. He'll receive a clear liquid diet for 12 to 24 hours before the test. As ordered, he's to stop taking medications for up to 24 hours before the test.
- Unless he's undergoing a barium swallow test, the patient will receive a laxative the afternoon before the test and up to three cleaning enemas the evening before or the morning of the test. Explain that the presence of food or fluid may obscure details of the structures being studied.
- Let the patient having a barium enema know that he will lie on his left side while the practitioner inserts a small, lubricated tube into his rectum. Instruct the patient to keep his anal sphincter tightly contracted against the tube to hold it in position and help prevent barium leakage. Stress the importance of retaining the barium.

Eliminating barium

- After the test, the patient may resume his normal diet and medication as ordered, and will receive a laxative to help expel the barium. Stress the importance of barium elimination because retained barium may harden, causing obstruction or impaction. The barium will lighten the color of his stools for 24 to 72 hours after the test.
- If the patient is having an oral cholangiogram, explain that, if ordered, he'll eat a meal containing fat at noon the day before the test and a fat-free meal that evening. After the evening meal, he can have only water but should continue any drug regimen, as ordered.
- Tell the patient that he'll be given a cleaning enema and, 2 to 3 hours before the test, he'll be asked to swallow six tablets, one at a time, at 5-minute intervals. The enema and tablets help outline the gallbladder on the X-ray film. He should immediately report any adverse reactions to the tablets, such as diarrhea, nausea, vomiting, abdominal cramps, and dysuria.
- Explain that he'll be asked to swallow barium several times during the test. Describe barium's thick consistency and chalky taste.

Virtual colonoscopy

Virtual colonoscopy is a nonsurgical approach to evaluate the colon. A soft-tipped catheter introduces air into the colon while a three-dimensional CT scan is performed. The scan takes about

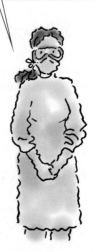

Virtual colonoscopy is a new, nonsurgical procedure that's useful for patients who refuse colonoscopy. I guess that means I don't have to prep for surgery either...

10 minutes. Images are assembled in a computer program that can be viewed on a screen. This test may be useful for the patient who refuses traditional colonoscopy.

Nursing considerations
• Tell the patient that he may feel discomfort when air is introduced into the colon.
• Instruct the patient to remain still while images are taken.
• Tell the patient that he'll have no restrictions after the test but that he may feel bloated from the air introduced into his colon.

Treatments

GI dysfunction presents many treatment challenges. After all, it stems from various pathophysiologic mechanisms that may exist separately or simultaneously. These mechanisms include tumors, hyperactivity and hypoactivity, malabsorption, infection and inflammation, vascular disorders, intestinal obstruction, and degenerative disease. Treatments for these disorders include drug therapy, surgery, and related measures that call for effective nursing care.

Drug therapy

The most commonly used GI drugs include antacids, digestants, histamine-2 (H_2) receptor antagonists, proton pump inhibitors, anticholinergics, antidiarrheal agents, laxatives, emetics, and antiemetics. Some of these drugs, such as antacids and antiemetics, provide relief immediately. Other drugs, such as laxatives and H_2-receptor antagonists, may take several days or longer to solve the problem.

Surgery

The patient who has undergone GI surgery may need special postoperative support because he may have to make permanent and difficult changes in his lifestyle. For example, besides teaching a colostomy patient about stoma care, you'll also have to help him adjust to changes in his body image and personal relationships. Another patient may have to endure a bowel training program for weeks or even months, which can be a frustrating and embarrassing experience. You'll have to draw on your own emotional strengths to help the patient come

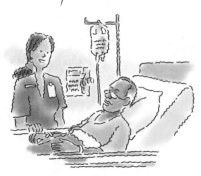

The patient who has undergone GI surgery may need special support because of the possible permanent and difficult lifestyle changes.

to terms with these feelings. Still another patient may have great difficulty complying with dietary restrictions. He'll need to be convinced of the firm link between such measures and a full recovery.

Esophageal surgeries

Surgery may be necessary to manage an emergency, such as acute constriction, or to provide palliative care for an incurable disease such as advanced esophageal cancer.

So many surgeries!

Major esophageal surgeries include cardiomyotomy, cricopharyngeal myotomy, Nissen fundoplication, esophagectomy, esophagogastrostomy, and esophagomyotomy. The surgical approach is through the neck, chest, or abdomen, depending on the location of the problem.

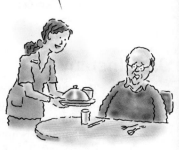

Help your patient understand the firm link between following dietary guidelines and making a full recovery.

Patient preparation

Explain the procedure to the patient. Tell him that, when he awakes from the anesthetic, he'll probably have an NG tube in place to aid feeding and relieve abdominal distention. Warn him of the risk of pneumonia and the importance of good pulmonary hygiene during recovery to prevent it. Demonstrate coughing and deep-breathing exercises, and show the patient how to splint his incision to protect it and minimize pain. Discuss possible postoperative complications and measures to prevent or minimize them.

Monitoring and aftercare

After surgery, follow these steps:
• Place the patient in semi-Fowler's position to help minimize esophageal reflux.
• Provide antacids as needed for symptomatic relief.
• If surgery involving the upper esophagus produces hypersalivation, the patient may be unable to swallow the excess saliva. Control drooling with gauze wicks or suctioning. Encourage the patient to spit into an emesis basin placed within his reach.

Head's up!

• To reduce the risk of aspiration pneumonia, elevate the head of the patient's bed and encourage him to turn frequently. Carefully monitor his vital signs and auscultate his lungs. Encourage coughing and deep-breathing exercises.
• Watch for developing mediastinitis, especially if surgery involved extensive thoracic invasion (as in esophagogastrostomy). Note and report fever, dyspnea, and complaints of substernal pain.

If ordered, administer antibiotics to help prevent or correct this complication.
• Watch for signs of leakage at the anastomosis site. Check drainage tubes for blood, test for occult blood in stool and drainage, and monitor hemoglobin levels for evidence of slow blood loss. If the patient has an NG tube in place, don't handle the tube because this may damage the internal sutures or anastomoses. For the same reason, avoid deep suctioning in a patient who has undergone extensive esophageal repair.

Home care instructions
Provide these instructions to the patient:
• Advise him to sleep with his head elevated to prevent reflux. Suggest that he raise the head of his bed on blocks.
• If the patient smokes, encourage him to stop. Explain that nicotine adversely affects the LES. Advise the patient to avoid alcohol, aspirin, and effervescent over-the-counter products (such as Alka-Seltzer) because they may damage the tender esophageal mucosa.
• Advise the patient to avoid heavy lifting, straining, and coughing, which could rupture the weakened mucosa.
• Tell him to report any respiratory signs and symptoms, such as wheezing, coughing, and nocturnal dyspnea.

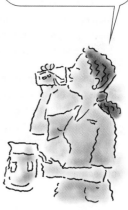

Tell the patient to avoid alcohol, which may damage the tender esophageal mucosa. I'll stick with water for now.

Gastric surgeries
If chronic ulcer disease doesn't respond to medication, diet, and rest, gastric surgery is used to remove diseased or malignant tissue, to prevent ulcers from recurring, or to relieve an obstruction or perforation.

Drastic gastric surgery
In an emergency, gastric surgery may be performed to control severe GI hemorrhage or perforation. Surgery may also be necessary when laser endoscopic coagulation for control of severe GI bleeding isn't possible.

Gastric surgery can take various forms, depending on the location and extent of the disorder. For example, a partial gastrectomy reduces the amount of acid-secreting mucosa. A bilateral vagotomy eliminates vagal nerve stimulation of gastric secretions and may help relieve ulcer symptoms. A pyloroplasty improves drainage and prevents obstruction. Most commonly, however, two gastric surgeries are combined, such as vagotomy with gastroenterostomy, or vagotomy with antrectomy. Although controversial in cases of morbid obesity, gastric reduction surgery may be performed to aid in weight loss. (See *Understanding common gastric surgeries*, page 448.)

Understanding common gastric surgeries

In addition to treating chronic ulcers, gastric surgeries help remove obstructions and malignant tumors. Names of gastric surgeries (other than vagotomy) usually refer to the stomach portion removed. Most procedures combine two surgery types.

Note: Keep in mind that *-ostomy* means "an opening into." If only one prefix precedes *-ostomy,* then the surgical opening is made from the exterior — for example, *gastrostomy.* Two prefixes indicate anastomosis — for example, *gastroenterostomy* means anastomosis of a stomach *(gastro-)* remnant with a small intestine *(entero-)* segment.

Make sure you're familiar with these commonly performed gastric surgeries.

Vagotomy with gastroenterostomy

In this procedure, the surgeon resects the vagus nerves and creates a stoma for gastric drainage. He'll perform selective, truncal, or parietal cell vagotomy, depending on the degree of decreased gastric acid secretion required.

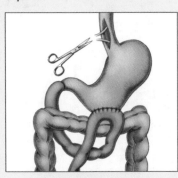

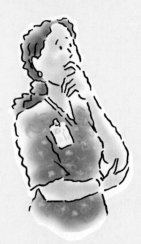

Vagotomy with antrectomy

After resecting the vagus nerves, the surgeon removes the antrum. Then he anastomoses the remaining stomach segment to the jejunum and closes the duodenal stump.

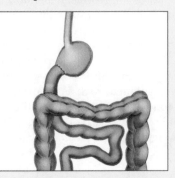

Billroth I

In this partial gastrectomy with a gastroduodenostomy, the surgeon excises the distal one-third to one-half of the stomach and anastomoses the remaining stomach to the duodenum.

Vagotomy with pyloroplasty

In this procedure, the surgeon resects the vagus nerves and refashions the pylorus to widen the lumen and aid gastric emptying.

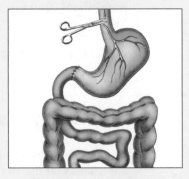

Billroth II

In this partial gastrectomy with a gastrojejunostomy, the surgeon removes the distal segment of the stomach and antrum. Then he anastomoses the remaining stomach and the jejunum and closes the duodenal stump.

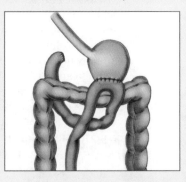

Patient preparation

Before surgery, implement these measures:
• Evaluate and begin stabilizing the patient's fluid and electrolyte balance and nutritional status — both of which may be severely compromised by chronic ulcer disease or other GI disorders.
• Monitor intake and output, and draw serum samples for hematologic studies.
• Prepare the patient for abdominal X-rays.
• On the night before surgery, administer laxatives and enemas as necessary.
• On the morning of surgery, insert an NG tube as ordered.

Monitoring and aftercare

Follow these steps after surgery:
• Place the patient in low or semi-Fowler's position. Either position will ease breathing and prevent aspiration if he vomits.
• Maintain tube feedings or total parenteral nutrition (TPN) and I.V. fluid and electrolyte replacement therapy as ordered. Monitor blood studies daily. If you perform gastric suctioning, watch for signs of dehydration, hyponatremia, and metabolic alkalosis. Weigh the patient daily, and monitor and record intake and output, including NG tube drainage.

When bowel sounds rebound

• Auscultate the abdomen frequently for bowel sounds. When they return, notify the practitioner, who will order clamping or removal of the NG tube and gradual resumption of oral feeding. During NG tube clamping, watch for nausea and vomiting; if they occur, unclamp the tube immediately and reattach it to suction.
• Throughout recovery, have the patient cough, deep-breathe, and change position frequently. Encourage incentive spirometry. Teach the patient to splint his incision while coughing to help reduce pain. Assess his breath sounds frequently to detect atelectasis.
• Assess the patient for other complications, including vitamin B_{12} deficiency, anemia (especially common in patients who have undergone total gastrectomy), and dumping syndrome, a potentially serious digestive complication marked by weakness, nausea, flatulence, and palpitations that occurs within 30 minutes of a meal.

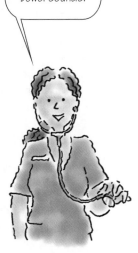

Auscultate the abdomen frequently for bowel sounds.

Home care instructions

Provide these instructions for the patient:
• Advise the patient to seek medical attention immediately if he develops any signs of life-threatening complications, such as hemorrhage, obstruction, and perforation.

• Explain dumping syndrome and how to avoid it. Advise the patient to eat small, frequent, nutritious meals evenly spaced throughout the day. He should chew his food thoroughly and drink fluids between meals rather than with them. In his diet, he should decrease intake of carbohydrates and salt while increasing fat and protein. After a meal, he should lie down for 20 to 30 minutes. If the patient is being discharged on tube feedings, teach him and his family how to give the feeding.
• If the practitioner has prescribed a GI anticholinergic to decrease motility and acid secretion, instruct the patient to take the drug 30 minutes to 1 hour before meals.
• Encourage the patient to avoid smoking because it alters pancreatic secretions that neutralize gastric acid in the duodenum.

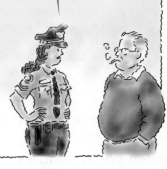

Encourage the patient not to smoke because it alters pancreatic secretions that neutralize gastric acid. Put that out!

Bowel surgery with ostomy

In bowel surgery with ostomy, the surgeon removes diseased colonic and rectal segments and creates a stoma on the outer abdominal wall to allow fecal elimination. This surgery is performed for such intestinal maladies as inflammatory bowel disease, familial polyposis, diverticulitis, and advanced colorectal cancer if conservative surgery and other treatments aren't successful or if the patient develops acute complications, such as obstruction, abscess, and fistula.

Take your pick

The surgeon can choose from several types of surgery, depending on the nature and location of the problem.
• Intractable obstruction of the ascending, transverse, descending, or sigmoid colon requires permanent colostomy and removal of the affected bowel segments.
• Cancer of the rectum and lower sigmoid colon commonly calls for abdominoperineal resection, which involves creation of a permanent colostomy and removal of the affected portion of the colon, rectum, and anus.
• Perforated sigmoid diverticulitis, Hirschsprung's disease, rectovaginal fistula, and penetrating trauma commonly require temporary colostomy to interrupt the intestinal flow and allow inflamed or injured bowel segments to heal. After healing occurs (usually within 8 weeks), the divided segments are anastomosed to restore bowel integrity and function.
• In a double-barrel colostomy, the transverse colon is divided and both ends are brought out through the abdominal wall to

create a proximal stoma for fecal drainage and a distal stoma leading to the nonfunctioning bowel.

• Loop colostomy, done to relieve acute obstruction in an emergency, involves creating proximal and distal stomas from a loop of intestine that has been pulled through an abdominal incision and supported with a plastic or glass rod.

• Severe, widespread colonic obstruction may require total or near-total removal of the colon and rectum and creation of an ileostomy from the proximal ileum. A permanent ileostomy requires that the patient wear a drainage pouch or bag over the stoma to receive the constant fecal drainage. In contrast, a continent, or Kock, ileostomy doesn't require an external pouch.

Patient preparation

Before surgery, implement these measures:

• Arrange for the patient to visit with an enterostomal therapist, who can provide more detailed information. The therapist can also help the patient select the best location for the stoma.

Sharing insights

• Try to have the patient meet with an ostomy patient (from a group such as the United Ostomy Association), who can share his personal insights into the realities of living with and caring for a stoma.

• Evaluate the patient's nutritional and fluid status. The patient may receive TPN to prepare him for the physiologic stress of surgery.

• Record the patient's fluid intake and output and weight daily, and watch for early signs of dehydration.

• Expect to draw periodic blood samples for hematocrit and hemoglobin determinations. Be prepared to transfuse blood if ordered.

Monitoring and aftercare

Follow these steps after surgery:

• Monitor intake and output, and weigh the patient daily. Maintain fluid and electrolyte balance, and watch for signs of dehydration (decreased urine output, poor skin turgor) and electrolyte imbalance.

• Provide analgesics as ordered. Be especially alert for pain in the patient with an abdominoperineal resection because of the extent and location of the incisions.

• Note and record the color, consistency, and odor of fecal drainage from the stoma. If the patient has a double-barrel colostomy, check for mucus drainage from the inactive (distal) stoma. The nature of fecal drainage is determined by the type of ostomy

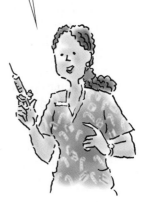

Before surgery, expect to draw periodic blood samples to measure hematocrit and hemoglobin, and be prepared to administer a blood transfusion, if necessary.

surgery; generally, the less colon tissue that's removed, the more closely drainage will resemble normal stool. For the first few days after surgery, fecal drainage probably will be mucoid (and possibly slightly blood-tinged) and mostly odorless. Report excessive blood or mucus content, which could indicate hemorrhage or infection.

Searching for sepsis

- Observe the patient for signs of peritonitis or sepsis, caused by bowel contents leaking into the abdominal cavity. Remember that immunocompromised patients or those receiving TPN are at an increased risk for sepsis.
- Provide meticulous wound care, changing dressings often. Check dressings and drainage sites frequently for signs of infection (purulent drainage, foul odor) or fecal drainage. If the patient has had an abdominoperineal resection, irrigate the perineal area as ordered.
- Regularly check the stoma and surrounding skin for irritation and excoriation, and take corrective measures. Also observe the stoma's appearance. The stoma should look smooth, cherry red, and slightly edematous; immediately report any discoloration or excessive swelling, which may indicate circulatory problems that could lead to ischemia.

Air those anxieties

- During the recovery period, encourage the patient to express his feelings and concerns; reassure an anxious or depressed patient that these common postoperative reactions should fade as he adjusts to the ostomy. Continue to arrange for visits by an enterostomal therapist.

Home care instructions

Provide these instructions to the patient:
- If the patient has a colostomy, teach him or a caregiver how to apply, remove, and empty the pouch. When appropriate, teach him how to irrigate the colostomy with warm tap water to gain some control over elimination. If appropriate, reassure him that he may be able to regain continence with dietary control and bowel retraining.
- Instruct the colostomy patient to change the stoma appliance as needed, to wash the stoma site with warm water and mild soap every 3 days, and to change the adhesive layer. These measures help prevent skin irritation and excoriation.

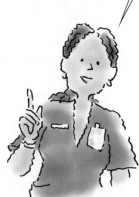

If the patient has had an abdominoperineal resection, irrigate the perineal area as ordered.

- If the patient has an ileostomy, instruct him to change the drainage pouch only when leakage occurs. Also, emphasize meticulous skin care and use of a protective skin barrier around the stoma site.
- Discuss dietary restrictions and suggestions to prevent stoma blockage, diarrhea, flatus, and odor. Tell the patient to stay on a low-fiber diet for 6 to 8 weeks and to add new foods to his diet gradually. Suggest that the patient use an ostomy deodorant or an odorproof pouch if he includes odor-producing foods in his diet.
- Trial and error will help the patient determine which foods cause gas. Gas-producing fruits include apples, melons, avocados, and cantaloupe; gas-producing vegetables include beans, corn, broccoli, and cabbage.

Bring on the bouillon

- The patient is especially susceptible to fluid and electrolyte losses. He must drink plenty of fluids, especially in hot weather or when he has diarrhea. Fruit juice and bouillon, which contain potassium, are particularly helpful.
- Warn the patient to avoid alcohol, laxatives, and diuretics, which increase fluid loss and may contribute to an imbalance.
- Tell the patient to report persistent diarrhea through the stoma, which can quickly lead to fluid and electrolyte imbalance.

A nice, warm bath...

- If the patient had an abdominoperineal resection, suggest sitz baths to help relieve perineal discomfort.

Bowel resection and anastomosis

Resection of diseased intestinal tissue (colectomy) and anastomosis of the remaining segments helps treat localized obstructive disorders, including diverticulosis, intestinal polyps, bowel adhesions, and malignant or benign intestinal lesions. This is the preferred surgical technique for localized bowel cancer but not for widespread carcinoma, which usually requires massive resection and a temporary or permanent colostomy or an ileostomy.

Unlike the patient who undergoes total colectomy or more extensive surgery, the patient who undergoes simple resection and anastomosis usually retains normal bowel function.

Patient preparation

Before surgery, as ordered, administer antibiotics to reduce intestinal flora and laxatives or enemas to remove fecal contents.

Monitoring and aftercare

Follow these steps after surgery:
• For the first few days after surgery, monitor the patient's intake, output, and weight daily. Maintain fluid and electrolyte balance through I.V. replacement therapy, and check regularly for signs of dehydration, such as decreased urine output and poor skin turgor.
• Keep the NG tube patent. Warn the patient that he should never attempt to reposition a dislodged tube himself because doing so could damage the anastomosis. Perform frequent mouth care.
• Observe the patient for signs of peritonitis or sepsis caused by leakage of bowel contents into the abdominal cavity. He's at increased risk for sepsis if he's immunosuppressed or receiving TPN.

An attack of hot flashes

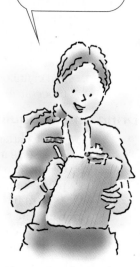

For the first few days after surgery, monitor the patient's intake, output, and weight daily.

• Provide meticulous wound care, changing dressings when needed. Check dressings and drainage sites frequently for signs of infection (purulent drainage, foul odor) and fecal drainage. Also, watch for sudden fever, especially when accompanied by abdominal pain and tenderness.
• Regularly assess the patient for signs of postresection obstruction. Examine the abdomen for distention and rigidity, auscultate for bowel sounds, and note the passage of any flatus or stool.
• After the patient regains peristalsis and bowel function, help him avoid constipation and straining during defecation, both of which can damage the anastomosis. Encourage him to drink plenty of fluids, and administer a stool softener or other laxative, as ordered. Note and record the frequency and amount of all bowel movements as well as characteristics of the stool.
• Encourage regular coughing and deep breathing to prevent atelectasis; remind the patient to splint the incision site as necessary.
• Assess pain and provide analgesics, as ordered.

Home care instructions

Provide these instructions to the patient:
• Instruct the patient to record the frequency and character of bowel movements and to tell the practitioner if he notices any changes in his normal pattern. Warn him against using laxatives without consulting his practitioner.

Feeling the strain

• Tell the patient to avoid abdominal straining and heavy lifting until the sutures are completely healed and the practitioner gives permission to do so.

• Encourage the patient to maintain the prescribed semibland diet until his bowel has healed completely (usually 4 to 8 weeks after surgery). Stress the need to avoid carbonated beverages and gas-producing foods.
• Because extensive bowel resection may interfere with the patient's ability to absorb nutrients, emphasize the importance of taking prescribed vitamin supplements.

Appendectomy

With rare exception, the only effective treatment for acute appendicitis is to remove the inflamed vermiform appendix. A common emergency surgery, an appendectomy aims to prevent imminent rupture or perforation of the appendix. When completed before these complications occur, an appendectomy is usually effective and uneventful. A perforated appendix carries a greater risk of mortality. If the appendix ruptures or perforates before surgery, its infected contents spill into the peritoneal cavity, possibly causing peritonitis. Most appendectomies are now done laparoscopically, except in cases where rupture is suspected.

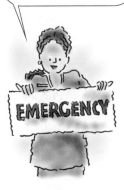

An appendectomy is commonly an emergency procedure, and it's virtually the only effective treatment for acute appendicitis.

Patient preparation

Before surgery, implement these measures:
• Reduce the patient's pain by placing him in Fowler's position.
• Avoid giving analgesics, which can mask the pain that heralds rupture.

Risking rupture

• Never apply heat to the abdomen, give cathartics or enemas, or palpate the abdomen; these measures could trigger rupture.

Monitoring and aftercare

Follow these steps after surgery:
• Carefully monitor vital signs and record intake and output for 2 days after surgery.
• Auscultate the abdomen for bowel sounds, which signal the return of peristalsis.
• Regularly check the wound dressing for drainage, and change it as necessary. If abdominal drains are in place, check and record the amount and nature of drainage, and maintain drain patency.
• Check drainage from the NG tube, and irrigate as needed.
• Encourage ambulation within 12 hours after surgery if possible. Assist the patient as needed.

• Encourage coughing, deep breathing, use of an incentive spirometer, and frequent position changes to prevent pulmonary complications.
• On the day after surgery, remove the NG tube and gradually resume oral foods and fluids as ordered.
• Assess the patient closely for signs of peritonitis. Watch for and report continuing pain and fever, excessive wound drainage, hypotension, tachycardia, pallor, weakness, and other signs of infection and fluid and electrolyte loss. If peritonitis develops, expect to assist with emergency treatment, including GI intubation, parenteral fluid and electrolyte replacement, and antibiotic therapy.

Home care instructions

Provide these instructions to the patient:
• Tell the patient to watch for and immediately report fever, chills, diaphoresis, nausea, vomiting, or abdominal pain and tenderness.
• Instruct the patient to avoid strenuous activity (heavy lifting, stooping, and pushing or pulling) for up to 1 month following surgery.
• Encourage the patient to keep scheduled follow-up appointments to monitor healing and diagnose complications.

Gallbladder surgery

When gallbladder and biliary disorders fail to respond to drugs, diet therapy, and supportive treatments, surgery may be required to restore biliary flow from the liver to the small intestine. Gallbladder removal, or *cholecystectomy*, restores biliary flow in gallstone disease (cholecystitis or cholelithiasis) and relieves symptoms. It's one of the most commonly performed surgeries. Conventional cholecystectomy requires an incision several inches long, produces considerable discomfort, and results in weeks of recovery time.

Laparoscope to the rescue

Laparoscopic laser cholecystectomy allows gallbladder removal without major abdominal surgery. This speeds recovery and reduces the risk of such complications as infection and herniation. Patients are usually discharged from the hospital and can resume a normal diet after 24 to 36 hours. Typically, patients can return to the workplace within 10 days. Laparoscopic laser cholecystectomy is contraindicated in pregnancy, acute cholangitis, septic peritonitis, and severe bleeding disorders. (See *Understanding cholecystectomy.*)

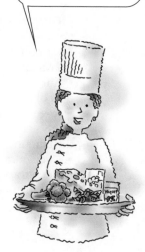

Laparoscopic laser cholecystectomy speeds recovery and allows patients to resume a normal diet after 24 to 36 hours.

Understanding cholecystectomy

Gallbladder surgeries include abdominal cholecystectomy and laparoscopic laser cholecystectomy as well as several less commonly performed procedures. The two more common procedures are described here.

Abdominal cholecystectomy

Performed under general anesthesia, abdominal cholecystectomy begins with a right subcostal or paramedial incision. The surgeon then surveys the abdomen and uses laparotomy packs to isolate the gallbladder from the surrounding organs. After identifying biliary tract structures, he may use cholangiography or ultrasonography to help identify gallstones. Using a choledocoscope, he directly visualizes the bile ducts and inserts a balloon-tipped catheter to clear the ducts of stones.

The surgeon ligates and divides the cystic duct and artery and removes the entire gallbladder. Typically, he performs a choledochotomy — the insertion of a T tube into the common bile duct to decompress the biliary tree and prevent bile peritonitis during healing. He may also insert a drain into the ducts.

Laparoscopic laser cholecystectomy

Several small entry points (1 to 3 cm) are made on the abdomen — at the umbilicus (for the laparoscope and attached camera) and at the upper midline, right lateral line, and right midclavicular line (for various grasping and dissecting forceps). The abdomen is insufflated with carbon dioxide, which allows viewing of the structures. The attached camera transmits images to a television monitor, allowing the surgical team to view the procedure. The cystic duct and artery are clipped and divided. Laser or cautery is used to cut and coagulate during removal of the gallbladder from its liver bed. Needle aspiration of bile facilitates gallbladder removal through the stab wound at the umbilicus.

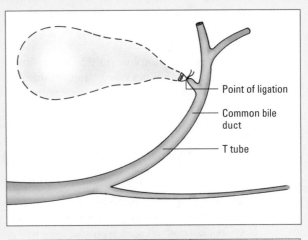

Point of ligation

Common bile duct

T tube

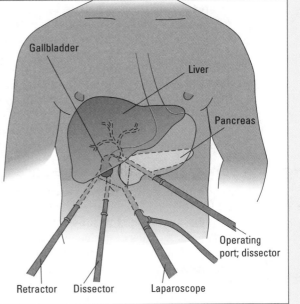

Gallbladder

Liver

Pancreas

Operating port; dissector

Retractor   Dissector   Laparoscope

A clean sweep

In patients who aren't good candidates for cholecystectomy, cholecystostomy (incision into the fundus of the gallbladder to remove and drain any retained gallstones or inflammatory debris) or choledochotomy (incision into the common bile duct to remove any gallstones or other obstructions) are sometimes performed.

Patient preparation

Before surgery, implement these measures:
• Monitor and, if necessary, help stabilize the patient's nutritional status and fluid balance. Such measures may include vitamin K administration, blood transfusions, and glucose and protein supplements.
• For 24 hours before surgery, give the patient clear liquids only.
• As ordered, administer preoperative medications and insert an NG tube.

Monitoring and aftercare

Follow these steps after laparoscopic surgery:
• Check the small stab wounds; they will be closed with staples or sutures and may have small dressings.
• Monitor for anesthesia-related nausea and vomiting.
• Apply heat to the patient's shoulder to alleviate right shoulder pain caused by phrenic irritation from carbon dioxide under the diaphragm. To decrease discomfort, place the patient in semi-Fowler's position. Early ambulation also helps.
• Tell the patient a light meal is usually permitted the same evening.
• The day after discharge, place a follow-up phone call to the patient's home to check on his progress.

Nothing conventional about this care

Follow these steps after conventional surgery:
• Place the patient in low Fowler's position. If the patient has an NG tube, attach it to low intermittent suction. Monitor the amount and characteristics of drainage from the NG tube as well as from any abdominal drains. Check the dressing frequently, and change it as necessary.
• If the patient has a T tube in place, frequently assess the position and patency of the tube and drainage bag. Make sure the bag is level with the abdomen to prevent excessive drainage. Also note the amount and characteristics of drainage; bloody or blood-tinged bile usually occurs for only the first few hours after surgery. Provide meticulous skin care around the tube insertion site to prevent irritation.

• After a few days, expect to remove the NG tube and begin introducing foods: first liquids, then gradually soft solids. As ordered, clamp the T tube for an hour before and an hour after each meal to allow bile to travel to the intestine to aid digestion.
• Watch for signs of postcholecystectomy syndrome (such as fever, abdominal pain, and jaundice) and other complications involving obstructed bile drainage. For several days after surgery, monitor vital signs and record intake and output every 8 hours. Report unusual signs and symptoms to the practitioner, and collect urine and stool specimens for laboratory analysis of bile content.

Home care instructions

After laparoscopic laser cholecystectomy, instruct the patient on the use of oral analgesics, how to clean the surgical stab sites, and when to call the practitioner. Also, include these instructions in your teaching:
• Recommend activity as tolerated, but tell the patient to avoid heavy lifting for about 2 weeks. Assure him that patients typically return to a normal schedule within 10 days.
• Tell the patient that he'll be given an appointment to see the practitioner or return to the clinic within 7 days for removal of the staples. Assure him that scarring is usually minimal.
• If the patient underwent the procedure as a same-day, outpatient procedure, tell him he may feel shoulder pain from the carbon dioxide used during surgery. Explain that he can relieve the pain by walking and applying heat to his shoulder.

Conventional wisdom

After conventional surgery, give these instructions:
• If the patient is being discharged with a T tube in place, stress the need for the patient to practice meticulous tube care.
• Tell him to immediately report any signs or symptoms of biliary obstruction: fever, jaundice, pruritus, pain, dark urine, and clay-colored stools.
• Encourage the patient to maintain a diet low in fats and high in carbohydrates and protein. Tell him that his ability to digest fats will improve as bile flow to the intestine increases. As this occurs — usually within 6 weeks — he may gradually add fats to his diet.

> Tell the same-day surgery patient that he can relieve shoulder pain from the carbon dioxide used during surgery by walking and applying heat to his shoulder.

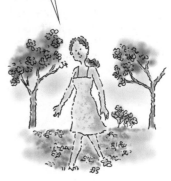

Liver transplantation

For the patient with a life-threatening liver disorder that doesn't respond to treatment, a liver transplant may seem the last best hope. Even so, transplant surgery is used infrequently because of its risks and high cost, as well as the shortage of suitable donor organs. Typically, it's used only in large teaching centers and is reserved for those terminally ill patients who have a realistic chance of surviving the surgery and withstanding postoperative complications. Candidates include patients with congenital biliary abnormalities, chronic hepatitis B or C, inborn errors of metabolism, or end-stage liver disease.

Meet the candidate

Careful identification of suitable candidates for referral to the transplant team is essential to the success of therapy. Criteria for referral for transplantation include:
• advanced hepatic failure with a predicted survival rate of less than 2 years
• unavailability of other medical or surgical therapies that offer long-term survival
• absence of contraindicated conditions, such as extrahepatic carcinoma, severe cardiac disease, and current active alcohol or drug addiction
• full understanding by the patient and his family of the physical, psychological, and financial aspects of the transplant process.

Waiting game

Many qualified transplant candidates are awaiting suitable donor organs, but few survive the wait. Also, even if a compatible healthy liver is located and transplantation performed, the patient faces many obstacles to recovery. Besides the complications accompanying extensive abdominal and vascular surgeries, liver transplantation carries a high risk of tissue rejection. Current 1-year survival rates range from 85% to 90%.

Patient preparation

Before surgery, implement these measures:
• As ordered, begin immunosuppressant therapy to decrease the risk of tissue rejection, using such drugs as cyclosporine and corticosteroids.
• Explain the need for lifelong therapy to prevent rejection.
• Address the emotional needs of the patient and his family. Discuss the typical stages of emotional adjustment to a liver transplant: overwhelming relief and elation at surviving the operation, followed by anxiety, frustration, and depression if complications occur.

Monitoring and aftercare

Focus your aftercare on four areas:
• maintaining immunosuppressant therapy to combat tissue rejection
• monitoring for early signs of rejection and other complications
• preventing opportunistic infections, which can lead to rejection
• providing emotional support to the patient throughout the prolonged recovery period.

Candidates for liver transplantation must not have any contraindicated conditions, including severe cardiac disease.

Home care instructions

Teach the patient and his family to:
• watch for early indications of tissue rejection — including fever, tachycardia, jaundice, changes in the color of urine or stool, and pain and tenderness in the right upper quadrant, right flank, or center of the back — and notify the practitioner immediately if any of these signs or symptoms develop
• watch for and report any signs or symptoms of liver failure, such as abdominal distention, bloody stool or vomitus, decreased urine output, abdominal pain and tenderness, anorexia, and altered level of consciousness (LOC)

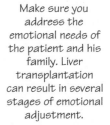

Make sure you address the emotional needs of the patient and his family. Liver transplantation can result in several stages of emotional adjustment.

A wave instead of a handshake

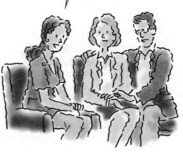

• reduce the risk of tissue rejection by avoiding contact with any person who has or may have a contagious illness and report any early signs or symptoms of infection, including fever, weakness, lethargy, and tachycardia
• keep follow-up appointments, which will include regular liver function tests, complete blood count (CBC), and blood cyclosporin levels, to evaluate the integrity of the surgical site and continued tissue compatibility
• strictly comply with the prescribed immunosuppressive drug regimen because noncompliance can trigger rejection, even of a liver that has been functioning well for years
• be aware of potential adverse effects of immunosuppressive therapy, such as infection, fluid retention, acne, glaucoma, diabetes, and cancer
• seek psychological counseling if necessary to help the patient and his family cope with the effects of the patient's long and difficult recovery.

Liver resection or repair

Resection or repair of diseased or damaged liver tissue may be indicated for various hepatic disorders, including cysts, abscesses, tumors, and lacerations or crush injuries from blunt or penetrating trauma. Usually, surgery is performed only after conservative measures prove ineffective. For instance, if aspiration fails to correct a liver abscess, resection may be necessary.

Liver resection procedures include a partial or subtotal hepatectomy (excision of a portion of the liver) and lobectomy (excision of an entire lobe). Lobectomy is the surgery of choice for primary liver tumors, but partial hepatectomy may be effective for small tumors.

Rarely resectable

Even so, because liver cancer is often advanced at diagnosis, few tumors are resectable. In fact, only single tumors confined to one lobe are usually considered resectable, and then only if the patient is free from complicating cirrhosis, jaundice, or ascites. Because of the liver's anatomic location, surgery is usually performed through a thoracoabdominal incision.

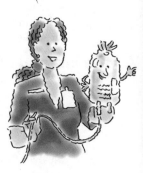

Tell the patient he'll be receiving I.V. fluid replacement when he wakes up from surgery.

Patient preparation

Before surgery, implement these measures:
• Encourage rest and good nutrition and provide vitamin supplements, as ordered, to help improve liver function.
• Prepare the patient for additional diagnostic tests, which may include liver scan, CT scan, ultrasonography, percutaneous needle biopsy, hepatic angiography, and cholangiography.
• Explain postoperative care measures. Tell the patient he'll awaken from surgery with an NG tube, a chest tube, and hemodynamic monitoring lines in place. Tell him to expect frequent checks of vital signs, fluid and electrolyte balance, and neurologic status as well as I.V. fluid replacement and possible blood transfusions and TPN. If possible, allow the patient to visit and familiarize himself with the intensive care unit.
• To reduce the risk of postoperative atelectasis, encourage the patient to practice coughing and deep-breathing exercises, and teach him how to use an incentive spirometer.

Monitoring and aftercare

Follow these steps after surgery:
• Frequently assess for complications, such as hemorrhage and infection. Monitor the patient's vital signs and evaluate fluid status every 1 to 2 hours. Report any signs of volume deficit, which could indicate intraperitoneal bleeding. Keep an I.V. line patent for possible emergency fluid replacement or blood transfusion. Provide analgesics as ordered.
• At least daily, check laboratory test results for hypoglycemia, increased PT, increased ammonia levels, azotemia (increased blood urea nitrogen [BUN] and creatinine levels), and electrolyte imbalances (especially potassium, sodium, and calcium imbalances). Promptly report adverse findings, and take corrective steps, as ordered. For example, give I.M. vitamin K to decrease PT, or infuse hypertonic glucose solution to correct hypoglycemia.
• Check wound dressings often and change them as needed. Note and report excessive bloody drainage on the dressings or in the drainage tube. Also note the amount and characteristics of NG tube drainage; keep in mind that excessive drainage could trigger metabolic alkalosis. If the patient has a chest tube in place,

maintain tube patency. Make sure the suction equipment is operating properly. Don't strip the tube because the increase in negative pressure could harm the patient.

Dazed and confused

- Watch for signs and symptoms of hepatic encephalopathy, including behavioral or personality changes, such as confusion, forgetfulness, lethargy or stupor, and hallucinations. Also observe for asterixis, apraxia, and hyperactive reflexes.

Home care instructions

Provide these instructions to the patient:
- Tell him that adequate rest and good nutrition conserve energy and reduce metabolic demands on the liver, thereby speeding healing. For the first 6 to 8 months after surgery, he should gradually resume normal activities, balance periods of activity and rest, and avoid overexertion.
- As ordered, instruct the patient to maintain a high-calorie, high-carbohydrate, and high-protein diet during this period to help restore the liver mass. However, if the patient had hepatic encephalopathy, advise him to follow a low-protein diet, with carbohydrates making up the balance of calorie intake.

Transjugular intrahepatic portosystemic shunt insertion

Intractable ascites resulting from chronic liver failure can be controlled by diverting blood flow from the portal vein to the venous circulation with a transjugular intrahepatic portosystemic shunt (TIPS). Using angiographic techniques and contrast dye, the surgeon places an expandable metal stent to form a connection between the intrahepatic portal vein and the hepatic vein. This reduces intravascular fluid pressure in the liver by allowing blood to return to the systemic circulation. The TIPS is extremely effective in reducing sodium retention, improving renal function, and reducing cirrhosis-related esophageal and gastric variceal bleeding. (See *How TIPS works*, page 464.)

Patient preparation

Before the procedure, implement these measures:
- Explain to the patient and his family how the TIPS works.
- Tell the patient that it may be necessary to withhold medications, such as aspirin and other NSAIDs and anticoagulants, for a period of time before the procedure.
- Assess the patient for contrast dye allergies.

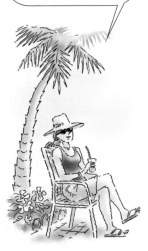

Tell your patient he should balance periods of activity and rest to avoid overexertion as he gradually resumes normal activities. I'm certainly avoiding overexertion right now!

How TIPS works

In this radiologic procedure, a catheter is inserted into the jugular vein. Under X-ray guidance, the practitioner then threads and places the transjugular intrahepatic porto-systemic shunt (TIPS) between the portal and hepatic veins. Once the TIPS is in place, it relieves portal hypertension by allowing blood to flow directly into general circulation.

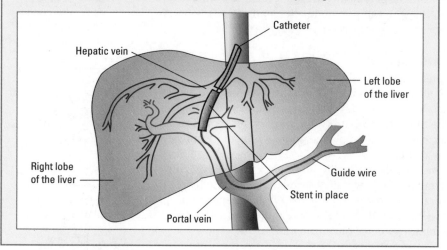

- Tell the patient that he'll receive a local anesthetic during the procedure to minimize discomfort at the internal jugular catheter insertion site; he may also receive sedation during the procedure.
- Measure and record the patient's weight and abdominal girth to serve as a baseline.
- Obtain a CBC; electrolyte, BUN, and creatinine levels; and coagulation laboratory studies to establish a baseline.

Monitoring and aftercare
Follow these steps after the procedure:
- Make the patient as comfortable as possible by placing him in low Fowler's or semi-Fowler's position; administer analgesics as ordered.
- Monitor the patient's vital signs, and watch for hypervolemia or hypovolemia. Be alert for signs of heart failure and infection. Monitor his electrolyte levels.

Toxic effects
- Because blood from the GI tract is shunted around the liver, the patient is at increased risk for hepatic encephalopathy from circulating toxins; monitor his mental status, and report changes to the practitioner immediately.

• Weigh the patient and measure his abdominal girth daily. Watch for signs of shunt failure, such as gastric bleeding or increases in abdominal girth.

Home care instructions

Provide these instructions to the patient:
• Instruct the patient to weigh himself daily and to keep a log. Tell him to report increases of 2 or more pounds to the practitioner.
• Tell him he'll need to have his shunt periodically assessed for placement and patency, typically with ultrasound.
• Explain that, if his shunt becomes stenosed, a stenting procedure can usually reestablish patency.
• Encourage the patient to keep regular follow-up appointments.

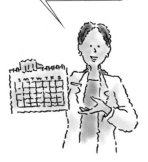

Encourage the patient to keep regular follow-up appointments.

Endoscopic retrograde sphincterotomy

First used to remove retained gallstones from the common bile duct after cholecystectomy, endoscopic retrograde sphincterotomy (ERS) is now also used to treat high-risk patients with biliary dyskinesia and to insert biliary stents for draining malignant or benign strictures in the common bile duct.

A-tisket, a-tasket, balloons or a basket

In this procedure, a fiber-optic endoscope is advanced through the stomach and duodenum to the ampulla of Vater. A papillotome is passed through the endoscope to make a small incision to widen the biliary sphincter. If the stone doesn't drop out into the duodenum on its own, the doctor may introduce a Dormia basket, a balloon, or a lithotriptor through the endoscope to remove or crush the stone.

Quick, painless, and safe

ERS allows treatment without general anesthesia or a surgical incision, ensuring a quicker and safer recovery. It may be performed on an outpatient basis for some patients, making it a cost-effective alternative to surgery.

Patient preparation

Explain the treatment to the patient:
• His throat will be sprayed with an anesthetic to prevent discomfort during the insertion and he may also receive a sedative to help him relax. Reassure him that the procedure should cause little or no discomfort.
• He'll be positioned on the fluoroscopy table in a left side-lying position, with his left arm behind him. Encourage him to relax.

Monitoring and aftercare

Follow these steps after treatment:
• Instruct the patient to cough, deep-breathe, and expectorate regularly to avoid aspirating secretions. Keep in mind that the anesthetic's effects may hinder expectoration and swallowing.
• Withhold food and fluids until the anesthesia wears off and the patient's gag reflex returns.
• Check the patient's vital signs frequently and monitor carefully for signs of hemorrhage: hematemesis, melena, tachycardia, and hypotension. If any of these signs develop, notify the practitioner immediately.

Home care instructions

Provide these instructions to the patient:
• Tell him to immediately report any signs of hemorrhage, sepsis, cholangitis, or pancreatitis.
• Encourage him to report any recurrence of the characteristic jaundice and pain of biliary obstruction. He may need repeat ERS to remove new stones or to replace a malfunctioning biliary stent.

> You don't have to be a judge to rule in favor of ERS. Any objection to a quicker, safer recovery is out of order.

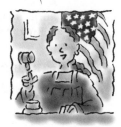

Nursing diagnoses

The following nursing diagnoses are commonly used in patients with GI disorders. For each diagnosis, you'll also find nursing interventions with rationales. See *NANDA-I taxonomy II by domain*, page 936, for the complete list of NANDA diagnoses.

Constipation

Related to inadequate intake of fluid and bulk, *Constipation* may pertain to all patients undergoing periods of restricted food or fluid intake.

Expected outcomes

• Patient expresses decreased feelings of constipation.
• Patient reports a more regular bowel elimination pattern.
• Patient identifies proper methods used to help promote a regular bowel pattern.

Nursing interventions and rationales

• Record intake and output accurately to ensure correct fluid replacement therapy.
• Note the color and consistency of stool and frequency of bowel movements to form the basis of an effective treatment plan.

• Promote ample fluid intake, if appropriate, to minimize constipation with increased intestinal fluid content.
• Encourage the patient to increase dietary intake of fiber to improve intestinal muscle tone and promote comfortable elimination.
• Discourage routine use of laxatives and enemas to avoid trauma to intestinal mucosa, dehydration, and eventual failure of defecation stimulus. (Bulk-adding laxatives aren't irritating and are usually permitted.)
• Encourage the patient to walk and exercise as much as possible to stimulate intestinal activity.
• Encourage the patient to take the time necessary each day to have a bowel movement to help promote a regular bowel pattern.

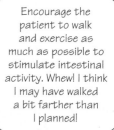

Encourage the patient to walk and exercise as much as possible to stimulate intestinal activity. Whew! I think I may have walked a bit farther than I planned!

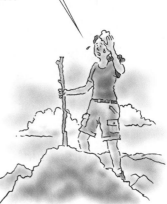

Diarrhea

Related to malabsorption, inflammation, or irritation of the bowel, *Diarrhea* may be associated with irritable bowel syndrome, colitis, Crohn's disease, and other conditions.

Expected outcomes

• Patient reports cessation of diarrhea as evidenced by formed stool.
• Patient identifies proper methods for treating diarrhea.

Nursing interventions and rationales

• Assess the patient's level of dehydration and electrolyte status. Fluid loss secondary to diarrhea can be life-threatening.
• Monitor the patient's weight daily to detect fluid loss or retention.
• Note the color and consistency of stool and frequency of bowel movements to monitor treatment effectiveness.
• Test stool for occult blood, and obtain stool for culture to help evaluate factors contributing to diarrhea.
• Assess for fecal impaction. Liquid stool may seep around an impaction.

Fluids are fine, but forget fiber

For acute diarrhea, provide the following dietary regimen:
• Give clear fluids, including glucose, electrolyte-containing beverages, and commercial rehydration preparations, orally. Clear fluids provide rapidly absorbed calories and electrolytes with minimal stimulation. After diarrhea has stopped for 24 to 48 hours, progress to a full fluid diet, then to a regular diet.

• Avoid milk, caffeine, and high-fiber foods for 1 week to avoid irritating the intestinal mucosa.
• In chronic diarrhea, encourage the patient to avoid foods and activities that may cause diarrhea. His awareness and self-regulation of contributing factors help manage chronic diarrhea.

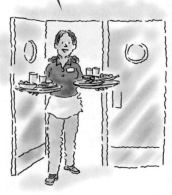

Patients with diarrhea should avoid milk, caffeine, and high-fiber foods for a week. Let me get you a cup of decaf!

Ineffective tissue perfusion: GI

Related to reduced blood flow, *Ineffective tissue perfusion: GI* may be associated with cirrhosis, hepatic failure, and other conditions.

Expected outcomes

• Patient maintains adequate blood flow to the intestinal mucosa.
• Patient identifies reportable symptoms such as pain after eating.

Nursing interventions and rationales

• Assess the patient for bowel sounds, increasing abdominal girth, pain, nausea and vomiting, and electrolyte imbalance. Acute changes may indicate a surgical emergency due to ischemia.
• If the patient has a chronic circulatory problem, provide small, frequent feedings of light, bland foods to promote digestion. Also, encourage rest after feedings to maximize blood flow available for digestion.

Bowel incontinence

Related to neuromuscular involvement, *Bowel incontinence* may be seen in patients who have had a hemorrhoidectomy, radical prostatectomy, or abdominal perineal resection.

Expected outcomes

• Patient remains continent of stool.
• Patient identifies measures to help maintain bowel schedule.

Nursing interventions and rationales

• Establish a schedule for defecation — $1/2$ hour after a meal works well for active peristalsis. A regular pattern encourages adaptation and routine physiologic function.
• Instruct the patient to use the bathroom or commode if possible to allow easy defecation without anxiety.

- If bedpan use is necessary, assist the patient to the most normal position possible for defecation to increase comfort and reduce anxiety.
- Instruct the patient to bear down or help him lean his trunk forward to increase intra-abdominal pressure.
- If necessary, use a glycerine suppository or gentle manual stimulation with a lubricated finger in the anal sphincter to encourage regular physiologic function, stimulate peristalsis, minimize infection, and promote comfort with elimination.
- Provide skin care to prevent infection and promote comfort.
- Refrain from commenting about "accidents" to avoid embarrassing the patient and help promote his self-image.

Common GI disorders

Below are several common GI disorders, along with their causes, pathophysiology, signs and symptoms, diagnostic test findings, treatments, and nursing interventions.

Appendicitis

Appendicitis occurs when the appendix becomes inflamed. It's the most common major surgical emergency. More precisely, this disorder is an inflammation of the vermiform appendix, a small, fingerlike projection attached to the cecum just below the ileocecal valve. The appendix may harbor good bacteria that protect the gut and play a role in the immune system.

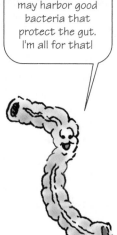

The appendix may harbor good bacteria that protect the gut. I'm all for that!

What causes it

Causes of appendicitis include:
- mucosal ulceration
- fecal mass (fecalith)
- stricture
- barium ingestion
- viral infection.

Pathophysiology

Mucosal ulceration triggers inflammation, which temporarily obstructs the appendix. The obstruction blocks mucus outflow. Pressure in the now-distended appendix increases, and the appendix contracts. Bacteria multiply, and inflammation and pressure continue to increase, restricting blood flow to the organ and causing severe abdominal pain.

Inflammation can lead to infection, clotting, tissue decay, and perforation of the appendix. If the appendix ruptures or perforates, the infected contents spill into the abdominal cavity, causing peritonitis, the most common and dangerous complication.

What to look for

Initially, the patient may manifest these signs and symptoms:
• abdominal pain, generalized or localized in the right upper abdomen, eventually localizing in the right lower abdomen (McBurney's point) (see *Eliciting McBurney's sign*)
• anorexia
• nausea and vomiting
• boardlike abdominal rigidity
• retractive respirations
• increasingly severe abdominal spasms and rebound spasms. (Rebound tenderness on the opposite side of the abdomen suggests peritoneal inflammation.)
  Later symptoms include:
• constipation (although diarrhea is also possible)
• fever of 99° to 102° F (37.2° to 38.9° C)
• tachycardia

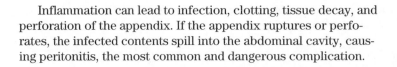

Memory jogger

When you have a patient with abdominal pain that's generalized or localized in the right upper abdomen or right lower abdomen (McBurney's point), you probably suspect appendicitis. To remember the other early signs and symptoms of appendicitis that may appear, always use your **BRAIN**:

Boardlike abdominal rigidity

Retractive respirations

Anorexia

Increasingly severe abdominal and rebound spasms

Nausea and vomiting.

Eliciting McBurney's sign

To elicit McBurney's sign, help the patient into a supine position, with his knees slightly flexed and his abdominal muscles relaxed. Then palpate deeply and slowly in the right lower quadrant over McBurney's point—located about 2″ (5 cm) from the right anterior superior spine of the ilium, on a line between the spine and the umbilicus. Point pain and tenderness, a positive McBurney's sign, indicates appendicitis.

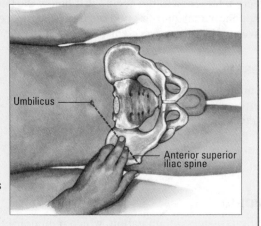

Umbilicus

Anterior superior iliac spine

• sudden cessation of abdominal pain (indicates perforation or infarction of the appendix).

What tests tell you
• White blood cell (WBC) count is moderately elevated, with increased immature cells.
• Ultrasound of the abdomen and pelvis can help diagnose a nonperforated appendix. CT scan can help to identify abscess.

How it's treated
An appendectomy is the only effective treatment for appendicitis. If peritonitis develops, treatment involves GI intubation, parenteral replacement of fluids and electrolytes, and administration of antibiotics.

What to do

For suspected appendicitis or to prepare for appendectomy
• Administer I.V. fluids to prevent dehydration. Never administer cathartics or enemas because they may rupture the appendix.
• Give the patient nothing by mouth, and administer analgesics judiciously because they may mask symptoms of rupture.
• Place the patient in Fowler's position to reduce pain. (This is also helpful postoperatively.) Never apply heat to the lower right abdomen or perform palpation; these actions may cause the appendix to rupture.

After an appendectomy
• Monitor the patient's vital signs and intake and output.
• Give analgesics, as ordered.
• Document bowel sounds, passing of flatus, or bowel movements — signs of peristalsis return. If these signs appear in a patient whose nausea and abdominal rigidity have subsided, he's ready to resume oral fluids.
• Watch closely for possible surgical complications. Continuing pain and fever may signal an abscess. The complaint that "something gave way" may mean wound dehiscence. If an abscess or peritonitis develops, incision and drainage may be necessary. Frequently assess the dressing for wound drainage.
• If peritonitis complicates appendicitis, the patient may need an NG tube to decompress the stomach and reduce nausea and vomiting. If so, record drainage, and provide good mouth and nose care.

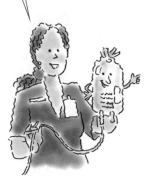

Administer I.V. fluids to prevent dehydration in suspected appendicitis or preparation for an appendectomy.

• Evaluate the patient. He should demonstrate appropriate activity restrictions, be able to resume a normal diet and bowel elimination pattern, and understand the importance of follow-up care. (See *Appendicitis teaching tips.*)

Gallbladder and biliary tract disorders

Gallbladder and biliary tract disorders, such as cholecystitis, cholelithiasis, choledocholithiasis, and cholangitis, are common, painful conditions that usually require surgery and may be life-threatening. They typically accompany calculus deposition and inflammation.

What causes it

The exact cause of cholecystitis is unknown; risk factors include:
• a high-calorie, high-cholesterol diet, associated with obesity
• elevated estrogen levels from hormonal contraceptives, postmenopausal therapy, pregnancy, or multiparity
• diabetes mellitus, ileal disease, hemolytic disorders, liver disease, or pancreatitis
• genetic factors
• weight-reduction diets with severe calorie restriction and rapid weight loss.

Pathophysiology

Certain conditions (such as age, obesity, and estrogen imbalance) cause the liver to secrete bile that's abnormally high in cholesterol or that lacks the proper concentration of bile salts. Excessive water and bile salts are reabsorbed, making the bile less soluble. Cholesterol, calcium, and bilirubin then precipitate into gallstones. (See *Understanding gallbladder and biliary tract disorders* and *Understanding gallstone formation*, page 474.)

What to look for

In acute cholecystitis, acute cholelithiasis, and choledocholithiasis, look for:
• the classic attack with severe midepigastric or right upper quadrant pain radiating to the back or referred to the right scapula, commonly after meals rich in fats
• recurring fat intolerance
• belching that leaves a sour taste in the mouth
• flatulence
• indigestion
• diaphoresis

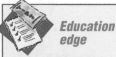

Education edge

Appendicitis teaching tips

• Explain what happens in appendicitis.
• Help the patient understand the required surgery and its possible complications. If time allows, provide preoperative teaching.
• Discuss postoperative activity limitations. Tell the patient to follow the practitioner's orders for driving, returning to work, and resuming physical activity.

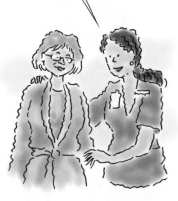

Age and estrogen imbalance can cause the liver to secrete bile that lacks the proper concentration of bile salts or is abnormally high in cholesterol.

Understanding gallbladder and biliary tract disorders

The five major disorders associated with the gallbladder and biliary tract are:

• *cholecystitis* — an acute or chronic inflammation of the gallbladder, usually associated with a gallstone impacted in the cystic duct, causing painful distention of the gallbladder. The acute form is most common during middle age; the chronic form, among elderly people. Prognosis is good with treatment.

• *cholangitis* — infection of the bile duct, commonly associated with choledocholithiasis; may follow percutaneous transhepatic cholangiography. Widespread inflammation may cause fibrosis and stenosis of the common bile duct and biliary radicles. Without liver transplantation, prognosis for this rare condition is poor.

• *cholelithiasis* — stones or calculi in the gallbladder (gallstones) resulting from changes in bile components. It's the leading biliary tract disease, affecting over 20 million Americans, and is the third most common surgical procedure performed in the United States (cholecystectomy). Prognosis is usually good with treatment unless infection occurs, in which case prognosis depends on the infection's severity and response to antibiotics.

• *choledocholithiasis* — gallstones passed out of the gallbladder lodge in the common bile duct, causing partial or complete biliary obstruction. Prognosis is good unless infection develops.

• *gallstone ileus* — involves small-bowel obstruction by a gallstone. Typically, the gallstone travels through a fistula between the gallbladder and small bowel and lodges at the ileocecal valve. This condition is most common in elderly people. Prognosis is good with surgery.

• nausea
• chills and low-grade fever
• possible jaundice and clay-colored stools with common duct obstruction.

The gist of cholangitis

In cholangitis, look for:
• abdominal pain
• high fever and chills
• possible jaundice and related itching
• weakness and fatigue.

Ileus ailments

In gallstone ileus, look for:
• nausea and vomiting
• abdominal distention
• absent bowel sounds (in complete bowel obstruction)
• intermittent colicky pain over several days.

Cholangitis can cause high fever and chills. What a miserable combination!

Understanding gallstone formation

Abnormal metabolism of cholesterol and bile salts plays an important role in gallstone formation. Bile is made continuously by the liver and is concentrated and stored in the gallbladder until the duodenum needs it to help digest fat. Changes in the composition of bile may allow gallstones to form. Changes to the absorptive ability of the gallbladder lining may also contribute to gallstone formation.

Too much cholesterol

Certain conditions, such as age, obesity, and estrogen imbalance, cause the liver to secrete bile that's abnormally high in cholesterol or lacking the proper concentration of bile salts.

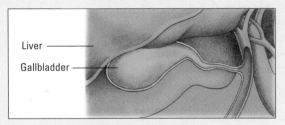

Inside the gallbladder

When the gallbladder concentrates this bile, inflammation may or may not occur. Excessive water and bile salts are reabsorbed, making the bile less soluble. Cholesterol, calcium, and bilirubin precipitate into gallstones.

Fat entering the duodenum causes the intestinal mucosa to secrete the hormone cholecystokinin, which stimulates the gallbladder to contract and empty. If a stone lodges in the cystic duct, the gallbladder contracts but can't empty.

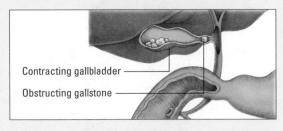

Jaundice, irritation, inflammation

If a stone lodges in the common bile duct, the bile flow into the duodenum becomes obstructed. Bilirubin is absorbed into the blood, causing jaundice.

Biliary narrowing and swelling of the tissue around the stone can also cause irritation and inflammation of the common bile duct.

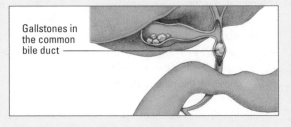

Up the biliary tree

Inflammation can progress up the biliary tree and cause infection of any of the bile ducts. This causes scar tissue, fluid accumulation, cirrhosis, portal hypertension, and bleeding.

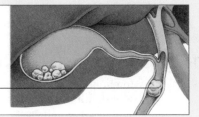

What tests tell you

• Ultrasonography reveals calculi in the gallbladder with 96% accuracy. PTHC distinguishes between gallbladder disease and cancer of the pancreatic head in patients with jaundice.

- CT scan may identify ductal stones.
- ERCP visualizes the biliary tree after endoscopic examination of the duodenum, cannulation of the common bile and pancreatic ducts, and injection of a contrast medium.
- Cholescintigraphy detects obstruction of the cystic duct.
- If stones are identified in the common bile duct by radiologic examination, a therapeutic ERCP may be performed before cholecystectomy to remove the stones.
- Oral cholecystography shows calculi in the gallbladder and biliary duct obstruction.
- Laboratory tests showing an elevated icteric index and elevated total bilirubin, urine bilirubin, and alkaline phosphatase levels support the diagnosis.
- WBC count is slightly elevated during a cholecystitis attack.
- Serum amylase levels distinguish gallbladder disease from pancreatitis.
- Serial enzyme tests and an electrocardiogram (ECG) should precede other diagnostic tests if heart disease is suspected.

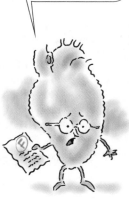

Serial enzyme tests and ECG should precede other tests if heart disease is suspected. Boy do I hate tests!

How it's treated

Several treatments exist for gallbladder and biliary tract disorders:
- Surgery, usually elective, is the treatment of choice for gallbladder and duct disease. Procedures may include cholecystectomy, cholecystectomy with operative cholangiography and, possibly, exploration of the common bile duct.
- A low-fat diet is prescribed to prevent attacks as well as vitamin K for itching, jaundice, and bleeding tendencies caused by vitamin K deficiency.
- During an acute attack, treatment may include insertion of an NG tube and I.V. line as well as antibiotic administration.
- A nonsurgical treatment for choledocholithiasis involves insertion of a flexible catheter, formed around a T tube, through the sinus tract into the common bile duct. Guided by fluoroscopy, the doctor directs the catheter toward the stone. A Dormia basket is threaded through the catheter to entrap the calculi.

That's really trippy — I mean, tripsy
- Lithotripsy, the ultrasonic breakup of gallstones, is usually unsuccessful and has a significant recurrence rate. The relative ease, short length of stay, and cost-effectiveness of laparoscopic cholecystectomy have made dissolution and lithotripsy less viable options.

What to do

• For information on preoperative and postoperative care of surgical patients, see "Gallbladder surgery," page 456.
• Evaluate the patient. He should return to normal nutrition and hydration status, be free from complications, and be able to tolerate normal activity and follow diet restrictions. (See *Gallbladder or biliary tract disorder teaching tips.*)

Cirrhosis

Cirrhosis, a chronic liver disease, is characterized by widespread destruction of hepatic cells, which are replaced by fibrous cells. This process is called *fibrotic regeneration*. Cirrhosis is a common cause of death in the United States and, among people ages 35 to 55, the fourth leading cause of death. It can occur at any age.

What causes it

There are many types of cirrhosis, and causes differ with each type:
• Laënnec's cirrhosis (also known as *portal, nutritional,* or *alcoholic cirrhosis*), the most common type of cirrhosis, results from malnutrition (especially of dietary protein) and chronic alcohol ingestion.
• Biliary cirrhosis results from bile duct diseases.
• Pigment cirrhosis may stem from disorders such as hemochromatosis.
• Other causes of cirrhosis include drug- or toxin-induced hepatic failure and chronic right-sided heart failure.
• In about 10% of patients, cirrhosis has no known cause.

Pathophysiology

Cirrhosis is characterized by irreversible chronic injury of the liver, extensive fibrosis, and nodular tissue growth. These changes result from:
• liver cell death (hepatocyte necrosis)
• collapse of the liver's supporting structure (the reticulin network)
• distortion of the vascular bed (blood vessels throughout the liver)
• nodular regeneration of the remaining liver tissue.

First one thing, then another

When the liver begins to malfunction, blood clotting disorders (coagulopathies), jaundice, edema, and many metabolic problems

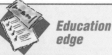

Gallbladder or biliary tract disorder teaching tips

• If a low-fat diet is prescribed, suggest ways to implement it. If necessary, ask the dietitian to reinforce your instructions. Make sure the patient understands how dietary changes help to prevent biliary colic.
• Reinforce the practitioner's explanation of the ordered treatment, such as surgery, endoscopic retrograde cholangiopancreatography, or lithotripsy. Make sure the patient fully understands the possible complications, if any, associated with his treatment.

develop. Fibrosis and the distortion of blood vessels may impede blood flow in the capillary branches of the portal vein and hepatic artery, leading to portal hypertension (elevated pressure in the portal vein). Increased pressure may lead to the development of esophageal varices — enlarged, tortuous veins in the lower part of the esophagus where it meets the stomach. Esophageal varices may easily rupture and leak large amounts of blood into the upper GI tract.

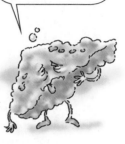

Collapse of my supporting structures can result in cirrhosis.

What to look for

Cirrhosis affects many body systems. Assess the patient for these signs and symptoms:
• GI (usually early and vague) — anorexia, indigestion, nausea and vomiting, constipation or diarrhea, dull abdominal ache
• respiratory — pleural effusion, limited thoracic expansion
• central nervous system — progressive signs and symptoms of hepatic encephalopathy, including lethargy, mental changes, slurred speech, asterixis (flapping tremor), peripheral neuritis, paranoia, hallucinations, extreme obtundation, coma
• hematologic — bleeding tendencies (nosebleeds, easy bruising, bleeding gums), anemia
• endocrine — testicular atrophy, menstrual irregularities, gynecomastia, loss of chest and axillary hair
• skin — severe pruritus, extreme dryness, poor tissue turgor, abnormal pigmentation, spider angiomas, palmar erythema, possibly jaundice
• hepatic — jaundice, hepatomegaly, ascites, edema of the legs
• miscellaneous — musty breath, enlarged superficial abdominal veins, muscle atrophy, pain in the right upper abdominal quadrant that worsens when the patient sits up or leans forward, palpable liver or spleen, temperature of 101° to 103° F (38.3° to 39.4° C), bleeding from esophageal varices.

What tests tell you

• Liver biopsy, the definitive test for cirrhosis, reveals destruction and fibrosis of hepatic tissue.
• A liver scan shows abnormal thickening and a liver mass.
• Cholecystography and cholangiography allow visualization of the gallbladder and the biliary duct system, respectively.
• Splenoportal venography allows visualization of the portal venous system.
• PTHC helps differentiate extrahepatic from intrahepatic obstructive jaundice and helps reveal hepatic disorders and gallstones.
• CT scan can show lobe enlargement, vascular changes, and nodules.

- WBC count, hematocrit, and hemoglobin, albumin, serum electrolyte, and cholinesterase levels are decreased.
- Globulin, serum ammonia, total bilirubin, alkaline phosphatase, alanine aminotransferase (ALT), aspartate aminotransferase (AST), and lactate dehydrogenase levels are increased.
- Anemia, neutropenia, and thrombocytopenia are present. PT and PTT are prolonged.

Vanishing vitamins

- Folic acid, iron levels, and vitamins A, B_{12}, C, and K are decreased.
- Glucose tolerance tests may be abnormal.
- Galactose tolerance and urine bilirubin tests are positive.
- Fecal and urine urobilinogen levels are elevated.

How it's treated

Therapy aims to remove or alleviate the underlying cause of cirrhosis, prevent further liver damage, and prevent or treat complications. In cases of active variceal bleeding, treatment aims to actively control blood loss through medication, surgery, or balloon tamponade. The patient may benefit from a high-protein diet, but this may be restricted by developing hepatic encephalopathy. Sodium is usually restricted to 200 to 500 mg/day and fluids to 1 to $1^{1}/_{2}$ qt (1 to 1.5 L)/day.

If the patient's condition continues to deteriorate, he may need tube feedings or TPN. Other supportive measures include:
- supplemental vitamins — A, B complex, C, and K — to compensate for the liver's inability to store them
- vitamin B_{12}, folic acid, and thiamine for anemia
- rest and moderate exercise and avoiding exposure to infections and toxic agents
- antiemetics, such as trimethobenzamide (Tigan) for nausea (when absolutely necessary)
- vasopressin for esophageal varices
- diuretics, such as furosemide (Lasix) and spironolactone (Aldactone), for edema with careful monitoring because fluid and electrolyte imbalance may precipitate hepatic encephalopathy
- paracentesis and infusions of salt-poor albumin to alleviate ascites
- insertion of a TIPS
- surgical procedures, including endoscopic sclerotherapy (or banding of varices), splenectomy, esophagogastric resection, and surgical shunts to relieve portal hypertension
- liver transplantation for the patient with advanced disease
- programs for preventing cirrhosis, which usually emphasize avoiding alcohol.

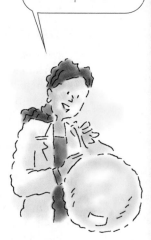

In cases of active variceal bleeding, control of blood loss is attempted through medication, surgery, or balloon tamponade.

What to do

• Check skin, gums, stool, and vomitus regularly for bleeding. Apply pressure to injection sites to prevent bleeding.
• Observe closely for signs of behavioral or personality changes. Report increasing stupor, lethargy, hallucinations, or neuromuscular dysfunction. Watch for asterixis, a sign of developing hepatic encephalopathy.
• To assess fluid retention, weigh the patient and measure abdominal girth daily, inspect his ankles and sacrum for dependent edema, and accurately record intake and output.

Handle with care

• To prevent skin breakdown associated with edema and pruritus, avoid using soap when you bathe the patient. Instead, use lubricating lotion or moisturizing agents. Handle him gently, and turn and reposition him frequently to keep skin intact.
• Evaluate the patient's response to therapy. Look for him to maintain normal nutrition and skin integrity. Note whether he has adapted his lifestyle and diet to his disorder and whether he understands the need for appropriate follow-up care. (See *Cirrhosis teaching tips*.)

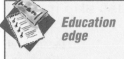

Education edge

Cirrhosis teaching tips

• Warn the patient against taking aspirin, straining during defecation, and blowing his nose or sneezing too vigorously. Suggest using an electric razor and a soft toothbrush.
• Tell the patient that rest and good nutrition will conserve energy and decrease metabolic demands on the liver. Urge him to eat frequent, small meals.
• Stress the need to avoid infections and abstain from alcohol.
• Instruct the patient to avoid drugs that may be toxic to the liver such as acetaminophen (Tylenol).

Crohn's disease

An inflammatory disorder, Crohn's disease can affect any part of the GI tract (usually the terminal ileum), extending through all layers of the intestinal wall. It may also involve regional lymph nodes and the mesentery.

Crohn's disease is most prevalent in adults ages 20 to 40, but a second peak incidence occurs between ages 55 and 65.

What causes it

The exact cause of Crohn's disease is unknown. Possible causes include allergies, immune disorders, lymphatic obstruction, infection, and genetic factors. Crohn's disease is most prevalent in adults ages 20 to 40, but a second peak incidence occurs between ages 55 and 65.

Pathophysiology

In Crohn's disease, inflammation spreads slowly and progressively. Here's what happens:
• Lymph nodes enlarge and lymph flow in the submucosa is blocked.

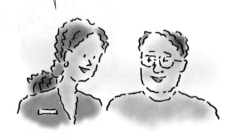

Just skip it

• Lymphatic obstruction causes edema, mucosal ulceration, fissures, abscesses and, sometimes, granulomas. Mucosal ulcerations are called *skipping lesions* because they aren't continuous as in ulcerative colitis.
• Oval, elevated patches of closely packed lymph follicles — called *Peyer's patches* — develop on the lining of the small intestine.
• Fibrosis occurs, thickening the bowel wall and causing stenosis, or narrowing of the lumen. (See *Changes to the bowel in Crohn's disease.*)

What to look for

Clinical effects vary according to the location and extent of inflammation and at first may be mild and nonspecific.

Changes to the bowel in Crohn's disease

As Crohn's disease progresses, fibrosis thickens the bowel wall and narrows the lumen. Narrowing — or *stenosis* — can occur in any part of the intestine and causes varying degrees of intestinal obstruction. At first, the mucosa may appear normal but, as the disease progresses, it takes on a "cobblestone" appearance, as shown here.

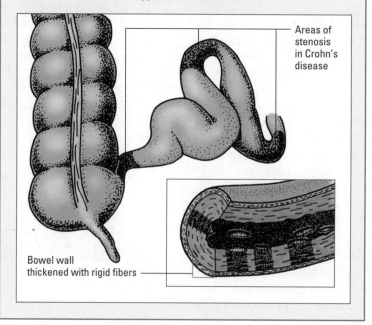

Areas of stenosis in Crohn's disease

Bowel wall thickened with rigid fibers

• In acute disease, look for right lower abdominal quadrant pain, cramping, tenderness, flatulence, nausea, fever, diarrhea, and bleeding (usually mild but may be massive).
• In chronic disease, look for diarrhea, four to six stools per day, right lower quadrant pain, steatorrhea, marked weight loss, possible weakness and, rarely, clubbing of fingers.

What tests tell you

• Laboratory findings typically indicate increased WBC count and erythrocyte sedimentation rate (ESR), hypokalemia, hypocalcemia, hypomagnesemia, and decreased hemoglobin levels.
• A barium enema showing the string sign (segments of stricture separated by normal bowel) supports this diagnosis.
• Sigmoidoscopy and colonoscopy may show patchy areas or inflammation, thus helping to rule out ulcerative colitis.
• Biopsy results confirm the diagnosis.
• Upper GI series with small-bowel examination helps determine disease in the ileum.

How it's treated

TPN helps to maintain nutrition while resting the bowel of a debilitated patient. Surgery can correct bowel perforation, massive hemorrhage, fistulas, or acute intestinal obstruction. The patient with extensive disease of the large intestine and rectum may require colectomy with ileostomy.

Take a pill

Effective drug therapy requires important changes in lifestyle: physical rest, a restricted-fiber diet (low in fruit and vegetables), and elimination of dairy products for lactose intolerance. Drug therapy may include:
• anti-inflammatory corticosteroids and antibacterials, such as sulfasalazine (Azulfidine) and mesalamine (Asacol)
• metronidazole (Flagyl)
• opium tincture and diphenoxylate (Lomotil) to help combat diarrhea (contraindicated in patients with significant intestinal obstruction)
• immunosuppressants, such as azathioprine (Imuran), cyclosporin (Sandimmune), and 6-mercaptopurine (Purinethol), for patients who can't be controlled on steroid therapy
• infliximab (Remicade), a tumor necrosis factor-alpha, to promote closure of fissures and treat refractory Crohn's disease

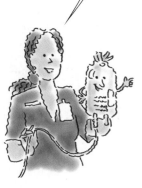

TPN helps maintain nutrition while resting the bowel of a debilitated patient.

flare-ups, given in a monitored setting by I.V. infusion in a cycle of three treatments (at weeks 1, 2, and 6).

What to do

• Record fluid intake and output (including the amount of stool), and weigh the patient daily.
• Watch for dehydration and maintain fluid and electrolyte balance.
• Be alert for signs of intestinal bleeding (bloody stool). Check stool daily for occult blood.
• If the patient is receiving steroids, watch for adverse reactions such as GI bleeding. Remember that steroids can mask signs of infection. Check hemoglobin levels and hematocrit regularly. Also check the WBC count if the patient is on immunomodulators. Give iron supplements, blood transfusions, and analgesics as ordered.
• Watch for fever and pain on urination, which may signal bladder fistula. Abdominal pain, fever, and a hard, distended abdomen may indicate intestinal obstruction.
• Before ileostomy, arrange for a visit by an enterostomal therapist. For postoperative care, see "Bowel surgery with ostomy," page 450.
• Evalate the patient. After successful treatment for Crohn's disease, he will maintain optimal nutrition, hydration, and skin integrity. He'll use positive coping mechanisms to deal with a changed body image. He should be able to identify and avoid foods likely to cause distress. Make sure he can demonstrate proper care of an ostomy, if required, and uses appropriate support groups. Evaluate his understanding of the need for follow-up care and when to seek immediate attention. (See *Crohn's disease teaching tips*.)

Education edge

Crohn's disease teaching tips

• Teach stoma care to the patient and his family. Realize that ileostomy changes the patient's body image; offer reassurance and emotional support.
• Stress the need for a severely restricted diet and bed rest, which may be difficult, particularly for the young patient. Encourage the patient to try to reduce tension. If stress is clearly an aggravating factor, refer him for counseling. Teach the patient to follow a low-residue diet, exercise, and seek family support.

Diverticular disease

In diverticular disease, bulging, pouchlike herniations (diverticula) in the GI wall push the mucosal lining through the surrounding muscle. Diverticula occur most commonly in the sigmoid colon, but they may develop anywhere, from the proximal end of the pharynx to the anus. Other typical sites are the duodenum, near the pancreatic border or the ampulla of Vater, and the jejunum.

Diverticular disease of the stomach is rare and is usually a precursor of peptic or neoplastic disease. Diverticular disease of the ileum (Meckel's diverticulum) is the most common congenital anomaly of the GI tract.

Diverticular disease has two clinical forms:
• diverticulosis — diverticula present but typically produces no symptoms
• diverticulitis — inflamed diverticula; may cause potentially fatal obstruction, infection, and hemorrhage.

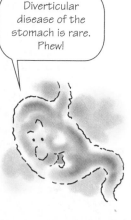

Diverticular disease of the stomach is rare. Phew!

What causes it

The exact cause is unknown, but it may result from:
• diminished colonic motility and increased intraluminal pressure
• defects in colon wall strength.

Pathophysiology

Diverticula probably result from high intraluminal pressure on an area of weakness in the GI wall where blood vessels enter. Diet may be a contributing factor because insufficient fiber reduces fecal residue, narrows the bowel lumen, and leads to high intra-abdominal pressure during defecation.

A sad sac

In diverticulitis, undigested food and bacteria accumulate in the diverticular sac. This hard mass cuts off the blood supply to the thin walls of the sac, making them more susceptible to attack by colonic bacteria. Inflammation follows and may lead to perforation, abscess, peritonitis, obstruction, or hemorrhage. Occasionally, the inflamed colon segment adheres to the bladder or other organs and causes a fistula.

What to look for

The different forms of diverticular disease result in different signs and symptoms:
• Meckel's diverticulum usually produces no symptoms.
• In diverticulosis, recurrent left lower abdominal quadrant pain is relieved by defecation or passage of flatus. Constipation and diarrhea alternate.
• In diverticulitis, the patient may have moderate left lower abdominal quadrant pain, mild nausea, gas, irregular bowel habits, low-grade fever, leukocytosis, rupture of the diverticuli (in severe diverticulitis), and fibrosis and adhesions (in chronic diverticulitis).

What tests tell you

• An upper GI series confirms or rules out diverticulosis of the esophagus and upper bowel.
• Barium enema confirms or rules out diverticulosis of the lower bowel. Biopsy rules out cancer; however, a colonoscopic biopsy isn't recommended during acute diverticular disease because of the strenuous bowel preparation it requires.
• Blood studies may show an elevated ESR in diverticulitis, especially if the diverticula are infected.

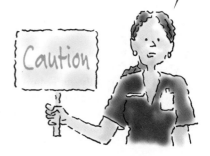

Colonoscopic biopsy isn't recommended during acute diverticular disease because of the strenuous bowel preparation required.

Caution

How it's treated

Diverticulosis that produces no symptoms usually doesn't require treatment. Treatment for diverticular disease depends on the type.
• Intestinal diverticulosis with pain, mild GI distress, constipation, or difficult defecation may respond to a liquid or bland diet, stool softeners, and occasional doses of mineral oil. These measures relieve symptoms, minimize irritation, and lessen the risk of progression to diverticulitis. After pain subsides, the patient also benefits from a high-residue diet and bulk-forming laxatives such as psyllium.

Mild measures

• Treatment of mild diverticulitis without signs of perforation seeks to prevent constipation and combat infection. It may include bed rest, a liquid diet, stool softeners, a broad-spectrum antibiotic, meperidine to control pain and relax smooth muscle, and an antispasmodic such as dicyclomine to control muscle spasms.

Major management

Diverticulitis unresponsive to medical treatment requires a colon resection to remove the involved segment.
• Complications that accompany diverticulitis may require a temporary colostomy to drain abscesses and rest the colon, followed by later anastomosis.
• Patients who hemorrhage need blood replacement and careful monitoring of fluid and electrolyte balance. Such bleeding usually stops spontaneously. If it continues, angiography for catheter placement and infusion of vasopressin into the bleeding vessel is effective. Rarely, surgery may be required.

What to do

• If the patient with diverticulosis is hospitalized, observe his stool carefully for frequency, color, and consistency.
• Keep accurate pulse and temperature charts because changes in pulse or temperature may signal developing inflammation or complications.
  Management of diverticulitis depends on the severity of symptoms.
• In mild disease, administer medications as ordered, explain diagnostic tests and preparations for such tests, observe stool carefully, and maintain accurate records of temperature, pulse rate, respiratory rate, and intake and output.
• Monitor carefully if the patient requires angiography and catheter placement for vasopressin infusion. Inspect the insertion site

frequently for bleeding, check pedal pulses frequently, and keep the patient from flexing his legs at the groin.
• Watch for signs and symptoms of vasopressin-induced fluid retention (apprehension, abdominal cramps, seizures, oliguria, and anuria) and severe hyponatremia (hypotension; rapid, thready pulse; cold, clammy skin; and cyanosis).
• For postsurgical care, see "Bowel resection and anastomosis," page 453.
• Evaluate the patient. After successful treatment and appropriate teaching, the patient will observe and report the character of the stool, modify his diet as needed, understand the need for follow-up care, and know when to seek immediate attention. (See *Diverticular disease teaching tips.*)

Gastroesophageal reflux disease

GERD is the backflow of gastric or duodenal contents, or both, past the LES, into the esophagus, without associated belching or vomiting. Reflux may or may not cause symptoms or abnormal changes. Persistent reflux may cause reflux esophagitis (inflammation of the esophageal mucosa).

What causes it

Reflux occurs when LES pressure is deficient or when pressure within the stomach exceeds LES pressure. Predisposing factors include:
• pyloric surgery (alteration or removal of the pylorus), which allows reflux of bile or pancreatic juice
• long-term NG intubation (more than 5 days)
• any agent that decreases LES pressure, such as food, alcohol, cigarettes, anticholinergics (atropine, belladonna, propantheline), and other drugs (morphine, diazepam, and meperidine)
• hiatal hernia (especially in children)
• any condition or position that increases intra-abdominal pressure.

Pathophysiology

Normally, the LES maintains enough pressure around the lower end of the esophagus to close it and prevent reflux. Typically, the sphincter relaxes after each swallow to allow food into the stomach. In GERD, the sphincter doesn't remain closed (usually due to deficient LES pressure or pressure within the stomach exceeding LES pressure), and stomach contents flow into the esophagus. The high acidity of the stomach contents causes pain and irritation in the esophagus, and stricture or ulceration can occur. If the

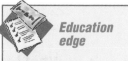

Education edge

Diverticular disease teaching tips

• Explain what diverticula are as well as how they form.
• Make sure the patient understands the importance of dietary fiber and the harmful effects of constipation and straining at stool. Encourage increased intake of foods high in digestible fiber. Advise the patient to relieve constipation with stool softeners or bulk-forming laxatives, but caution against taking bulk-forming laxatives without plenty of water.
• As needed, teach colostomy care, and arrange for a visit by an enterostomal therapist.

gastric contents enter the throat and are aspirated, chronic pulmonary disease may result.

What to look for

Gastroesophageal reflux doesn't always cause symptoms, and in patients showing clinical effects, physiologic reflux isn't always confirmable.

Achy, breaky heartburn

The most common feature of gastroesophageal reflux is heartburn, which may become more severe with vigorous exercise, bending, or lying down and may be relieved by antacids or sitting upright. The pain of esophageal spasm resulting from reflux esophagitis tends to be chronic and may mimic angina pectoris, radiating to the neck, jaws, and arms. Other symptoms include:
• odynophagia (pain when swallowing), which may be followed by a dull substernal ache from severe, long-term reflux
• dysphagia from esophageal spasm, stricture, or esophagitis and bleeding (bright red or dark brown)
• rarely, nocturnal regurgitation wakes the patient with coughing, choking, and a mouthful of saliva.

Don't hold your breath

Pulmonary symptoms, which result from reflux of gastric contents into the throat and subsequent aspiration include:
• chronic pulmonary disease or nocturnal wheezing
• bronchitis
• asthma
• morning hoarseness and cough.

What tests tell you

• In children, barium esophagography under fluoroscopic control can show reflux. Recurrent reflux after age 6 weeks is abnormal.
• An acid perfusion (Bernstein) test can show that reflux is the cause of symptoms.
• Endoscopy and biopsy allow visualization and confirmation of any abnormal changes in the mucosa.
• An ambulatory pH test measures the acidity of the esophagus.
• Manometry indicates the strength and activity of the lower esophageal sphincter.

How it's treated

Effective management relieves symptoms by reducing reflux through gravity, strengthening the LES with drug therapy,

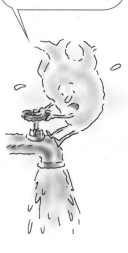

The most common feature of gastroesophageal reflux is heartburn. Maybe this will cool things down.

neutralizing gastric contents, and reducing intra-abdominal pressure. Specific treatments include the following:
• To reduce intra-abdominal pressure, the patient should sleep in a reverse Trendelenburg position (with the head of the bed elevated) and should avoid lying down after meals and late-night snacks as well as wearing tight-fitting clothing around the abdomen. In uncomplicated cases, positional therapy is especially useful in infants and children.

Neutralize the problem

• Antacids given 1 hour and 3 hours after meals and at bedtime help control intermittent reflux. A nondiarrheal antacid containing aluminum carbonate or aluminum hydroxide (rather than magnesium) may be preferred, depending on the patient's bowel status.
• Proton pump inhibitors are now a mainstay of therapy for GERD and erosive esophagitis. Other helpful drug treatments include metoclopramide (Reglan) and H_2-blockers.
• If possible, the patient should have NG intubation for no more than 5 days because the tube interferes with sphincter integrity and itself allows reflux, especially when the patient lies flat.
• Surgery may be necessary to control severe and refractory symptoms, such as pulmonary aspiration, hemorrhage, obstruction, severe pain, perforation, incompetent LES, and associated hiatal hernia. Surgery is also preferred in some young patients with severe GERD (rather than a lifetime of pharmacologic therapy).

What to do

After surgery using a thoracic approach, follow these steps:
• Carefully watch and record chest tube drainage and respiratory status.
• If needed, give chest physiotherapy and oxygen.
• Position the patient with an NG tube in semi-Fowler's position to help prevent reflux.
• Evaluate the patient; assess for optimal hydration and nutritional levels, diet modification, positioning, appropriate activity levels, and increased comfort as the patient complies with therapy. (See *GERD teaching tips*.)

Hepatic encephalopathy

Hepatic encephalopathy, also known as *portosystemic encephalopathy* or *hepatic coma*, is a neurologic syndrome that develops as a complication of chronic liver disease. It commonly occurs in patients with cirrhosis, resulting primarily from cerebral ammonia intoxication. It may be acute and self-limiting or chronic and

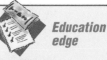
Education edge

GERD teaching tips

• Teach the patient what causes reflux; how to avoid it with medication, diet, and positional therapy; and what symptoms to watch for and report.
• Instruct the patient to avoid circumstances that increase intra-abdominal pressure (bending, coughing, vigorous exercise, tight clothing, and constipation). The patient should also avoid substances that reduce sphincter control (tobacco, alcohol, fatty foods, peppermint, caffeine, and certain drugs).
• Advise the patient to sit upright, particularly after meals, and to eat small, frequent meals.
• Tell him to avoid highly seasoned food, acidic juices, alcoholic drinks, caffeine, bedtime snacks, and foods high in fat or carbohydrates, which reduce lower esophageal sphincter pressure. He should eat meals at least 2 hours before lying down.

progressive. In advanced stages, the prognosis is poor despite vigorous treatment.

What causes it

Rising blood ammonia levels may result from:
- cirrhosis
- excessive protein intake
- sepsis
- constipation or GI hemorrhage, resulting in excessive accumulation of nitrogenous body wastes
- bacterial action on protein and urea to form ammonia.

Pathophysiology

Hepatic encephalopathy follows rising blood ammonia levels. Normally, the protein breakdown in the bowel is metabolized to urea in the liver. However, when portal blood shunts past the liver, ammonia directly enters the systemic circulation and is carried to the brain. Such shunting may result from the collateral venous circulation that develops in portal hypertension or from surgically created portosystemic shunts.

What to look for

Although clinical manifestations of hepatic encephalopathy vary (depending on the severity of neurologic involvement), they develop in four stages:

> All the world's a stage, but hepatic encephalopathy develops in only four stages.

In the *prodromal stage*, early symptoms are usually overlooked because they're subtle. They include slight personality changes (disorientation, forgetfulness, slurred speech), sleep disturbance, diminished affect, and slight tremor.

During the *impending stage*, tremor progresses into asterixis, the hallmark of hepatic coma. Asterixis is characterized by quick, irregular extensions and flexions of the wrists and fingers when the wrists are held out straight and the hands flexed upward. Lethargy, aberrant behavior, and apraxia also occur.

Hyperventilation occurs in the *stuporous stage*, and the patient is stuporous, but noisy and abusive when aroused.

In the *comatose stage*, signs include hyperactive reflexes, a positive Babinski's sign, fetor hepaticus (musty, sweet breath odor), and coma.

What tests tell you

• Elevated venous and arterial ammonia levels, clinical features, and a positive history of liver disease confirm the diagnosis.
• Arterial blood gas (ABG) analysis shows respiratory alkalosis with central hyperventilation.
• EEG shows slow waves as the disease progresses.
• Other test results that suggest the disorder include elevated serum bilirubin levels and prolonged PT.

How it's treated

• Treatment aims to improve hepatic function and correct underlying liver disease. Specific steps include the following:
• Adequate calorie intake (1,800 to 2,400 cal/day) in the form of glucose or carbohydrates helps prevent protein catabolism. Protein may be restricted to 40 g/day and advanced to up to 100 g/day as symptoms improve.
• Correction of electrolyte imbalances and management of GI bleeding are also essential.
• Effective treatment stops advancing encephalopathy by reducing blood ammonia levels. Ammonia-producing substances are removed from the GI tract by administering neomycin to suppress bacterial ammonia production, using sorbitol to induce catharsis to produce osmotic diarrhea, continuously aspirating blood from the stomach, reducing dietary protein intake, and administering lactulose to reduce blood ammonia levels.
• Potassium supplements help correct alkalosis (from increased ammonia levels), especially if the patient is taking diuretics.

Toxic cleanup

• Hemodialysis may temporarily clear toxic blood. Exchange transfusions may provide dramatic but temporary improvement; however, these require a particularly large amount of blood.
• Salt-poor albumin may be used to maintain fluid and electrolyte balance, replace depleted albumin levels, and restore plasma.

What to do

• Frequently assess and record the patient's LOC.
• Continually orient him to place and time.
• Keep a daily record of the patient's handwriting to monitor the progression of neurologic involvement.
• Monitor intake, output, and fluid and electrolyte balance. Check daily weight and measure abdominal girth.
• Watch for and immediately report signs of anemia (decreased hemoglobin levels), infection, alkalosis (increased serum bicarbonate levels), and GI bleeding (melena, hematemesis).

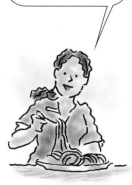

The patient will need adequate calorie intake in the form of glucose or carbohydrates to prevent protein catabolism.

• Provide the specified low-protein diet, with carbohydrates supplying most of the calories. Provide good mouth care.
• Promote rest, comfort, and a quiet atmosphere. Discourage stressful exercise.
• Protect the comatose patient's eyes from corneal injury by using artificial tears or eye patches.
• Provide emotional support for the patient's family in the terminal stage of hepatic coma.
• Evaluate the patient. He should have adequate hydration and intact skin. His family should have adequate support to deal with his condition. (See *Hepatic encephalopathy teaching tips*.)

Hepatitis, nonviral

Nonviral hepatitis is an inflammation of the liver that usually results from exposure to certain chemicals or drugs. Most patients recover from nonviral hepatitis, although a few develop fulminating hepatitis or cirrhosis.

What causes it

Causes of nonviral hepatitis include:
• hepatotoxic chemicals, such as carbon tetrachloride, trichloroethylene, and vinyl chloride
• hepatotoxic drugs such as acetaminophen (Tylenol)
• poisonous mushrooms.

Pathophysiology

After exposure to a hepatotoxin, hepatic cellular necrosis, scarring, Kupffer's cell hyperplasia, and infiltration by mononuclear phagocytes occur with varying severity. Alcohol, anoxia, and preexisting liver disease exacerbate the effects of some toxins.

Unlike toxic hepatitis, which appears to affect all exposed people indiscriminately, drug-induced hepatitis may begin with a hypersensitivity reaction unique to the individual. Symptoms usually manifest after 2 to 5 weeks of therapy.

What to look for

Look for these signs and symptoms:
• anorexia, nausea, and vomiting
• jaundice
• dark urine
• hepatomegaly
• possibly, abdominal pain
• possibly, clay-colored stools and pruritus (in cholestatic form).

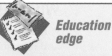

Education edge

Hepatic encephalopathy teaching tips

• Teach the patient, if he's still able to understand, and his family about hepatic encephalopathy and its treatment. Repeat explanations of each treatment before you perform it. Be sure to explain all procedures even if the patient is comatose.
• If the patient has chronic encephalopathy, be sure that he and his family understand the mental and physical effects that the illness will eventually have on the patient. Alert them to signs of complications or worsening symptoms. Advise them when to notify the practitioner.
• As the patient begins to recover, inform him about the low-protein diet. Emphasize that recovery from a severe illness takes time. Review how to use medications.

What tests tell you

• Liver biopsy may help identify the underlying disorder, especially if it shows infiltration with WBCs and eosinophils.
• Elevated serum transaminase levels (ALT and AST), total and direct serum bilirubin levels (with cholestasis), alkaline phosphatase levels, and WBC count can all occur in nonviral hepatitis.
• Increased eosinophil levels may occur in drug-induced nonviral hepatitis.

How it's treated

Effective treatment aims to remove the causative agent by lavage, catharsis, or hyperventilation, depending on the route of exposure. Dimercaprol (BAL in Oil) may serve as an antidote for toxic hepatitis caused by gold or arsenic poisoning, but it doesn't prevent drug-induced hepatitis caused by other substances. Corticosteroids may be ordered for patients with the drug-induced type of the disorder.

What to do

• Monitor closely for complications of liver failure (bleeding and hepatic coma).
• Ensure adequate hydration and nutrition.
• Relieve the patient's nausea, pruritus, and abdominal pain.
• Evaluate the patient. He should be able to maintain normal nutrition and hydration, make lifestyle and dietary changes, and seek follow-up care as needed. (See *Nonviral hepatitis teaching tips.*)

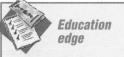

Education edge

Nonviral hepatitis teaching tips

• Instruct the patient about the proper use of drugs.
• Instruct the patient about proper handling of cleaning agents and solvents, which can trigger a toxic reaction.

Hepatitis, viral

The viral form of hepatitis is an acute inflammation of the liver marked by liver-cell destruction, necrosis, and autolysis. In most patients, hepatic cells eventually regenerate with little or no residual damage. However, old age and serious underlying disorders make complications more likely. The prognosis is poor if edema and hepatic encephalopathy develop.

Types of hepatitis

Five major forms of viral hepatitis are currently recognized, each caused by a different virus:

Type A is transmitted almost exclusively by the fecal-oral route, and outbreaks are common in areas of overcrowding and poor sanitation. Day-care centers and other institutional settings are common sources of outbreaks.

Type B accounts for 5% to 10% of posttransfusion hepatitis cases in the United States. Vaccinations are available and are now required for health care workers and school children in many states.

 Type C accounts for about 20% of all viral hepatitis as well as most cases that follow transfusion.

 Type D, in the United States, is confined to people frequently exposed to blood and blood products, such as I.V. drug users and hemophiliacs.

 Type E was formerly grouped with type C under the name non-A, non-B hepatitis. In the United States, this type mainly occurs in people who have visited an endemic area, such as India, Africa, Asia, or Central America. (See *Viral hepatitis from A to E.*)

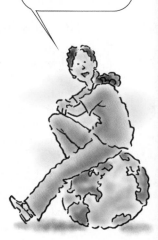

In the U.S., type E hepatitis mainly occurs in people who have visited an endemic area, such as India, Africa, Asia, or Central America.

What causes it

All forms of viral hepatitis are caused by hepatitis viruses A, B, C, D, or E.

Pathophysiology

Despite the different causative viruses, changes to the liver are usually similar in each type of viral hepatitis. Varying degrees of liver cell injury and necrosis occur. These changes in the liver are completely reversible when the acute phase of the disease subsides.

A fairly common complication is chronic persistent hepatitis, which prolongs recovery up to 8 months. Some patients also suffer relapses. A few may develop chronic active hepatitis, which destroys part of the liver and causes cirrhosis. In rare cases, severe and sudden (fulminant) hepatic failure and death may result from massive tissue loss.

What to look for

In the preicteric phase, look for:
- fatigue, malaise, arthralgia, myalgia, photophobia, and headache
- loss of appetite, nausea, and vomiting
- altered sense of taste and smell
- fever, possibly with liver and lymph node enlargement.
    The icteric phase lasts 1 to 2 weeks. Signs and symptoms include:
- mild weight loss
- dark urine and clay-colored stools
- yellow sclera and skin
- continued hepatomegaly with tenderness.

Viral hepatitis from A to E

This chart compares the features of each type of viral hepatitis.

Feature	Hepatitis A	Hepatitis B	Hepatitis C	Hepatitis D	Hepatitis E
Incubation	15 to 45 days	30 to 180 days	15 to 160 days	14 to 64 days	14 to 60 days
Onset	Acute	Insidious	Insidious	Acute and chronic	Acute
Age-group most affected	Children, young adults	Any age	More common in adults	Any age	Ages 20 to 40
Transmission	Fecal-oral, sexual (especially oral-anal contact), nonpercutaneous (sexual, maternal-neonatal), percutaneous (rare)	Blood-borne; parenteral route, sexual, maternal-neonatal; virus is shed in all body fluids	Blood-borne; parenteral route	Parenteral route; most people infected with hepatitis D are also infected with hepatitis B	Primarily fecal-oral
Severity	Mild	Commonly severe	Moderate	Can be severe and lead to fulminant hepatitis	Mild unless patient is pregnant; in pregnant patients, can be highly virulent
Prognosis	Generally good	Worsens with age and debility	Moderate	Fair; worsens in chronic cases; can lead to chronic hepatitis D and chronic liver disease	Good unless pregnant
Progression to chronicity	None	Occasional	10% to 50% of cases	Occasional	None

    The convalescent phase lasts 2 to 12 weeks or longer. Signs and symptoms include:
- continued fatigue
- flatulence, abdominal pain or tenderness, and indigestion.

What tests tell you

- The presence of hepatitis B surface antigens and hepatitis B antibodies confirms a diagnosis of type B hepatitis.
- Detection of an antibody to type A hepatitis confirms past or present infection with type A hepatitis.
- Detection of an antibody to type C confirms a diagnosis of type C hepatitis. Viral load is measured by quantitative polymerase chain reaction assay and is useful in determining need for treatment and monitoring therapy.
- PT is prolonged (more than 3 seconds longer than normal indicates severe liver damage).
- Serum transaminase levels (ALT and AST) are elevated.
- Serum alkaline phosphatase levels are slightly elevated.
- Serum and urine bilirubin levels are elevated (with jaundice).
- Serum albumin levels are low, and serum globulin levels are high.
- Liver biopsy and scan show patchy necrosis.

How it's treated

The patient should rest in the early stages of the illness and combat anorexia by eating small meals high in calories and protein. (Protein intake should be reduced if signs of precoma — lethargy, confusion, mental changes — develop.) Large meals are usually better tolerated in the morning. Other measures include the following:

- Chronic hepatitis B with liver inflammation is treated with interferon alfa-2b for 16 weeks. Monitoring of blood counts is essential during treatment.
- Lamivudine (Epivir) is another hepatitis B therapy that decreases the viral load of hepatitis B.
- Current therapy for hepatitis C includes interferon or a combined interferon and ribavirin therapy. The decision on how to treat the individual is made after laboratory tests and liver biopsy confirm hepatic inflammation or early cirrhosis. Treatment lasts from 6 to 18 months, based on the outcome and genotype of the virus. The patient needs instruction on self-injection and adverse effects.
- Laboratory tests — including CBC with differential, thyroid studies, liver function tests, and hepatitis quantitative studies — help determine the effectiveness of therapy and prevent complications during treatment. Drug dosages may be reduced if WBC count, hemoglobin level, or hematocrit drop below normal.
- Adverse effects of medication include depression, flulike syndrome, fatigue, malaise, and GI disturbance.

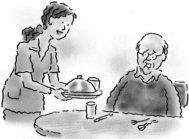

In the early stages of hepatitis, the patient should combat anorexia by eating small meals high in calories and protein.

Patients, take charge!

- Patients need to be proactive in their treatment to properly monitor and succeed in taking their medication. Current eradication rates of combined therapy in patients with hepatitis C range from 30% to 40%.
- Antiemetics, such as trimethobenzamide or benzquinamide, given 30 minutes before meals can help relieve nausea and prevent vomiting; the patient shouldn't take phenothiazines, which have a cholestatic effect. If vomiting persists, the patient needs I.V. infusions.
- In severe hepatitis, corticosteroids may give the patient a sense of well-being and may stimulate the appetite while decreasing itching and inflammation; however, their use in hepatitis is controversial.

What to do

- Observe enteric and blood and body fluid precautions for all types of hepatitis. Inform visitors about isolation precautions.
- Give the patient plenty of fluids (at least 4,000 ml/day). Encourage the anorexic patient to drink fruit juices. Also, offer chipped ice and effervescent soft drinks to promote adequate hydration without inducing vomiting.
- Record weight daily, and keep accurate intake and output records.
- Observe the patient's stool for color, consistency, frequency, and amount.
- Watch for signs of hepatic coma, dehydration, pneumonia, vascular problems, and pressure ulcers.
- Report all cases of hepatitis to health officials. Ask the patient to name anyone he came in contact with recently.
- Evaluate the patient. He should be able to maintain adequate hydration and nutrition, follow appropriate isolation precautions, modify his diet and lifestyle as needed, and obtain appropriate follow-up care. His close contacts also should seek evaluation and possible vaccination. (See *Viral hepatitis teaching tips.*)

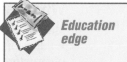

Education edge

Viral hepatitis teaching tips

- Before discharge, emphasize the importance of having regular medical checkups for at least 1 year. Warn the patient not to drink any alcohol during this period, and teach him how to recognize signs of recurrence. Refer the patient for follow-up care as needed.
- Advise a hepatitis carrier to prevent exchange of body fluids during sexual relations. Tell the patient to avoid contact sports for as long as his liver is enlarged; he should also abstain from alcohol.
- If the patient is a female of child-bearing age, caution her not to become pregnant during the course of therapy or for 6 months after treatment.

Intestinal obstruction

In an intestinal obstruction, the lumen of the small or large bowel becomes partly or fully blocked. Small-bowel obstruction is far more common (affecting 90% of patients) and usually more serious. If left untreated, complete obstruction in any part of the bowel can cause death within hours from shock and vascular collapse. Intestinal obstruction is most likely to occur after abdominal surgery or in persons with congenital bowel deformities.

What causes it

Mechanical obstruction can result from:
• adhesions and strangulated hernias (usually small-bowel obstruction)
• carcinomas (usually large-bowel obstruction)
• foreign bodies (fruit pits, gallstones, worms)
• compression
• stenosis
• intussusception
• volvulus of the sigmoid colon or cecum
• tumors
• atresia.

Not mechanically obstructed

Nonmechanical obstruction can result from:
• electrolyte imbalances
• toxicity
• neurogenic abnormalities
• thrombosis or embolism of mesenteric vessels
• paralytic ileus (see *A closer look at paralytic ileus*).

Pathophysiology

Intestinal obstruction develops in three forms:

In a *simple* obstruction, blockage prevents intestinal contents from passing, with no other complications.

In a *strangulated* obstruction, the blood supply to part or all of the obstructed section is cut off, in addition to blockage of the lumen.

When a *close-looped* obstruction occurs, both ends of a bowel section are occluded, isolating it from the rest of the intestine.

Cause and effect

All three forms of obstruction cause similar physiologic effects. When intestinal obstruction occurs, fluid, air, and gas collect near the site. Peristalsis increases temporarily as the bowel tries to force its contents through the obstruction, injuring intestinal mucosa and causing distention at and above the site of the obstruction. Distention blocks the flow of venous blood and halts normal absorptive processes. As a result, the bowel begins to secrete water, sodium, and potassium into the fluid pooled in the lumen.

A closer look

A closer look at paralytic ileus

Paralytic ileus is a physiologic form of intestinal obstruction that usually develops in the small bowel after abdominal surgery. It causes decreased or absent intestinal motility that usually disappears spontaneously after 2 to 3 days.

Signs and symptoms
• Severe abdominal distention
• Extreme distress
• Vomiting
• Severe constipation
• Passage of flatus and small, liquid stools
• Dimished or absent bowel sounds

Causes
• Trauma
• Toxemia
• Peritonitis
• Electrolyte deficiencies (especially hypokalemia)

• Drugs, such as ganglionic blocking agents and anticholinergics
• Vascular causes, such as thrombosis and embolism
• Excessive air swallowing (rarely lasts more than 24 hours from this factor alone)

Treatment
• Intubation for decompression and nasogastric suctioning (if lasts longer than 48 hours)
• Miller-Abbott tube in the patient with severe abdominal distention (used with caution to avoid additional trauma to the bowel)
• Cholinergic agents, such as neostigmine (Prostigmin) and bethanechol (Myotonachol) (when resulting from surgical manipulation of the bowel)
• Patient teaching to explain effects of cholinergics, such as intestinal cramps and diarrhea
• Monitoring for cardiovascular adverse effects of neostigmine, such as bradycardia and hypotension
• Frequent checks for returning bowel sounds

What to look for

To help detect small-bowel obstruction, take the following steps:
• Assess the patient for colicky pain, nausea, vomiting, and constipation.
• Auscultate for high-pitched, loud, musical, or tinkling bowel sounds; borborygmi; and rushes (occasionally loud enough to be heard without a stethoscope).
• Palpate for abdominal tenderness with moderate distention. Rebound tenderness may occur when obstruction has caused strangulation with ischemia.
• Assess for vomiting of fecal contents in complete obstruction.

Significant signs: Blockage this way

In large-bowel obstruction, take these steps:
• Assess for constipation in the first few days.
• Look for other signs and symptoms, including colicky abdominal pain, nausea (usually without vomiting at first), and abdominal distention. Eventually, pain becomes continuous and the patient may vomit fecal contents.

> To help detect small-bowel obstruction, listen for high-pitched, loud, musical, or tinkling bowel sounds.

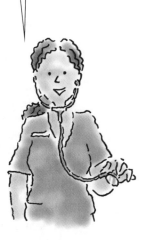

What tests tell you

• Abdominal X-rays confirm the diagnosis. They show the presence and location of intestinal gas or fluid. In small-bowel obstruction, a typical "stepladder" pattern emerges, with alternating fluid and gas levels apparent in 3 to 4 hours.
• CT scans rule out obstruction or identify perforation or volvulus.
• In large-bowel obstruction, barium enema reveals a distended, air-filled colon or a closed loop of sigmoid colon with extreme distention (in sigmoid volvulus).
• Early in diagnosis, laboratory results might be normal.

Lab levels: The highs and the lows

The following laboratory results support a diagnosis of intestinal obstruction:
• Sodium, chloride, and potassium levels are decreased (from vomiting).
• WBC count is slightly elevated (with necrosis, peritonitis, or strangulation).
• Serum amylase level is increased (possibly from irritation of the pancreas).
• ABG analysis indicates metabolic alkalosis, a result of prolonged vomiting.

How it's treated

Preoperative treatment aims to correct fluid and electrolyte imbalances, decompress the bowel to relieve vomiting and distention, and alleviate shock and peritonitis. Specific treatments might include these measures:
• Strangulated obstruction usually requires blood replacement as well as I.V. fluid administration. Passage of a Levin tube, followed by use of the longer, weighted Miller-Abbott tube, usually accomplishes decompression, especially in small-bowel obstruction.
• Esophagogastroduodenoscopy may be performed to remove obstructive lesions.
• Close monitoring of the patient's condition determines the duration of treatment. If the patient fails to improve or his condition deteriorates, he'll require surgery.
• In large-bowel obstruction, surgical resection with anastomosis, colostomy, or ileostomy commonly follows decompression with a Levin tube.
• TPN may be appropriate if the patient suffers a protein deficit from chronic obstruction, postoperative or paralytic ileus, or infection.
• Drug therapy includes analgesics or sedatives, such as meperidine (Demerol) — not opiates, which inhibit GI motility — and antibiotics for peritonitis caused by bowel strangulation or infarction.

• For intussusception, hydrostatic reduction may be attempted by infusing barium into the rectum. If this fails, manual reduction or bowel resection is performed.

What to do

• Monitor the patient's vital signs frequently. Decreased blood pressure may indicate reduced circulating blood volume due to blood loss from a strangulated hernia. Remember, as much as 10 L of fluid can collect in the small bowel, drastically reducing plasma volume. Observe closely for signs of shock (such as pallor, decreased urine output, rapid pulse, and hypotension).

• Stay alert for signs and symptoms of metabolic alkalosis (including changes in sensorium, hypertonic muscles, tetany, and slow, shallow respirations) or acidosis (including shortness of breath on exertion, disorientation and, later, deep, rapid breathing, weakness, and malaise). Also watch for signs and symptoms of secondary infection, such as fever and chills.

• Monitor urine output carefully to assess renal function and possible urine retention from bladder compression by the distended intestine. If you suspect bladder compression, catheterize the patient for residual urine immediately after he has voided. Also, measure abdominal girth frequently to detect progressive distention.

• Provide thorough mouth and nose care if the patient has undergone decompression by intubation or if he has vomited. Look for signs of dehydration (such as a thick, swollen tongue; dry, cracked lips; and dry oral mucous membranes).

• Record the amount and color of drainage from the decompression tube. If necessary, irrigate the tube with normal saline solution to maintain patency.

• If a weighted tube has been inserted, check periodically to make sure it's advancing. Help the patient turn from side to side (or walk around, if he can) to promote passage of the tube.

• Keep the patient in Fowler's position as much as possible to promote pulmonary ventilation and ease respiratory distress from abdominal distention.

• Auscultate for bowel sounds, and watch for signs of returning peristalsis (passage of flatus and mucus through the rectum).

• Evaluate the patient. He should have normal fluid and electrolyte status, adequate oral intake, normal bowel sounds, and regular bowel elimination patterns. He should also be free from abdominal distention and complications. (See *Intestinal obstruction teaching tips*.)

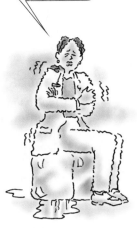

Watch for signs of secondary infection, such as fever and — brrr — chills.

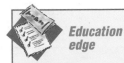

Education edge

Intestinal obstruction teaching tips

• Provide emotional support and positive reinforcement after surgery.

• Arrange for an enterostomal therapist to visit the patient who has had a colostomy.

Irritable bowel syndrome

Also referred to as *spastic colon* or *spastic colitis*, irritable bowel syndrome (IBS) is marked by chronic symptoms of abdominal pain, alternating constipation and diarrhea, excess flatulence, a sense of incomplete evacuation, and abdominal distention. IBS is a common, stress-related disorder. About 20% of patients never seek medical attention for this benign condition that has no anatomic abnormality or inflammatory component. It's twice as common in women as in men.

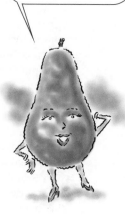

In addition to stress, IBS may result from ingestion of raw fruits and vegetables.

What causes it

IBS is usually associated with psychological stress but may also result from physical factors, such as:
- ingestion of irritants (coffee, raw fruits or vegetables)
- lactose intolerance
- abuse of laxatives
- hormonal changes (menstruation). (See *IBS: Quality of life takes a hit.*)

Pathophysiology

IBS appears to reflect motor disturbances of the entire colon in response to stimuli. Some muscles of the small bowel are particularly sensitive to motor abnormalities and distention; others are particularly sensitive to certain foods and drugs. The patient may

---

Weighing the evidence

IBS: Quality of life takes a hit

Irritable bowel syndrome (IBS) can seriously disrupt a patient's life, and it seems that psychological factors can play a major role. To investigate the connection, researchers looked at the relationship between dysfunctional thought patterns, anxiety, and depression and daily IBS symptoms and overall quality of life in a group of 268 IBS patients.

Painful conclusions

The researchers found that not only did about a third of the patients have anxiety and depression, but that patients with dysfunctional thought patterns had more severe symptoms and a lower quality of life. The study confirms the key role psychological factors play in influencing quality of life for IBS patients.

Source: Thijssen, A., et al. (2010). Dysfunctional cognitions, anxiety and depression in irritable bowel syndrome. *Journal of Clinical Gastroenterology, 44*(10), e236–e241.

be hypersensitive to the hormones gastrin and cholecystokinin. The pain of IBS seems to result from abnormally strong contractions of the intestinal smooth muscle as it reacts to distention, irritants, or stress.

What to look for

These signs and symptoms alternate with constipation or normal bowel function:
• lower abdominal pain (usually relieved by defecation or passage of gas)
• diarrhea (typically occurring during the day)
• small stools that contain visible mucus
• possible dyspepsia
• abdominal distention.

What tests tell you

• Stool examination for blood, parasites, and bacteria can rule out other disorders.
• Other tests may include sigmoidoscopy, colonoscopy, barium enema, and rectal biopsy.

How it's treated

• Counseling helps the patient understand the relationship between stress and her illness.
• Strict dietary restrictions don't help, but food irritants should be investigated and the patient should be instructed to avoid them.
• Rest can also help, as can judicious use of sedatives and antispasmodics (such as diphenoxylate with atropine sulfate or dicyclomine). With chronic use, however, the patient may become dependent on these drugs.
• If IBS results from chronic laxative abuse, the patient may need bowel retraining to help correct the condition.

What to do

Evaluate the patient. She should modify her diet and lifestyle to control or avoid symptoms, demonstrate a regular bowel elimination pattern, understand the need for follow-up care, and know when to seek immediate attention. However, because the patient with IBS isn't hospitalized, focus your care on patient teaching. (See *Irritable bowel syndrome teaching tips.*)

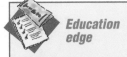

Education edge

Irritable bowel syndrome teaching tips

• Tell the patient to avoid irritating foods, and encourage her to develop regular bowel habits.
• Teach her to keep a food diary to identify food irritants.
• Help her deal with stress, and warn against dependence on sedatives or antispasmodics.
• Encourage her to increase her fiber intake and drink plenty of fluids to promote regular stools.

Pancreatitis

Pancreatitis — inflammation of the pancreas — occurs in acute and chronic forms and may result from edema, necrosis, or hemorrhage. The prognosis is good when pancreatitis follows biliary tract disease but poor when it's a complication of alcoholism. Mortality reaches 60% when pancreatitis causes tissue destruction or hemorrhage.

What causes it

Most commonly caused by biliary tract disease and alcoholism, pancreatitis also results from:
• pancreatic cancer
• possibly, peptic ulcer, mumps, or hypothermia
• certain drugs, such as glucocorticoids, zidovudine (Retrovir), didanosine (Videx), sulfonamides, chlorothiazide (Diuril), and azathioprine (Imuran)
• less commonly, from stenosis or obstruction of Oddi's sphincter, hyperlipidemia, metabolic and endocrine disorders, vascular disease, viral infections, mycoplasmal pneumonia, or pregnancy
• iatrogenic causes, including diagnostic or therapeutic ERCP, which increases the risk of pancreatitis by 3% to 6%.

Pathophysiology

Chronic pancreatitis is a persistent inflammation that produces irreversible changes in the structure and function of the pancreas. It sometimes follows an episode of acute pancreatitis. Here's what probably happens:
• Protein precipitates block the pancreatic duct and eventually harden or calcify.
• Structural changes lead to fibrosis and atrophy of the glands.
• Growths called *pseudocysts*, containing pancreatic enzymes and tissue debris, form.
• An abscess results if these growths become infected.

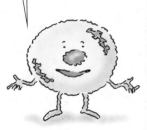

Necrotizing acute pancreatitis causes tissue damage and cell death. I don't like the sound of that...

The acute angle

Acute pancreatitis occurs in two forms:

edematous (interstitial), causing fluid accumulation and swelling

necrotizing, causing cell death and tissue damage.
    The inflammation that occurs with both types is caused by premature activation of enzymes, which causes tissue damage. Normally, the acini in the pancreas secrete enzymes in an inactive form.

Interesting theories...

Two theories explain why enzymes become prematurely activated:

A toxic agent, such as alcohol, alters the way the pancreas secretes enzymes. This agent increases pancreatic secretion, alters the metabolism of the acinar cells, and encourages duct obstruction by causing pancreatic secretory proteins to precipitate.

A reflux of duodenal contents containing activated enzymes enters the pancreatic duct, activating other enzymes and setting up a cycle of more pancreatic damage.

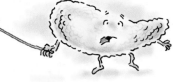

When pancreatitis results from alcoholism, the prognosis is poor. No alcohol for me, thanks!

What to look for

Steady epigastric pain centered close to the umbilicus, that radiates between the 10th thoracic and 6th lumbar vertebrae and is unrelieved by vomiting may be the first and only symptom of mild pancreatitis. A severe attack may cause:

- extreme pain
- persistent vomiting
- abdominal rigidity
- diminished bowel activity (suggesting peritonitis)
- crackles at lung bases
- left pleural effusion
- extreme malaise
- restlessness
- mottled skin
- tachycardia
- low-grade fever (100° to 102° F [37.8° to 38.9° C])
- cold, sweaty extremities
- possible ileus.

What tests tell you

- Dramatically elevated serum amylase levels — commonly more than 500 Somogyi units/dl — confirm pancreatitis and rule out perforated peptic ulcer, acute cholecystitis, appendicitis, and bowel infarction or obstruction. Dramatic elevations of amylase levels also occur in urine, ascites, and pleural fluid. Characteristically, amylase levels return to normal 48 hours after the onset of pancreatitis, despite continuing signs and symptoms.
- Serum lipase levels are increased but rise more slowly than serum amylase levels.
- Serum calcium levels are low from fat necrosis and formation of calcium soaps.

• Glucose levels are elevated and may be as high as 900 mg/dl, indicating severe hyperglycemia.
• WBC counts range from 8,000 to 20,000/µl, with increased polymorphonuclear leukocyte levels.
• Hematocrit occasionally exceeds 50% concentrations.
• Abdominal X-rays may show dilation of the small or large bowel or calcification of the pancreas.
• A GI series indicates extrinsic pressure on the duodenum or stomach caused by edema of the pancreas head.
• An ultrasound isn't usually helpful in providing diagnosis because the pancreas is poorly visualized.
• An abdominal CT scan can help distinguish between cholelithiasis and pancreatitis.

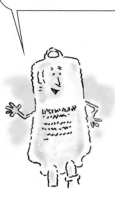

After the emergency phase, I.V. therapy should continue for 5 to 7 days with solutions that don't stimulate the pancreas.

How it's treated

Treatment must maintain circulation and fluid volume, relieve pain, and decrease pancreatic secretions.
• Emergency treatment for shock (the most common cause of death in early-stage pancreatitis) consists of vigorous I.V. replacement of electrolytes and proteins. Metabolic acidosis secondary to hypovolemia and impaired cellular perfusion requires vigorous fluid volume replacement.
• Hypocalcemia requires infusion of 10% calcium gluconate; serum glucose levels greater than 300 mg/dl require insulin therapy.
• After the emergency phase, continuing I.V. therapy for 5 to 7 days should provide adequate electrolytes and protein solutions that don't stimulate the pancreas.

Whenever you're ready...

• If the patient isn't ready to resume oral feedings by then, he may need TPN.
• Nonstimulating elemental gavage feedings may be safer because of the decreased risk of infection and overinfusion.
• In extreme cases, the patient may require laparotomy to drain the pancreatic bed, 95% pancreatectomy, or a combination of cholecystostomy-gastrostomy, feeding jejunostomy, and drainage.

What to do

• Give plasma or albumin, if ordered, to maintain blood pressure.
• Record fluid intake and output, check urine output hourly, and monitor electrolyte levels.
• For bowel decompression, maintain constant NG suctioning and give nothing by mouth. Perform good mouth and nose care.
• Watch for signs of calcium deficiency — tetany, cramps, carpopedal spasm, and seizures. If you suspect hypocalcemia, keep airway and suction apparatus handy and pad the side rails.

- Administer analgesics as needed to relieve the patient's pain and anxiety.

A case of dry mouth

- Don't confuse thirst caused by hyperglycemia (indicated by serum glucose levels of up to 350 mg/dl and glucose and acetone in urine) with dry mouth caused by NG intubation and anticholinergics.
- Watch for complications due to TPN, such as sepsis, hypokalemia, overhydration, and metabolic acidosis.
- Evaluate the patient. He should have normal nutrition and hydration levels, balanced electrolyte levels, and an improved comfort level. He also should understand the need for lifestyle modifications and adjust lifestyle factors that aggravate his disease. (See *Pancreatitis teaching tips.*)

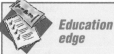

Education edge

Pancreatitis teaching tips

- Emphasize the importance of avoiding factors that precipitate acute pancreatitis, especially alcohol.
- Refer the patient and his family to a dietitian. Stress the need for a diet high in carbohydrates and low in protein and fats. Caution the patient to avoid beverages with caffeine and irritating foods.

Peptic ulcers

Appearing as circumscribed lesions in the gastric mucosal membrane, peptic ulcers can develop in the lower esophagus, stomach, pylorus, duodenum, or jejunum from contact with gastric juice (especially hydrochloric acid and pepsin). About 80% of all peptic ulcers are duodenal ulcers.

What causes it

The precise cause of peptic ulcer is unknown but may include:
- *H. pylori* infection
- use of NSAIDs or salicylates
- inadequate protection of mucous membranes
- pathologic hypersecretory disorders.

Factor it in

Factors that predispose a person to peptic ulcer include:
- blood type (gastric ulcers and type A; duodenal ulcers and type O) and other genetic factors
- exposure to irritants, such as alcohol, coffee, and tobacco
- emotional stress
- physical trauma
- normal aging.

Pathophysiology

In a peptic ulcer due to *H. pylori*, acid adds to the effects of the bacterial infection. *H. pylori* releases a toxin that destroys the stomach's mucus coat, promoting mucosal inflammation and ulceration. Salicylates and other NSAIDs encourage ulcer formation by inhibiting the secretion of prostaglandins (substances that block ulceration). (See *A close look at peptic ulcers*.)

What to look for

Patients with duodenal ulcers may experience attacks about 2 hours after meals, whenever the stomach is empty, or after consuming orange juice, coffee, aspirin, or alcohol. Exacerbations tend to recur several times a year, then fade into remission. Such

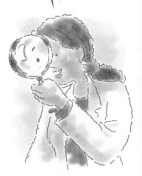

Note that acute and chronic ulcers extend beyond the mucosal lining.

A closer look

A close look at peptic ulcers

This illustration shows different degrees of peptic ulceration. Lesions that don't extend below the mucosal lining (epithelium) are called *erosions*. Lesions of acute and chronic ulcers can extend through the epithelium and may perforate the stomach wall. Chronic ulcers also have scar tissue at the base.

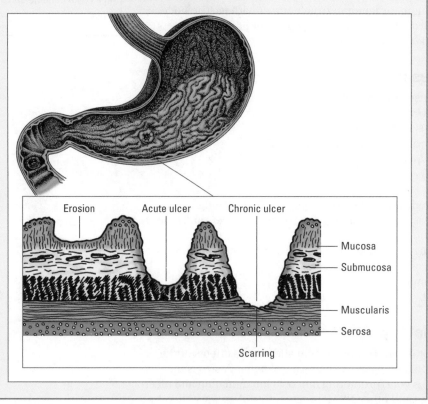

patients may report heartburn and localized midepigastric pain, which is relieved after eating.

What tests tell you

- Upper GI tract X-rays show abnormalities in the mucosa.
- Gastric secretory studies show hyperchlorhydria.
- Upper GI endoscopy confirms the presence of an ulcer.
- Serologic or breath urea test shows presence of *H. pylori*.
- Biopsy rules out cancer.
- Stool may test positive for occult blood.

How it's treated

Treatment is essentially symptomatic and emphasizes drug therapy and rest:

- Antacids reduce gastric acidity. Proton pump inhibitors, such as omeprazole (Prilosec) or lansoprazole (Prevacid), or H_2-receptor antagonists, such as cimetidine (Tagamet) or ranitidine (Zantac), reduce gastric secretion in short-term therapy (up to 8 weeks).
- Anticholinergics, such as propantheline, inhibit the vagus nerve effect on the parietal cells and reduce gastrin production and excessive gastric activity in duodenal ulcers.
- Physical rest promotes healing.
- Gastroscopy can promote coagulation of the bleeding site by cautery or laser therapy.
- If GI bleeding occurs, emergency treatment begins with passage of an NG tube to allow for iced saline lavage, possibly containing norepinephrine. Sclerotherapy with epinephrine is used to ligate active vessels. Angiography assists placement of an intra-arterial catheter, followed by infusion of vasopressin to constrict blood vessels and control bleeding. This type of therapy allows postponement of surgery until the patient's condition stabilizes.
- Surgery is indicated for perforation unresponsive to conservative treatment and suspected cancer. Surgical procedures for peptic ulcers include vagotomy and pyloroplasty or distal subtotal gastrectomy. (For more information, see "Gastric surgeries," page 447.)

What to do

- Administer medications as ordered, and watch for adverse effects of cimetidine (dizziness, rash, mild diarrhea, muscle pain, leukopenia, and gynecomastia) and anticholinergics (dry mouth, blurred vision, headache, constipation, and urine retention). Anticholinergics are usually most effective when given 30 minutes before meals. Give sedatives and tranquilizers as needed.

• Evaluate the patient. After successful treatment for peptic ulcers, he should understand the disease process and comply with the treatment regimen. He should recognize the need to avoid factors that may exacerbate his condition and modify his diet and lifestyle to do so. He should also understand the need for follow-up care and know when to seek immediate attention. (See *Peptic ulcer disease teaching tips.*)

Peritonitis

An acute or chronic inflammation, peritonitis may extend throughout the peritoneum, the membrane that lines the abdominal cavity and covers the visceral organs, or it may be localized as an abscess. Peritonitis commonly reduces intestinal motility and causes intestinal distention with gas. Mortality is 10%. Death usually results from sepsis and progressive organ faiure.

What causes it

• Peritonitis results from bacterial inflammation due to a ruptured appendix, perforated bowel, a strangulated obstruction, an abdominal neoplasm, or a stab wound.
• It may also result from chemical inflammation, as in ruptured fallopian tubes or bladder, perforated gastric ulcer, or released pancreatic enzymes.

Pathophysiology

Although the GI tract normally contains bacteria, the peritoneum is sterile. When bacteria or chemical irritants invade the peritoneum because of inflammation and perforation of the GI tract, peritonitis results. In chemical and bacterial inflammation, accumulated fluids containing protein and electrolytes make the transparent peritoneum opaque, red, inflamed, and edematous. Because the peritoneal cavity is so resistant to contamination, infection is commonly localized as an abscess.

What to look for

The main symptom of peritonitis is sudden, severe, diffuse abdominal pain that tends to intensify and localize in the area of the underlying disorder. Also assess the patient for:
• weakness, pallor, excessive sweating, and cold skin
• decreased intestinal motility and paralytic ileus
• abdominal distention
• an acutely tender abdomen associated with rebound tenderness
• shallow breathing

Education edge

Peptic ulcer disease teaching tips

• Instruct the patient to take antacids 1 hour after meals. Advise the patient who has a history of cardiac disease or one who's on a sodium-restricted diet to take only low-sodium antacids. Also warn him that antacids may cause some changes in bowel habits (diarrhea with magnesium-containing antacids and constipation with aluminum-containing antacids).
• Warn the patient to avoid aspirin-containing drugs, nonsteroidal anti-inflammatory drugs, reserpine, and phenylbutazone because they irritate the gastric mucosa. Also warn him against excessive intake of coffee, exposure to stressful situations, and consumption of alcoholic beverages during exacerbations. Advise him to stop smoking and to avoid milk products because these stimulate gastric secretion.

- diminished movement by the patient to minimize pain
- hypotension, tachycardia, and signs of dehydration
- fever of 103° F (39.4° C) or higher
- possible shoulder pain and hiccups.

What tests tell you

- Abdominal X-rays showing edematous and gaseous distention of the small and large bowel support the diagnosis. With perforation of a visceral organ, the X-ray shows air in the abdominal cavity.
- Chest X-rays may show an elevated diaphragm.
- Blood studies show leukocytosis (more than 20,000 leukocytes/μl).
- Paracentesis reveals bacteria, exudate, blood, pus, or urine.
- Laparotomy may be necessary to identify the underlying cause.

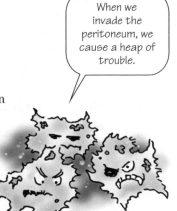

When we invade the peritoneum, we cause a heap of trouble.

How it's treated

Early treatment of GI inflammatory conditions and preoperative and postoperative antibiotic therapy prevent peritonitis. After peritonitis develops, emergency treatment aims to stop infection, restore intestinal motility, and replace fluids and electrolytes:

- Massive antibiotic therapy usually includes administration of cephalosporins with an aminoglycoside according to the infecting organisms. Quinolones may also be used.
- To decrease peristalsis and prevent perforation, the patient should be given nothing by mouth and should receive supportive fluids and electrolytes parenterally.
- Supplementary treatment measures include preoperative and postoperative analgesics, such as meperidine; NG intubation to decompress the bowel; and possible use of a rectal tube to help passage of flatus.
- When peritonitis results from perforation, surgery is performed as soon as the patient can tolerate it. Surgery aims to eliminate the infection source by evacuating the spilled contents and inserting drains.
- Occasionally, paracentesis may be needed to remove accumulated fluid.
- Irrigation of the abdominal cavity with antibiotic solutions during surgery may be appropriate.

Placing the patient in semi-Fowler's position helps him deep-breathe with less pain.

What to do

• Regularly monitor vital signs, fluid intake and output, and the amount of NG drainage or vomitus.
• Place the patient in semi-Fowler's position to help him deep-breathe with less pain, which helps to prevent pulmonary complications.

Evacuation procedures

After surgery to evacuate the peritoneum:
• Watch for signs and symptoms of dehiscence (the patient may complain that "something gave way") and abscess formation (continued abdominal tenderness and fever).
• Frequently assess peristaltic activity by listening for bowel sounds and checking for gas, bowel movements, and a soft abdomen.
• When peristalsis returns and temperature and pulse rate are normal, gradually decrease parenteral fluids and increase oral fluids. If the patient has an NG tube in place, clamp it for short intervals. If neither nausea nor vomiting results, begin oral fluids as ordered and tolerated.
• Evaluate the patient by assessing for normal fluid and electrolyte balance, normal body temperature and WBC count, lack of bowel obstruction or other complications, and normal oral intake and bowel elimination patterns. (See *Peritonitis teaching tips.*)

Ulcerative colitis

An inflammatory, typically chronic disease, ulcerative colitis affects the mucosa and submucosa of the colon. It usually begins in the rectum and sigmoid colon and commonly extends upward into the entire colon. It rarely affects the small intestine, except for the terminal ileum. Severity ranges from a mild, localized disorder to a fulminant disease that may cause a perforated colon, progressing to potentially fatal peritonitis and toxemia.

What causes it

The cause of ulcerative colitis is unknown. Risk factors include a family history of the disease; bacterial infection; allergic reaction to food, milk, or other substances that release inflammatory histamine in the bowel; overproduction of enzymes that break down the mucous membranes; and emotional stress. Autoimmune disorders, such as rheumatoid arthritis, hemolytic anemia, erythema nodosum, and uveitis, may heighten the risk.

Education edge

Peritonitis teaching tips

• Teach the patient about peritonitis, its cause (in his case), and necessary treatments. If time allows before surgery, reinforce the surgeon's explanation of the procedure and its possible complications. Tell him how long he can expect to be hospitalized; many patients remain hospitalized for 2 weeks or more after surgery.
• Review diet and activity limitations (depending on the type of surgery). Typically, the patient must avoid lifting for at least 6 weeks postoperatively.

Pathophysiology

Ulcerative colitis damages the large intestine's mucosal and sub-mucosal layers. Here's how it progresses:

1. Usually, the disease originates in the rectum and lower colon. Then it spreads to the entire colon.

2. The mucosa develops diffuse ulceration with hemorrhage, congestion, edema, and exudative inflammation. Unlike Crohn's disease, ulcerations are continuous.

3. Abscesses formed in the mucosa drain purulent pus, become necrotic, and ulcerate.

4. Sloughing occurs, causing bloody, mucus-filled stools.

Close-up on the colon

As ulcerative colitis progresses, the colon undergoes changes:

1. Initially, the colon's mucosal surface becomes dark, red, and velvety.

2. Abscesses form and coalesce into ulcers.

3. Necrosis of the mucosa occurs.

4. As abscesses heal, scarring and thickening may appear in the bowel's inner muscle layer.

5. As granulation tissue replaces the muscle layer, the colon narrows, shortens, and loses its characteristic pouches (haustral folds).

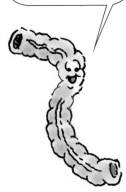

As ulcerative colitis progresses, the colon undergoes changes.

What to look for

Recurrent bloody diarrhea and symptom-free remissions are the hallmarks of ulcerative colitis. The stool typically contains pus and mucus. Assess the patient for other signs and symptoms, such as:

- spastic rectum and anus
- abdominal pain
- irritability
- weight loss
- weakness
- anorexia
- nausea and vomiting
- fever
- occasional constipation (in elderly patients).

What tests tell you

- Sigmoidoscopy shows increased mucosal friability, decreased mucosal detail, and thick inflammatory exudate. Biopsy during sigmoidoscopy helps confirm the diagnosis.
- Colonoscopy helps determine the extent of disease and evaluate strictured areas, pseudopolyps, and precancerous changes.
- A barium enema helps to assess the extent of the disease and to detect complications, such as strictures and carcinoma.
- A stool specimen may reveal leukocytes, ova, and parasites.
- The ESR will be increased in proportion to the severity of the attack.
- Decreased serum levels of potassium, magnesium, hemoglobin, and albumin as well as leukocytosis and increased PT support the diagnosis.

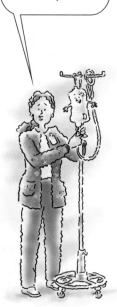

Supportive treatment for ulcerative colitis includes bed rest, I.V. fluid replacement, and a clear liquid diet.

How it's treated

Treatment seeks to control inflammation, replace nutritional losses and blood volume, and prevent complications.
- Supportive treatment includes bed rest, I.V. fluid replacement, and a clear liquid diet.
- For a patient awaiting surgery or showing signs of dehydration and debilitation from excessive diarrhea, TPN is administered to rest the intestinal tract, decrease stool volume, and restore positive nitrogen balance. The patient may also need blood transfusions or iron supplements to correct anemia.
- Drug therapy to control inflammation includes adrenocorticotropic hormone and adrenal corticosteroids, such as prednisone, prednisolone (Prelone), hydrocortisone (Cortef), and budesonide (Entocort EC).
- If disease is limited to the left side of the colon, topical mesalamine suppositories or enemas or hydrocortisone enemas may be effective.
- Sulfasalazine and mesalamine (Asacol), which have anti-inflammatory and antimicrobial properties, may also be used.

Don't spaz out

- Antispasmodics, such as tincture of belladonna, and antidiarrheals, such as diphenoxylate, are used only for patients whose ulcerative colitis is under control but who have frequent, troublesome diarrheal stools. These drugs may precipitate massive dilation of the colon (toxic megacolon) and are usually contraindicated.
- Immunomodulatory agents, such as azathioprine and 6-mercaptopurine, may be effective for patients who have frequent flare-ups of symptoms despite continuous steroid therapy. Patients with severe disease have also been treated with cyclosporine.

These medications require careful monitoring along with serial CBC with differential counts.

• Surgery is the treatment of last resort if the patient has toxic megacolon, fails to respond to drugs and supportive measures, or finds symptoms unbearable. The most common surgical technique is proctocolectomy with ileostomy. Total colectomy with ileorectal anastomosis is done less often because of its associated mortality (2% to 5%).

• In pouch ileostomy, a pouch is created from a small loop of the terminal ileum and a nipple valve formed from the distal ileum. The resulting stoma opens just above the pubic hairline; the pouch empties through a catheter inserted in the stoma several times each day.

• Colectomy to prevent colon cancer is controversial in treatment for ulcerative colitis. (For more information, see "Bowel surgery with ostomy," page 450.)

What to do

• Accurately record intake and output, particularly the frequency and volume of stools. Watch for signs of dehydration (poor skin turgor, furrowed tongue) and electrolyte imbalances, especially signs of hypokalemia (muscle weakness, paresthesia) and hypernatremia (tachycardia, flushed skin, fever, dry tongue).

• Monitor hemoglobin level and hematocrit, and give blood transfusions as ordered.

• Provide good mouth care for the patient who's allowed nothing by mouth.

• After each bowel movement, thoroughly clean the skin around the rectum.

• Provide an air mattress or a sheepskin to help prevent skin breakdown.

• Watch for adverse effects of prolonged corticosteroid or immunomodulator therapy (hyperglycemia, hypertension, hirsutism, edema, gastric irritation). Be aware that such therapy may mask infection.

• Watch closely for signs of complications, such as a perforated colon and peritonitis (fever, severe abdominal pain, abdominal rigidity and tenderness, cool, clammy skin) and toxic megacolon (abdominal distention, decreased bowel sounds).

• Do a bowel preparation, as ordered. This usually involves keeping the patient on a clear liquid diet, using enemas, and administering antimicrobials such as neomycin.

• Evaluate the patient. He should maintain optimal nutrition and hydration, report his feelings about his changed body image, identify and avoid foods likely to cause distress, demonstrate proper ostomy care, use appropriate support groups, understand the need for follow-up care, and know when to seek immediate attention. (See *Ulcerative colitis teaching tips.*)

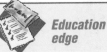

Education edge

Ulcerative colitis teaching tips

• Prepare the patient for surgery and inform him about ileostomy. Encourage him to verbalize his feelings and provide emotional support.

• After a proctocolectomy and ileostomy, teach good stoma care. After a pouch ileostomy, also teach the patient how to insert the catheter.

• Instruct the patient about his disease, and teach him to watch for signs of increased activity and flare-ups. Discuss adverse effects of medications, especially immunomodulators.

• Include instruction on self-administration of enemas and topical creams.

• Explain the importance of a healthy, low-residue diet and an adequate intake of protein, calcium, folate, and vitamin D.

• Encourage the patient to have regular physical examinations because he's at risk for developing colorectal cancer.

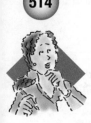

Quick quiz

1. When performing an abdominal assessment, do the four basic steps in which order?
  A. Inspection, percussion, palpation, auscultation
  B. Inspection, auscultation, percussion, palpation
  C. Palpation, inspection, percussion, auscultation
  D. Percussion, auscultation, palpation, inspection

Answer: B. In an abdominal assessment, auscultation is performed before percussion and palpation because the latter can alter intestinal activity.

2. When performing a urine bilirubin test or a urobilinogen test, the specimen must be tested within:
  A. 5 minutes.
  B. 10 minutes.
  C. 30 minutes.
  D. 1 hour.

Answer: C. Both tests must be conducted within 30 minutes of specimen collection before the specimen deteriorates.

3. Your patient has severe midepigastric or right upper quadrant pain radiating to the back or referred to the right scapula, belching that leaves a sour taste in the mouth, and flatulence. She most likely has:
  A. appendicitis.
  B. acute cholecystitis, acute cholelithiasis, or choledocholithiasis.
  C. diverticular disease.
  D. acute gastritis.

Answer: B. These signs and symptoms suggest your patient has acute cholecystitis, acute cholelithiasis, or choledocholithiasis.

4. In a patient with suspected appendicitis, which of these interventions are appropriate?
  A. Give I.V. fluids, give the patient nothing by mouth, and apply heat to his abdomen for comfort.
  B. Give I.V. fluids, give the patient nothing by mouth, and give an enema to clean his bowel before surgery.
  C. Give I.V. fluids; give the patient nothing by mouth, but give analgesics judiciously; and place him in Fowler's position to reduce pain.
  D. Give clear liquids only along with heat applied to the abdomen for comfort.

Answer: C. Never apply heat to the right lower abdomen or give cathartics or enemas because they may cause the appendix to rupture. Give analgesics judiciously because they may mask symptoms of rupture.

5. Which statement about hepatitis is true?
   A. Type A hepatitis can lead to fulminant hepatitis.
   B. Type B hepatitis is transmitted via blood products, urine, and other body fluids.
   C. Type C hepatitis is transmitted via the fecal-oral route only.
   D. Type D hepatitis is mild in severity.

Answer: B. Type B hepatitis is transmitted via serum, blood, blood products, and all other body fluids. Type A hepatitis is mild in severity and won't lead to fulminant hepatitis. Type C hepatitis is transmitted via blood and other parenteral means. Type D hepatitis can be severe and lead to fulminant hepatitis.

6. When assessing a patient in the early stages of cirrhosis of the liver, what sign would be anticipated?
   A. Jaundice
   B. Peripheral edema
   C. Ascites
   D. Anorexia

Answer: D. Early manifestations of cirrhosis are vague and usually include GI symptoms such as anorexia, indigestion, nausea, vomiting, or bowel pattern problems

7. Which measure should the patient with diverticulitis be taught to integrate into his daily routine at home?
   A. Eating a diet high in digestible fiber
   B. Limiting fluid intake
   C. Using enemas to relieve constipation
   D. Straining with each bowel movement

Answer: A. A diet high in digestible fiber is recommended to increase stool volume, decrease colonic transit time, and reduce intraluminal pressure.

Scoring

⭐⭐⭐   If you answered all seven questions correctly, excellent! You've fully digested this GI information.

⭐⭐   If you answered five or six questions correctly, super! You're full steam ahead in your knowledge of the alimentary canal.

⭐   If you answered fewer than five questions correctly, relax. Chew on this chapter a bit more, and it should go down smoothly.

Endocrine disorders

12

Just the facts

In this chapter, you'll learn:

♦ the functions of hormones in the body

♦ techniques for assessing the endocrine system

♦ causes, pathophysiology, diagnostic tests, and nursing interventions for common endocrine system disorders.

A look at endocrine disorders

Endocrine disorders alter a patient's health and self-image. These disorders may affect the patient's growth and development, reproductive system, energy level, metabolic rate, or ability to adapt to stress. Some disorders, such as Cushing's syndrome and goiter, profoundly alter the body. Others, such as diabetes mellitus, require the patient to follow a stringent drug regimen and meal plan.

Anatomy and physiology

The endocrine system consists of three major components:

glands, which are specialized cell clusters or organs

hormones, which are chemical substances secreted by glands in response to stimulation

receptors, which are protein molecules that trigger specific physiologic changes in a target cell in response to hormonal stimulation.

Glands

The major glands of the endocrine system are:
- pituitary gland
- thyroid gland
- parathyroid glands
- adrenal glands
- pancreas
- thymus
- pineal gland
- gonads (ovaries and testes). (See *Endocrine system components*.)

Pituitary gland

The pea-sized pituitary gland, located on the inferior aspect of the brain, is called the "master gland" because it regulates many key processes. It has two lobes: the posterior lobe, which stores and releases oxytocin and antidiuretic hormone produced by the hypothalamus, and the anterior lobe, which produces at least six hormones.

growth hormone (GH), or somatotropin

thyroid-stimulating hormone (TSH), or thyrotropin

corticotropin

follicle-stimulating hormone (FSH)

luteinizing hormone (LH)

prolactin.

Thyroid gland

The thyroid gland lies directly below the larynx, partially in front of the trachea. Its two lateral lobes — one on either side of the trachea — join with a narrow tissue bridge, called the *isthmus*, to give the gland its butterfly shape. The two lobes of the thyroid function as one unit to produce two hormones:
- Triiodothyronine (T_3) and thyroxine (T_4), collectively referred to as *thyroid hormone*, are the body's major metabolic hormones.
- Calcitonin maintains the blood calcium level by inhibiting the release of calcium from bone.

Parathyroid glands

Four parathyroid glands lie embedded on the posterior surface of the thyroid, one in each corner. Like the thyroid lobes, the parathyroid glands work together as a single gland, producing

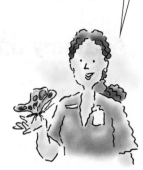

The two lateral lobes of the thyroid gland join with a narrow tissue bridge to give the gland its characteristic butterfly shape.

A closer look

Endocrine system components

Endocrine glands secrete hormones directly into the bloodstream to regulate body function. This illustration shows the location of the major endocrine glands.

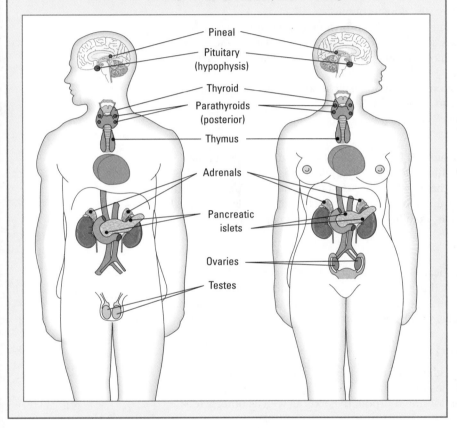

Pineal

Pituitary (hypophysis)

Thyroid

Parathyroids (posterior)

Thymus

Adrenals

Pancreatic islets

Ovaries

Testes

parathyroid hormone (PTH), which helps regulate the blood's calcium balance.

Adrenal glands

The two adrenal glands sit atop the two kidneys. Each gland contains two distinct structures — the adrenal cortex and the adrenal medulla — that function as separate endocrine glands. The adrenal medulla, the inner portion, produces catecholamines. Because catecholamines play an important role in the autonomic nervous system, the adrenal medulla is considered a neuroendocrine structure.

Zoning in on the outer layer

The adrenal cortex is the large outer layer. It has three zones, or cell layers:
• The zona glomerulosa, the outermost zone, produces mineralo-corticoids, primarily aldosterone.
• The zona fasciculata, the middle and largest zone, produces the glucocorticoids cortisol (hydrocortisone), cortisone, and corticos-terone as well as small amounts of the sex hormones androgen and estrogen.
• The zona reticularis, the innermost zone, produces mainly glu-cocorticoids and some sex hormones.

Pancreas

The pancreas, nestled in the curve of the duodenum, stretches horizontally behind the stomach and extends to the spleen. The islets of Langerhans, which perform the endocrine function of this gland, contain alpha, beta, and delta cells. Alpha cells produce glu-cagon; beta cells, insulin; and delta cells, somatostatin.

Thymus

The thymus is located below the sternum and contains lymphatic tissue. Although this gland produces the hormones thymosin and thymopoietin, its major role seems related to the immune system; it produces T cells, which are important in cell-mediated immunity.

Pineal gland

The tiny pineal gland lies at the back of the third ventricle of the brain. It produces the hormone melatonin, which may play a role in the neuroendocrine reproductive axis as well as other wide-spread actions.

Gonads

The gonads include the ovaries (in females) and the testes (in males). The ovaries promote development and maintenance of the female sex characteristics, regulate the menstrual cycle, maintain the uterus for pregnancy and, along with other hormones, pre-pare the mammary glands for lactation. The testes produce spermatozoa and the male sex hormone testosterone. Testosterone stimulates and main-tains male sex characteristics.

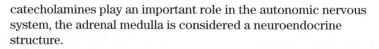

Testosterone stimulates and maintains male sex characteristics.

Yeah, but can it find the remote?

Hormones

Structurally, hormones can be classified into three types:

🤚 amines

✌️ polypeptides

🤟 steroids.

Amenable amines

Amines are derived from tyrosine, an essential amino acid found in most proteins. They include the thyroid hormones (T_3 and T_4) and the catecholamines (epinephrine, norepinephrine, and dopamine).

Poly want a peptide?

Polypeptides are protein compounds made of many amino acids that are connected by peptide bonds. They include anterior pituitary hormones (GH, TSH, corticotropin, FSH, LH, interstitial cell-stimulating hormone, and prolactin), posterior pituitary hormones (antidiuretic hormone [ADH] and oxytocin), PTH, and pancreatic hormones (insulin and glucagon).

Steroids: So sexy

Steroids, derived from cholesterol, include the adrenocortical hormones secreted by the adrenal cortex (aldosterone and cortisol) and the sex hormones (estrogen and progesterone in females and testosterone in males) secreted by the gonads.

Hormonal release and transport

Although all hormone release results from endocrine gland stimulation, their release patterns vary greatly.
• Corticotropin (secreted by the anterior pituitary) and cortisol (secreted by the adrenal cortex) are released in irregular spurts in response to body rhythm cycles, with levels peaking in the early morning.
• Secretion of PTH (by the parathyroid gland) and prolactin (by the anterior pituitary) occurs fairly evenly throughout the day.
• Secretion of insulin by the pancreas has both steady and sporadic release patterns.

Hormonal action

When a hormone reaches its target site, it binds to a specific receptor on the cell membrane or within the cell. Polypeptides and some amines bind to membrane receptor sites. The smaller, more lipid-soluble steroids and thyroid hormones diffuse through the cell membrane and bind to intracellular receptors.

When a hormone reaches its target site, it binds to a specific receptor on or in the cell.

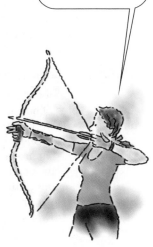

Right on target!

After binding occurs, each hormone produces unique physiologic changes, depending on its target site and its specific action at that site. A particular hormone may have different effects at different target sites.

Hormonal regulation

A complex feedback mechanism involving hormones, the central nervous system (CNS), and blood chemicals and metabolites helps maintain the body's delicate equilibrium by regulating hormone synthesis and secretion. Feedback refers to information sent to endocrine glands that signals the need for changes in hormone levels, either increasing or decreasing hormone production and release. (See *The feedback loop.*)

Assessment

To thoroughly assess the endocrine system, you must take an accurate health history and conduct a physical examination.

History

Because the endocrine system interacts with all other body systems, it's important to ask the patient about his health history and current patterns of health and illness.

Current health status

Ask the patient to describe his chief complaint. Common complaints associated with endocrine disorders include fatigue, weakness, weight changes, mental status changes, polyuria, polydipsia, and abnormalities of sexual maturity and function.

Asking the tough questions

Conduct a complete body systems review. Here are some examples of questions you might include:
• Have you noticed changes in your skin? If so, what kind?
• Do you feel tired?
• What are your sleep patterns?
• Have you noticed changes in your skin or changes in the amount or distribution of your body hair?
• Do your eyes burn or feel gritty when you close them?
• How good is your sense of smell?

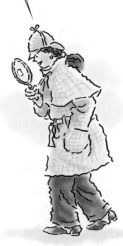

Information about current and previous health, family history, and lifestyle provide the clues you need for a thorough assessment.

The feedback loop

This diagram shows the negative feedback mechanism that helps regulate the endocrine system.

From simple…

Simple feedback occurs when the level of one substance regulates the secretion of hormones (simple loop). For example, a low serum calcium level stimulates the parathyroid gland to release parathyroid hormone (PTH). PTH, in turn, promotes resorption of calcium. A high serum calcium level inhibits PTH secretion.

…to complex

When the hypothalamus receives negative feedback from target glands, the mechanism is more complicated (complex loop). *Complex feedback* occurs through an axis established between the hypothalamus, pituitary gland, and target organ. For example, secretion of corticotropin-releasing hormone from the hypothalamus stimulates release of corticotropin by the pituitary, which in turn stimulates cortisol secretion by the adrenal gland (the

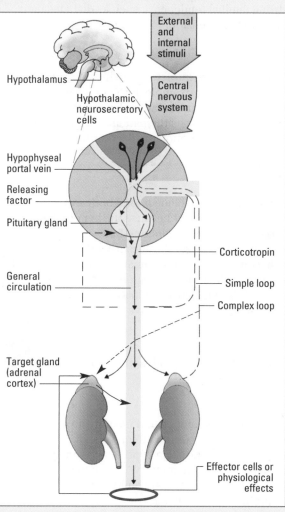

target organ). The cortisol goes through the bloodstream to effector cells, which cause physiologic effects. A rise in serum cortisol levels inhibits corticotropin secretion by decreasing corticotropin-releasing hormone.

Simple feedback occurs when the level of one substance regulates the secretion of hormones.

Complex feedback occurs through an axis established between the hypothalamus, pituitary gland, and target organ.

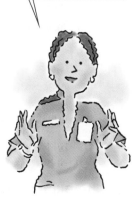

Previous health status

Ask about the patient's medical history. You may identify insidious and vague symptoms of endocrine dysfunction by asking if the patient has had a skull fracture, surgery, complications of surgery, or brain infection, such as meningitis or encephalitis.

Family history

Ask about family history because certain endocrine disorders are inherited or have strong familial tendencies, such as diabetes mellitus, thyroid disease, and hypertension.

Lifestyle patterns

Ask the patient about temperature intolerance, which may indicate certain thryoid disorders. For example, intolerance to cold may indicate hypothyroidism, and intolerance to warmth, hyperthyroidism. Also ask what medications the patient is taking. Some medications can alter hormone secretion or receptor response.

Physical examination

Your physical examination should include a total body evaluation and a complete neurologic assessment because the hypothalamus plays an important role in regulating endocrine function through the pituitary gland. Begin by measuring the patient's vital signs, height, and weight. Compare the findings with normal expected values and the patient's baseline measurements, if available. Then inspect, palpate, and auscultate the patient to obtain the most objective findings.

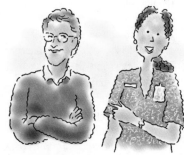

Note the patient's physical appearance, including appropriateness and neatness of dress.

Inspection

Systematically inspect the patient's overall appearance and examine all areas of his body.

Appearances are revealing

Assess the patient's physical appearance and mental and emotional status. Note such factors as overall affect, speech, level of consciousness (LOC) and orientation, appropriateness and neatness of dress and grooming, and activity level. Evaluate general body development, including posture, body build, proportionality of body parts, and distribution of body fat.

Get the skinny on the skin

Assess the patient's overall skin color, temperature, thickness, and turgor, and inspect his skin and mucous membranes for lesions, bruising, or areas of increased, decreased, or absent pigmentation. As you do so, be sure to consider racial and ethnic variations. In a dark-skinned patient, color variations are best assessed in the sclera, conjunctiva, mouth, nail beds, and palms. Next, assess the patient's skin texture and hydration.

A hairy situation

Inspect the hair for amount, distribution, condition, and texture. Observe scalp and body hair for abnormal patterns of growth or hair loss. Again, remember to consider normal racial and ethnic — as well as gender — differences in hair growth and texture. Next, check the patient's fingernails for cracking, peeling, separation from the nail bed (onycholysis), or clubbing; observe the toenails for fungal infection, ingrown nails, discoloration, length, and thickness.

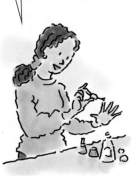

Check nail beds for cracking, peeling, separation from the nail bed, or clubbing. Looking good!

Eyeing the head

Assess the patient's face for overall color and the presence of erythematous areas, especially in the cheeks. Note facial expression. Is it pained and anxious, dull and flat, or alert and interested? Note the shape and symmetry of the patient's eyes, and look for eyeball protrusion, incomplete eyelid closure, or periorbital edema. Have the patient extend his tongue, and inspect it for color, size, lesions, positioning, and tremors or unusual movements.

Stick your neck out

While standing in front of the patient, examine his neck — first with it held straight, then slightly extended, and finally while the patient swallows water. Check for neck symmetry and midline positioning and for symmetry of the trachea. Use tangential lighting directed downward from the patient's chin to help you see the thyroid gland. An enlarged thyroid may be diffuse and asymmetrical.

Test the chest

Evaluate the overall size, shape, and symmetry of the patient's chest, noting deformities. In females, assess the breasts for size, shape, symmetry, pigmentation (especially on the nipples and in skin creases), and nipple discharge (galactorrhea). In males, observe for bilateral or unilateral breast enlargement (gynecomastia) and nipple discharge.

Inspect the patient's external genitalia — particularly the testes and clitoris — for normal development.

Extreme inspection

Inspect the patient's extremities. Check the arms and hands for tremors. To do so, have the patient hold both arms outstretched in front with the palms down and fingers separated. Place a sheet of paper on the outstretched fingers and watch for trembling. Note any muscle wasting, especially in the upper arms, and have the patient grasp your hands to assess the strength and symmetry of his grip.

Next, inspect the legs for muscle development, symmetry, color, and hair distribution. Then assess muscle strength by having the patient sit on the edge of the examination table and extend his legs horizontally. A patient who can maintain this position for 2 minutes exhibits normal strength. Examine the feet for size, and note lesions, corns, calluses, or marks from socks or shoes. Inspect the toes and the spaces between them for maceration and fissures.

> Examine the patient's feet for size, and note lesions, corns, calluses, or marks from socks or shoes.

Palpation

Palpate the thyroid gland and testes, the only endocrine glands accessible to palpation. You won't be able to palpate the thyroid gland in every patient. However, when you can examine the gland, it should be smooth, finely lobulated, nontender, and either soft or firm. You should be able to feel the gland's sections. (See *Palpating the thyroid.*)

A thyroid nodule feels like a knot, protuberance, or swelling; a firm, fixed nodule may be a tumor. Be careful not to confuse thick neck musculature with an enlarged thyroid or a goiter.

The testes should be firm to palpation and about $3/4''$ (2 cm) long before puberty. By age 16, the testes should be about $1 3/4''$ (4.5 cm) long (normal range is $1 3/8''$ to $2 1/8''$ [3.5 to 5.5 cm]). Palpate the spermatic cord while the patient is standing.

Signs, signs, everywhere a sign

Attempt to elicit Chvostek's sign and Trousseau's sign if you suspect a patient has hypocalcemia (low serum calcium levels) related to deficient or ineffective PTH secretion from hypoparathyroidism or surgical removal of the parathyroid glands. To elicit Chvostek's sign, tap the facial nerve in front of the ear with a finger; if the facial muscles contract toward the ear, the test is positive for hypocalcemia. To elicit Trousseau's sign, place a blood pressure cuff on the patient's arm and inflate it above his systolic pressure. In a positive test, the patient will exhibit carpal spasm (ventral contraction of the thumb and digits) within 3 minutes.

Auscultation

If you palpate an enlarged thyroid, auscultate the gland for systolic bruits, a sign of hyperthyroidism. Bruits occur when

Palpating the thyroid

To palpate the thyroid from the front, as shown, stand in front of the patient and place your index and middle fingers below the cricoid cartilage on both sides of the trachea. Palpate for the thyroid isthmus as he swallows. Then ask the patient to flex his neck toward the side being examined as you gently palpate each lobe. In most cases, you'll feel only the isthmus connecting the two lobes. However, if the patient has a thin neck, you may feel the whole gland. If he has a short, stocky neck, you may have trouble palpating even an enlarged thyroid.

Locating the lobes

To locate the right lobe, use your right hand to displace the thyroid cartilage slightly to your left. Hook your left index and middle fingers around the sternocleidomastoid muscle to palpate for thyroid enlargement. Then examine the left lobe, using your left hand to displace the thyroid cartilage and your right hand to palpate the lobe.

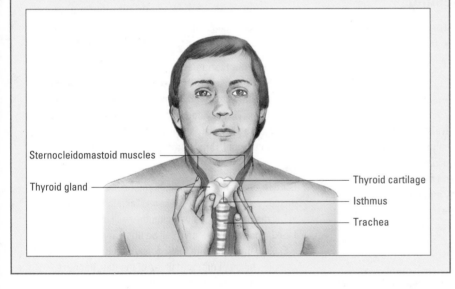

Sternocleidomastoid muscles

Thyroid gland

Thyroid cartilage

Isthmus

Trachea

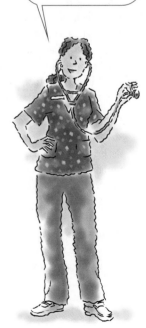

Auscultate for bruits by placing the stethoscope's bell over one of the thyroid's lateral lobes and listening for a low, soft, rushing sound.

accelerated blood flow through the thyroid arteries produces vibrations. To auscultate for bruits, place the bell of the stethoscope over one of the lateral lobes of the thyroid and then listen carefully for a low, soft, rushing sound. To ensure that tracheal sounds don't obscure bruits, have the patient hold his breath while you auscultate.

To distinguish an arterial bruit from a venous hum, first listen for the rushing sound; then gently occlude the jugular vein with your fingers on the side you're auscultating and listen again. A venous hum (produced by jugular blood flow) disappears during venous compression; an arterial bruit doesn't.

Diagnostic tests

Endocrine function is tested by direct, indirect, and provocative testing as well as radiographic studies.

Direct testing

The most common method, direct testing measures hormone levels in the blood or urine. However, accurate measurement requires special techniques because the body contains only minute hormone amounts. (See *Methods of direct testing*.)

Methods of direct testing

Methods of direct testing used to measure hormone levels in the blood or urine are:
• immunoradiometric assays (IRMAs)
• radioimmunoassay (RIA)
• 24-hour urine testing.

Immunoradiometric assays
IRMAs are used to measure levels of peptide and protein hormones. These tests use a receptor antiserum labeled with radioiodine. Immunochemiluminometric assays (ICMAs) use a chemical reagent that emits a specific light wavelength when activated by a particular substance. IRMAs and ICMAs are more specific, stable, precise, and easier than RIAs. Tests called *radioreceptor assays* measure the activity of a hormone.

Radioimmunoassay
RIA, the technique used to determine many hormone levels, incubates blood or urine (or a urine extract) with the hormone's antibody and a radiolabeled hormone tracer (antigen). Antibody-tracer complexes are then measured. For example, charcoal absorbs and removes a hormone not bound to its antibody-antigen complex. Measuring the remaining radiolabeled complex indicates the extent to which the sample hormone blocks binding, compared with a standard curve showing reactions with known hormone quantities. Although the RIA method provides reliable results, it doesn't measure every hormone.

24-hour urine testing
A 24-hour urine test measures hormones and their metabolites. Metabolite measurement helps evaluate hormones excreted in virtually undetectable amounts. The patient's health care provider usually orders 24-hour urine tests to confirm adrenal, renal, and gonadal disorders.

Nursing considerations
For all types of direct testing, hormone measurement may include serum or urine collection. Take the following steps:
• Tell the patient that a venipuncture will be done to collect blood, and explain when it will be done and who will do it
• Explain that accurate testing may require several blood samples taken at different times of the day, because physiologic factors — such as stress, diet, episodic secretions, and body rhythms — can alter circulating hormone levels.
• Explain that his urine will be collected for 24 hours with the appropriate collection device provided and that if a specimen is accidentally discarded, the collection must be restarted.
• For best results, keep a 24-hour urine specimen on ice during the collection period.

Indirect testing

Indirect testing measures the substance a particular hormone controls but not the hormone itself. For instance, glucose measurements help evaluate insulin, and calcium measurements help assess PTH activity. Although radioimmunoassays measure these substances directly, indirect testing is easier and less costly.

Glucose levels obtained indirectly will accurately reflect insulin's effectiveness, but various factors unrelated to an endocrine problem may affect calcium levels. For example, abnormal protein levels can lead to seemingly abnormal calcium levels because nearly one-half of calcium binds to plasma proteins. Therefore, rule out other possibilities before you assume that an abnormal calcium level reflects a PTH imbalance.

Provocative testing

Provocative testing helps determine an endocrine gland's reserve function when other tests show borderline hormone levels or can't quite pinpoint the abnormality's site. For instance, an abnormally low cortisol level may indicate adrenal hypofunction or indirectly reflect pituitary hypofunction.

Provocative testing works on this principle: Stimulate an underactive gland and suppress an overactive gland, depending on the patient's suspected disorder. A hormone level that doesn't increase with stimulation confirms primary hypofunction. Hormone secretion that continues after suppression confirms hyperfunction.

Radiographic studies

Radiographic studies are done with or after other tests. Computed tomography (CT) scans and magnetic resonance imaging (MRI) studies assess an endocrine gland by providing high-resolution, tomographic, three-dimensional images of the gland's structure, whereas nuclear imaging studies help determine the cause of hyperthyroidism.

Routine X-rays help evaluate how an endocrine dysfunction affects body tissues, although they don't reveal endocrine glands. For example, a bone X-ray, routinely ordered for a suspected parathyroid disorder, can show the effects of a calcium imbalance.

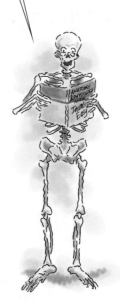

A bone X-ray, routinely ordered for a suspected parathyroid disorder, can show the effects of a calcium imbalance. Very interesting...

Treatments

Here is practical information about treatments for patients with endocrine disorders. You'll play a crucial role in preparing these patients for treatment, monitoring them during and after treatment, and teaching various aspects of self-care.

Drug therapy

Commonly used drugs to treat endocrine disorders include:
- corticosteroids for inflammation and adrenal insufficiency
- antidiabetics to lower blood glucose levels for type 1 and type 2 diabetes mellitus and diabetic ketoacidosis
- glucagon for hypoglycemia
- drugs that affect calcium levels for Paget's disease and hypocalcemia
- pituitary hormones for some forms of diabetes insipidus and pituitary growth hormone deficiency
- thyroid hormone antagonists for hyperthyroidism
- thyroid hormone for hypothyroidism.

Nonsurgical treatments

Nonsurgical treatments for endocrine disorders include meal planning for diabetes and radioactive iodine (^{131}I) administration.

Diabetic meal planning

Diabetes specialists regard meal planning as the cornerstone of diabetes care because it directly controls the body's major glucose source. Your patient's food intake can be carefully controlled to prevent widely fluctuating blood glucose levels. If he's taking insulin or sulfonylureas, he'll have to adhere to his meal plan even more carefully to avoid hypoglycemia.

In balance

Your patient's nutritional requirements include a well-balanced diet containing all the necessary nutrients. However, to avoid wide blood glucose variations, he needs to closely regulate his protein, fat and, especially, carbohydrate intake. Currently, the American Dietetic Association and the American Diabetes Association recommend an individual nutritional assessment to determine appropriate medical nutrition therapy. Carbohydrate and protein composition will vary, depending on therapeutic goals, and fat

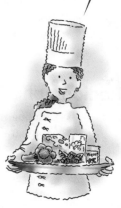

A patient's nutritional requirements include a well-balanced diet containing all the necessary nutrients.

should be less than 30% of total calories. The relatively low fat content may also help reduce the risk of cardiovascular disease.

Patient preparation

If your patient requires a meal plan, take the following steps:
- Explain to the patient that his meal plan will help control his blood glucose levels.
- Take a thorough dietary history, keeping in mind that difficulty with the diabetic meal plan may result from unnecessarily limiting the patient's food preferences and habits. Considering not only what he eats but also when he eats will help you and the patient to set up appropriate meal and snack times.
- Determine what your patient knows about diabetic meal planning. If he will be using the exchange system, explain that he needs to keep track of all the foods he eats and categorize them according to food exchanges. Mention that no foods can be exempted — even so-called dietetic foods.

Concentrating on sweets

- Make sure you discuss concentrated sweets (foods high in simple sugars) with the patient. Old-fashioned diabetic diets forbid such foods as ice cream, cookies, candies, and pastries. Studies that categorize foods according to their glycemic index (the blood glucose level after ingestion) show that complete restriction may not be necessary. Baked potatoes, for instance, have a higher glycemic index than ice cream. Findings such as these challenge researchers to investigate diabetic meal plans more closely. However, encourage your patient to remain cautious about concentrated sweets, particularly if weight loss is a goal. He still may need to avoid them unless his diabetes is well controlled.
- Arrange for a dietitian to teach your patient how to plan his meals. The dietitian may recommend the food exchange system. This method, based on the carbohydrate, fat, and protein content of six basic food groups, allows greater flexibility in meal planning. Exchange groups include milk products, vegetables, fruits, breads, meats, and fats.

Monitoring and aftercare

If your patient has newly diagnosed diabetes with extremely high blood glucose levels, he may require hospitalization while his blood glucose levels are monitored and insulin therapy is initiated. During his stay, take the following steps:
- Monitor for signs of hypoglycemia, such as nervousness, diaphoresis, tremors, dizziness, fatigue, faintness and, possibly, seizures or coma.

Old-fashioned diabetic diets forbid concentrated sweets, although glycemic index studies show that complete restriction may not be needed.

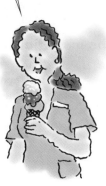

• Also watch for signs of hyperglycemia, such as polyuria, polydipsia, and dehydration.
• Finally, be on guard for signs of ketoacidosis, such as a fruity breath odor, dehydration, weak and rapid pulse, and Kussmaul's respirations. Be sure to monitor urine ketones if his blood glucose levels are over 400 mg/dl.

Home care instructions

Teach the patient how to adjust his meal plan when he engages in extra activity or exercise. If he eats many meals in restaurants, have the dietitian show him how to select a meal that fits his plan. If appropriate, tell him how to obtain nutrient composition lists from fast-food restaurants.

For an overweight patient, implement weight-reduction measures as ordered, and explain the reduced-calorie meal plan. Suggest a support group, such as Weight Watchers and Overeaters Anonymous, if necessary.

^{131}I administration

A form of radiation therapy, the administration of ^{131}I treats hyperthyroidism, particularly Graves' disease, and is an adjunctive treatment of thyroid cancer. It shrinks functioning thyroid tissue, decreasing circulating thyroid hormone levels and destroying malignant cells.

The incredible shrinking thyroid

After oral ingestion, ^{131}I is rapidly absorbed and concentrated in the thyroid as if it were normal iodine, resulting in acute radiation thyroiditis and gradual thyroid atrophy. ^{131}I causes symptoms to subside after about 3 weeks and exerts its full effect only after 3 to 6 months.

> ^{131}I doesn't exert its full effect until 3 to 6 months after therapy.

Patient preparation

Take the following steps before ^{131}I administration:
• Explain the procedure to the patient and check his history for allergies to iodine.
• Unless contraindicated, instruct the patient to stop thyroid hormone antagonists 4 to 7 days before ^{131}I administration because these drugs reduce the sensitivity of thyroid cells to radiation.
• Tell the patient to fast overnight because food may delay ^{131}I absorption.
• Make sure the patient isn't taking lithium carbonate, which may interact with ^{131}I to cause hypothyroidism.

• Inform the patient that ^{131}I won't be administered if he develops severe vomiting or diarrhea because these conditions reduce absorption.

Monitoring and aftercare

After ^{131}I administration, the patient is usually discharged with appropriate instructions. However, he may stay in the hospital for monitoring if he received an unusually large dose or if treatment was for cancer. In such cases, observe radiation precautions for 3 days.

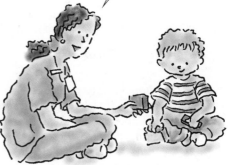

Tell the patient to avoid close contact with young children and pregnant women for 7 days after ^{131}I therapy.

Home care instructions

Before discharge, instruct the patient to:
• drink plenty of fluids for 48 hours to speed excretion of ^{131}I
• urinate into a lead-lined container for 48 hours
• use disposable eating utensils and avoid close contact with young children and pregnant women for 7 days after therapy (If you're pregnant, arrange for another nurse to care for this patient.)
• dispose of urine, saliva, and vomitus properly because urine and saliva will be slightly radioactive for 24 hours and vomitus will be highly radioactive for 6 to 8 hours after therapy
• expect to see improvement in several weeks, although the maximum effects won't occur for 3 to 6 months
• report pain, swelling, fever, and other signs and symptoms that could result from radiation treatment because these signs and symptoms are easily treated when reported
• avoid conception for several months after therapy (if patient is a female of childbearing age).

Surgery

Surgical treatment of endocrine disorders includes adrenalectomy, hypophysectomy, and thyroidectomy.

Adrenalectomy

Adrenalectomy — the resection or removal of one or both adrenal glands — is the treatment of choice for adrenal hyperfunction and hyperaldosteronism. It's also used to treat adrenal tumors, such as adenomas and pheochromocytomas, and has been used to aid treatment of breast and prostate cancer. The prognosis is good when adrenalectomy is used to treat adrenal adenomas. However, it's less favorable for adrenal carcinomas.

Patient preparation

Before adrenalectomy, take these steps:
• Expect to give oral or I.V. potassium supplements to correct low serum potassium levels. Monitor for muscle twitching and a positive Chvostek's sign (indications of alkalosis).
• Keep the patient on a low-sodium, high-potassium diet as ordered to help correct hypernatremia.
• Give aldosterone antagonists as ordered for blood pressure control.
• Explain to the patient that surgery may cure his hypertension if it results from an adenoma.

A soothing setting

• Give the patient with adrenal hyperfunction emotional support and a controlled environment to offset his emotional lability. If ordered, give a sedative to help him rest.
• Expect to administer medications to control his hypertension, edema, diabetes, and cardiovascular signs and symptoms as well as his increased tendency to develop infections.
• As ordered, give glucocorticoids the morning of surgery to help prevent acute adrenal insufficiency during surgery.

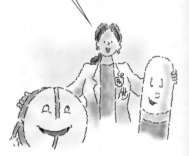

Expect to administer medications to control the patient's hypertension, edema, diabetes, and cardiovascular signs and symptoms as well as his increased tendency to develop infections.

Monitoring and aftercare

After adrenalectomy, take these steps:
• Monitor the patient's vital signs carefully, observing for indications of shock from hemorrhage.
• Keep in mind that postoperative hypertension is common because handling the adrenal glands stimulates catecholamine release.
• Watch for weakness, nausea, and vomiting, which may signal hyponatremia.
• Use sterile technique when changing dressings to minimize the risk of infection.
• Administer analgesics for pain, and give replacement steroids as ordered.

Crisis control

• Remember, glucocorticoids from the adrenal cortex are essential to life and must be replaced to prevent adrenal crisis until the hypothalamic, pituitary, and adrenal axis resumes functioning.
• If the patient had primary hyperaldosteronism, he'll have had preoperative renin suppression with resulting postoperative hypoaldosteronism. Monitor his serum potassium levels carefully; he may develop hyperkalemia if he's receiving spironolactone (Aldactone), a potassium-sparing diuretic for control of postoperative hypertension. Fludrocortisone may be indicated.

Home care instructions

Before discharge, take these steps:
• Explain the importance of taking prescribed medications as directed. If the patient had a unilateral adrenalectomy, explain that he may be able to taper his medications in a few months, when his remaining gland resumes function and his pituitary resumes secreting corticotropin.
• Make sure the patient understands that sudden withdrawal of steroids can precipitate adrenal crisis and that he needs continued medical follow-up to adjust his steroid dosage appropriately during stress or illness.

Sign language

• Describe the signs of adrenal insufficiency, and make sure the patient understands how this can progress to adrenal crisis if not treated. Explain that he should consult his practitioner if he develops such adverse reactions as weight gain, acne, headaches, fatigue, and increased urinary frequency, which can indicate steroid overdose. Advise him to take his steroids with meals or antacids to minimize gastric irritation.
• If the patient had adrenal hyperfunction, explain that he'll see a reversal of the physical characteristics of his disease over the next few months. However, caution him that his improved physical appearance doesn't mean he can stop his medications.
• Advise the patient to wear medical identification jewelry to ensure adequate medical care in an emergency.

Hypophysectomy

Microsurgical techniques have dramatically reversed the high mortality previously associated with removal of pituitary and sella turcica tumors. Transsphenoidal hypophysectomy is now the treatment of choice for pituitary tumors, which can cause acromegaly, gigantism, and Cushing's disease. The surgery also serves as a palliative measure for patients with metastatic breast or prostate cancer to relieve pain and reduce the hormonal secretions that spur neoplastic growth.

Risky business

Hypophysectomy may be performed subfrontally (approaching the sella turcica through the cranium) or transsphenoidally (entering from the inner aspect of the upper lip through the sphenoid sinus). (See *Transsphenoidal hypophysectomy*, page 536.) The subfrontal approach carries a high risk of mortality or complications, such as loss of smell and taste and permanent, severe diabetes insipidus. As a result, this approach is used only

Transsphenoidal hypophysectomy

When a pituitary tumor is confined to the sella turcica, the doctor performs transsphenoidal hypophysectomy. For the procedure, the patient is placed in a semirecumbent position and given a general anesthetic. The doctor incises the upper lip's inner aspect so that he can enter the sella turcica through the sphenoid sinus to remove the tumor.

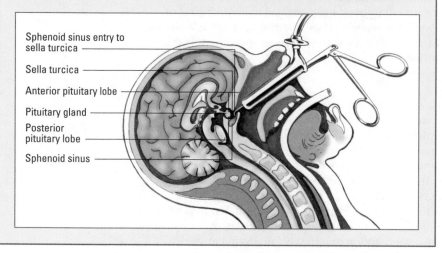

Sphenoid sinus entry to
sella turcica

Sella turcica

Anterior pituitary lobe

Pituitary gland

Posterior
pituitary lobe

Sphenoid sinus

rarely — in cases where a tumor causes marked subfrontal or subtemporal extension and with optic chiasm involvement.

Patient preparation

Before hypophysectomy, take these steps:
• Tell the patient that he'll receive a general anesthetic and may go to the intensive care unit (ICU) postoperatively for up to 48 hours for careful monitoring.
• Explain that he'll have a nasal catheter and packing in place for at least 1 day after surgery as well as an indwelling urinary catheter.
• Arrange for appropriate tests and examinations as ordered. For example, if the patient has acromegaly, he'll need a thorough cardiac evaluation because he may have incipient myocardial ischemia. If he has Cushing's disease, he'll need blood pressure and serum potassium level checks.
• Arrange for a visual field test to serve as a baseline for the patient.
• Review the patient's preoperative medication regimen if appropriate. If he has hypothyroidism, he may need hormone replacement therapy (HRT). Many patients receive I.V. hydrocortisone (Solu-Cortef) preoperatively and postoperatively.

Monitoring and aftercare

After hypophysectomy, take these steps:
• Keep the patient on bed rest for 24 hours after surgery and then encourage ambulation.
• Keep the head of his bed elevated to avoid placing tension or pressure on the suture line.
• Tell him not to sneeze, cough, blow his nose, or bend over for several days to avoid disturbing the suture line.
• Give mild analgesics as ordered for headache caused by cerebrospinal fluid loss during surgery or for paranasal pain. Paranasal pain typically subsides when the catheters and packing are removed — usually 24 to 72 hours after surgery.
• Anticipate that the patient may develop transient diabetes insipidus, usually 24 to 48 hours after surgery. Be alert for increased thirst and increased urine volume with a low specific gravity.
• If diabetes insipidus occurs, replace fluids and administer aqueous or sublingual desmopressin acetate (DDAVP), as ordered. With these measures, diabetes insipidus usually resolves within 72 hours.
• Arrange for visual field testing as soon as possible and compare the results to the patient's baseline because new vision defects can indicate hemorrhage.
• Collect a serum sample to measure pituitary hormone levels and evaluate the need for hormone replacement.

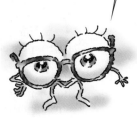

Arrange for visual field testing as soon as possible and compare the results to the patient's baseline. New vision defects can indicate hemorrhage.

Home care instructions

Before discharge, take these steps:
• Instruct the patient to report signs of diabetes insipidus immediately. Explain that he may need to limit fluid intake or take prescribed medications.
• Tell the patient with hyperprolactinemia that she'll need follow-up visits for several years because relapse is possible. Explain that she may be placed on bromocriptine (Parlodel), which inhibits secretion of prolactin, if relapse occurs.
• Advise the patient to brush teeth gently using a fingertip soft brush and to avoid suture line disruption. Tell the patient that using a mouthwash is acceptable.
• Explain to the patient that she may need HRT as a result of decreased pituitary secretion of tropic hormones. If cortisol or thyroid hormone replacement becomes necessary, teach the patient to recognize the signs of excessive or insufficient dosage.
• Advise the patient to wear medical identification jewelry.

Thyroidectomy

Thyroidectomy (removal of all or part of the thyroid gland) is performed to treat hyperthyroidism, respiratory obstruction from goiter, and thyroid cancer. Subtotal thyroidectomy, which reduces secretion of thyroid hormone, is used to correct hyperthyroidism when drug therapy fails or radiation therapy is contraindicated. It may also effectively treat diffuse goiter. After surgery, the remaining thyroid tissue usually supplies enough thyroid hormone for normal function, although hypothyroidism may occur later.

Patient preparation

Before thyroidectomy, take these steps:
• Explain to the patient that thyroidectomy will remove diseased thyroid tissue or, if necessary, the entire gland.
• Tell him that he'll have an incision in his neck and a drain and dressing in place after surgery and that he may experience some hoarseness and a sore throat from intubation and anesthesia. Reassure him that he'll receive analgesics to relieve his discomfort.
• Make sure that the patient has followed his preoperative drug regimen, which will render the gland euthyroid (having a normally functioning thyroid gland) to prevent thyrotoxicosis during surgery. He probably will have received either propylthiouracil or methimazole (Tapazole), usually starting 4 to 6 weeks before surgery.
• Expect him to receive iodine for 10 to 14 days before surgery to reduce the gland's vascularity and thus prevent excess bleeding. He may also take propranolol (Inderal) to reduce excess sympathetic effects. Notify the practitioner immediately if the patient hasn't followed his medication regimen.
• If necessary, arrange for an electrocardiogram (ECG) to evaluate cardiac status.

Monitoring and aftercare

After thyroidectomy, take these steps:
• Watch for signs of respiratory distress. Tracheal collapse, mucus accumulation in the trachea, laryngeal edema, and vocal cord paralysis can all cause respiratory obstruction with sudden stridor and restlessness. Keep a tracheostomy tray at the patient's bedside for 24 hours after surgery, and be prepared to assist with emergency tracheotomy if necessary.
• Be alert for indications of thyroid storm (a sudden and dangerous increase of the signs of thyrotoxicosis), a rare but serious complication. In thyroid storm, pulse and respirations rise to dangerous levels and temperature increases rapidly.
• Keep the patient in high semi-Fowler's position to promote venous return from the head and neck and to decrease oozing into the incision.

Be alert for indications of thyroid storm, a rare but serious condition.

• Check for laryngeal nerve damage by asking the patient to speak as soon as he wakes from anesthesia.
• Assess for signs of hemorrhage, which may cause shock, tracheal compression, and respiratory distress. Check the patient's dressing and palpate the back of his neck, where drainage tends to flow. Expect about 50 ml of drainage in the first 24 hours; if you find no drainage, check for drain kinking or the need to reestablish suction. Expect only scant drainage after 24 hours.

A pain in the neck

• As ordered, administer an analgesic to relieve a sore neck or throat. Reassure the patient that his discomfort should resolve within a few days.
• Assess for hypocalcemia, which may occur when bones depleted of calcium from hyperthyroidism begin to heal, rapidly taking up calcium from the blood, or if the parathyroid glands are injured or destroyed. Test for positive Chvostek's and Trousseau's signs, indicators of neuromuscular irritability from hypocalcemia. Keep calcium gluconate available for emergency I.V. administration.

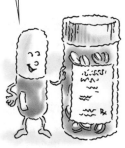

If parathyroid damage occurred during surgery, the patient may need to take calcium supplements.

Home care instructions
Before discharge, take these steps:
• If the patient has had a subtotal or total thyroidectomy, or if the parathyroid glands are injured or destroyed, explain the importance of regularly taking his prescribed thyroid hormone replacement. Teach him to recognize and report signs of hypothyroidism and hyperthyroidism.
• If parathyroid damage occurred during surgery, explain to the patient that he may need to take calcium supplements. Teach him to recognize the warning signs of hypocalcemia.
• Tell the patient to keep the incision site clean and dry.
• Arrange follow-up appointments as necessary, and explain to the patient that the practitioner needs to check the incision and serum thyroid hormone levels.

Fashion tips

• Help the patient cope with concerns about appearance. Suggest loosely buttoned collars, high-necked blouses and shirts, jewelry, or scarves, which can hide the incision until it heals. The practitioner may recommend a mild body lotion to soften the healing scar and improve its appearance.

Nursing diagnoses

When caring for patients with endocrine disorders, you'll typically use several nursing diagnoses. These appear below, along with appropriate nursing interventions and rationales. See *NANDA-I taxonomy II by domain*, page 936, for the complete list of NANDA diagnoses.

> Encourage activity and exercise based on the patient's physical ability and limitations. Cartwheels might be a bit much, though.

Imbalanced nutrition: More than body requirements

Related to increased appetite, high calorie intake, inability to use nutrients, and inactivity, *Imbalanced nutrition: More than body requirements* is associated with many disorders, including Cushing's syndrome and diabetes mellitus.

Expected outcomes
- Patient expresses feelings about weight.
- Patient plans menus appropriate to prescribed diet.
- Patient adheres to prescribed diet.

Nursing interventions and rationales
- Obtain the patient's dietary history. Permanent weight change begins with examination of contributing factors. Provide the patient with a written copy of a calorie-based meal plan. Obtain dietary consultation as needed. Evaluate the patient's eating habits and include preferred foods in his meal plan.
- Provide support and encouragement as the patient attempts to change his calorie intake. Encouragement provides positive reinforcement and reduces frustration.
- Encourage activity and exercise based on the patient's physical ability and limitations. Exercise not only helps the patient lose weight, it also reduces stress and helps curb stress-related eating.
- Refer the patient to community resources as needed and available.

Insomnia

Related to anxiety or hormone imbalance, *Insomnia* is associated with such disorders as hyperthyroidism, diabetes insipidus, and diabetes mellitus.

Expected outcomes
- Patient identifies factors that prevent or disrupt sleep.
- Patient sleeps ___ hours per night.
- Patient expresses a feeling of being well rested.

Nursing interventions and rationales

• Promote usual sleep and rest practices. Decrease environmental stimuli. Provide a quiet, darkened, private room.
• Encourage frequent, short periods of ambulation.
• Administer antihormone medications as ordered and sedatives as needed.
• Instruct the patient and his family to eliminate caffeine-containing foods — such as coffee, tea, cola, and chocolate — from his diet.
• Provide and encourage quiet diversionary activities to promote rest and sleep.

Common endocrine disorders

Endocrine dysfunction takes one of two forms: hyperfunction, which results in excessive hormone production or response, or hypofunction, which results from a relative or absolute hormone deficiency. Hormonal imbalance can also be classified according to the disease site. Disease within an endocrine gland causes *primary dysfunction*. Disease caused by dysfunction outside a particular endocrine gland, but affecting that gland or its hormone or hormones, is termed *secondary dysfunction*.

Addison's disease

The most common form of adrenal hypofunction, Addison's disease occurs when more than 90% of the adrenal gland is destroyed. With early diagnosis and adequate replacement therapy, the prognosis for adrenal hypofunction is good. Acute adrenal insufficiency, or adrenal crisis (addisonian crisis), is a medical emergency requiring immediate, rigorous treatment.

What causes it

Although autoimmune causes are the most common causes of Addison's disease, it can also result from:
• tuberculosis
• bilateral adrenalectomy
• hemorrhage into the adrenal gland
• neoplasms
• fungal infections.
    Secondary adrenal hypofunction can be caused by:
• hypopituitarism
• abrupt withdrawal of long-term corticosteroid therapy
• removal of a nonendocrine, corticotropin-secreting tumor.

Pathophysiology

In the autoimmune process of Addison's disease, circulating antibodies react specifically against the adrenal tissue, leading to decreased secretion of androgens, glucocorticoids, and mineralocorticoids. Adrenal hypofunction may also result from a disorder outside the gland, in which case aldosterone secretion commonly continues. In a patient with adrenal hypofunction, adrenal crisis occurs when the body's stores of glucocorticoids are exhausted by trauma, infection, surgery, or other physiologic stressors.

What to look for

When trying to determine the presence of Addison's disease, look for:
- weakness or fatigue
- anorexia and weight loss
- nausea and vomiting
- chronic constipation or diarrhea
- conspicuous bronze skin coloration, especially in hand creases and over the metacarpophalangeal joints, elbows, and knees
- darkening of scars and areas of vitiligo (absence of pigmentation)
- increased pigmentation of the mucous membranes, especially the buccal mucosa
- cardiovascular abnormalities, such as orthostatic hypotension, decreased heart size and cardiac output, and a weak, irregular pulse
- decreased tolerance for even minor stress
- poor coordination
- fasting hypoglycemia
- a craving for salty food
- amenorrhea.

The clinical effects of secondary adrenal hypofunction resemble those of Addison's disease but without hyperpigmentation, hypotension, and electrolyte abnormalities. Adrenal crisis is characterized by profound weakness and fatigue, shock, severe nausea and vomiting, hypotension, dehydration and, occasionally, high fever.

What tests tell you

- Decreased plasma cortisol and serum sodium levels and increased corticotropin, serum potassium, and blood urea nitrogen (BUN) levels confirm adrenal hypofunction.
- Metyrapone and corticotropin stimulation tests are special provocative studies that determine whether adrenal hypofunction is primary or secondary.

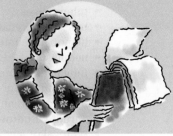

Hmmm... decreased plasma cortisol and serum sodium and increased corticotropin, serum potassium, and BUN. I suspect adrenal hypofunction!

How it's treated

Corticosteroid replacement, usually with cortisone or hydrocortisone (both also have a mineralocorticoid effect), is the primary lifelong treatment for patients with primary or secondary adrenal hypofunction. Drug therapy may also include fludrocortisone, which acts as a mineralocorticoid to prevent dehydration and hypotension.

Adrenal crisis requires prompt administration of dexamethasone, hydrocortisone, or both. The patient receives later doses of hydrocortisone I.V. until his condition stabilizes. With proper treatment, the crisis usually subsides quickly, blood pressure stabilizes, and fluid and sodium levels return to normal. Subsequent oral maintenance doses of hydrocortisone preserve stability.

What to do

• In an adrenal crisis, monitor vital signs carefully for hypotension, volume depletion, and other signs of shock (decreased LOC and urine output). Watch for hyperkalemia before treatment and for hypokalemia after treatment (from excessive mineralocorticoid effect).
• If the patient also has diabetes, check blood glucose levels frequently because steroid replacement may necessitate changing the insulin dosage. Carefully record weight and intake and output, because the patient may have volume depletion. Force fluids to replace excessive fluid loss until the onset of mineralocorticoid effects.

The dish on diet

• Arrange for a diet that maintains sodium and potassium balance. If the patient is anorectic, suggest six small meals per day to increase calorie intake. Ask the dietitian to provide a diet high in protein and carbohydrates.
• Observe the patient receiving steroids for cushingoid signs such as fluid retention around the eyes and face. Watch for fluid and electrolyte imbalance, especially if the patient receives mineralocorticoids.
• Evaluate the patient's understanding of his condition and treatment. He should maintain a proper diet; maintain normal serum sodium, potassium, and plasma cortisol levels; understand the need to take his medication routinely; and make necessary adjustments in times of stress. (See *Addison's disease teaching tips*.)

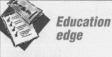

Education edge

Addison's disease teaching tips

• Explain to the patient that he'll need lifelong cortisone replacement therapy.
• Advise the patient about signs and symptoms of overdose and underdose, and explain that he'll need to increase the dosage during times of stress (when he has a cold, for example).
• Warn that infection, injury, or profuse sweating in hot weather may precipitate a crisis.
• Instruct the patient to always carry a medical identification card and wear a bracelet stating the name and dosage of the steroid he takes.
• Teach the patient how to give himself a hydrocortisone injection.
• Tell him to keep an emergency kit containing hydrocortisone in a prepared syringe for use in times of stress.
• Warn that he may need additional cortisone to prevent a crisis after any type of stress.

Cushing's syndrome

A disorder of adrenal hyperfunction, Cushing's syndrome results from excessive levels of adrenocortical hormones (particularly cortisol) or related corticosteroids and, to a lesser extent, androgens and aldosterone. Its unmistakable signs include adiposity of the face (moon face), neck, and trunk and purple striae on the skin, especially the abdomen. Cushing's syndrome is more common in females than males by a 5:1 margin. Prognosis depends on the underlying cause; it's poor in untreated persons and in those with untreatable ectopic corticotropin-secreting carcinoma or metastatic adrenal carcinoma.

What causes it

Cushing's syndrome can stem from:
• pituitary hypersecretion of corticotropin (Cushing's disease)
• corticotropin-secreting tumor in another organ (particularly bronchogenic or pancreatic carcinoma)
• administration of synthetic glucocorticoids
• adrenal tumor, which is usually benign in adults (less common cause).

Pathophysiology

A loss of normal feedback inhibition by cortisol occurs in Cushing's syndrome. Elevated levels of cortisol don't suppress hypothalamic and anterior pituitary secretion of corticotropin-releasing hormone and corticotropin. The result is excessive levels of circulating cortisol.

What to look for

The patient who has some or all of these signs and symptoms might have Cushing's syndrome:
• weight gain
• muscle weakness
• fatigue
• buffalo hump
• thinning extremities with muscle wasting and fat mobilization
• thin, fragile skin
• moon face and ruddy complexion
• hirsutism
• truncal obesity
• broad purple striae
• bruising
• impaired wound healing.

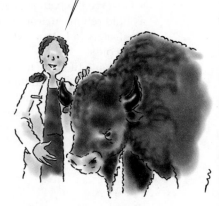

Buffalo hump is a sign of Cushing's syndrome — in humans, that is.

What tests tell you

• A low-dose (overnight) dexamethasone suppression test, elevated 24-hour urinary free cortisol levels, and high nighttime cortisol levels (indicating loss of circadian rhythm) confirm the diagnosis of Cushing's syndrome.
• A plasma corticotropin test and high-dose dexamethasone suppression test can determine the cause of Cushing's syndrome.
• With an adrenal tumor, corticotropin levels aren't detectable and steroid levels aren't suppressed. Ectopic corticotropin syndrome shows elevated corticotropin or unsuppressed steroid levels. Normal to elevated corticotropin with steroid suppressed to less than 50% of baseline indicates Cushing's disease.
• Ultrasonography, CT scan, or angiography localizes adrenal tumors.
• CT scan or MRI of the head helps localize pituitary tumors.

How it's treated

The patient may require radiation, drug therapy, or surgery to restore hormone balance and reverse Cushing's syndrome. For example:
• Transsphenoidal resection of the corticotropin-secreting pituitary microadenoma is the therapy of choice for pituitary tumors that cause Cushing's disease.
• Adrenal tumor is treated by unilateral adrenalectomy with good prognosis, but the patient will require glucocorticoid therapy perioperatively and postoperatively.
• Nonendocrine corticotropin-secreting tumors require excision. Drug therapy with etomidate (Amidate), ketoconazole (Nizoral), metyrapone (Demser), or mitotane (Lysodren) decreases cortisol levels if signs and symptoms persist or the tumor is inoperable.
• Before surgery, the patient with cushingoid signs and symptoms needs special management to control hypertension, edema, diabetes, and cardiovascular manifestations and to prevent infection. Glucocorticoid administration on the morning of surgery can help prevent acute adrenal insufficiency during surgery.

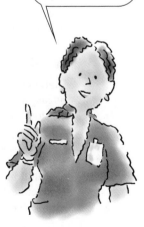

Patients with Cushing's syndrome require painstaking assessment and supportive care.

What to do

• Provide painstaking assessment and supportive care to the patient with Cushing's syndrome. Implement these measures:
– Frequently monitor vital signs, especially blood pressure. Carefully observe the hypertensive patient who also has cardiac disease.

– Check laboratory reports for hypernatremia, hypokalemia, hyperglycemia, and glycosuria.

– Because the cushingoid patient is likely to retain sodium and water, check for edema and carefully monitor daily weight, intake, and output. To minimize weight gain, edema, and hypertension, ask the dietitian to provide a diet high in protein and potassium but low in calories, carbohydrates, and sodium.

– Watch for infection — a significant problem in Cushing's syndrome.

– Carefully perform passive range-of-motion exercises for the patient who has osteoporosis and is bedridden.

– Cushing's syndrome produces emotional lability. Record incidents that upset the patient, and try to prevent such situations if possible. Help the patient get the necessary physical and mental rest — by sedation if necessary. Offer emotional support throughout the difficult testing period.

– Evaluate the patient. After successful therapy, the patient will take medication as prescribed, recognize signs and symptoms of steroid underdose and overdose, and carry medical identification. Fluid, electrolyte, and plasma cortisol levels will be within normal limits and the patient will seek counseling for stress as needed. (See *Cushing's syndrome teaching tips.*)

Diabetes insipidus

Diabetes insipidus results from a deficiency of circulating ADH, or vasopressin. It's an uncommon condition but occurs equally in men and women. The prognosis is good with uncomplicated diabetes insipidus and, with adequate water replacement, patients usually lead normal lives. The prognosis varies in cases complicated by an underlying disorder such as metastatic cancer.

What causes it

Diabetes insipidus may be familial, acquired, or idiopathic. It can be acquired as the result of intracranial neoplastic or metastatic lesions. Other causes may include:
- hypophysectomy or other neurosurgery
- head trauma, which damages the neurohypophyseal structures
- infection
- granulomatous disease
- vascular lesions
- autoimmune disorders.

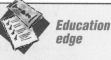

Education edge

Cushing's syndrome teaching tips

- Advise the postoperative Cushing's syndrome patient to take replacement steroids with antacids or meals to minimize gastric irritation. (It can help to take two-thirds of the dose in the morning and the remaining one-third in the late afternoon to mimic diurnal adrenal secretion.)
- Instruct the patient to use I.M. cortisol when ill or unable to keep food down, and provide guidelines for when the patient should contact the practitioner.
- Have the patient carry medical identification and immediately report physiologically stressful situations, which require increased dosage.
- Instruct the patient to recognize signs and symptoms of steroid underdose (fatigue, weakness, dizziness) and overdose (severe edema, weight gain).
- Warn the patient that discontinuing steroid dosage abruptly may produce a fatal adrenal crisis.

Pathophysiology

Normally, ADH is synthesized in the hypothalamus and then stored by the posterior pituitary gland. When it's released into the general circulation, ADH increases the water permeability of the distal and collecting tubules of the kidneys, causing water reabsorption. If ADH is absent, the filtered water is excreted in the urine instead of being reabsorbed, and the patient excretes large quantities of dilute urine.

What to look for

The cardinal sign of diabetes insipidus is extreme polyuria — usually 4 to 16 L/day of dilute urine but sometimes as much as 30 L/day, with a low specific gravity (less than 1.005). Other symptoms include:
• polydipsia, particularly for cold, iced drinks
• nocturia
• fatigue (in severe cases)
• dehydration, characterized by weight loss, poor tissue turgor, dry mucous membranes, constipation, muscle weakness, dizziness, tachycardia, and hypotension.

What tests tell you

• Urinalysis reveals almost colorless urine of low osmolality (less than 200 mOsm/kg) and low specific gravity (less than 1.005).
• A water deprivation test confirms the diagnosis by demonstrating renal inability to concentrate urine (evidence of ADH deficiency).
• Subcutaneous injection of 5 units of vasopressin produces decreased urine output with increased specific gravity if the patient has central diabetes insipidus.

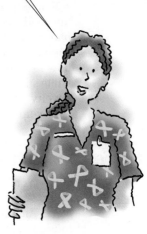

Until the cause of diabetes insipidus can be identified, vasopressin or a vasopressin stimulant can help control fluid balance and prevent dehydration.

How it's treated

Until the cause of diabetes insipidus can be identified and eliminated, administering various forms of vasopressin or a vasopressin stimulant controls fluid balance and prevents dehydration. Thiazide diuretics may be prescribed to reduce urine volume by creating mild salt depletion.

What to do

• Record fluid intake and output carefully. Maintain the patient's fluid intake to prevent severe dehydration.
• Watch for signs of hypovolemic shock, and monitor blood pressure and heart and respiratory rates regularly, especially during the water deprivation test.
• Check weight daily.
• Remember to keep the bed's side rails up and assist with walking if the patient is dizzy or has muscle weakness.
• Monitor urine specific gravity between doses. Watch for decreased specific gravity with increased urine output, indicating an inability to concentrate urine and the need for the next dose or a dosage increase.

Bulking up

• Add more bulk foods and fruit juices to the diet if constipation develops. If necessary, obtain an order for a mild laxative such as milk of magnesia.
• Provide meticulous skin and mouth care, and apply a lubricant to cracked or sore lips.
• Make sure caloric intake is adequate and the meal plan is low in sodium.
• Watch for decreased urine output and increased specific gravity between doses of medication.
• Monitor electrolyte levels and watch for hyponatremia.
• Evaluate the patient. He should maintain an adequate fluid volume and electrolyte balance and resume his normal elimination pattern. If diabetes insipidus hasn't been eliminated, the patient should also know how to administer his medication correctly and how to record his intake and output; preferably he'll self-medicate while still an inpatient. He should wear medication identification jewelry, carry a wallet identification card, and schedule regular follow-up appointments. (See *Diabetes insipidus teaching tips.*)

Diabetes mellitus

Diabetes mellitus is characterized by disturbances in carbohydrate, protein, and fat metabolism. A leading cause of death in North America, diabetes is a major risk factor for myocardial infarction (MI), stroke, renal failure, and peripheral vascular disease. It's also the leading cause of blindness in adults.

Taking form

Two forms exist: type 1 and the more prevalent type 2 diabetes mellitus. Type 1 diabetes usually occurs before age 30 (although it may occur at any age); the patient is usually thin and will require

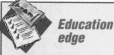

Education edge

Diabetes insipidus teaching tips

• Teach the patient to monitor fluid intake and output and restrict sodium in his meal plan if he's taking a thiazide diuretic.
• Instruct him to administer desmopressin by nasal insufflation or by mouth. Advise the patient about possible adverse drug effects such as headaches. Tell him to report weight gain because it may mean the dosage is too high. Recurrence of polyuria, as reflected on the intake and output sheet, indicates that the dosage is too low.
• Advise the patient to wear medical identification jewelry and carry his medication with him at all times.
• Provide written instructions on how and when to use his medication and what signs and symptoms he should report to his practitioner.

exogenous insulin and dietary management to achieve control. Conversely, type 2 most commonly occurs in obese adults after age 40; it's usually treated with exercise, meal planning, and antidiabetic drugs. Treatment may include insulin therapy. An increasing number of adolescents and young people are being diagnosed with type 2 diabetes.

Shocking results

In hyperosmolar hyperglycemic nonketotic syndrome (HHNS), dehydration may cause hypovolemia and shock. Long-term diabetes may lead to retinopathy, nephropathy, atherosclerosis, and peripheral and autonomic neuropathy. Peripheral neuropathy usually affects the legs and may cause numbness.

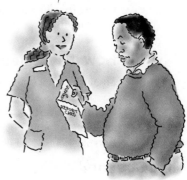

Type 2 diabetes most commonly occurs in obese adults after age 40, and treatment usually includes meal planning. Let's check out the menu!

What causes it

Type 1 is an autoimmune disease strongly associated with human leukocyte antigens DR 3 and 4. It may also be associated with certain viral infections.

Type 2 may result from:
• impaired insulin secretion
• peripheral insulin resistance
• increased basal hepatic glucose production.
   Other associated factors include:
• obesity
• insulin antagonists (such as excess counter-regulatory hormones and phenytoin)
• hormonal contraceptives
• pregnancy.

Pathophysiology

The effects of diabetes mellitus result from insulin deficiency or resistance to endogenous insulin. Normally, insulin allows glucose transport into the cells for use as energy or storage as glycogen. Insulin also stimulates protein synthesis and free fatty acid storage in adipose tissue. Insulin deficiency compromises the body tissues' access to essential nutrients for fuel and storage.

What to look for

Assess the patient for:
• fatigue
• polyuria related to hyperglycemia
• polydipsia
• nocturia
• dry mucous membranes

- poor skin turgor
- weight loss
- blurred vision
- polyphagia.

What tests tell you

- Two fasting plasma glucose tests above 126 mg/dl or, with normal fasting glucose, two blood glucose levels above 200 mg/dl during a 2-hour glucose tolerance test confirm the diagnosis.
- Ophthalmologic examination may show diabetic retinopathy.
- Other tests include plasma insulin level determination, urine testing for glucose and acetone, and glycosylated hemoglobin (hemoglobin A_{1C} [Hb A_{1C}]) determination.

How it's treated

Meal planning, exercise and, sometimes, insulin or oral antidiabetic agents are prescribed to normalize carbohydrate, fat, and protein metabolism and avert long-term complications while avoiding hypoglycemia. (See *Treatment of type 1 diabetes mellitus*, pages 552 and 553.)

All about food

All types of diabetes require strict adherence to carefully planned meals to meet nutritional needs, control blood glucose levels, and reach and maintain appropriate body weight. The American Diabetes Association recommends an individualized nutritional assessment and medical nutrition therapy to achieve therapeutic goals. Therapy works best when the patient consistently follows the meal plan. Aerobic exercise is also generally prescribed at least three times per week for a minimum of 45 to 60 minutes. Patients are asked to exercise five or six times per week when weight loss is a therapeutic goal. (See *Standards of care for diabetes*.)

Insulin deficiency? Absolutely!

Patients with type 1 diabetes must take insulin daily because of their absolute insulin deficiency. Patients with type 2 diabetes may require insulin to control blood glucose levels unresponsive to diet and oral antidiabetic agents, or during periods of acute stress. Patients with other types of diabetes commonly require daily insulin therapy to achieve blood glucose control. (See *Insulin therapy*, page 554.)

Weighing the evidence

Standards of care for diabetes

The American Diabetes Association has issued standards of care to help practitioners care for patients with diabetes. Here are some examples:

• Patients diagnosed with diabetes should receive medical care from a doctor-coordinated team that includes doctors, nurse practitioners, nurses, dietitians, and pharmacists who have expertise and a special interest in diabetes.

• Patients should receive individualized medical nutritional therapy from a registered dietitian.

• Patients capable of participating in regular physical activity programs should take part in individualized programs adapted to their needs.

• Educational plans should recognize the importance of diabetes self-management and ongoing support.

• All patients with diabetes, regardless of age, should receive pneumococcal and influenza vaccines.

Source: American Diabetes Association. (2010). Standards of medical care in diabetes. *Diabetes Care, 33,* 511–561.

Adding drugs to the mix

Patients with type 2 diabetes who can't achieve their target blood glucose levels with meal planning and exercise may require antidiabetic medications. Used in combination with one another or with insulin, these medications help patients with type 2 diabetes maintain normal glucose levels. Several types of medications are used to treat type 2 diabetes.

• Insulin secretagogues enhance pancreatic insulin secretion and include:
– first generation — the sulfonylureas, tolazamide, tolbutamide
– second generation — glyburide (DiaBeta), glipizide (Glucotrol), and glimepiride (Amaryl).

In addition, repaglinide (Prandin) enhances insulin secretion but acts more quickly.

• Biguanides (metformin [Glucophage] is the only one currently available) prevent inappropriate hepatic gluconeogenesis.

• Alpha-glucosidase inhibitors acarbose (Precose) and miglitol (Glyset) delay the intestinal absorption of carbohydrates.

(Text continues on page 554.)

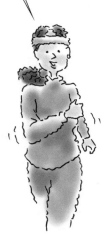

Patients with type 2 diabetes may need antidiabetic drugs in addition to meal planning and exercise.

Treatment of type 1 diabetes mellitus

This algorithm shows the pathophysiologic process of diabetes and indicates points for treatment intervention.

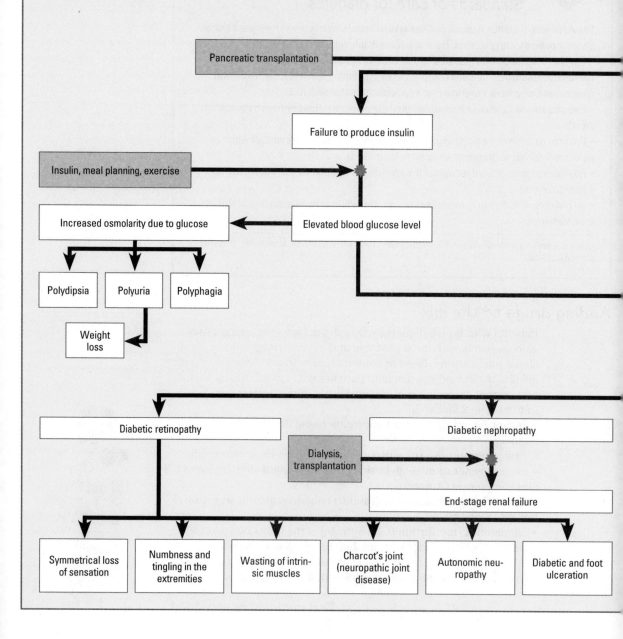

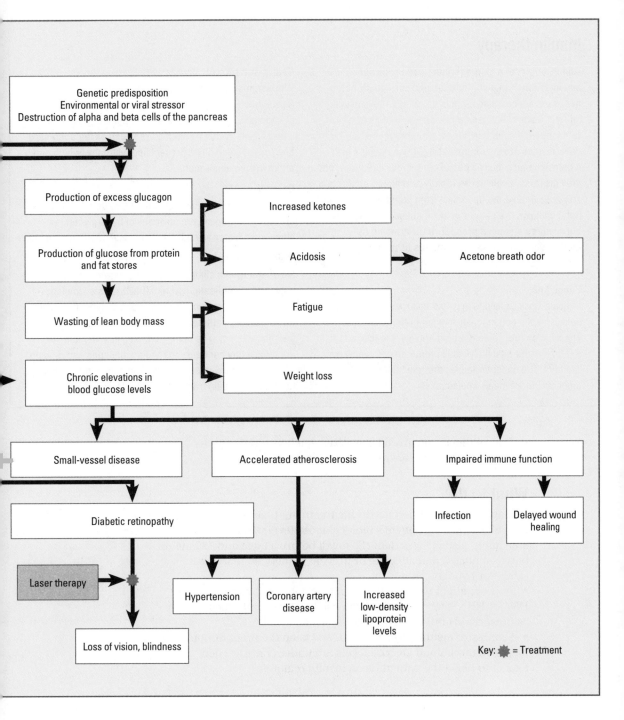

Genetic predisposition
Environmental or viral stressor
Destruction of alpha and beta cells of the pancreas

Production of excess glucagon

Increased ketones

Production of glucose from protein and fat stores

Acidosis → Acetone breath odor

Wasting of lean body mass

Fatigue

Chronic elevations in blood glucose levels

Weight loss

Small-vessel disease

Accelerated atherosclerosis

Impaired immune function

Infection

Delayed wound healing

Diabetic retinopathy

Laser therapy

Hypertension

Coronary artery disease

Increased low-density lipoprotein levels

Loss of vision, blindness

Key: ✱ = Treatment

Insulin therapy

Administer insulin as prescribed, usually by subcutaneous injection with a standard insulin syringe. Subcutaneous insulin can also be given with a penlike insulin injector device that uses a disposable needle and replaceable insulin cartridges, eliminating the need to draw insulin into a syringe. Jet-injection devices are expensive and require special cleaning procedures, but they disperse insulin more rapidly and speed absorption. These devices draw up insulin from standard containers (which allows the patient to mix insulins, if necessary, but requires a special procedure for drawing up) and deliver it into the subcutaneous tissue with a pressure jet.

Pump it up

Multiple-dose regimens may use an insulin pump to deliver insulin continuously into subcutaneous tissue. The infusion rate selector automatically releases about one-half of the total daily insulin requirement evenly over 24 hours. The patient releases the remainder in bolus amounts before meals and snacks.

Ready, set, rotate!

When administering subcutaneous insulin injections, rotate the injection sites. Because absorption rates differ at each site, diabetic educators recommend rotating the injection site within a specific area such as the abdomen. Site rotation also helps prevent lipodystrophy, which can affect insulin absorption.

Only I.V. or I.M.

Regular insulin or insulin lispro may also be administered I.M. or I.V. during severe episodes of hyperglycemia. Never administer any other type of insulin by these routes.

Grand experiment

Now undergoing clinical trials, the programmable implantable medication system (PIMS) has an implantable infusion pump unit that holds and delivers the insulin and a delivery catheter that feeds insulin directly into the peritoneal cavity. The pump, encased in a titanium shell, contains a tiny computer to regulate dosages and runs on a battery with a 5-year life span. The patient uses a handheld external radio transmitter to control insulin release.

• Thiazolidinedione insulin sensitizers such as pioglitazone (Actos) enhance the sensitivity of peripheral cells to insulin.

What to do

• Emphasize that adherence to the treatment plan is essential. It's crucial to bring the patient's blood glucose level within an acceptable range (usually less than 120 mg/dl before a meal and 180 mg/dl between meals) and alleviate or prevent diabetic ketoacidosis (DKA) or hypoglycemia.
• For the patient with unstable diabetes who isn't experiencing DKA or HHNS, monitor blood glucose levels several times per day as prescribed until they stabilize.
• Administer insulin as prescribed, and keep the practitioner informed until blood glucose levels are under control. Then expect to begin the patient on an insulin regimen.

- If the patient has type 2 diabetes, he may need an oral antidiabetic or a trial period with diet therapy.

Dinner is at 6 sharp!

- Make sure meals are on time for the patient receiving insulin or an insulin secretagogue.
- Monitor the patient closely for signs and symptoms of DKA or HHNS as well as for hypoglycemia (caused by too rapid reduction in blood glucose level). Suspect DKA or HHNS if your patient begins to exhibit Kussmaul's respirations, develops a fruity odor to his breath, and shows signs and symptoms of severe dehydration. If these indications occur, immediately notify the practitioner.
- If the patient has DKA or HHNS, treatment may include fluid and electrolyte replacement, increased insulin therapy, and therapy to reduce acidosis. Administer doses of I.V. insulin as prescribed. Monitor the patient's blood glucose levels frequently during insulin infusion. Alert the practitioner when the glucose level reaches 250 to 300 mg/dl so that the insulin dosage can be decreased to prevent hypoglycemia. Typically, insulin decreases blood glucose levels by about 75 to 100 mg/dl each hour. Patients with HHNS have a greater insulin sensitivity than patients with DKA, so expect to give less insulin.
- After the crisis, expect to resume the patient's usual insulin regimen. Infuse I.V. fluids rapidly at the prescribed rate. Hypotonic or isotonic saline solution will be administered, depending on the patient's condition. When the glucose level is slightly above normal, the practitioner may switch to a glucose solution to prevent hypoglycemia and reduce the risk of cerebral edema.

Preserving potassium

- Monitor an elderly patient closely for evidence of fluid overload. Monitor the patient's electrolyte levels closely and administer potassium replacement therapy as ordered. Patients with an extremely low pH level may require bicarbonate therapy to treat acidosis, but fluid and insulin replacement alone usually correct metabolic acidosis.
- The meal plan is the cornerstone of diabetes care because it directly controls the body's major glucose source. Your patient can prevent widely fluctuating blood glucose levels by controlling his food intake. If he takes insulin or sulfonylureas, he'll need to adhere to his meal plan even more carefully to avoid hypoglycemia.
- Monitor the patient for complications related to insulin therapy, which include hypoglycemia, the dawn phenomenon (early morning rise in blood glucose), insulin lipodystrophy (usually caused by continually using the same injection site), insulin allergy, and insulin resistance.

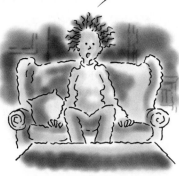

The dawn phenomenon refers to an early morning rise in glucose. This horror movie is giving me a late-night rise in adrenaline!

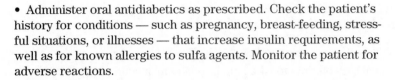
• Administer oral antidiabetics as prescribed. Check the patient's history for conditions — such as pregnancy, breast-feeding, stressful situations, or illnesses — that increase insulin requirements, as well as for known allergies to sulfa agents. Monitor the patient for adverse reactions.

Keying in on ketones

• If necessary, check your patient's urine for ketones. Urine testing is sometimes used to monitor blood glucose control, but it's rapidly being replaced with blood glucose monitoring. Despite their convenience, urine tests don't always reflect blood glucose levels accurately. However, only urine testing can detect ketone bodies — particularly important for the ketosis-prone patient with type 1 diabetes.

• Demonstrate to the patient how to check his blood glucose. Because blood glucose changes may cause misleading signs and symptoms — or none at all — the patient with diabetes must measure his glucose level often. Capillary blood glucose monitoring allows the patient (and the nurse) to determine metabolic status quickly, receive feedback on problems with the diet or medication regimen, and make immediate adjustments. It's especially useful for the patient on a tightly controlled regimen. Recent research shows that good glycemic control (Hb A_{1C} level less than 7%) reduces the risk of long-term complications from diabetes.

• Blood glucose monitoring equipment varies greatly, so it's important to carefully follow the manufacturer's instructions. The health care provider may order blood glucose testing before meals, after meals, and at bedtime, or less frequently for a patient who has established stable control.

• Monitor the patient's Hb A_{1C} as ordered to assess long-term diabetes control. The amount of glycosylation directly correlates with blood glucose levels. Ideally, the patient's Hb A_{1C} should measure no more than $1^{1}/_{2}$ times the normal level, which ranges from 3% to 6%. A high Hb A_{1C} value with any blood glucose level suggests hyperglycemia over several weeks; a low value coupled with a high blood glucose level suggests recent onset of hyperglycemia.

Vital records

• Keep accurate records of vital signs, weight, fluid intake, urine output, and caloric intake in addition to monitoring serum glucose and urine ketone levels.

• Monitor the patient closely for signs and symptoms of hyperglycemia and hypoglycemia. If a hypoglycemic reaction occurs, obtain a blood glucose level and immediately give carbohydrates in the form of fruit juice, hard candy, or honey. Give glucagon or

I.V. dextrose if the patient is unconscious. Notify the practitioner of a significant change in the patient's blood glucose levels.

• Provide meticulous skin care, especially to the feet and legs, to avert problems associated with peripheral vascular disease and neuropathy. Even a tiny skin break can produce complications that lead to amputation. Avoid constricting hose, slippers, or bed linens. Refer the patient to a podiatrist if indicated.

• Evaluate the patient. He should have normal blood glucose levels, maintain an adequate nutritional intake, understand his drug regimen, monitor himself for complications of the disease, and obtain medical identification jewelry and a wallet identification card. (See *Diabetes mellitus teaching tips*.)

Hyperparathyroidism

Hyperparathyroidism is characterized by excess activity of one or more of the four parathyroid glands, resulting in excessive secretion of PTH. Such hypersecretion of PTH promotes bone resorption and leads to hypercalcemia and hypophosphatemia. Increased renal and GI absorption of calcium also occurs.

What causes it

Primary hyperparathyroidism may result from a single adenoma, a genetic disorder, or multiple endocrine neoplasias. Secondary hyperparathyroidism may be caused by rickets, vitamin D deficiency, chronic renal failure, or phenytoin (Dilantin) or laxative abuse.

Pathophysiology

Hyperparathyroidism may be primary or secondary. In primary hyperparathyroidism, one or more of the parathyroid glands enlarge, leading to increased PTH secretion and elevated serum calcium levels.

A close second

In secondary hyperparathyroidism, a hypocalcemia-producing abnormality outside the parathyroid gland doesn't respond to the metabolic action of PTH, leading to excessive compensatory production of PTH.

What to look for

Hyperparathyroidism may produce symptoms. Secondary hyperparathyroidism may produce the same clinical features as primary hyperparathyroidism, with possible skeletal deformities of the

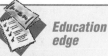

Education edge

Diabetes mellitus teaching tips

• Review the prescribed meal plan with the patient, and teach him when to adjust his diet.

• Advise the patient about aerobic exercise programs. Explain how exercise affects blood glucose levels, and provide safety guidelines.

• Instruct the patient on insulin administration, if prescribed, including type, peak times, dosage, drawing up the insulin, mixing (if applicable), administration technique, and site rotation.

• Teach the patient about oral antidiabetic therapy, if prescribed.

• Instruct the patient to keep a log of his blood glucose levels and insulin administration. Tell him to take the log to his practitioner visits.

• Teach the patient to inspect all the skin of both feet daily and to report any open areas to his practitioner at once.

long bones (for example, rickets) as well as other symptoms of the underlying disease. Symptoms include:

• *CNS* — psychomotor and personality disturbances, loss of memory for recent events, depression, overt psychosis, stupor and, possibly, coma

• *GI* — anorexia, nausea, vomiting, dyspepsia, and constipation

• *neuromuscular* — fatigue and marked muscle weakness and atrophy, particularly in the legs

• *renal* — signs and symptoms of recurring nephrolithiasis, which may lead to renal insufficiency

• *skeletal and articular* — chronic lower back pain and easy fracturing from bone degeneration, bone tenderness, and joint pain

• *other* — skin pruritus, vision impairment from cataracts, and subcutaneous calcification.

What tests tell you

• Immunoradiometric assay reveals elevated serum PTH levels. This finding, in conjunction with increased serum calcium and decreased phosphorus levels, confirms the diagnosis of hyperparathyroidism.

• X-rays may show diffuse demineralization of bones, bone cysts, outer cortical bone resorption, and subperiosteal erosion of the radial aspect of the middle fingers.

• Laboratory tests reveal elevated urine and serum calcium, chloride, and alkaline phosphatase levels and decreased serum phosphorus levels.

• Secondary hyperparathyroidism is confirmed when serum calcium levels are normal or slightly decreased, with variable serum phosphorus and bicarbonate levels.

How it's treated

Treatment varies, depending on the cause of the disease. Surgery to remove the adenoma or all but one-half of one gland (the remaining part of the gland is needed to maintain normal PTH levels) is commonly the treatment of choice. Although surgery can relieve bone pain within 3 days, the patient's renal damage may be irreversible.

Control the calcium

Less invasive treatments are used to decrease calcium levels preoperatively or when surgery isn't an option. These include:

• forcing fluids

• limiting dietary calcium intake

• promoting sodium and calcium excretion through forced diuresis

• using normal saline solution (up to 6 L in life-threatening situations)

- furosemide (Lasix), or ethacrynic acid (Edecrin)
- administering oral sodium or potassium phosphate, or calcitonin.

Uncover the underlying cause

Treatment for secondary hyperparathyroidism must correct the underlying cause of parathyroid hypertrophy. It includes vitamin D therapy or aluminum hydroxide for hyperphosphatemia in the patient with renal disease. In the patient with chronic secondary hyperparathyroidism, the enlarged glands may not revert to normal size and function even after calcium levels have been controlled; if so, they should be surgically removed.

What to do

- Record intake and output as the patient receives hydration to reduce serum calcium levels.
- Strain urine to check for calculi.
- Monitor sodium, potassium, and magnesium levels frequently.

Listen closely...

- Auscultate for breath sounds often, and be alert for pulmonary edema in the patient receiving large amounts of I.V. saline solution — especially in the presence of pulmonary or cardiac disease.
- Take precautions to avoid falls because the patient is predisposed to pathologic fractures.
- Evaluate the patient. He should understand the need for regular serum calcium level studies, the signs and symptoms of hypercalcemia and hypocalcemia and which ones to report, the reasons for drug therapy and adequate hydration, and possible adverse drug effects. (See *Hyperparathyroidism teaching tips.*)

Hypoparathyroidism

Hypoparathyroidism stems from a deficiency of PTH. Because PTH primarily regulates calcium balance, hypoparathyroidism leads to hypocalcemia and produces neuromuscular signs and symptoms ranging from paresthesia to tetany. The clinical effects are usually correctable with replacement therapy. However, some complications of this disorder, such as cataracts and basal ganglion calcifications, are irreversible.

What causes it

The three major causes of hypoparathyroidism are:
- congenital absence or malfunction of the parathyroid glands
- autoimmune destruction
- removal of or injury to one or more parathyroid glands during neck surgery.

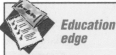

Education edge

Hyperparathyroidism teaching tips

- Teach the patient about the possible adverse effects of drug therapy.
- Emphasize the need for periodic follow-up through laboratory blood tests.
- If hyperparathyroidism isn't corrected surgically, warn the patient to avoid prolonged periods of immobilization, to maintain adequate hydration, and to avoid calcium-containing antacids and thiazide diuretics.
- Instruct the patient to contact his practitioner if he experiences significant diarrhea or vomiting.

Other causes include:
• ischemic infarction of the parathyroids during surgery or from disease, such as amyloidosis or neoplasms
• suppression of normal gland function caused by hypercalcemia (reversible)
• hypomagnesemia-induced impairment of hormone secretion (reversible)
• massive thyroid radiation therapy (rare).

Pathophysiology

PTH usually maintains serum calcium levels by increasing bone resorption and by stimulating renal conversion of vitamin D to its active form, which enhances GI absorption of calcium and bone resorption. PTH also maintains the inverse relationship between serum calcium and phosphate levels by inhibiting phosphate reabsorption in the renal tubules and enhancing calcium reabsorption. Abnormal PTH production in hypoparathyroidism disrupts this delicate balance.

What to look for

Hypoparathyroidism may not produce symptoms in mild cases. Otherwise, signs and symptoms include:
• neuromuscular irritability
• increased deep tendon reflexes
• positive Chvostek's and Trousseau's signs
• dysphagia
• paresthesia
• psychosis.

Other indications include tetany; seizures; arrhythmias; cataracts; abdominal pain; dry, lusterless hair; spontaneous hair loss; brittle fingernails that develop ridges or fall out; possibly dry, scaly skin; and weakened tooth enamel that may cause teeth to stain, crack, and decay easily.

What tests tell you

• Test results that confirm hypoparathyroidism include decreased PTH and serum calcium levels and elevated serum phosphorus levels.
• X-rays reveal increased bone density.
• An ECG shows prolonged QT intervals and QRS-complex and ST-segment changes that are caused by hypocalcemia and may be mistaken for acute MI or conduction abnormalities.

X-rays reveal increased bone density in the patient with hypoparathyroidism.

How it's treated

Therapy includes vitamin D, usually with supplemental calcium. Such therapy is usually lifelong, except for patients with the reversible form of the disease. Types of vitamin D given include dihydrotachysterol if renal function is adequate and calcitriol if renal function is severely compromised.

Call in the calcium cavalry

Acute life-threatening tetany calls for immediate I.V. administration of calcium to raise serum calcium levels. Sedatives and anticonvulsants are given to control spasms until calcium levels rise. Chronic tetany calls for vitamin D and possibly oral calcium supplements to maintain normal serum calcium levels.

What to do

- While awaiting diagnosis of hypoparathyroidism in a patient with a history of tetany, maintain a patent I.V. line and keep 10% calcium gluconate solution available.
- Institute seizure precautions because the patient is at risk for seizures.
- Keep a tracheostomy tray and an endotracheal tube at the bedside because laryngospasm may result from hypocalcemia.
- Monitor for Chvostek's and Trousseau's signs.
- For the patient with tetany, prepare to administer 10% calcium gluconate by slow I.V. infusion and maintain a patent airway. Prepare the patient for transport to the ICU according to facility policy because the patient may also require intubation and sedation with I.V. diazepam (Valium). Monitor vital signs often, especially if the patient received I.V. diazepam, to make sure his blood pressure and heart rate return to normal.
- When caring for the patient with hypoparathyroidism, stay alert for minor muscle twitching (especially in the hands) and for signs of laryngospasm (respiratory stridor or dysphagia). These effects may signal the onset of tetany.

Toxic trouble

- Because the patient with chronic disease has prolonged QT intervals on an ECG, watch for ventricular arrhythmias, heart block, and signs of decreased cardiac output. Closely monitor the patient who receives digoxin (Lanoxin) and calcium because calcium potentiates the effect of digoxin. Watch for signs and symptoms of digoxin toxicity (arrhythmias, nausea, fatigue, changes in vision).
- Evaluate the patient. He shouldn't develop tetany, and his serum calcium levels should be normal. The patient should understand the signs and symptoms of hypocalcemia and hypercalcemia and

state which ones to report; identify high-calcium, low-phosphorus foods; and understand the importance of good nail grooming and the need for emollient creams to soften the skin. (See *Hypoparathyroidism teaching tips.*)

Hyperthyroidism

Hyperthyroidism is a metabolic imbalance that results from excessive thyroid hormone. The most common form of hyperthyroidism is Graves' disease (thyrotoxicosis), which increases T_4 production, enlarges the thyroid gland (goiter), and causes multisystem changes. With treatment, most patients can lead normal lives. However, thyroid storm — an acute exacerbation of hyperthyroidism — is a medical emergency that may lead to heart failure. (See *Understanding forms of hyperthyroidism.*)

What causes it

Graves' disease is an autoimmune disease and is usually familial. Thyroid receptor antibodies occur in most patients with this disorder.

Pathophysiology

In Graves' disease, thyroid-stimulating antibodies bind to and stimulate the TSH receptors of the thyroid gland. The trigger for this autoimmune response is unclear. Graves' disease is also associated with the production of several autoantibodies formed because of a defect in suppressor T-lymphocyte function.

What to look for

Classic signs and symptoms of Graves' disease include:
- diffusely enlarged thyroid
- nervousness
- heat intolerance
- weight loss despite increased appetite
- sweating
- diarrhea
- tremor
- palpitations
- possibly exophthalmos.

Hypoparathyroidism teaching tips

- Instruct the patient with scaly skin to use creams to soften his skin.
- Tell him to keep his nails trimmed to prevent them from splitting.
- Advise him to follow a high-calcium, low-phosphorus diet, and tell him which foods are permitted.
- If he's on drug therapy, emphasize the importance of checking serum calcium levels at least three times per year. Instruct him to watch for signs of hypercalcemia and to keep medications away from light.

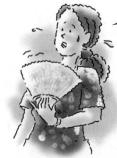

Heat intolerance and sweating are two classic signs of Graves' disease. Is it just me, or is it gravely hot in here?

Understanding forms of hyperthyroidism

In addition to Graves' disease, hyperthyroidism occurs in several other forms:

• *Toxic multinodular goiter* — a small, benign nodule in the thyroid gland that secretes thyroid hormone — is the second most common cause of hyperthyroidism. The cause of this type of goiter is unknown; incidence is highest among elderly patients. Clinical effects are essentially similar to those of Graves' disease, but they're milder and may have cardiovascular predominance. This condition doesn't induce ophthalmopathy, pretibial myxedema, or acropachy. Toxic multinodular goiter is confirmed by radioactive iodine (^{131}I) uptake and thyroid scan, which shows at least one hyperfunctioning nodule that may suppress the rest of the gland. Treatment includes ^{131}I therapy or surgery to remove the goiter after antithyroid drugs achieve a euthyroid state.

• *Thyrotoxicosis factitia* results from chronic ingestion of thyroid hormone for thyrotropin suppression in patients with thyroid carcinoma, or from thyroid hormone abuse by persons who are trying to lose weight.

• *Functioning metastatic thyroid carcinoma* is a rare disease that causes excess production of thyroid hormone.

• *Thyroid-stimulating hormone-secreting pituitary tumor* causes overproduction of thyroid hormone.

• *Subacute thyroiditis* is a virus-induced granulomatous inflammation of the thyroid, producing transient hyperthyroidism associated with fever, pain, pharyngitis, and tenderness in the thyroid gland.

• *Silent thyroiditis* is a self-limiting, transient form of hyperthyroidism with histologic thyroiditis but no inflammatory signs and symptoms.

Weathering the storm

In thyroid storm, these signs and symptoms can be accompanied by extreme irritability, hypertension, tachycardia, vomiting, temperature up to 106° F (41.1° C), delirium, and coma. Other signs and symptoms include:

• *cardiovascular system* — tachycardia; full, bounding pulse; wide pulse pressure; cardiomegaly; increased cardiac output and blood volume; a visible point of maximal impulse; paroxysmal supraventricular tachycardia and atrial fibrillation (found especially in elderly patients); occasionally, a systolic murmur at the left sternal border

• *CNS* — difficulty concentrating, excitability or nervousness, fine tremor, shaky handwriting, clumsiness, and mood swings ranging from occasional outbursts to overt psychosis

• *eyes* — exophthalmos; occasional inflammation of conjunctivae, corneas, or eye muscles; diplopia; increased tearing; lid lag; lid retraction

• *GI* — increased appetite but occasional anorexia, especially in elderly patients; increased defecation; soft stools or, with severe disease, diarrhea; liver enlargement

• *musculoskeletal system* — weakness, fatigue, and proximal muscle atrophy; periodic paralysis, especially in Asian and Latino males; occasional acropachy (soft-tissue swelling), accompanied by underlying bone changes where new bone formation occurs

- *reproductive system* — in females, oligomenorrhea or amenorrhea, decreased fertility, higher incidence of spontaneous abortions; in males, gynecomastia
- *respiratory system* — dyspnea on exertion and, possibly, at rest
- *skin, hair, and nails* — smooth, warm, flushed paper-thin skin; pretibial myxedema (dermopathy), producing thickened skin, accentuated hair follicles, and raised red patches of skin that are itchy and sometimes painful, with occasional nodule formation; fine, soft hair; premature graying and increased hair loss in both sexes; friable nails and Plummer's nails (distal nail separated from the bed).

What tests tell you

- Radioimmunoassay test shows elevated T_4 levels.
- Thyroid scan reveals increased ^{131}I uptake.
- Immunometric assay shows suppressed sensitive TSH levels.
- Orbital sonography and CT scan show subclinical ophthalmopathy.

How it's treated

The primary forms of treatment for hyperthyroidism are antithyroid drugs, ^{131}I, beta-adrenergic blockers, sedation, and surgery. Appropriate treatment depends on the size of the goiter, the causes, the patient's age and parity, and how long surgery (if planned) will be delayed. Treatment includes:
- Antithyroid drug therapy with propylthiouracil (PTU) and methimazole blocks thyroid hormone synthesis. It's used for pregnant women and patients who refuse surgery or ^{131}I treatment.
- Another major form of therapy for hyperthyroidism is a single oral dose of ^{131}I. After ablative treatment with ^{131}I or surgery, patients require regular, frequent medical supervision for the rest of their lives. They usually develop hypothyroidism, sometimes several years after treatment.

Rein in those hormones

- Partial thyroidectomy is indicated for the patient with a very large goiter, whose hyperthyroidism has repeatedly relapsed after drug therapy. Subtotal thyroidectomy removes part of the thyroid gland, decreasing its size and capacity for hormone production and storage.
- Before surgery, the patient may receive iodides (Lugol's solution or saturated solution of potassium iodide), antithyroid drugs, or high doses of propranolol, a beta-adrenergic blocker, to help prevent thyroid storm. If euthyroidism isn't achieved, surgery is delayed and the patient receives propranolol to decrease systemic effects (such as cardiac arrhythmias) caused by hyperthyroidism.
- During pregnancy, PTU is the preferred therapy. In pregnant patients, antithyroid medication should be limited to the minimum

Memory jogger

Grave's disease—the most common form of hyperthyroidism—causes a collection of classic signs and symptoms. You'll take big strides toward remembering them all when you're **STEPN' WIDE:**

Sweating

Tremor

Enlarged thyroid (diffusely enlarged)

Palpitations

Nervousness

Weight loss (despite increased appetite)

Intolerance to heat

Diarrhea

Exophthalmos (possible).

dosage required to keep maternal thyroid function testing at high-normal or slightly elevated levels. About 1% of infants born to mothers receiving antithyroid medication have hypothyroidism.

Steroid injections

• Therapy for hyperthyroid ophthalmopathy includes local applications of topical medications but may also require high doses of corticosteroids given systemically or, in severe cases, injected into the retrobulbar area.

• A patient with severe exophthalmos that causes pressure on the optic nerve may require surgical decompression to lessen pressure on the orbital contents.

• Treatment for thyroid storm includes an antithyroid drug such as PTU, I.V. propranolol to block sympathetic effects, a corticosteroid to replace depleted cortisol levels, and an iodide to block release of thyroid hormone. Supportive measures include nutrients, vitamins, fluid administration, and sedation, as necessary.

What to do

• Provide vigilant care to prevent acute exacerbations and complications:
– Record vital signs and weight.
– Monitor serum electrolyte levels and check periodically for hyperglycemia and glycosuria.
– Carefully monitor cardiac function.
– Check LOC and urine output.

• If the patient is in her first trimester of pregnancy, report signs and symptoms of spontaneous abortion (spotting and occasional mild cramps) to the doctor immediately.

• Remember, extreme nervousness may produce bizarre behavior. Reassure the patient and his family that such behavior subsides with treatment. Provide sedatives as necessary.

• To promote weight gain, provide a high-protein, high-calorie diet, with six meals per day and vitamin supplements. Suggest a low-sodium diet for the patient with edema.

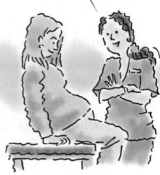

Antithyroid drug therapy with PTU and methimazole to block thyroid hormone synthesis is used for pregnant patients with hyperthyroidism.

Storm watch

• Watch for signs of thyroid storm. Check intake and output carefully to ensure adequate hydration and fluid balance. Closely monitor blood pressure, cardiac rate and rhythm, and body temperature. If the patient has a high fever, reduce it with appropriate hypothermic measures (sponging, hypothermia blankets, and aceta-minophen); avoid aspirin because it raises T_4 levels. Maintain an I.V. line and give drugs, as ordered.

• If iodine is part of the treatment, mix it with water or juice to prevent GI distress, and administer it through a straw to prevent tooth discoloration.

• If the patient underwent thyroidectomy, provide meticulous postoperative care to prevent complications.

• Evaluate the patient. He should maintain adequate fluid volume and electrolyte balance, normal cardiac function, normal body temperature, and adequate weight (preferably, he'll gain weight); his eyes should be as comfortable as possible and free from corneal damage; thyroid storm should be prevented. He will understand the need for regular medical follow-up and will schedule return appointments. If he takes an antithyroid drug or is on ^{131}I therapy, he'll know which signs and symptoms to report to his practitioner and will have a sheet that lists them. (See *Hyperthyroidism teaching tips*.)

Hypothyroidism

A state of low serum thyroid hormone levels or cellular resistance to thyroid hormone, hypothyroidism results from hypothalamic, pituitary, or thyroid insufficiency. Hypothyroidism is most prevalent in women and can progress to life-threatening myxedema coma — usually precipitated by infection, exposure to cold, or sedatives.

What causes it

Hypothyroidism may result from:
• thyroidectomy
• radiation therapy
• chronic autoimmune thyroiditis (Hashimoto's disease)
• inflammatory conditions, such as amyloidosis and sarcoidosis
• pituitary failure to produce TSH
• hypothalamic failure to produce thyrotropin-releasing hormone (TRH)
• inborn errors of thyroid hormone synthesis
• inability to synthesize thyroid hormone because of iodine deficiency (usually dietary)
• use of antithyroid medications such as PTU.

Pathophysiology

In primary hypothyroidism, a decrease in thyroid hormone production is a result of the loss of thyroid tissue. This results in an increased secretion of TSH that leads to a goiter. In secondary hypothyroidism, typically the pituitary fails to synthesize or

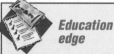

Education edge

Hyperthyroidism teaching tips

• If the patient has exophthalmos or another ophthalmopathy, suggest sunglasses or eye patches to protect his eyes from light. Moisten the conjunctivae often with artificial tears. Warn the patient with severe lid retraction to avoid sudden physical movements that might cause the lid to slip behind the eyeball. Elevate the head of the bed to reduce periorbital edema.

• Stress the importance of regular medical follow-up after discharge because hypothyroidism may develop from 2 to 4 weeks postoperatively. Drug therapy and ^{131}I therapy require careful monitoring and comprehensive patient teaching.

• If the patient is pregnant, tell her to watch closely during the 1st trimester for signs and symptoms of spontaneous abortion (spotting, occasional mild cramps) and to report such signs to the practitioner immediately.

What do I do?

Managing myxedema coma

Myxedema coma is a medical emergency that commonly has a fatal outcome. Progression is usually gradual, but when stress aggravates severe or prolonged hypothyroidism, coma may develop abruptly. Examples of severe stress are infection, exposure to cold, and trauma. Other precipitating factors include thyroid medication withdrawal and the use of sedatives, narcotics, or anesthetics.

Patients in myxedema coma have significantly depressed respirations, so their partial pressure of carbon dioxide in arterial blood may increase. Decreased cardiac output and worsening cerebral hypoxia may also occur. The patient is stuporous and hypothermic, and her vital signs reflect bradycardia and hypotension.

Lifesaving interventions

If the patient becomes comatose, begin these interventions as soon as possible:
- Maintain airway patency with ventilatory support if necessary.
- Maintain circulation through I.V. fluid replacement.
- Provide continuous electrocardiogram monitoring.

- Monitor arterial blood gas measurements to detect hypoxia and metabolic acidosis.
- Warm the patient by wrapping her in blankets. Don't use a warming blanket because it might increase peripheral vasodilation, causing shock.
- Monitor the patient's body temperature until stable with a low-reading thermometer.
- Replace thyroid hormone by administering large I.V. levothyroxine doses as ordered. Monitor vital signs because rapid correction of hypothyroidism can cause adverse cardiac effects.
- Monitor intake and output and daily weight. With treatment, urine output should increase and body weight should decrease; if not, report this to the doctor.
- Replace fluids and other substances such as glucose. Monitor serum electrolyte levels.
- Administer corticosteroids as ordered.
- Check for possible sources of infection, such as blood, sputum, or urine, which may have precipitated coma. Treat infections or other underlying illnesses as ordered.

secrete adequate amounts of TSH, or target tissues fail to respond to normal blood levels of thyroid hormone. Either type may progress to myxedema, which is clinically more severe and considered a medical emergency. (See *Managing myxedema coma.*)

What to look for

Signs and symptoms of hypothyroidism include:
- weakness, fatigue
- forgetfulness
- cold intolerance
- unexplained weight gain
- constipation
- goiter
- slow speech
- decreasing mental stability
- cool, dry, coarse, flaky, inelastic skin

> Unexplained weight gain is one sign of hypothyroidism.

- puffy face, hands, and feet; periorbital edema
- dry, sparse hair
- thick, brittle nails.

    Other indications include a slow pulse rate, anorexia, abdominal distention, menorrhagia, decreased libido, infertility, ataxia, intention tremor, nystagmus, and delayed reflex relaxation time (especially in the Achilles tendon).

    Clinical effects of myxedema coma include progressive stupor, hypoventilation, hypoglycemia, hyponatremia, hypotension, and hypothermia.

What tests tell you

- Radioimmunoassay tests showing low T_3 and T_4 levels indicate hypothyroidism.
- The TSH level increases with primary hypothyroidism and decreases in secondary hypothyroidism. The TRH level is decreased in hypothalamic insufficiency.
- Serum cholesterol, carotene, alkaline phosphatase, and triglyceride levels are increased.
- In myxedema coma, laboratory tests may also show low serum sodium levels and decreased pH and increased partial pressure of carbon dioxide in arterial blood, indicating respiratory acidosis.

How it's treated

Therapy for hypothyroidism consists of gradual thyroid replacement with levothyroxine (Synthroid). Effective treatment of myxedema coma supports vital functions while restoring euthyroidism. To support blood pressure and pulse rate, the patient receives I.V. levothyroxine, plus hydrocortisone in cases of pituitary or adrenal insufficiency. Hypoventilation requires oxygenation and vigorous respiratory support. Other supportive measures include careful fluid replacement and antimicrobial medications for infection.

What to do

- Provide a high-bulk, low-calorie diet and encourage activity.
- Administer cathartics and stool softeners as needed.
- After thyroid replacement therapy begins, watch for signs of hyperthyroidism, such as restlessness, sweating, and excessive weight loss.
- Advise the patient how to obtain medical identification jewelry.
- Evaluate the patient. She should have a normal bowel elimination pattern and adequate cardiac function, know which cardiac

symptoms to report, and understand the need for lifelong thyroid replacement and regular medical care to monitor replacement therapy. She should have medical identification jewelry and a wallet identification card. She should show signs of adequate cardiac output and function, including normal blood pressure and pulse rate, adequate urine output, intact skin, adequate fluid volume and electrolyte balance, and adequate gas exchange. (See *Hypothyroidism teaching tips.*)

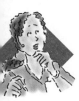

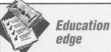

Quick quiz

1. After ^{131}I administration, urine and saliva will be slightly radioactive for how many hours?
   A. Fewer than 2 hours
   B. 6 to 8 hours
   C. 24 hours
   D. 36 hours

Answer: C. Urine and saliva will be slightly radioactive for 24 hours and vomitus will be highly radioactive for 6 to 8 hours after therapy.

2. Which statement should be stressed in home care instructions after adrenalectomy?
   A. The patient can stop taking his medication when his physical appearance improves.
   B. The patient should take his steroids on an empty stomach.
   C. The patient should take prescribed medications as directed.
   D. The patient won't need any medication.

Answer: C. The patient should take his prescribed medication as directed. Sudden withdrawal of steroids can precipitate adrenal crisis.

3. An adrenal crisis is characterized by all of these signs and symtoms except:
   A. weakness and fatigue.
   B. nausea and vomiting.
   C. hypotension.
   D. sodium and fluid retention.

Answer: D. Sodium and fluid retention are characteristics of Cushing's syndrome; adrenal crisis causes decreased sodium levels and hypotension.

4. Which statement about diabetes mellitus is false?
A. Type 2 diabetes commonly occurs in adults after age 40.
B. Type 1 diabetes usually occurs before age 30.
C. Type 1 diabetes is treated primarily with exercise and meal planning.
D. An increasing number of adolescents are being diagnosed with type 2 diabetes.

Answer: C. Type 1 diabetes is treated with insulin and dietary management.

Scoring

☆☆☆ If you answered all four questions correctly, zowee! You've got all the energy you need to master endocrine disorders.

☆☆ If you answered three questions correctly, yahoo! Your receptors are doing a great job of triggering correct endocrine information.

☆ If you answered fewer than three questions correctly, don't stress! With a quick infusion of endocrine information, you'll achieve a regular release of correct answers.

13

Renal and urologic disorders

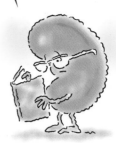

Just the facts

In this chapter, you'll learn:

♦ the role of the renal and urinary systems and their effects on other body systems

♦ techniques for assessing renal and urologic function

♦ causes, signs and symptoms, diagnostic tests, and nursing interventions for common renal and urologic disorders.

A look at renal and urologic disorders

The renal and urinary systems retain useful materials and excrete foreign or excessive materials and wastes. Through these basic functions, they profoundly affect other body systems and the patient's overall health. Renal and urologic disorders can affect fluid and electrolyte balance and other important body functions.

Anatomy and physiology

> Ooh, I'm highly vascular. That sounds impressive.

The renal system consists of two kidneys, two ureters, one bladder, and one urethra. Working together, these structures remove wastes from the body, regulate acid-base balance by retaining or excreting hydrogen ions, and regulate fluid and electrolyte balance. (See *Renal system*, page 572.)

The kidneys

The kidneys are bean-shaped and highly vascular. Located retroperitoneally on either side of the vertebral column, they lie between the 12th thoracic and 3rd lumbar vertebrae. Abdominal contents, muscles attached to the vertebral column, and a

A closer look

Renal system

As this frontal view suggests, the kidneys constitute the major portion of the renal system. These bean-shaped organs lie near and on either side of the spine at the small of the back, with the left kidney positioned slightly higher than the right. The *adrenal glands,* perched atop the kidneys, influence blood pressure as well as sodium and water retention by the kidneys.

Filtration station

The kidneys receive blood from the *renal arteries,* which branch off the *abdominal aorta.* After passing through a complicated network of smaller blood vessels and nephrons, the filtered blood recirculates through the *renal veins,* which empty into the *inferior vena cava.*

Excrete to complete

The kidneys excrete waste products that the nephrons remove from the blood, along with other fluids that constitute the formed urine. Urine passes, by peristalsis, through the *ureters* to the *urinary bladder.* As the bladder fills, nerves in the bladder wall relax the *sphincter* (an action known as the *micturition reflex*); then a voluntary stimulus occurs, and the urine passes into the urethra and is expelled from the body.

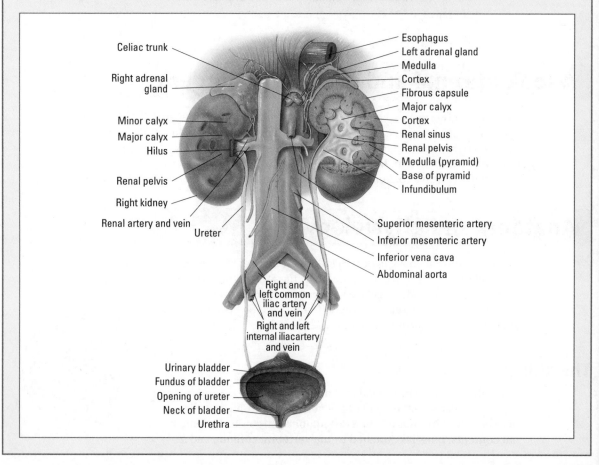

perirenal fat layer protect them. The kidneys consist of the renal cortex, central renal medulla, internal calyces, and renal pelvis as well as the nephron, which serves as the kidney's functional unit. (See *A close look at the kidney*, page 574.)

Down and out

The structures of the renal system, extending downward from the kidneys, include:

• *ureters* — tubes that act as ducts channeling urine to the bladder via peristaltic waves that occur about one to five times per minute; they measure about 10″ to 12″ (25.5 to 30.5 cm) in adults and have a diameter varying from 2 to 8 mm, with the narrowest portion being at the ureteropelvic junction

• *urinary bladder* — a hollow, spherical, muscular organ in the pelvis that serves to store urine delivered by the ureters; bladder capacity ranges from 500 to 600 ml in a normal adult (less in children and elderly people)

• *urethra* — a small duct that channels urine outside the body from the bladder; it has an exterior opening known as the *urinary (urethral) meatus*; in the female, the urethra ranges from 1″ to 2″ (2.5 to 5 cm) long, with the urethral meatus located anterior to the vaginal opening; in the male, the urethra is about 8″ (20 cm) long, with the urethral meatus located at the end of the glans penis; the male urethra serves as a passageway for semen as well as urine.

Urine formation

The kidneys collect and eliminate wastes from the body in a three-step process:

In *glomerular filtration*, the kidney's blood vessels, or glomeruli, filter the blood that flows through them. (See *Understanding GFR*, page 575.)

During *tubular reabsorption*, the minute canals (tubules) that make up the kidney reabsorb filtered fluid.

In *tubular secretion*, the tubules release the filtered substance.

Results may vary

Varying with fluid intake and climate, total daily urine output averages 720 to 2,400 ml. For example, after a patient drinks a large volume of fluid, urine output increases as the body rapidly excretes excess water. If a patient restricts water intake or has an excessive intake of such solutes as sodium, urine output declines as the body retains water to maintain normal fluid concentration.

Total daily urine output varies with fluid intake and climate. I could use a nice, cool drink right now.

A close look at the kidney

Illustrated here is a kidney along with an enlargement of a nephron, the kidney's functional unit. Major structures of the kidney include:
- medulla — inner portion of the kidney, made up of renal pyramids and tubular structures
- renal artery — supplies blood to the kidney
- renal pyramid — channels output to renal pelvis for excretion
- renal calyx — channels formed urine from the renal pyramids to the renal pelvis
- renal vein — about 99% of filtered blood is circulated through the renal vein back to the general circulation; the remaining 1%, which contains waste products, undergoes further processing in the kidney
- renal pelvis — after blood that contains waste products is processed in the kidney, formed urine is channeled to the renal pelvis
- ureter — tube that terminates in the urinary bladder; urine then enters the urethra for excretion
- cortex — outer layer of the kidney.

Note the nephron

The nephron is the functional and structural unit of the kidney. Each kidney contains about 1 million nephrons. The nephron's two main activities are selective reabsorption and secretion of ions and mechanical filtration of fluids, wastes, electrolytes, and acids and bases.

Components of the nephron include:
- glomerulus — a network of twisted capillaries that acts as a filter for the passage of protein-free and red blood cell–free filtrate to the proximal convoluted tubules
- Bowman's capsule — contains the glomerulus and acts as a filter for urine
- proximal convoluted tubule — site of reabsorption of glucose, amino acids, metabolites, and electrolytes from filtrate; reabsorbed substances return to circulation
- loop of Henle — a U-shaped nephron tubule located in the medulla and extending from the proximal convoluted tubule to the distal convoluted tubule, site for further concentration of filtrate through reabsorption
- distal convoluted tubule — site from which filtrate enters the collecting tubule
- collecting tubule — releases urine.

Kidney

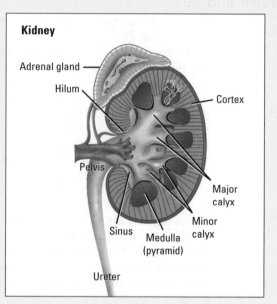

Nephron

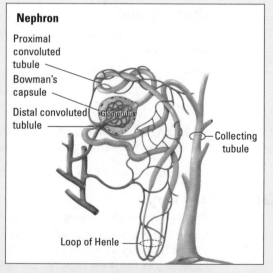

Understanding GFR

Glomerular filtration rate (GFR) is the rate at which the glomeruli filter blood. The normal GFR is 90 to 120 ml/minute. GFR depends on:
- permeability of capillary walls
- vascular pressure
- filtration pressure.

GFR and clearance

Clearance is the complete removal of a substance from the blood. The most accurate measure of glomerular filtration is creatinine clearance because creatinine is filtered by the glomeruli but not reabsorbed by the tubules.

Equal to, greater than, or less than

Here's more about how the GFR affects clearance measurements for a substance in the blood:
- If the tubules neither reabsorb nor secrete the substance — as happens with creatinine — clearance equals the GFR.
- If the tubules reabsorb the substance, clearance is less than the GFR.
- If the tubules secrete the substance, clearance exceeds the GFR.
- If the tubules reabsorb and secrete the substance, clearance may be equal to, greater than, or less than the GFR.

Hormones and the kidneys

Two hormones help regulate tubular reabsorption and secretion:

Antidiuretic hormone (ADH), which is produced by the pituitary gland, acts in the distal tubule and collecting ducts to increase water reabsorption and urine concentration. ADH deficiency decreases water reabsorption, causing dilute urine.

Aldosterone, which is produced by the adrenal gland, affects tubular reabsorption by regulating sodium retention and helping control potassium secretion by tubular epithelial cells.

Other hormonal functions of the kidneys include:
- *secretion of the hormone erythropoietin.* In response to low arterial oxygen tension, the kidneys produce erythropoietin, which travels to the bone marrow and stimulates red blood cell (RBC) production.
- *regulation of calcium and phosphorus balance.* To help regulate calcium and phosphorus balance, the kidneys filter and reabsorb about one-half of unbound serum calcium and activate vitamin D_3, a compound that promotes intestinal calcium absorption and regulates phosphate excretion.

Renin's role

The kidneys help regulate blood pressure by producing and secreting the enzyme renin in response to an actual or perceived decline in extracellular fluid volume. Renin, in turn, forms angiotensin I, which is converted to the more potent angiotensin II.

Potassium regulation

The distal tubules of the kidneys regulate potassium excretion. Responding to an elevated serum potassium level, the adrenal cortex increases aldosterone secretion. Aldosterone regulates potassium secretion into distal tubules so it can be eliminated from the body. If the body fails to produce enough aldosterone, potassium is reabsorbed and serum potassium levels increase.

Assessment

Assessing the urinary system may uncover clues to problems in any body system.

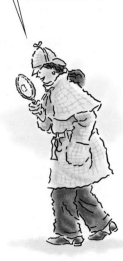

Assessing the urinary system may uncover clues to problems in any body system.

History

Begin your assessment with a thorough history, including current and past health, family history, and lifestyle patterns.

Current health status

To determine the patient's chief complaint, ask "What made you seek medical help?" Document the reason for seeking care in the patient's own words. When a patient has a renal disorder, expect these common complaints:
- urinary frequency and urgency
- pain on urination
- difficulty urinating
- flank pain.

Previous health status

Explore all of the patient's previous major illnesses, recurrent minor illnesses, accidents or injuries, surgical procedures, and allergies. Ask about a history of urologic-related disorders such as hypertension.

Other questions to ask include:
- Have you ever had a urinary infection?
- Are you taking herbal medications or prescription, over-the-counter, or recreational drugs?
- Do you have pain or burning on urination?
- Is initiating urination difficult?
- What color is your urine?

- Are you allergic to drugs, foods, or other products? If yes, describe the reaction you experienced.
- Have you ever had a sexually transmitted disease (STD)?

Family history

For clues to risk factors, ask if blood relatives have ever been treated for renal or cardiovascular disorders, diabetes, cancer, or other chronic illness.

Lifestyle patterns

Investigate psychosocial factors that may affect the way the patient deals with his condition. Marital problems, unstable living conditions, job insecurity, and other stresses can strongly affect how he feels.

Self-reflection

Also, find out how the patient views himself. Try to determine what concerns he has about his condition. For example, does he fear that the disease or therapy, such as hemodialysis, will affect his quality of life? If he can express his fears and concerns, you can develop appropriate nursing interventions more easily.

> Stressors such as marital problems and job insecurity can affect how the patient deals with his condition.

Physical examination

Begin the physical examination by documenting baseline vital signs and weighing the patient. Ask the patient to urinate into a specimen cup. Assess the specimen for color, odor, and clarity. Because the renal system affects many body functions, a thorough assessment includes examination of multiple related body systems using inspection, auscultation, percussion, and palpation techniques.

Inspection

Renal system inspection includes examination of the abdomen and urethral meatus.

Abdomen

Help the patient assume a supine position with his arms relaxed at his sides. Expose the patient's abdomen from the xiphoid process to the symphysis pubis, and inspect the abdomen for gross enlargements or fullness by comparing the left and right sides, noting asymmetrical areas. In a normal adult, the abdomen is smooth, flat or scaphoid (concave), and symmetrical. Ask about scars, lesions, bruises, or discolorations found on abdominal skin.

Urethral meatus

Help the patient feel more at ease during your inspection by examining the urethral meatus last and by explaining beforehand how you'll assess this area. Be sure to wear gloves.

Auscultation

Auscultate the renal arteries in the left and right upper abdominal quadrants by pressing the stethoscope bell lightly against the abdomen and instructing the patient to exhale deeply. Begin auscultating at the midline and work to the left. Then return to the midline and work to the right. Systolic bruits (whooshing sounds) or other unusual sounds are potentially significant abnormalities.

Percussion

After auscultating the renal arteries, percuss the patient's kidneys to detect any tenderness or pain and percuss the bladder to evaluate its position and contents. (See *Percussing the urinary organs*.)

Palpation

Palpation of the kidneys and bladder is next. Through palpation, you can detect any lumps, masses, or tenderness. To achieve optimal results, ask the patient to relax his abdomen by taking deep breaths through his mouth. (See *Palpating the urinary organs*, page 580.)

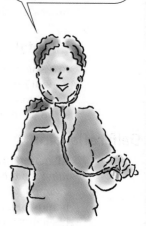

Auscultate the renal arteries by pressing the bell lightly against the abdomen and telling the patient to exhale deeply.

Diagnostic tests

Advanced technology — including improved computer processing and imaging techniques — allows noninvasive assessment of renal and urologic problems that were previously detectable only by invasive techniques. These diagnostic tests can help evaluate the patient's renal and urologic status.

Blood studies

When considered with urinalysis findings, blood studies help the doctor diagnose genitourinary disease and evaluate kidney function. Blood studies include blood urea nitrogen (BUN) and serum creatinine.

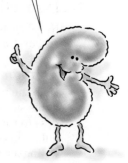

When considered with urinalysis findings, blood studies evaluate my function.

Percussing the urinary organs

Percuss the kidneys and bladder using the techniques described below.

Kidney percussion

With the patient upright, percuss each costovertebral angle (the angle over each kidney whose borders are formed by the lateral and downward curve of the lowest rib and the vertebral column). To perform mediate percussion, place your left palm over the costovertebral angle and gently strike it with your right fist. To perform immediate percussion, gently strike your fist over each costovertebral angle. Usually, the patient will feel a thudding sensation or pressure during percussion.

Bladder percussion

Using mediate percussion, percuss the area over the bladder, beginning 2″ (5 cm) above the symphysis pubis. To detect differences in sound, percuss toward the bladder's base. Percussion usually produces a tympanic sound. (Over a urine-filled bladder, it produces a dull sound.)

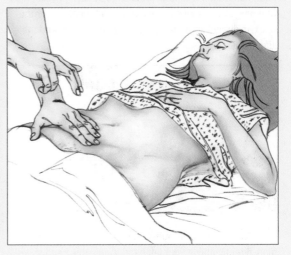

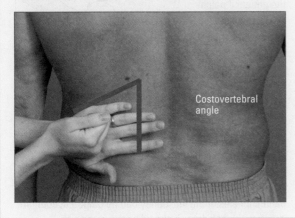

Costovertebral angle

BUN

Urea, the chief end product of protein metabolism, constitutes 40% to 50% of the blood's nonprotein nitrogen. It's formed from ammonia in the liver, filtered by the glomeruli, reabsorbed (to a limited degree) in the tubules, and finally excreted. Insufficient urea excretion elevates the BUN level.

Normal BUN levels range from 7 to 20 mg/dl for adults. For the most accurate interpretation of test results, examine BUN levels in conjunction with serum creatinine levels and in light of the patient's underlying condition.

Nursing considerations

• Tell the patient that the test requires a blood sample.
• Check the patient's medication history for drugs that may influence BUN levels. (Chloramphenicol may depress levels; aminoglycosides and amphotericin B can elevate levels.)

Palpating the urinary organs

In a normal adult, the kidneys usually aren't palpable because they're located deep within the abdomen. However, they may be palpable in a thin patient or in one with reduced abdominal muscle mass, and the right kidney, slightly lower than the left, may be easier to palpate altogether. Keep in mind that both kidneys descend with deep inhalation. An adult's bladder may not be palpable either. However, if it's palpable, it usually feels firm and relatively smooth. When palpating urinary organs, use bimanual palpation, beginning on the patient's right side and proceeding as follows.

Kidney palpation

Help the patient to a supine position, and expose the abdomen from the xiphoid process to the symphysis pubis. Standing at the right side, place your left hand under the back, midway between the lower costal margin and the iliac crest.

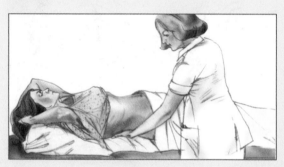

Next, place your right hand on the patient's abdomen, directly above your left hand. Angle this hand slightly toward the costal margin. To palpate the right lower edge of the right kidney, press your right fingertips about 1¹/₂″ (4 cm) above the right iliac crest at the midinguinal line; press your left fingertips upward into the right costovertebral angle.

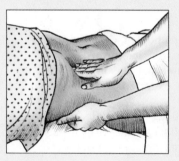

Instruct the patient to inhale deeply so that the lower portion of the right kidney can move down between your hands. If it does, note its shape and size. Usually, it feels smooth, solid, and firm, yet elastic. Ask the patient if palpation causes tenderness. (*Note:* Avoid using excessive pressure to palpate the kidney because this may cause intense pain.)

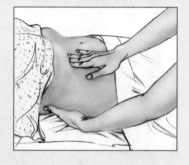

To assess the left kidney, move to the patient's left side, and position your hands as described above, but with this change: Place your right hand 2″ (5 cm) above the left iliac crest. Then apply pressure with both hands as the patient inhales. If the left kidney can be palpated, compare it with the right kidney; it should be the same size.

Bladder palpation

Before palpating the bladder, make sure the patient has voided. Then locate the edge of the bladder by pressing deeply in the midline 1″ to 2″ (2.5 to 5 cm) above the symphysis pubis. As the bladder is palpated, note its size and location, and check for lumps, masses, and tenderness. The bladder normally feels firm and relatively smooth. During deep palpation, the patient may report the urge to urinate — a normal response.

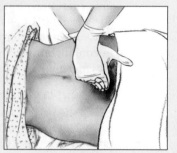

- If a hematoma develops at the venipuncture site, apply warm soaks.

Serum creatinine

Creatinine, another nitrogenous waste, results from muscle metabolism of creatine. Normal serum creatinine values for adult males range from 0.6 to 1.2 mg/dl; for adult females, 0.4 to 1 mg/dl. Diet and fluid intake don't affect serum creatinine levels, but muscle mass does.

This test measures renal damage more reliably than BUN level measurements because severe, persistent renal impairment is virtually the only reason that creatinine levels rise significantly. Creatinine levels greater than 1.5 mg/dl indicate 66% or greater loss of renal function; levels greater than 2 mg/dl indicate renal insufficiency.

Nursing considerations

- Tell the patient that the test requires a blood sample.
- Check the patient's medication history for drugs that may influence serum creatinine levels (ascorbic acid, barbiturates, and diuretics may raise serum creatinine levels).
- If a hematoma develops at the venipuncture site, apply warm soaks.

Clearance tests

Clearance tests for filtration, reabsorption, and secretion permit a precise evaluation of renal function. These tests measure the volume of plasma that can be cleared of a substance (such as creatinine) per unit of time, thus helping evaluate urine-forming mechanisms. They also measure renal blood flow, which renal disease may reduce.

Creatinine clearance

The creatinine clearance test, commonly used to assess glomerular filtration rate (GFR), determines how efficiently the kidneys clear creatinine from the blood. Normal values depend on the patient's age.

Nursing considerations

- Tell the patient the test requires a timed urine specimen and at least one blood sample.

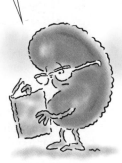

If I don't study hard for these clearance tests, I'll never pass!

- A high-protein diet before the test and strenuous physical exercise during the collection period may increase creatinine excretion. Inform the patient that he shouldn't eat an excessive amount of meat before the test and should avoid strenuous physical exercise during the collection period.

Urea clearance

The urea clearance test measures urine levels of urea, the chief end product of protein metabolism and the chief nitrogenous component of urine. The urea clearance rate usually ranges from 64 to 100 ml/minute at a urine flow rate of 2 ml/minute or more. At flow rates of less than 2 ml/minute, the normal range decreases to 40 to 70 ml/minute.

Nursing considerations
- Tell the patient that the test requires two timed urine specimens and one blood sample.
- Instruct him to fast after midnight before the test and to abstain from exercise before and during the test.

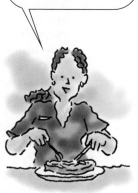

Before a creatinine clearance test, the patient shouldn't eat an excessive amount of meat.

Radiologic and imaging studies

Radiologic and imaging studies help screen for renal and urologic abnormalities. These studies include computed tomography (CT) scan, excretory urography, kidney-ureter-bladder (KUB) radiography, magnetic resonance imaging (MRI), radionuclide renal scans, renal angiography, ultrasonography, and voiding cystourethrography.

CT scan

In a renal CT scan, the image's density reflects the amount of radiation absorbed by renal tissue, thus permitting identification of masses and other lesions.

Nursing considerations
- If contrast enhancement isn't scheduled, inform the patient that he need not restrict food or fluids. If a contrast medium will be used, instruct him to fast for 4 hours before the test.
- If contrast enhancement is ordered, check the patient's history for an allergy to iodine, shellfish, or previous contrast media.
- Inform the patient that he'll be positioned on an X-ray table and that a scanner will take films of his kidneys. Warn him that he may hear loud, clacking sounds as the scanner rotates around his body.

• Just before the procedure, instruct the patient to put on a hospital gown and to remove any metallic objects that could interfere with the scan.

Excretory urography

After I.V. administration of a contrast medium, this common procedure (also known as *I.V. pyelography*) allows visualization of the renal parenchyma, calyces, pelvises, ureters, bladder and, in some cases, the urethra.

Picture perfect

In the 1st minute after injection (the nephrographic stage), the contrast medium delineates the size and shape of the kidneys. After 3 to 5 minutes (the pyelographic stage), the contrast medium moves into the calyces and pelvises, allowing visualization of cysts, tumors, and other obstructions.

Nursing considerations
• Check the patient's history for hypersensitivity to iodine, iodine-containing foods, or contrast media containing iodine.
• Check the patient's laboratory results for elevated BUN and creatinine levels. Excretory urography is contraindicated in patients with renal insufficiency.
• Ensure that the patient is well hydrated, and instruct him to fast for 8 hours before the test.
• Inform the patient that he may experience a transient burning sensation and metallic taste when the contrast medium is injected.

KUB radiography

KUB radiography is the main radiologic study used for the urinary system. The KUB study, consisting of plain, contrast-free X-rays, shows kidney size, position, and structure as well as calculi and other lesions. Before performing a renal biopsy, the doctor may use this test to determine kidney placement. For diagnostic purposes, however, the KUB study provides limited information.

Nursing considerations
• Inform the patient that he need not restrict food or fluids before the test.
• No specific posttest care is necessary.

MRI

MRI provides tomographic images that reflect the differing hydrogen densities of body tissues. Physical, chemical, and cellular

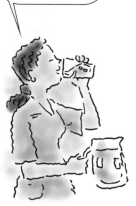

Ensure that the patient is well hydrated before excretory urography.

microenvironments modify these densities, as do the fluid characteristics of tissues. MRI can provide precise images of anatomic detail and important biochemical information about the tissue examined and can efficiently visualize and stage kidney, bladder, and prostate tumors.

Nursing considerations

• Before the patient enters the MRI chamber, make sure he has removed all metal objects, such as earrings, watch, necklace, bracelets, and rings. Patients with internal metal objects, such as pacemakers or aneurysm clips, can't undergo MRI testing.
• If you're accompanying the patient, be sure to remove metal objects from your pockets, such as scissors, forceps, a penlight, metal pens, and your credit cards (the magnetic field will erase the numerical information in the code strips).
• Tell the patient that he must remain still throughout the test, which takes about 45 minutes. If the patient complains of claustrophobia, reassure him and provide emotional support.

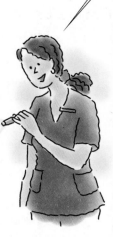

If you're accompanying the patient for an MRI, be sure to remove metal objects from your pockets, such as scissors, forceps, and penlights.

Radionuclide renal scan

A radionuclide renal scan, which may be substituted for excretory urography in patients who are hypersensitive to contrast media, involves I.V. injection of a radionuclide, followed by scintiphotography. Observation of the uptake concentration and radionuclide transit during the procedure allows assessment of renal blood flow, nephron and collecting system function, and renal structure.

Nursing considerations

• Inform the patient that he'll receive an injection of a radionuclide and may experience transient flushing and nausea. Emphasize that he'll receive only a small amount of radionuclide, which is usually excreted within 24 hours.
• After the test, instruct the patient to flush the toilet immediately every time he urinates for 24 hours as a radiation precaution.

Renal angiography

Renal angiography permits radiographic examination of the renal vasculature and parenchyma after arterial injection of a contrast medium. Renal venography (angiography of the veins) may be performed to detect renal vein thrombosis and venous extension of renal cell carcinoma.

Nursing considerations

• Check the patient's history for hypersensitivity to iodine-based contrast media or iodine-containing foods such as shellfish.

- Instruct him to fast for 8 hours before the test and drink extra fluids the day before and after the test to maintain adequate hydration (or start an I.V. line if needed).
- Keep the patient flat in bed after the procedure; keep the leg on the affected side straight for at least 6 hours or as ordered.

Ultrasonography

Ultrasonography uses high-frequency sound waves to reveal internal structures. The pulse-echo transmission technique of this test determines the kidney's size, shape, and position. It also reveals internal structures and perirenal tissue and helps the practitioner diagnose complications after kidney transplantation. Doppler ultrasonography allows the evaluation of the speed, direction, and patterns of blood flow.

Nursing considerations
- Tell the patient that he'll either be prone or supine during the test.
- Explain that a technician will apply a water-based conductive gel on the patient's skin and then press a probe or transducer against the skin and move it across the area being tested.

Voiding cystourethrography

In voiding cystourethrography, a urinary catheter inserted into the bladder allows instillation of a contrast medium by gentle syringe pressure or gravity. Fluoroscopic films or overhead radiographs demonstrate bladder filling and then show excretion of the contrast medium as the patient voids.

Nursing considerations
- Check the patient's history for hypersensitivity to contrast media or iodine-containing foods such as shellfish.
- Inform the patient that a catheter will be inserted into his bladder and a contrast medium will be instilled through the catheter. Tell him he may experience a feeling of fullness and an urge to void when the contrast is instilled.
- After the test, instruct the patient to drink lots of fluids to reduce burning on urination and to flush out any residual contrast dye.
- Monitor for chills and fever related to extravasation of contrast material or urinary sepsis.

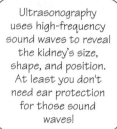

Ultrasonography uses high-frequency sound waves to reveal the kidney's size, shape, and position. At least you don't need ear protection for those sound waves!

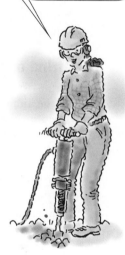

Urine studies

Urine studies, such as urinalysis and urine osmolality, can indicate urinary tract infection (UTI) and other disorders.

Urinalysis

Performed on a urine specimen of at least 10 ml, urinalysis can indicate urinary or systemic disorders, warranting further investigation.

Nursing considerations
• Collect a random urine specimen, preferably the first-voided morning specimen. Send the specimen to the laboratory immediately.
• Refrigerate the specimen if analysis will be delayed longer than 1 hour.

Urine osmolality

Urine osmolality evaluates the diluting and concentrating ability of the kidneys. It may aid in the differential diagnosis of polyuria, oliguria, or syndrome of inappropriate antidiuretic hormone secretion. To gather more information about the patient's renal function, compare the urine specific gravity with urine osmolality.

Nursing considerations
• Obtain a random urine specimen.
• Keep in mind that urine osmolality typically ranges from 50 to 1,400 mOsm/kg, with the average being 300 to 800 mOsm/kg.

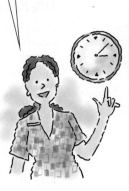

Refrigerate the urine specimen if analysis will be delayed longer than 1 hour.

Other tests

Further diagnostic tests can help evaluate urologic structure and function. These include cystometry, percutaneous renal biopsy, and uroflowmetry.

Cystometry

Used to help determine the cause of bladder dysfunction, cystometry assesses the bladder's neuromuscular function by measuring the efficiency of the detrusor muscle reflex, intravesicular pressure and capacity, and the bladder's reaction to thermal stimulation. Abnormal test results may indicate a lower urinary tract obstruction.

Nursing considerations
• Explain to the patient the different steps of the test and what will happen in each. Let him know that a urinary catheter will need to be inserted.

• Tell the patient that, if no more tests are needed, the catheter will be removed after the test. Warn him that he may experience transient burning or urinary frequency after the test but that a sitz bath may alleviate discomfort.

Percutaneous renal biopsy

Histologic examination can help differentiate glomerular from tubular renal disease, monitor the disorder's progress, and assess the effectiveness of therapy. It can also reveal a malignant tumor such as Wilms' tumor. Histologic studies can help the doctor diagnose disseminated lupus erythematosus, amyloid infiltration, acute and chronic glomerulonephritis, renal vein thrombosis, and pyelonephritis. (See *Assisting with percutaneous renal biopsy*.)

> Histologic examination can help differentiate glomerular from tubular renal disease. I feel ill just thinking about it.

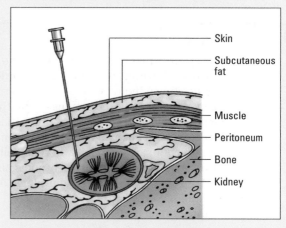

Assisting with percutaneous renal biopsy

To prepare a patient for percutaneous renal biopsy, position him on his abdomen. To stabilize his kidneys, place a sandbag beneath his abdomen as shown.

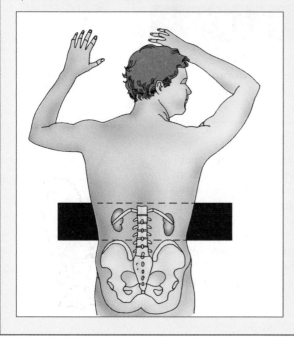

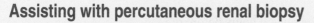

After administering a local anesthetic, the doctor instructs the patient to hold his breath and remain immobile. Then the doctor inserts a needle with the obturator between the patient's last rib and the iliac crest as shown below. After asking the patient to breathe deeply, the doctor removes the obturator and inserts cutting prongs, which gather blood and tissue samples. This test is commonly performed in the radiology department so that special radiographic procedures may be used to help guide the needle.

Skin

Subcutaneous fat

Muscle

Peritoneum

Bone

Kidney

Nursing considerations
• Instruct the patient to restrict food and fluids for 8 hours before the test. Inform him that he'll receive a mild sedative before the test to help him relax.
• After the test, tell him that pressure will be applied to the biopsy site to stop superficial bleeding and then a pressure dressing will be applied.
• Instruct him to lie flat on his back without moving for at least 12 hours to prevent bleeding.
• Tell him he should avoid strenuous activity for at least 2 weeks.

Uroflowmetry

Uroflowmetry measures the volume of urine expelled from the urethra in milliliters per second (urine flow rate) and determines the urine flow pattern. This test is performed to evaluate lower urinary tract function and demonstrate bladder outlet obstruction. Normal flow rate for males is 20 to 25 ml/second; for females, 25 to 30 ml/second.

Nursing considerations
• Advise the patient not to urinate for several hours before the test and to increase his fluid intake so that he'll have a full bladder and a strong urge to void.

Treatments

If uncorrected, renal and urologic disorders can adversely affect virtually every body system. Treatments for these disorders include drug therapy, dialysis, nonsurgical procedures, and surgery.

Drug therapy

Ideally, drug therapy should be effective and not impair renal function. However, because renal disorders alter the chemical composition of body fluids and the pharmacokinetic properties of many drugs, standard regimens of some drugs may require adjustment. For instance, dosages of drugs that are mainly excreted by the kidneys unchanged or as active metabolites may require adjustment to avoid toxicity. In renal failure, potentially toxic drugs should be used cautiously and sparingly.

Drug therapy for renal and urologic disorders can include:
• antibiotics
• urinary tract antiseptics

> Renal disorders can alter chemical composition of body fluids and pharmacokinetic properties of drugs, so many drug regimens require adjustment.

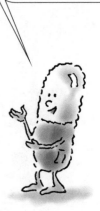

- electrolytes and replacements
- diuretics.

Dialysis

Depending on the patient's condition and, at times, his preference, dialysis may take the form of hemodialysis or peritoneal dialysis.

Hemodialysis

Hemodialysis removes toxic wastes and other impurities from the blood of a patient with renal failure. In this technique, the blood is removed from the body through a surgically created access site, pumped through a dialyzing unit to remove toxins, and then returned to the body. The extracorporeal dialyzer works through a combination of osmosis, diffusion, and filtration.

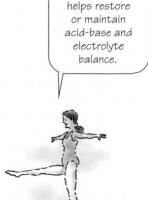

Hemodialysis helps restore or maintain acid-base and electrolyte balance.

Balancing act

By extracting by-products of protein metabolism — notably urea and uric acid — as well as creatinine and excess water, hemodialysis helps restore or maintain acid-base and electrolyte balance and prevent the complications associated with uremia. (See *How hemodialysis works*, page 590.)

Patient preparation

Before hemodialysis, take these steps:
- If the patient is undergoing hemodialysis for the first time, explain its purpose and what to expect during and after treatment. Explain that he first will undergo surgery to create vascular access.
- Assess the access site for the presence of a bruit and thrill, and keep the vascular access site supported and resting on a sterile drape or sterile barrier shield.

Monitoring and aftercare

After hemodialysis, take these steps:
- Monitor the vascular access site for bleeding. If bleeding is excessive, maintain pressure on the site and notify the practitioner.
- To prevent clotting or other problems with blood flow, make sure that the arm used for vascular access isn't used for any other procedure, including I.V. line insertion, blood pressure monitoring, and venipuncture.
- At least four times per day, assess circulation at the access site by auscultating for bruits and palpating for thrills. Unlike most other circulatory assessments, bruits and thrills should be present here. Lack of a bruit at a venous access site for dialysis may indicate a blood clot, which requires immediate surgical attention.

How hemodialysis works

Within the dialyzer, the patient's blood flows between coils, plates, or hollow fibers of semi-permeable material, depending on the machine being used. Simultaneously, the dialysis solution is pumped around the other side under hydrostatic pressure.

Pressure and concentration

Pressure and concentration gradients between blood and the dialysis solution remove toxic wastes and excess water. The dialysis solution is an aqueous solution typically containing low concentrations of sodium, potassium, calcium, and magnesium cations and chloride anions as well as high concentrations of acetate (which the

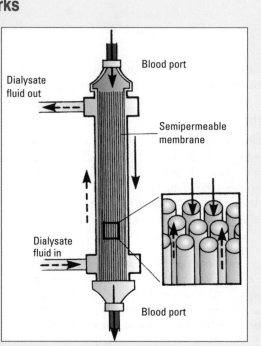

body readily converts to bicarbonate) and glucose. Because blood has higher concentrations of hydrogen ions and other electrolytes than dialysis solution, these solutes diffuse across the semipermeable material into the solution. Conversely, glucose and acetate are more highly concentrated in the dialysis solution and so diffuse back across the semipermeable material into the blood. Through this mechanism, hemodialysis removes excess water and toxins, reverses acidosis, and amends electrolyte imbalances.

Home care instructions

Before discharge, instruct the patient to:
• care for his vascular access site by keeping the incision clean and dry
• notify the practitioner of pain, swelling, redness, or drainage in the accessed arm
• palpate the site for thrills
• refuse treatments or procedures on the accessed arm, including blood pressure monitoring or needle punctures
• avoid putting excessive pressure on the arm (such as sleeping on it, wearing constricting clothing on it, and lifting heavy objects or straining with it), showering, bathing, or swimming for several hours after dialysis.

Peritoneal dialysis

Like hemodialysis, peritoneal dialysis removes toxins from the blood of a patient with acute or chronic renal failure that doesn't respond to other treatments. Unlike hemodialysis, it uses the patient's peritoneal membrane as a semipermeable dialyzing membrane.

Waste away

In this technique, a hypertonic dialyzing solution (dialysate) is instilled through a catheter inserted into the peritoneal cavity. Then, by diffusion, excessive concentrations of electrolytes and uremic toxins in the blood move across the peritoneal membrane into the dialysis solution. Next, through osmosis, excessive water in the blood does the same. After an appropriate dwelling time, the dialysate is drained, taking toxins and wastes with it.

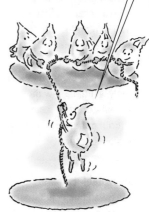

In peritoneal dialysis, osmosis causes excessive water in the blood to move through the peritoneal membrane into the dialysis solution. Hold on, I'm coming!

Patient preparation

Before dialysis, take these steps:
• For the first-time peritoneal dialysis patient, explain the purpose of the treatment and what he can expect during and after the procedure.
• Tell him that first the doctor will insert a catheter into his abdomen to allow instillation of dialysate. Explain the appropriate insertion procedure. (See *Comparing catheters for peritoneal dialysis*, page 592.)

Monitoring and aftercare

After dialysis, take these steps:
• Using sterile technique, change the catheter dressing every 24 hours or whenever it becomes soiled or wet.
• Watch closely for developing complications. Peritonitis can cause fever, persistent abdominal pain and cramping, slow or cloudy dialysis drainage, swelling and tenderness around the catheter, and increased white blood cell (WBC) count.

Home care instructions

Before discharge, instruct the patient to:
• participate in a training program before beginning treatment on his own
• wear medical identification jewelry or carry a card identifying him as a dialysis patient and keep the phone number of the dialysis center on hand at all times in case of an emergency
• watch for and report signs and symptoms of infection and fluid imbalance
• follow up regularly with the practitioner and dialysis team to evaluate the success of treatment and detect any problems.

Comparing catheters for peritoneal dialysis

The first step in any type of peritoneal dialysis is the insertion of a catheter to allow instillation of dialyzing solution. The surgeon may insert one of three different catheters, as described below.

Tenckhoff catheter

The Tenckhoff catheter is the most commonly used peritoneal catheter. To implant a Tenckhoff catheter, the surgeon inserts the first $6^3/_4''$ (17.1 cm) of the catheter into the patient's abdomen. The next $2^3/_4''$ (7-cm) segment, which has a Dacron cuff at each end, is imbedded subcutaneously. Within a few days of insertion, the patient's tissues grow around these Dacron cuffs, forming a tight barrier

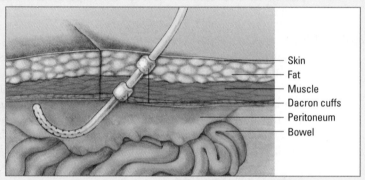

against bacterial infiltration. The remaining $3^7/_8''$ (9.8 cm) of the catheter extends outside of the abdomen and is equipped with a metal adapter at the tip to allow connection to dialyzer tubing.

Swan neck catheter

The Swan neck catheter has an inverted U-shaped arc (170 to 180 degrees) between the deep and superficial cuffs. This arc allows the catheter to exit the skin pointing downward. At the same time, the catheter enters the peritoneum pointing toward the pelvis. This catheter must be implanted in a tunnel the same shape as the catheter.

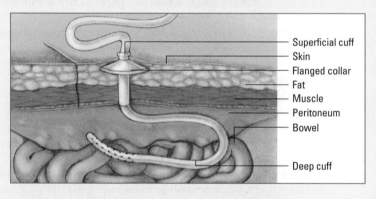

TWH catheter

The Toronto-Western Hospital (TWH) catheter has silicone discs perpendicular to the catheter. The discs' purpose is to hold the omentum and the bowel away from the exit holes and maintain their position in the pelvis, minimizing catheter tip migration. This catheter is more difficult to insert and remove than the Tenckhoff catheter.

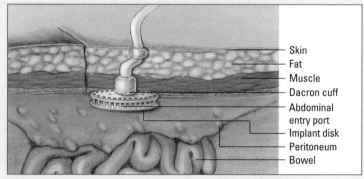

Nonsurgical procedures

Several nonsurgical procedures may be employed to treat renal or urologic disorders, including calculi basketing, catheterization, and extracorporeal shock-wave lithotripsy (ESWL).

Calculi basketing

When ureteral calculi are too large for normal elimination, removal with a basketing instrument is the treatment of choice, helping to relieve pain and prevent infection and renal dysfunction. In this technique, a basketing instrument inserted through a cystoscope or ureteroscope into the ureter captures the calculus and then is withdrawn to remove it.

Patient preparation

Before the procedure, take these steps:
• Tell the patient that after calculi removal, he'll have an indwelling urinary catheter inserted to ensure normal urine drainage; the catheter will probably remain in place for 24 to 48 hours.
• Tell him that he'll receive I.V. fluids during and immediately after the procedure to maintain urine output and prevent complications, such as hydronephrosis and pyelonephritis.

Monitoring and aftercare

After the procedure, take these steps:
• Promote fluids to maintain a urine output of 3 to 4 L/day. Observe the color of urine drainage from the indwelling urinary catheter; it should be slightly blood-tinged at first, gradually clearing within 24 to 48 hours. Irrigate the catheter as ordered using sterile technique.
• Administer analgesics as ordered.
• Observe for and report any signs or symptoms of septicemia, which may result from ureteral perforation during basketing.

Home care instructions

Before discharge, instruct the patient to:
• follow prescribed dietary and medication regimens to prevent recurrence of calculi
• drink 3 to 4 qt (3 to 4 L) of fluid per day, unless contraindicated
• take prescribed analgesics as needed
• immediately report signs and symptoms of recurrent calculi (such as flank pain, hematuria, nausea, fever, and chills) or acute ureteral obstruction (such as severe pain and inability to void).

> Tell the patient to drink 3 to 4 quarts of fluid per day unless contraindicated. It takes some juggling to drink all that!

Catheterization

The insertion of a drainage device into the urinary bladder, catheterization may be intermittent or continuous. Intermittent catheterization drains urine remaining in the bladder after voiding. It's used for patients with urinary incontinence, urethral strictures, cystitis, prostatic obstruction, neurogenic bladder, or other disorders that interfere with bladder emptying. It may also be used postoperatively.

Catheterization helps relieve bladder distention caused by such conditions as urinary tract obstruction and neurogenic bladder. It allows continuous urine drainage in patients with a urinary meatus swollen from local trauma or childbirth as well as from surgery. Catheterization also can provide accurate monitoring of urine output when normal voiding is impaired.

Patient preparation

Before catheterization, take these steps:
• Thoroughly review the procedure with the patient and reassure him that although catheterization may produce slight discomfort, it shouldn't be painful. Explain that you'll stop the procedure if he experiences severe discomfort.
• Assemble the necessary equipment, preferably a sterile catheterization package.

Monitoring and aftercare

During catheterization, note the difficulty or ease of insertion, any patient discomfort, and the amount and nature of urine drainage.

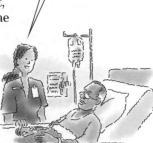

Reassure the patient that catheterization may produce slight discomfort but shouldn't be painful.

Keep fluids flowing

During urine drainage, monitor the patient for pallor, diaphoresis, and painful bladder spasms. If these occur, clamp the catheter tubing and call the practitioner.

In the thick of it

During the procedure, take these steps:
• Frequently assess the patient's intake and output. Encourage fluid intake to maintain continuous urine flow through the catheter and decrease the risk of infection and clot formation.
• Maintain good catheter care throughout the course of treatment. Clean the urinary meatus and catheter junction at least daily, more often if you note a buildup of exudate.
• To help prevent infection, maintain a closed drainage system and discontinue the catheter as soon as possible.

Home care instructions

Before discharge, instruct the patient to:
• drink at least 2 qt (2 L) of water per day, unless the practitioner orders otherwise
• perform daily periurethral care to minimize the risk of infection
• perform thorough hand washing before and after handling the catheter and collection system
• take showers but avoid tub baths while the catheter is in place
• notify the practitioner if he notices urine leakage around the catheter or any signs and symptoms of UTI, such as fever, chills, flank or urinary tract pain, and cloudy or foul-smelling urine.

> ESWL uses high-energy shock waves to break up calculi and allow their normal passage. I think I'll stick with these waves for now.

ESWL

A noninvasive technique for removing obstructive renal calculi, ESWL uses high-energy shock waves to break up calculi and allow their normal passage.

Patient preparation

Before the procedure, tell the patient that he may receive a general or epidural anesthetic, depending on the type of lithotriptor and the intensity of shock waves needed. Also explain that he'll have an I.V. line and an indwelling urinary catheter in place after ESWL.

Monitoring and aftercare

After treatment, take these steps:
• Encourage ambulation as early as possible and increase fluid intake as ordered to aid passage of calculi fragments.
• Strain all urine for calculi fragments and send these to the laboratory for analysis.
• Report frank or persistent bleeding to the practitioner. Keep in mind, however, that slight hematuria usually occurs for several days after ESWL.

Home care instructions

Before discharge, instruct the patient to:
• drink 3 to 4 qt (3 to 4 L) of fluid each day for about 1 month after treatment.
• strain all urine for the 1st week after treatment, save all fragments in the container provided, and bring the container with him on his first follow-up appointment
• report severe, unremitting pain; persistent hematuria; inability to void; fever and chills; or recurrent nausea and vomiting

- comply with any special dietary or drug regimen designed to reduce the risk of new calculi formation.

Surgery

Surgery may be necessary when conservative treatments fail to control the patient's renal or urologic disorder. Common surgeries include cystectomy, kidney transplantation, nephrectomy, suprapubic catheterization, transurethral resection of the bladder tumor (TURBT), and urinary diversion.

Cystectomy

Partial or total removal of the urinary bladder and surrounding structures may be necessary to treat advanced bladder cancer or, rarely, other bladder disorders such as interstitial cystitis. In most patients with bladder cancer, the combined use of chemotherapy, radiation therapy, and surgery yields the best results. In metastatic bladder cancer, cystectomy and radiation therapy may provide palliative benefits and prolong life.

Take three

Cystectomy may be partial, simple, or radical.

Partial, or segmental, cystectomy involves resection of cancerous bladder tissue. Typically preserving bladder function, this surgery is most commonly indicated for a single, easily accessible tumor.

Simple, or total, cystectomy involves resection of the entire bladder, with preservation of surrounding structures. It's indicated for multiple or extensive carcinoma, advanced interstitial cystitis, and related disorders.

Radical cystectomy is usually indicated for muscle-invading, primary bladder carcinoma. In men, the bladder, prostate, and seminal vesicles are removed. In women, the bladder, urethra and, usually, the uterus, fallopian tubes, ovaries, and a segment of the vaginal wall are excised. This procedure may involve bilateral pelvic lymphadenectomy. Because this surgery is so extensive, it typically produces impotence in men and sterility in women.

Diversionary tactics

A permanent urinary diversion is needed in both radical and simple cystectomy. A *cutaneous* diversion allows urine to drain through a newly created opening in the abdominal wall. In a *continent* diversion, a portion of the intestine is used to create a urinary reservoir.

Patient preparation

Before surgery, take these steps:
• If the patient will be undergoing simple or radical cystectomy, reassure him that urinary diversion need not interfere with his normal activities and arrange for a visit by an enterostomal therapist, who can provide further information.
• If the patient is scheduled for radical cystectomy, you'll need to address concerns about the loss of sexual or reproductive function. As appropriate, refer the patient for psychological and sexual counseling.
• If the bowel will be used as a reservoir, perform bowel preparation before surgery.

> If the patient is scheduled for radical cystectomy, address concerns about the loss of sexual or reproductive function.

Monitoring and aftercare

After surgery, take these steps:
• Periodically inspect the stoma and incision for bleeding, and observe urine drainage for frank hematuria and clots. Slight hematuria commonly occurs for several days after surgery but should clear thereafter.
• Observe the wound site and all drainage for signs of infection. Change abdominal dressings frequently, using sterile technique.
• Periodically ask the patient about incisional pain and, if he has had a partial cystectomy, ask about bladder spasms. Provide analgesics and an antispasmodic such as oxybutynin (Ditropan) as ordered.
• To prevent pulmonary complications associated with prolonged immobility, encourage frequent position changes, coughing and deep breathing and, if possible, early ambulation.

Home care instructions

Before discharge, instruct the patient to:
• watch for and report signs or symptoms of UTI and persistent hematuria
• learn how to care for his stoma and where to obtain needed supplies
• contact the local chapter of the United Ostomy Association for support
• follow up with the practitioner as recommended.

Kidney transplantation site and vascular connections

With kidney transplantation, the donated organ is implanted in the iliac fossa. The organ's vessels are then connected to the common iliac vein and common iliac artery, as shown below. Unless it will cause infection or high blood pressure, the diseased kidney is left in place.

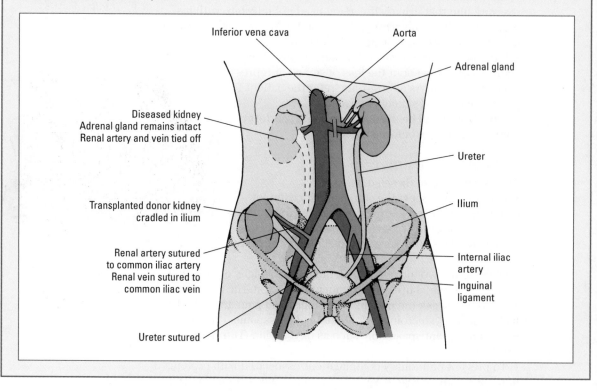

Inferior vena cava

Aorta

Adrenal gland

Diseased kidney
Adrenal gland remains intact
Renal artery and vein tied off

Ureter

Transplanted donor kidney
cradled in ilium

Ilium

Renal artery sutured
to common iliac artery
Renal vein sutured to
common iliac vein

Internal iliac
artery

Inguinal
ligament

Ureter sutured

Kidney transplantation

Ranking among the most commonly performed and most successful of all organ transplantations, kidney transplantation represents an attractive alternative to dialysis for many patients with otherwise unmanageable end-stage renal disease. It also may be necessary to sustain life in a patient who has suffered traumatic loss of kidney function or for whom dialysis is contraindicated. (See *Kidney transplantation site and vascular connections.*)

Patient preparation

The patient will understandably find the prospect of kidney transplantation confusing and frightening. Help him cope with such emotions by preparing him thoroughly for transplantation and a prolonged recovery period and by offering ongoing emotional support. To do so, take these steps:

• Describe the routine preoperative measures. Point out that he may need dialysis for a few days after surgery if his transplanted kidney doesn't start functioning immediately.
• Review the transplantation procedure itself, supplementing and clarifying the practitioner's explanations as necessary.
• Discuss the immunosuppressant drugs the patient will be taking and explain their possible adverse effects. Point out that these drugs increase his susceptibility to infection; as a result, he'll be kept temporarily isolated after surgery.

Monitoring and aftercare

After surgery, take these steps:
• First and foremost, take special precautions to reduce the risk of infection. For instance, use strict sterile technique when changing dressings and performing catheter care. Also, limit the patient's contact with staff, other patients, and visitors and have all people in the patient's room wear surgical masks for the first 2 weeks after surgery.

Feeling rejected

• Throughout the recovery period, watch for signs and symptoms of tissue rejection. Observe the transplantation site for redness, tenderness, and swelling.
• Monitor the patient for signs of diabetes mellitus. (See *Kidney transplantation and PTDM: Reducing the risk for complications*.)

> Have all people in the transplant patient's room wear surgical masks for the first 2 weeks after surgery.

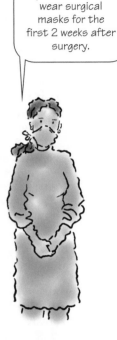

Weighing the evidence

Kidney transplantation and PTDM: Reducing the risk for complications

After kidney transplantation, some patients develop posttransplant diabetes mellitus (PTDM)—a complication that, in turn, increases the risk for graft rejection, infections, and cardiovascular disease. To identify the type of patient most at risk for developing PTDM, researchers reviewed the records of over 200 kidney transplant patients.

A triple threat

The researchers found three significant risk factors for PTDM: being age 40 or older, having a body mass index of 30 or greater, and having elevated triglyceride levels. They concluded that aggressive identification and treatment of patients at risk for PTDM can minimize further complications.

Source: Siraj, E., et al. (2010). Risk factors and outcomes associated with posttransplant diabetes mellitus in kidney transplant recipients. *Transplant Procedures, 42*(5), 1685–1689.

• Carefully monitor urine output; promptly report output of less than 100 ml/hour. A sudden decrease in urine output could indicate thrombus formation at the renal artery anastomosis site.

Home care instructions

Before discharge, instruct the patient to:
• carefully measure and record intake and output to monitor kidney function
• weigh himself at least twice per week and report any rapid gain (any gain of $2^1/_2$ lb [1.1 kg] or more in a single day)
• watch for and promptly report signs and symptoms of infection or transplant rejection, including redness, warmth, tenderness, or swelling over the kidney; fever; decreased urine output; and elevated blood pressure
• avoid crowds and contact with people with known or suspected infections for at least 3 months after surgery
• continue immunosuppressant therapy for as long as he has the transplanted kidney to prevent rejection.

Nephrectomy

Nephrectomy is the surgical removal of a kidney. It's the treatment of choice for advanced renal cell carcinoma that's refractory to chemotherapy and radiation, although radiofrequency ablation can treat small renal masses. (See *Radiofrequency ablation: Effective treatment for small renal masses.*) It's also used to harvest a healthy kidney for transplantation. When conservative treatments fail, nephrectomy may be used to treat renal trauma,

Weighing the evidence

Radiofrequency ablation: Effective treatment for small renal masses

An alternative to surgery for treating small renal masses, radiofrequency ablation (RFA) appears to be an effective treatment. But how effective is it over time? To answer that question, researchers looked at over 200 patients who had undergone RFA over a 7.5-year period, assessing both intermediate and long-term oncologic outcomes. They found RFA to be a successful treatment, with both a low rate of tumor recurrence as well as a posttreatment cancer-free survival rate of 5 years.

Tracy, C., et al. (2010). Durable oncologic outcomes after radiofrequency ablation: Experience from treating 243 small renal masses over 7.5 years. *Cancer, 116*(13), 3135–3142.

infection, hypertension, hydronephrosis, and inoperable renal calculi.

One kidney or two?

Nephrectomy may be unilateral or bilateral. Unilateral nephrectomy, the more commonly performed procedure, usually doesn't interfere with renal function as long as one healthy kidney remains. However, bilateral nephrectomy (or the removal of a lone kidney) requires lifelong dialysis or transplantation to support renal function.

Four major types of nephrectomy are performed:

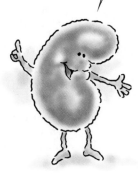

partial nephrectomy — resection of only a portion of the kidney

simple nephrectomy — removal of the entire kidney

radical nephrectomy — resection of the entire kidney and the surrounding fat tissue

nephroureterectomy — removal of the entire kidney, the perinephric fat, and the entire ureter.

> Unilateral nephrectomy places the weight of renal function all on my shoulders — but I can handle it!

Patient preparation

If the patient is having unilateral nephrectomy, reassure him that one healthy kidney is all he'll need for adequate function. If the surgery is bilateral or will remove the patient's only kidney, prepare him for radical changes in his lifestyle, most notably the need for regular dialysis.

Monitoring and aftercare

After nephrectomy, take these steps:
• Carefully monitor the rate, volume, and type of I.V. fluids. Keep in mind that mistakes in fluid therapy can be particularly devastating for a patient who has only one kidney.
• Check the patient's dressing and drain every 4 hours for the first 24 to 48 hours, then once every shift to assess the amount and nature of drainage. Maintain drain patency.

Home care instructions

Before discharge, instruct the patient to:
• monitor intake and output; explain how this helps assess renal function
• follow the practitioner's guidelines on fluid intake and dietary restrictions
• attend follow-up examinations to evaluate kidney function and assess for possible complications

- notify the practitioner immediately if he detects any significant decrease in urine output or develops fever, chills, hematuria, or flank pain
- avoid strenuous exercise or heavy lifting and sexual activity until his practitioner grants permission.

Suprapubic catheterization

Suprapubic catheterization is a type of urinary diversion connected to a closed drainage system that involves transcutaneous insertion of a catheter through the suprapubic area into the bladder.

A diverting procedure

Typically, suprapubic catheterization provides temporary urinary diversion after certain gynecologic procedures, bladder surgery, or prostatectomy and relieves obstruction from calculi, severe urethral strictures, or pelvic trauma. Less commonly, it may be used to create a permanent urinary diversion, thereby relieving obstruction from an inoperable tumor.

Patient preparation

Explain the procedure to the patient. Tell him that the doctor will insert a soft plastic tube through the skin of the abdomen and into the bladder and then connect the tube to an external collection bag. Also explain that the procedure is done under local anesthesia, causes little or no discomfort, and takes 15 to 45 minutes.

Monitoring and aftercare

After the procedure, take these steps:
- To ensure adequate drainage and tube patency, check the suprapubic catheter at least hourly for the first 24 hours after insertion. Make sure the collection bag is below bladder level to enhance drainage and prevent backflow, which can lead to infection.
- Tape the catheter securely in place on the abdominal skin to reduce tension and prevent dislodgment. To prevent kinks in the tube, curve it gently but don't bend it.
- Check dressings often and change them at least once per day or as ordered. Observe the skin around the insertion site for signs of infection and encrustation.

Home care instructions

Before discharge, instruct the patient to:
- change the dressing, and empty and reattach the collection bag
- drink plenty of fluids
- follow up with the practitioner as recommended
- meet with the enterostomal therapist to help manage the urinary diversion

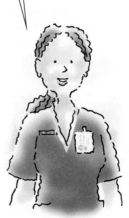

Suprapubic catheterization provides temporary or, less commonly, permanent urinary diversion.

• notify the practitioner promptly of signs or symptoms of infection or encrustation, such as discolored or foul-smelling discharge, impaired drainage, and swelling, redness, and tenderness at the tube insertion site.

TURBT

A relatively quick and simple procedure, TURBT involves insertion of a resectoscope through the urethra and into the bladder to remove lesions. (It can also be performed using an Nd:YAG laser.) Most commonly performed to treat superficial and early bladder carcinoma, TURBT may also be used to remove benign papillomas or to relieve fibrosis of the bladder neck. This treatment isn't indicated for large or infiltrating tumors or for metastatic bladder cancer.

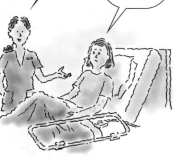

If the patient is scheduled to receive a local anesthetic, she'll be awake during treatment.

Lucky me!

Patient preparation

Tell the patient that he'll receive either a local or general anesthetic. If he receives a local anesthetic, explain that he'll be awake during treatment. Also inform him that he'll have an indwelling urinary catheter in place for 1 to 5 days after the procedure to ensure urine drainage.

Monitoring and aftercare

After TURBT, take these steps:
• Maintain adequate fluid intake and provide meticulous catheter care, including frequent irrigation. (The practitioner may prescribe continuous or intermittent irrigation, especially if the removal of a large vascular lesion has compromised hemostasis).
• Observe urine drainage for blood. Remember that slight hematuria usually occurs directly after TURBT. However, notify the practitioner immediately of any frank bleeding or if the hematuria seems excessive.
• Assess for signs and symptoms of bladder perforation, including abdominal pain and rigidity, fever, and decreased urine output despite adequate hydration.

Home care instructions

Before discharge, instruct the patient to:
• report bleeding or hematuria that lasts longer than several weeks, fever, chills, or flank pain, which may indicate UTI
• drink plenty of water (10 glasses daily) and void every 2 to 3 hours to reduce the risk of clot formation, urethral obstruction, and UTI
• heed the urge to urinate
• refrain from sexual or other strenuous activity, avoid lifting anything heavier than 10 lb (4.5 kg), and continue taking a stool softener or other laxative until the practitioner orders otherwise
• follow up with the practitioner as recommended.

Common urinary diversions

Various urinary diversions may be done for bladder cancer patients. Two of the most commonly performed types are the ileal conduit and the continent ileal diversion.

Ileal conduit
An ileal conduit is the preferred procedure for diverting urine through a segment of the ileum to a stoma on the abdomen (as shown). In this procedure, a segment of the ileum is excised, and the two ends of the ileum that result from the excision of the segment are sutured closed. Then the ureters are dissected from the bladder and anastomosed to the ileal segment. One end of the ileal segment is closed with sutures; the opposite end is brought through the abdominal wall, thereby forming a stoma. Because urine empties continuously, the patient must wear a collecting device (or pouch).

Continent ileal diversion
One continent ileal diversion, called the *Kock pouch*, is an alternative to the ileal conduit. In this procedure, the ureters are transplanted to a reservoir created from an isolated segment of the right colon or small bowel. A stoma is then created that connects the reservoir to the skin. Accumulated urine is drained by inserting a catheter into the stoma.

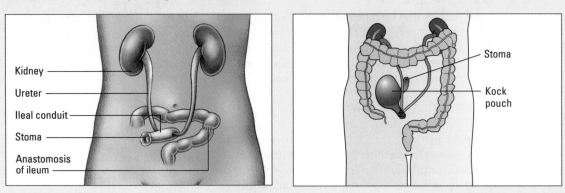

Kidney
Ureter
Ileal conduit
Stoma
Anastomosis of ileum

Stoma
Kock pouch

Urinary diversion

A urinary diversion provides an alternate route for urine excretion when a disorder or abnormality impedes normal flow through the bladder. Most commonly performed in patients who have undergone total or partial cystectomy, diversion surgery may also be performed in patients with a congenital urinary tract defect or a severe, unmanageable UTI that threatens renal function; an injury to the ureters, bladder, or urethra; an obstructive malignant tumor; or a neurogenic bladder.

Several types of urinary diversion surgery can be performed. The two most common are ileal conduit and continent ileal diversion. (See *Common urinary diversions.*)

Patient preparation

Before the procedure, take these steps:
• Prepare the patient for the appearance and general location of the stoma. If he's scheduled for an ileal conduit, explain that the stoma will be located somewhere in the lower abdomen, probably below the waistline. If he's scheduled for a continent vesicostomy, explain that the exact stoma site is commonly chosen during surgery, based on the length of the patent ureter available.
• Review the enterostomal therapist's explanation of the urine collection device that the patient will use after surgery.

Monitoring and aftercare

After the procedure, take these steps:
• Carefully check and record urine output. Report any decrease, which could indicate obstruction from postoperative edema or ureteral stenosis.
• Perform routine ostomy maintenance. Make sure the collection device fits closely around the stoma; allow no more than a $^1/_8''$ (0.3 cm) margin of skin between the stoma and the device's faceplate. Regularly check the appearance of the stoma and peristomal skin.

Home care instructions

Before discharge, instruct the patient to:
• properly perform stoma care or ostomy self-catheterization
• watch for and report signs and symptoms of complications, such as fever, chills, abdominal pain, and pus or blood in the urine
• keep scheduled follow-up appointments with the practitioner and enterostomal therapist to evaluate stoma care and make any necessary changes in equipment
• contact a support group such as the United Ostomy Association.

Before discharge, instruct the patient to contact a support group such as the United Ostomy Association.

Nursing diagnoses

When caring for patients with renal or urologic disorders, you'll find that several nursing diagnoses can be commonly used. These nursing diagnoses appear here, along with appropriate nursing interventions and rationales. See *NANDA-I taxonomy II by domain*, page 936, for the complete list of NANDA diagnoses.

Deficient fluid volume

Related to actual loss, *Deficient fluid volume* can be associated with dialysis, ingestion of large amounts of diuretics, renal failure, or metabolic acidosis.

Expected outcomes

- Patient exhibits normal skin color and temperature.
- Patient produces adequate urine volume.
- Patient's urine specific gravity remains between 1.005 and 1.030.

Nursing interventions and rationales

- Monitor and record vital signs every 2 hours, or as often as necessary until stable. Then monitor and record vital signs every 4 hours. Tachycardia, dyspnea, or hypotension may indicate deficient fluid volume or electrolyte imbalance.
- Measure intake and output every 1 to 4 hours. Record and report significant changes. Include urine, stools, vomitus, wound drainage, and any other output. Low urine output and high specific gravity indicate hypovolemia.
- Administer fluids, blood or blood products, or plasma expanders to replace fluids and whole blood loss and to promote fluid movement into vascular space. Monitor and record effectiveness and any adverse effects.
- Weigh the patient at the same time daily to give more accurate and consistent data. Weight loss or gain is a good indicator of fluid status.
- Assess skin turgor and oral mucous membranes every 8 hours to check for dehydration. Give meticulous mouth care every 4 hours to avoid dehydrating mucous membranes.

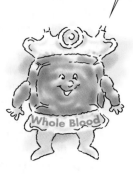

> Patients with deficient fluid volume may receive fluids, blood or blood products, or plasma expanders.

Excess fluid volume

Related to compromised regulatory mechanisms, *Excess fluid volume* can be associated with acute glomerulonephritis, acute or chronic renal failure, pyelonephritis, or other renal diseases.

Expected outcomes

- Patient's blood pressure is no higher than 130/80 mm Hg.
- Patient demonstrates no signs of hyperkalemia on electrocardiogram (ECG).
- Patient maintains fluid intake as directed by practitioner.

Nursing interventions and rationales

- Monitor blood pressure, pulse rate, cardiac rhythm, temperature, and breath sounds at least once every 4 hours; record and report changes. Changed parameters may indicate altered fluid or electrolyte status.

• Carefully monitor intake, output, and urine specific gravity at least once every 4 hours. Intake greater than output and elevated specific gravity may indicate fluid retention or overload.
• Monitor BUN, creatinine, electrolyte, and hemoglobin (Hb) levels, as well as hematocrit (HCT). BUN and creatinine levels indicate renal function; electrolyte levels, Hb levels, and HCT reflect fluid status.

Weighing in

• Weigh the patient daily before breakfast, as ordered, to provide consistent readings. Check for signs of fluid retention, such as dependent edema, sacral edema, or ascites.
• Give fluids as ordered. Monitor I.V. flow rate carefully because excess I.V. fluids can worsen the patient's condition.
• If oral fluids are allowed, help the patient create a schedule for fluid intake. Patient involvement encourages compliance.
• Assess skin turgor to monitor for dehydration.

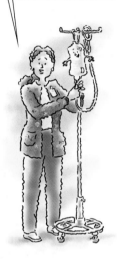

Monitor I.V. flow rate carefully because excess I.V. fluids can worsen the patient's condition.

Urge urinary incontinence

Related to decreased bladder capacity, *Urge urinary incontinence* may be associated with such conditions as acute bladder infection, bladder obstruction, and interstitial cystitis.

Expected outcomes

• Patient has decreased frequency of incontinence episodes.
• Patient states increased comfort.
• Patient demonstrates skill in managing incontinence.

Nursing interventions and rationales

• Observe voiding pattern and document intake and output to ensure correct fluid replacement therapy and provide information about the patient's ability to void adequately.
• Provide appropriate care for existing urologic conditions, monitor progress, and report the patient's responses to treatment. The patient should receive adequate and qualified care as well as understand and participate in care as much as possible.
• Unless contraindicated, maintain fluid intake of 3 qt (3 L)/day to moisten mucous membranes and ensure hydration; limit the patient to 5 oz (150 ml) after supper to reduce the need to void at night.
• Explain the urologic condition to the patient and his family; include instructions on preventive measures and the established bladder schedule.

Common renal and urologic disorders

This section discusses the most common renal and urologic disorders, including their causes, assessment findings, diagnostic tests, treatment, nursing interventions, patient-teaching recommendations, and evaluation criteria.

Acute poststreptococcal glomerulonephritis

Acute poststreptococcal glomerulonephritis is a bilateral inflammation of the glomeruli, commonly following a streptococcal infection. It's most common in boys ages 3 to 10 but can occur at any age. Up to 95% of children and up to 70% of adults fully recover; the rest may progress to chronic renal failure within months.

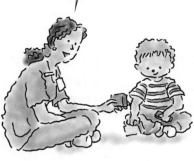

Acute poststreptococcal glomerulonephritis is most common in boys ages 3 to 10 but can occur at any age.

What causes it

Causes of the disorder include:
- streptococcal infection of the respiratory tract
- impetigo
- immunoglobulin (Ig) A nephropathy (Berger's disease)
- lipoid nephrosis.

Pathophysiology

Acute poststreptococcal glomerulonephritis results from entrapment and collection of antigen-antibody complexes in the glomerular capillary membranes after infection with group A hemolytic streptococci. The antigens stimulate the formation of antibodies. Circulating antigen-antibody complexes become lodged in the glomerular capillaries.

Complex process

Glomerular injury occurs when complexes initiate the release of immunologic substances that break down cells and increase membrane permeability. The severity of glomerular damage and renal insufficiency depends on the size, number, location, duration of exposure, and type of antigen-antibody complexes.

What to look for

Typically, this disorder begins 1 to 3 weeks after untreated pharyngitis. The most common symptoms are:
- mild to moderate edema
- azotemia
- hematuria (smoke- or coffee-colored urine)

- oliguria (less than 400 ml/day)
- fatigue
- mild to severe hypertension
- sodium or water retention.

What tests tell you

- Blood studies reveal elevated electrolyte, BUN, and creatinine levels.
- Urine studies reveal RBCs, WBCs, mixed cell casts, and protein.
- Elevated antistreptolysin-O titers (in 80% of patients), elevated streptozyme and anti-DNase B titers, and low serum complement levels verify recent streptococcal infection.
- A throat culture may also show group A beta-hemolytic streptococci.
- KUB X-rays show bilateral kidney enlargement.

How it's treated

The goals of treatment are the relief of symptoms and the prevention of complications. Vigorous supportive care includes bed rest, fluid and dietary sodium restrictions, and correction of electrolyte imbalances (possibly with dialysis, although this is rarely necessary). Therapy may include diuretics such as furosemide (Lasix) to reduce extracellular fluid overload and an antihypertensive such as hydralazine. The use of antibiotics to prevent secondary infection or transmission to others is controversial.

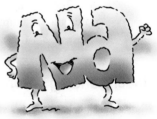

Vigorous supportive care includes bed rest, sodium restrictions, and correction of electrolyte imbalances.

What to do

- Promote bed rest during the acute phase. Allow the patient to resume normal activities gradually as symptoms subside; the disorder usually resolves within 2 weeks.
- Monitor vital signs, electrolyte values, intake and output, and daily weight.
- Assess renal function daily through serum creatinine and BUN levels, and urine creatinine clearance.
- Watch for and immediately report signs of acute renal failure (such as oliguria, azotemia, and acidosis).

Keep the calories coming

- Consult the dietitian to provide a diet high in calories and low in protein, sodium, potassium, and fluids.
- Evaluate the patient. After successful treatment, the patient has normal serum creatinine and BUN levels and a normal urine creatinine clearance and is free from complications. He's prepared

to follow a diet high in calories and low in protein and obtain the necessary follow-up examination. (See *Acute poststreptococcal glomerulonephritis teaching tips*.)

Acute pyelonephritis

One of the most common renal diseases, acute pyelonephritis is a sudden bacterial inflammation. It primarily affects the interstitial area, the renal pelvis and, less commonly, the renal tubules. With treatment and continued follow-up care, the prognosis is good. Extensive permanent damage is rare. (See *Understanding chronic pyelonephritis*.)

What causes it

Causes of chronic pyelonephritis include:
- infection
- hematogenous or lymphatic spread.

Factoring in risk

Risk factors include:
- diagnostic and therapeutic use of instruments, as in catheterization, cystoscopy, or urologic surgery
- inability to empty the bladder

Understanding chronic pyelonephritis

Chronic pyelonephritis, or persistent inflammation of the kidneys, can scar the kidneys and may lead to chronic renal failure. Its cause may be bacterial, metastatic, or urogenous. This disease occurs most commonly in patients who are predisposed to recurrent acute pyelonephritis, such as those with urinary obstructions or vesicoureteral reflux.

specific gravity, proteinuria, leukocytes in urine and, especially in late stages, hypertension. Uremia rarely develops from chronic pyelonephritis, unless structural abnormalities exist in the urinary system. Bacteriuria may be intermittent. When no bacteria are found in the urine, diagnosis depends on excretory urography (where the renal pelvis may appear small and flattened) and renal biopsy.

Signs and symptoms

Patients with chronic pyelonephritis may have a childhood history of unexplained fevers or bed-wetting. Signs and symptoms include flank pain, anemia, low urine

Treatment

Treatment requires control of hypertension, elimination of the existing obstruction (when possible), and long-term antimicrobial therapy.

Acute post-streptococcal glomerulonephritis teaching tips

- Stress to the patient the need for regular blood pressure, urine protein, and renal function assessments during the convalescent months to detect recurrence.
- Tell the patient that he'll need follow-up examinations to detect chronic renal failure. After the disorder resolves, hematuria may recur during nonspecific viral infections; abnormal urinary findings may persist for years.
- Advise the patient with a history of chronic upper respiratory tract infections to report immediately signs and symptoms of infection (such as fever or sore throat).
- Encourage a pregnant woman with a history of the disorder to have frequent medical evaluations because pregnancy further stresses the kidneys and increases the risk of chronic renal failure.

- urinary stasis
- urinary obstruction
- sexual activity (in women)
- use of diaphragms and condoms with spermicidal gel
- pregnancy
- diabetes
- other renal diseases.

Pathophysiology

Typically, the infection spreads from the bladder to the ureters, then to the kidneys. Bacteria refluxed to intrarenal tissues may create colonies of infection within 24 to 48 hours.

What to look for

Signs and symptoms of pyelonephritis include:
- urinary urgency and frequency
- burning during urination
- dysuria, nocturia, and hematuria
- cloudy urine with an ammonia or fish odor
- temperature of 102° F (38.9° C) or higher
- shaking chills
- flank pain
- anorexia
- general fatigue.

What tests tell you

- Urinalysis reveals pyuria and, possibly, a few RBCs; low specific gravity and osmolality; slightly alkaline pH; and, possibly, proteinuria, glycosuria, and ketonuria.
- Urine culture reveals more than 100,000 organisms/µl of urine.
- KUB radiography may reveal calculi, tumors, or cysts in the kidneys and the urinary tract.
- Excretory urography may show asymmetrical kidneys.

How it's treated

Treatment centers on antibiotic therapy appropriate to the specific infecting organism, after identification by urine culture and sensitivity studies.

A broader approach

When the infecting organism can't be identified, therapy usually consists of a broad-spectrum antibiotic. If the patient is pregnant, antibiotics must be prescribed cautiously. Analgesics are also appropriate.

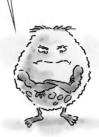

Those kidneys would have been all mine if it weren't for those pesky antibiotics!

Signs and symptoms may disappear after several days of antibiotic therapy. Although urine usually becomes sterile within 48 to 72 hours, the course of such therapy is 10 to 14 days. Follow-up treatment includes reculturing urine 1 week after drug therapy stops, then periodically for the next year to detect residual or recurring infection. Most patients with uncomplicated infections respond well to therapy and don't suffer reinfection.

Infection from obstruction or vesicoureteral reflux may not respond as well to antibiotics. The patient may then need surgery to relieve the obstruction or correct the anomaly. Patients at high risk for recurring UTIs and kidney infections, such as those using an indwelling urinary catheter for a prolonged period and those on maintenance antibiotic therapy, require long-term follow-up care.

What to do

- Administer antipyretics for fever.
- Encourage increased fluid intake to achieve a urine output of more than 2,000 ml (2 qt)/day. Don't encourage intake of more than 2 to 3 qt (2 to 3 L) because this may decrease the effectiveness of antibiotics.
- Evaluate the patient. The recovering patient has a normal temperature, has no urinary discomfort or flank pain, forces fluids, and takes antibiotics as prescribed. (See *Acute pyelonephritis teaching tips*.)

Acute renal failure

Acute renal failure (ARF) is the sudden interruption of kidney function from obstruction, reduced circulation, or renal parenchymatous disease. It's usually reversible with treatment. Otherwise, it can progress to end-stage renal disease, uremic syndrome, or death.

What causes it

ARF may be classified as prerenal, intrarenal, or postrenal. Each type has separate causes. (See *Causes of ARF.*)

Pathophysiology

Prerenal failure results from conditions that damage blood flow to the kidneys (hypoperfusion). When renal blood flow is interrupted, so is oxygen delivery. The ensuing hypoxemia and ischemia can rapidly and irreversibly damage the kidney. The tubules are most susceptible to the effects of hypoxemia.

Intrarenal failure results from damage to the filtering structures of the kidneys. Causes of intrarenal failure are classified

Education edge

Acute pyelonephritis teaching tips

- Teach the patient proper technique for collecting a clean-catch urine specimen. Tell him to be sure to refrigerate the specimen within 30 minutes of collection to prevent overgrowth of bacteria.
- Stress the need to complete the prescribed antibiotic therapy even after signs and symptoms subside.
- Advise routine check-ups for a patient with chronic urinary tract infections. Teach the patient to recognize signs and symptoms of infection, such as cloudy urine, burning on urination, and urinary urgency and frequency, especially when accompanied by a low-grade fever.
- Encourage long-term follow-up care for high-risk patients.

Causes of ARF

Acute renal failure (ARF) is classified as prerenal, intrarenal, or postrenal. All conditions that lead to prerenal failure impair blood flow to the kidneys (renal perfusion), resulting in decreased glomerular filtration rate and increased tubular reabsorption of sodium and water. Intrarenal failure results from damage to the kidneys themselves; postrenal failure, from obstructed urine flow. This table shows the causes of each type of ARF.

Prerenal failure

Cardiovascular disorders
- Arrhythmias
- Cardiac tamponade
- Cardiogenic shock
- Heart failure
- Myocardial infarction

Hypovolemia
- Burns
- Dehydration
- Diuretic overuse
- Hemorrhage
- Hypovolemic shock
- Trauma

Peripheral vasodilation
- Antihypertensive drugs
- Sepsis

Renovascular obstruction
- Arterial embolism, stenosis, or occlusion
- Arterial or venous thrombosis
- Tumor

Severe vasoconstriction
- Disseminated intravascular coagulation
- Eclampsia
- Malignant hypertension
- Vasculitis

Intrarenal failure

Acute tubular necrosis
- Ischemic damage to renal parenchyma from unrecognized or poorly treated prerenal failure
- Nephrotoxins, including anesthetics such as methoxyflurane, antibiotics such as gentamicin, and heavy metals, such as lead, radiographic contrast media, and organic solvents
- Obstetric complications, such as eclampsia, postpartum renal failure, septic abortion, and uterine hemorrhage
- Pigment release, such as crush injury, myopathy, sepsis, and transfusion reaction

Other parenchymal disorders
- Acute glomerulonephritis
- Acute interstitial nephritis
- Acute pyelonephritis
- Bilateral renal vein thrombosis
- Malignant nephrosclerosis
- Papillary necrosis
- Periarteritis nodosa (inflammatory disease of the arteries)
- Renal myeloma
- Sickle cell disease
- Systemic lupus erythematosus
- Vasculitis

Postrenal failure

Bladder obstruction
- Anticholinergic drugs
- Autonomic nerve dysfunction
- Infection
- Tumor

Ureteral obstruction
- Blood clots
- Calculi
- Edema or inflammation
- Necrotic renal papillae
- Retroperitoneal fibrosis or hemorrhage
- Surgery (accidental ligation)
- Tumor
- Uric acid crystals

Urethral obstruction
- Prostatic hyperplasia or tumor
- Strictures

as nephrotoxic, inflammatory, or ischemic. When the damage is caused by nephrotoxicity or inflammation, the delicate layer under the epithelium (the basement membrane) becomes irreparably damaged, typically leading to chronic renal failure. Severe or prolonged lack of blood flow by ischemia may lead to renal damage (ischemic parenchymal injury) and excess nitrogen in the blood (intrinsic renal azotemia).

Postrenal failure is a consequence of bilateral obstruction of urine outflow. The cause may be in the bladder, ureters, or urethra.

What to look for

Signs and symptoms of acute renal failure include:
- oliguria (usually the earliest sign)
- anorexia
- nausea and vomiting
- diarrhea or constipation
- stomatitis
- GI bleeding
- hematemesis
- dry mucous membranes
- uremic breath
- hypotension.

What tests tell you

- Blood studies reveal elevated BUN, creatinine, and potassium levels as well as low pH, bicarbonate levels, Hb levels, and HCT.
- Urine specimens show casts, cellular debris, decreased specific gravity and, in glomerular diseases, proteinuria and urine osmolality close to serum osmolality. Urine sodium level is less than 20 mEq/L if oliguria results from decreased perfusion; greater than 40 mEq/L if it results from an intrinsic problem.
- A creatinine clearance test measures the GFR and is used to estimate the number of remaining functioning nephrons.

Picturing the problem

- Other studies include ultrasonography of the kidneys, renal scan, CT scan, retrograde pyelography, MRI, and plain films of the abdomen, kidneys, ureters, and bladder.

How it's treated

The major goals for ARF are to reestablish effective renal function, if possible, and to maintain the constancy of the internal environment despite transient renal failure. Supportive measures include a diet high in calories and low in protein, sodium, and potassium, with supplemental vitamins and restricted fluids. Meticulous electrolyte monitoring is essential to detect hyperkalemia.

If hyperkalemia occurs, acute therapy may include dialysis, sodium bicarbonate, and hypertonic glucose and insulin infusions,

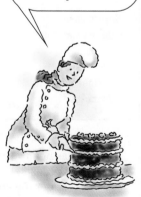

Supportive measures for ARF include a diet high in calories and low in protein, sodium, and potassium. Cake, anyone?

all administered I.V. Sodium polystyrene sulfonate (Kayexalate) can be administered by mouth or by enema to remove potassium from the body. If these measures fail to control uremic symptoms, the patient may require hemodialysis or peritoneal dialysis.

What to do

• Measure and record intake and output, including all body fluids, such as wound drainage, nasogastric output, and diarrhea. Weigh the patient daily.
• Assess HCT and Hb level and replace blood components as ordered. Don't use whole blood if the patient is prone to heart failure and can't tolerate extra fluid volume.
• Monitor vital signs.
• Watch for and report any signs or symptoms of pericarditis (such as pleuritic chest pain, tachycardia, and pericardial friction rub), inadequate renal perfusion (such as hypotension), or acidosis.
• Maintain the patient's nutritional status. Provide a high-calorie, low-protein, low-sodium, and low-potassium diet, with vitamin supplements. Give the anorectic patient small, frequent meals.

Days with malaise

• Maintain electrolyte balance. Strictly monitor potassium levels. Watch for symptoms of hyperkalemia (such as malaise, anorexia, paresthesia, and muscle weakness) and ECG changes (including tall, peaked T waves; widening QRS segment; and disappearing P waves) and report them immediately. Don't administer medications that contain potassium.
• Assist with peritoneal dialysis or hemodialysis as needed.
• Evaluate the patient. After successful treatment, the patient has no weight gain, has stable vital signs, exhibits no complications or signs of infection, talks openly about his illness, and has normal blood values. The patient is prepared to follow his diet and any necessary medical regimen at home. (See *ARF teaching tips*.)

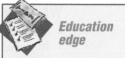

Education edge

ARF teaching tips

• Instruct the patient to follow a high-calorie, low-protein, low-sodium, and low-potassium diet with vitamin supplements.
• If the patient requires dialysis, explain what equipment is used during treatment and the monitoring that's involved with any type of dialysis.
• Explain the importance of fluid restriction and the need for daily weight measurements.

Chronic glomerulonephritis

Chronic glomerulonephritis, a slowly progressive, noninfectious disease, is characterized by inflammation of the renal glomeruli. It remains subclinical until the progressive phase begins. By the time it produces symptoms, it's usually irreversible. It results in eventual renal failure.

By the time glomerulonephritis produces symptoms, it can't be readily fixed.

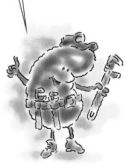

What causes it

- Membranoproliferative glomerulonephritis
- Membranous glomerulopathy
- Focal glomerulosclerosis
- Poststreptococcal glomerulonephritis

Blame the system

Systemic causes include:
- lupus erythematosus
- Goodpasture's syndrome
- hemolytic uremic syndrome.

Pathophysiology

The inflammation of the glomeruli that occurs with this condition results in sclerosis, scarring, and eventual renal failure.

What to look for

This disease usually develops insidiously and without producing symptoms, commonly over many years. At any time, however, it may suddenly become progressive. The initial stage includes:
- nephrotic syndrome
- hypertension
- proteinuria
- hematuria.

Late-stage findings include azotemia, nausea, vomiting, pruritus, dyspnea, malaise, fatigability, mild to severe anemia, and severe hypertension, which may cause cardiac hypertrophy, leading to heart failure.

What tests tell you

- Urinalysis reveals proteinuria, hematuria, cylindruria, and RBC casts.
- Blood tests reveal rising BUN and serum creatinine levels, indicating advanced renal insufficiency.
- X-ray or ultrasound examinations show small kidneys.

How it's treated

Treatment is essentially nonspecific and symptomatic. The goals are to control hypertension with antihypertensives and a sodium-restricted diet, correct fluid and electrolyte imbalances through restrictions and replacement, reduce edema with diuretics such as furosemide, and prevent heart failure. Treatment may also include antibiotics (for symptomatic UTIs), dialysis, or transplantation.

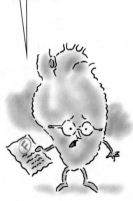

Treatment goals for glomerulonephritis include preventing heart failure. You know how I hate to fail!

What to do

• Provide supportive patient care, focusing on continual observation and sound patient teaching.
• Monitor vital signs, intake and output, and daily weight to evaluate fluid retention. Observe for signs of fluid, electrolyte, and acid-base imbalances.
• Consult the dietitian to plan low-sodium, high-calorie meals with adequate protein.
• Administer medications as ordered, and provide good oral hygiene and skin care (because of pruritus and edema).
• Evaluate the patient. After successful treatment, the patient has normal vital signs and hasn't gained weight after complying with his diet and medication regimen. He shows no signs of complications, is prepared to follow dietary and medical regimens at home, openly expresses his feelings about his illness, and exhibits good understanding of necessary procedures. (See *Chronic glomerulonephritis teaching tips*.)

Chronic renal failure

Typically the result of a gradually progressive loss of renal function, chronic renal failure occasionally results from a rapidly progressive disease of sudden onset. Few signs and symptoms develop until after more than 75% of glomerular filtration is lost. Then the remaining normal parenchyma deteriorate progressively, and signs and symptoms worsen as renal function decreases. If this condition continues unchecked, uremic toxins accumulate and produce potentially fatal physiologic changes in all major organ systems.

What causes it

Causes of chronic renal failure include:
• chronic glomerular disease such as glomerulonephritis
• chronic infections, such as chronic pyelonephritis and tuberculosis
• congenital anomalies such as polycystic kidney disease
• vascular diseases, such as renal nephrosclerosis and hypertension
• obstructive processes such as calculi
• collagen diseases such as systemic lupus erythematosus
• nephrotoxic agents such as long-term aminoglycoside therapy
• endocrine diseases such as diabetic neuropathy
• acute renal failure that fails to respond to treatment.

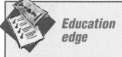

Education edge

Chronic glomerulonephritis teaching tips

• Instruct the patient to continue taking prescribed antihypertensives as scheduled, even if he's feeling better, and to report any adverse effects.
• Advise the patient to take diuretics in the morning so that sleep won't be disrupted to void. Teach the patient how to assess ankle edema.
• Warn the patient to report signs of infection, particularly urinary tract infection, and to avoid contact with infectious people.
• Urge follow-up examinations to assess renal function. Help the patient adjust to this illness by encouraging him to express his feelings.
• Explain all necessary procedures beforehand and answer the patient's questions about them.

Pathophysiology

Nephron damage is progressive. When nephrons are damaged, they can't function. Healthy nephrons compensate for damaged nephrons by enlarging and increasing their clearance capacity. The kidneys can maintain relatively normal function until about 75% of the nephrons are nonfunctional.

Unbearable burden

Eventually, the healthy glomeruli are so overburdened they become sclerotic and stiff, leading to their destruction as well. If this condition continues unchecked, toxins accumulate and produce potentially fatal changes in all major organ systems.

What to look for

The degree of renal failure partly determines the frequency and severity of clinical manifestations. (See *Effects of chronic renal failure.*)

What tests tell you

• Creatinine clearance tests can identify the stage of chronic renal failure. Reduced renal reserve occurs when the creatinine clearance GFR is 40 to 70 ml/minute. Renal insufficiency occurs at a GFR of 20 to 40 ml/minute, renal failure at a GFR of 10 to 20 ml/minute, and end-stage renal disease at a GFR of less than 10 ml/minute.
• Blood studies show elevated BUN, creatinine, and potassium levels; decreased arterial pH and bicarbonate levels; and a low Hb level and HCT.
• Urine specific gravity becomes fixed at 1.010; urinalysis may show proteinuria, glycosuria, erythrocytes, leukocytes, and casts, depending on the cause.
• X-ray studies include KUB films, excretory urography, nephrotomography, renal scan, and renal arteriography.
• Kidney biopsy allows histologic identification of the underlying abnormality.

How it's treated

The major goal of treatment early in the disease is to preserve existing kidney function and to correct specific symptoms. Conservative measures include a low-protein diet to reduce the production of end products of protein metabolism that the kidneys can't excrete. However, a patient receiving continuous peritoneal dialysis should have a high-protein diet. The patient should also consume enough calories to prevent weight loss and catabolism.

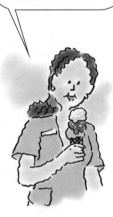

Consuming adequate calories prevents ketoacidosis in the patient with chronic renal failure. I'm not sure if that excuses a triple-scoop ice cream cone...

Effects of chronic renal failure

Chronic renal failure can affect every major body system.

Renal and urologic system
- Initially, hypotension, dry mouth, loss of skin turgor, listlessness, fatigue, and nausea from salt wasting and consequent hyponatremia
- Later, somnolence and confusion
- Salt retention and overload due to the decrease in functioning nephrons and the kidneys' subsequent inability to excrete sodium
- Muscle irritability, then weakness from accumulation of potassium
- Fluid overload from sodium retention and metabolic acidosis from loss of bicarbonate
- Decreased urine output with dilute urine that contains casts and crystals

Cardiovascular system
- Hypertension
- Arrhythmias (including life-threatening ventricular tachycardia and fibrillation)
- Cardiomyopathy
- Uremic pericarditis
- Pericardial effusion with possible cardiac tamponade
- Heart failure and peripheral edema

Respiratory system
- Reduced pulmonary macrophage activity
- Increased susceptibility to infection, pulmonary edema, pleuritic pain, pleural friction rub and effusions, uremic pleuritis and uremic lung (or uremic pneumonitis), dyspnea from heart failure, and Kussmaul's respirations as a result of acidosis

GI system
- Inflammation and ulceration of GI mucosa causing stomatitis, gum ulceration and bleeding and, possibly, parotitis, esophagitis, gastritis, duodenal ulcers, lesions on the small and large bowel, uremic colitis, pancreatitis, and proctitis
- Metallic taste in the mouth
- Uremic fetor (ammonia smell on breath)
- Anorexia
- Nausea and vomiting

Skin
- Typically, pallid, yellowish bronze, dry, and scaly skin
- Severe itching
- Purpura
- Ecchymoses
- Petechiae
- Uremic frost (usually in critically ill or terminally ill patients)
- Thin, brittle fingernails with characteristic lines
- Dry, brittle hair that may change color and fall out easily

Neurologic system
- Restless leg syndrome, one of the first signs of peripheral neuropathy, causing pain, burning, and itching in the legs and feet, which may be relieved by voluntarily shaking, moving, or rocking
- Eventually, paresthesia and motor nerve dysfunction (usually bilateral footdrop) unless dialysis is initiated
- Muscle cramping and twitching
- Shortened memory and attention span
- Apathy, drowsiness, irritability, and confusion
- Coma
- Seizures

- EEG changes that indicate metabolic encephalopathy

Endocrine system
- Stunted growth patterns in children (even with elevated growth hormone levels)
- Infertility and decreased libido in both sexes
- Amenorrhea and cessation of menses in women
- Impotence and decreased sperm production in men
- Increased aldosterone secretion
- Impaired carbohydrate metabolism

Hematopoietic system
- Anemia
- Decreased red blood cell survival time
- Blood loss from dialysis and GI bleeding
- Mild thrombocytopenia
- Platelet defects
- Increased bleeding and clotting disorders, demonstrated by purpura, hemorrhage from body orifices, easy bruising, ecchymoses, and petechiae

Musculoskeletal system
- Muscle and bone pain, skeletal demineralization, pathologic fractures, and calcifications in the brain, eyes, gums, joints, myocardium, and blood vessels caused by calcium-phosphorus imbalance and consequent parathyroid hormone imbalances
- Coronary artery disease due to arterial calcification
- Renal osteodystrophy in children

He should restrict sodium and potassium consumption as well. Maintaining fluid balance requires careful monitoring of vital signs, weight changes, and urine output.

Send in the drugs

Drug therapy commonly relieves associated signs and symptoms, but medications excreted by the kidneys may require dosage adjustments. Avoid using antacids or laxatives that contain magnesium to prevent magnesium toxicity. Drugs commonly used to treat chronic renal failure include:
• antipruritics, such as diphenhydramine (Benadryl) to relieve itching, and calcium carbonate to lower serum phosphate levels
• vitamin supplements (particularly B vitamins and vitamin D) and essential amino acids to relieve deficiencies caused by inadequate intake (from anorexia or dietary restrictions), altered metabolism (from uremia and medications), or increased losses of vitamins during dialysis
• loop diuretics, such as furosemide (if some renal function remains), along with fluid restriction to reduce fluid retention
• digoxin (Lanoxin) to mobilize edema fluids
• antihypertensives to control blood pressure and associated edema
• antiemetics taken before meals to relieve nausea and vomiting
• famotidine (Pepcid) or nizatidine (Axid) to decrease gastric irritation.

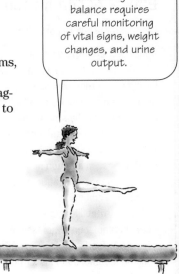

Maintaining fluid balance requires careful monitoring of vital signs, weight changes, and urine output.

Anemia ailments

Anemia necessitates iron and folate supplements; severe anemia requires infusion of fresh frozen packed cells or washed packed cells. Even so, transfusions only temporarily relieve anemia. Epoetin alfa may be administered to increase RBC production. Treatment may also include cleaning enemas to remove blood from the GI tract detected through regular stool analysis (guaiac test).

Dialysis dilemmas

Hemodialysis or peritoneal dialysis — particularly such techniques as continuous ambulatory peritoneal dialysis and continuous cyclic peritoneal dialysis — can help control most manifestations of end-stage renal disease. Altering dialyzing bath fluids can correct fluid and electrolyte disturbances. However, anemia, peripheral neuropathy, cardiopulmonary and GI complications, sexual dysfunction, and skeletal defects may persist. Also, maintenance dialysis may produce complications, such as protein wasting, refractory ascites, dialysis dementia, and hepatitis B from numerous blood transfusions.

What to do
- Monitor potassium levels.
- Assess hydration status carefully. Check for jugular vein distention and auscultate the lungs for crackles. Measure daily intake and output carefully. Record daily weight and the presence or absence of thirst, axillary sweat, dry tongue, hypertension, and peripheral edema.
- Observe for signs of bleeding.
- If the patient requires dialysis, explain the procedure fully and watch for complications during and after the procedure.
- Evaluate the patient. After successful therapy, the patient verbalizes an understanding of the disease process and medical regimen, exhibits no signs of complications, and has his signs and symptoms controlled by dialysis or transplantation. He has normal BUN, creatinine, and electrolyte levels and maintains a satisfactory diet with normal bowel function. (See *Chronic renal failure teaching tips.*)

Lower UTIs

Lower UTIs commonly respond readily to treatment, but recurrence and resistant bacterial flare-up during therapy are possible. Lower UTIs are nearly 10 times more common in women than in men and affect 1 in 5 women at least once. Lower UTIs also occur in relatively large percentages in sexually active teenage girls. Lower UTIs fall into two types:

☝ cystitis, which is an inflammation of the bladder that usually results from an ascending infection

✌ urethritis, which is an inflammation of the urethra.

What causes it
Causes of lower UTIs include:
- infection by gram-negative enteric bacteria, such as *Escherichia coli, Klebsiella, Proteus, Enterobacter, Pseudomonas,* or *Serratia*
- simultaneous infection with multiple pathogens in a patient with neurogenic bladder
- an indwelling urinary catheter
- fistula between the intestine and bladder.

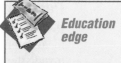

Education edge

Chronic renal failure teaching tips

- Instruct the outpatient to avoid foods high in sodium, potassium, and phosphate.
- Encourage adherence to fluid and protein restrictions.
- To prevent constipation, stress the need for exercise and sufficient dietary bulk.
- Encourage deep breathing and coughing to prevent pulmonary congestion.
- Refer the patient and his family for appropriate counseling and support.

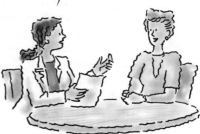

Lower UTIs are nearly 10 times more common in women than in men.

Pathophysiology

Recent studies suggest that infection results from a breakdown in local defense mechanisms in the bladder that allows bacteria to invade the bladder mucosa and multiply. These bacteria can't be readily eliminated by normal micturition.

What to look for

Characteristic signs and symptoms include:
- urinary urgency and frequency
- dysuria
- bladder cramps or spasms
- itching
- feeling of warmth during urination
- nocturia
- possibly hematuria
- fever
- urethral discharge in males.

   Other common features include lower back pain, malaise, confusion, nausea, vomiting, abdominal pain or tenderness over the bladder, chills, and flank pain.

What tests tell you

- Microscopic urinalysis showing RBC and WBC levels greater than 10/high-power field points to UTI. A clean midstream urine specimen revealing a bacterial count of more than 100,000/ml confirms it. Sensitivity testing suggests the appropriate therapeutic antimicrobial agent.
- A blood test or stained smear rules out venereal disease.
- Voiding cystourethrography or excretory urography may detect congenital anomalies.

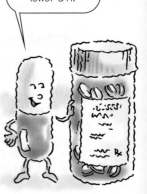

A 7- to 10-day course of antibiotics usually takes care of a lower UTI.

How it's treated

A 7- to 10-day course of an appropriate antibiotic is usually the treatment of choice for initial lower UTI. After 3 days of antibiotic therapy, a urine culture should show no organisms. If the urine isn't sterile, bacterial resistance has probably occurred, requiring a different antimicrobial. Single-dose antibiotic therapy with amoxicillin or ciprofloxacin may be effective in women with acute noncomplicated UTI. A urine culture taken 1 to 2 weeks later indicates whether the infection has been eradicated.

It's back...

Recurrent infections caused by renal calculi, chronic prostatitis, or a structural abnormality may require surgery. If the patient has no predisposing conditions, she will most likely receive long-term, low-dose antibiotic therapy.

What to do

• Collect all urine specimens for culture and sensitivity testing carefully and promptly.
• Watch for GI disturbances from antibiotic therapy. Nitrofurantoin macrocrystals, taken with milk or a meal, prevent such distress.
• Evaluate the patient. After successful treatment, the patient can explain the relation between personal hygiene and UTIs. She can describe hygiene practices to prevent UTIs and has completed the prescribed course of antibiotic therapy. (See *Lower UTI teaching tips*.)

Nephrotic syndrome

Nephrotic syndrome (NS) is a condition characterized by marked proteinuria, hypoalbuminemia, hyperlipidemia, and edema. Although NS isn't a disease itself, it results from a specific glomerular defect and indicates renal damage.

What causes it

• Primary (idiopathic) glomerulonephritis (affecting children and adults)
• Diabetes mellitus
• Collagen vascular disorders
• Circulatory diseases
• Nephrotoxins
• Allergic reactions
• Infection
• Pregnancy
• Hereditary nephritis
• Multiple myeloma and other neoplastic diseases

Pathophysiology

Regardless of the cause, the injured glomerular filtration membrane allows the loss of plasma proteins, especially albumin and immunoglobulin. Hypoalbuminemia results not only from urine loss but also from decreased hepatic synthesis of replacement albumin. Hypoalbuminemia stimulates the liver to synthesize lipoprotein (with consequent hyperlipidemia) and clotting factors.

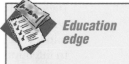

Education edge

Lower UTI teaching tips

• Explain the nature and purpose of antibiotic therapy to the patient. Emphasize the importance of completing the prescribed course of therapy and, with long-term prophylaxis, of adhering strictly to the ordered dosage.
• Urge the patient to drink plenty of water (at least eight glasses per day). Instruct the patient to avoid alcohol while taking antibiotics. Fruit juices, especially cranberry juice, and oral doses of vitamin C may help acidify the urine and enhance the action of the medication.
• Suggest warm sitz baths for relief of perineal discomfort. Advise the patient to apply heat sparingly and carefully to the perineum if baths aren't effective.

Decreased dietary intake (as with anorexia, malnutrition, or concomitant disease) further contributes to decreased plasma albumin levels. Loss of immunoglobulin also increases susceptibility to infection.

Runnin' on empty

Extensive proteinuria (more than 3.5 g/day) and a low serum albumin level lead to low serum colloid osmotic pressure and edema. The low serum albumin level also leads to hypovolemia and compensatory salt and water retention. Consequent hypertension may precipitate heart failure in compromised patients. (See *What happens in nephrotic syndrome*.)

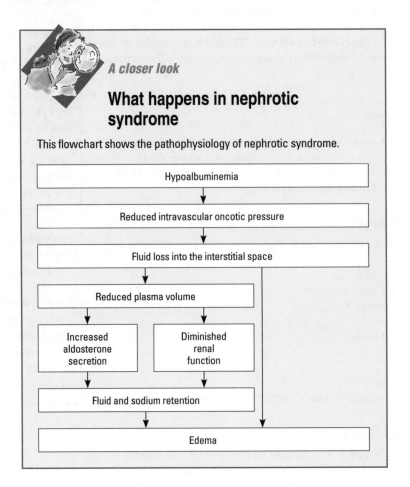

A closer look

What happens in nephrotic syndrome

This flowchart shows the pathophysiology of nephrotic syndrome.

Hypoalbuminemia

↓

Reduced intravascular oncotic pressure

↓

Fluid loss into the interstitial space

↓

Reduced plasma volume

↓

| Increased aldosterone secretion | Diminished renal function |

↓

Fluid and sodium retention

↓

Edema

What to look for

The dominant clinical feature in NS is mild to severe dependent edema of the ankles or sacrum or (especially in children) periorbital edema. It may lead to ascites, pleural effusion, and swollen external genitalia. Other signs and symptoms include:
• foamy urine
• orthostatic hypotension
• lethargy
• anorexia
• depression
• pallor.

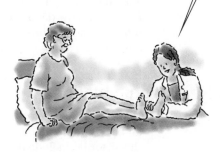

The dominant clinical feature of nephrotic syndrome is dependent edema of the ankles or sacrum.

What tests tell you

• Urine testing that reveals consistent proteinuria in excess of 3.5 g/day; an increased number of hyaline, granular, and waxy, fatty casts; and oval fat bodies strongly suggests NS.
• Increased cholesterol, phospholipid, and triglyceride levels and decreased albumin levels support the diagnosis.
• Histologic identification of the lesion requires kidney biopsy.

How it's treated

Effective treatment necessitates correction of the underlying cause if possible. Supportive treatment consists of:
• protein replacement with a nutritional diet of 1 g of protein per kilogram of body weight
• restricted sodium intake
• diuretics for edema
• antibiotics for infection.

Some patients respond to an 8-week course of corticosteroid therapy (such as prednisone), followed by a maintenance dose. Others respond better to a combination course of prednisone and azathioprine (Imuran) or cyclophosphamide (Cytoxan).

What to do

• Frequently check urine for protein. (Urine that contains protein appears frothy.)
• Measure blood pressure while the patient is supine and while he's standing; immediately report a drop in blood pressure that exceeds 20 mm Hg.
• Monitor intake and output, and check weight at the same time each morning.
• Ask the dietitian to plan a moderate-protein, low-sodium diet.

• Provide good skin care because the patient with NS usually has edema.
• To avoid thrombophlebitis, encourage activity and exercise and provide antiembolism stockings as ordered.
• To prevent GI complications, administer steroids with an antacid or with cimetidine (Tagamet) or ranitidine (Zantac).
• Evaluate the patient. After successful therapy, the patient is prepared to follow dietary and medical regimens at home, has no proteinuria, and exhibits no signs of complications. (See *Nephrotic syndrome teaching tips.*)

Neurogenic bladder

Neurogenic bladder refers to any bladder dysfunction caused by an interruption of normal bladder innervation. Other names for this disorder include neuromuscular dysfunction of the lower urinary tract, neurologic bladder dysfunction, and neuropathic bladder.

What causes it

Neurogenic bladder appears to stem from a host of underlying conditions, including:
• interstitial cystitis, cerebral disorders (such as stroke), brain tumor (such as meningioma and glioma), Parkinson's disease, multiple sclerosis, dementia, and incontinence from aging
• spinal cord disease or trauma (such as spinal stenosis and arachnoiditis), cervical spondylosis, myelopathies from hereditary disorders or nutritional deficiencies and, rarely, tabes dorsalis
• disorders of peripheral innervation, including autonomic neuropathies resulting from endocrine disturbances such as diabetes mellitus (most common)
• metabolic disturbances such as hypothyroidism
• heavy metal toxicity
• chronic alcoholism
• collagen diseases such as lupus erythematosus
• vascular diseases such as atherosclerosis
• distant effects of cancer such as primary oat cell carcinoma of the lung
• herpes zoster.

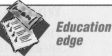

Education edge

Nephrotic syndrome teaching tips

• Watch for and teach the patient and his family how to recognize adverse effects of drug therapy, such as bone marrow toxicity from cytotoxic immunosuppressants and cushingoid symptoms from long-term steroid therapy.
• Because a steroid crisis may occur if the drug is discontinued abruptly, explain that steroid-related adverse effects will subside when therapy stops.
• Refer the patient and his family to appropriate counseling and support groups.

Pathophysiology

An upper motor neuron lesion (at or above T12) causes spastic neurogenic bladder. A lower motor neuron lesion (at or below S2 to S4) affects the spinal reflex that controls voiding, with a resulting flaccid neurogenic bladder. Mixed neurogenic bladder results from an incomplete upper motor neuron, the result of cortical damage from some disorder or trauma.

What to look for

Neurogenic bladder produces a wide range of clinical effects depending on the underlying cause and its effect on the structural integrity of the bladder. All types of neurogenic bladder are associated with:
• some degree of incontinence
• changes in initiation or interruption of micturition
• an inability to empty the bladder completely.
  Vesicoureteral reflux, deterioration or infection in the upper urinary tract, and hydroureteral nephrosis may also result.

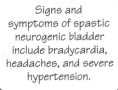

Signs and symptoms of spastic neurogenic bladder include bradycardia, headaches, and severe hypertension.

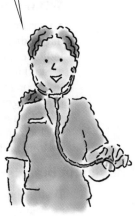

Spastic signs

Spastic neurogenic bladder signs and symptoms depend on the site and extent of the spinal cord lesion. They may include:
• involuntary, frequent, scant urination without a feeling of bladder fullness
• spontaneous spasms of the arms and legs
• increased anal sphincter tone
• voiding and spontaneous contractions of the arms and legs with tactile stimulation of the abdomen, thighs, or genitalia
• severe hypertension, bradycardia, and headaches, with bladder distention if cord lesions are in the upper thoracic (cervical) level.

Flaccid features

Clinical features of flaccid neurogenic bladder include:
• overflow incontinence
• diminished anal sphincter tone
• greatly distended bladder (evident on percussion or palpation) without the accompanying feeling of bladder fullness because of sensory impairment.

Memory jogger

All types of neurogenic bladder share three characteristic signs. So when you assess patients for this disorder, keep your eye on the ball by remembering these three I's:

Incontinence (degree varies)

Initiation changes in or interruption of micturition

Inability to empty the bladder completely.

In the mix

Signs and symptoms of mixed neurogenic bladder include:
• dulled perception of bladder fullness and a diminished ability to empty the bladder
• urgency to void without control of the bladder.

What tests tell you

• Cerebrospinal fluid analysis showing increased protein levels may indicate cord tumor; increased gamma globulin levels may indicate multiple sclerosis.
• Skull and vertebral column X-rays may show fracture, dislocation, congenital anomalies, or metastasis.
• Myelography may show spinal cord compression.
• EEG may be abnormal if a brain tumor exists.
• Electromyelography can confirm peripheral neuropathy.
• Brain and CT scans can localize and identify brain masses.

Check the bladder

Tests specifically to assess bladder function include the following:
• Cystometry evaluates bladder nerve supply and detrusor muscle tone.
• A urethral pressure profile determines urethral function.
• Uroflowmetry shows diminished or impaired urine flow.
• Retrograde urethrography reveals strictures and diverticula.
• Voiding cystourethrography evaluates bladder neck function and continence.
• A postvoid residual determination test measures the amount of urine remaining in the bladder using a catheter or bladder ultrasonography.

How it's treated

Bladder evacuation, drug therapy, surgery or, less commonly, neural blocks and electrical stimulation aim to maintain the integrity of the upper urinary tract, control infection, and prevent urinary incontinence.

Drug therapy may include oxybutynin, bethanechol, and phenoxybenzamine to promote bladder emptying and propantheline, flavoxate, dicyclomine, and imipramine (Tofranil) to facilitate urine storage. When drug therapy fails, the patient may require transurethral resection of the bladder neck, urethral dilation, external sphincterotomy, or a urinary diversion procedure to correct structural impairment. If permanent incontinence follows surgery, the patient may need an artificial urinary sphincter implanted.

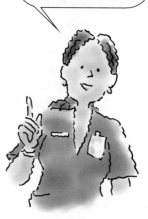

Treatment of neurogenic bladder aims to maintain upper urinary tract integrity, control infection, and prevent urinary incontinence.

What to do

• Watch for signs of infection (such as fever and cloudy or foul-smelling urine).
• Encourage the patient to drink plenty of fluids to prevent calculus formation and infection from urinary stasis. Try to keep the patient as mobile as possible.
• If the patient will undergo a urinary diversion procedure, arrange for consultation with an enterostomal therapist and coordinate the plans of care.
• Evaluate the patient. After successful therapy, the patient is free from infection, is continent, and verbalizes an understanding of his condition and the treatment techniques. (See *Neurogenic bladder teaching tips*.)

Renal calculi

Renal calculi may form anywhere in the urinary tract but usually develop in the renal pelvis or calyces. Such formation follows precipitation of substances normally dissolved in the urine (calcium oxalate, calcium phosphate, magnesium ammonium phosphate or, occasionally, urate or cystine). Renal calculi vary in size and may be solitary or multiple. They may remain in the renal pelvis or enter the ureter and may damage renal parenchyma. Large calculi cause pressure necrosis. In certain locations, calculi cause obstruction (with resultant hydronephrosis) and tend to recur. (See *Understanding renal calculi*, page 630.)

What causes it

Renal calculi may result from several causes:
• Decreased urine production from dehydration concentrates calculus-forming substances.
• An infection can result in damaged tissue that serves as a site for calculus development. Infected calculi (usually magnesium ammonium phosphate or staghorn calculi) may develop if bacteria serve as the nucleus in calculus formation. Such infections may promote destruction of renal parenchyma.
• Consistently acidic or alkaline urine provides a favorable medium for calculus formation.
• Urinary stasis (as in immobility from spinal cord injury) allows calculus constituents to collect and adhere, forming calculi. Obstruction also promotes infection which, in turn, compounds the obstruction.
• Increased intake of calcium or oxalate-rich foods encourage calculus formation.

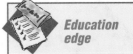

Education edge

Neurogenic bladder teaching tips

• Assure the patient that the lengthy diagnostic process is necessary to identify the most effective treatment plan.
• Explain the treatment plan to the patient in detail, and teach him and his family bladder evacuation techniques.
• Counsel the patient about sexual activities. Remember, the incontinent patient feels embarrassed and distressed. Provide emotional support.

Understanding renal calculi

Renal calculi vary in size and type. Small calculi, as shown in the first illustration, may remain in the renal pelvis or pass down the ureter. A staghorn calculus, shown in the second illustration, is a cast of the innermost part of the kidney — the calyx and renal pelvis. This type of calculus may develop from a small calculus that stays in the kidney.

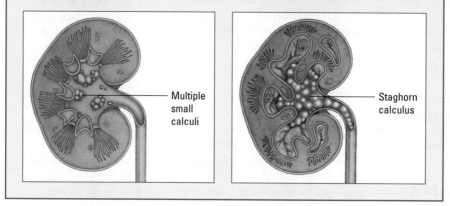

Multiple small calculi

Staghorn calculus

- Immobility from spinal cord injury or other disorders allows calcium to be released into the circulation and, eventually, filtered by the kidneys.
- Metabolic factors — including hyperparathyroidism, renal tubular acidosis, elevated uric acid levels (usually with gout), defective metabolism of oxalate, genetically defective metabolism of cystine, and excessive intake of vitamin D, protein, or dietary calcium — may predispose a patient to renal calculi.

Pathophysiology

Calculi form when substances normally dissolved in the urine, such as calcium oxalate and calcium phosphate, precipitate. Large, rough calculi may occlude the opening to the ureteropelvic junction. The frequency and force of peristaltic contractions increase, causing pain.

What to look for

Clinical effects vary with the size, location, and cause of the calculus. Pain is the key symptom. The pain of

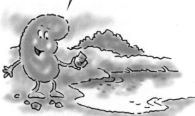

Renal calculi vary in size and may be solitary or multiple. I'll just toss this one in the pond and see what kind of splash it makes.

classic renal colic travels from the costovertebral angle to the flank, the suprapubic region, and the external genitalia. The pain fluctuates in intensity and may be excruciating at its peak. If calculi are in the renal pelvis and calyces, pain may be more constant and dull. Back pain occurs from calculi that produce an obstruction within a kidney. Nausea and vomiting usually accompany severe pain.

Other signs and symptoms include:
• abdominal distention
• fever and chills
• hematuria, pyuria and, rarely, anuria.

What tests tell you
• KUB X-rays reveal most renal calculi.
• Calculus analysis shows mineral content.
• Excretory urography confirms the diagnosis and determines the size and location of calculi.
• Renal ultrasonography may detect obstructive changes such as hydronephrosis.
• Urine culture of a midstream specimen may indicate UTI.
• Urinalysis results may be normal or may show increased specific gravity and acid or alkaline pH suitable for different types of calculus formation. Other urinalysis findings include hematuria (gross or microscopic), crystals (urate, calcium, or cystine), casts, and pyuria with or without bacteria and WBCs. A 24-hour urine collection is evaluated for calcium oxalate, phosphorus, and uric acid excretion levels.
• Other laboratory results support the diagnosis. Serial blood calcium and phosphorus levels detect hyperparathyroidism and show increased calcium levels in proportion to normal serum protein levels. Blood protein levels determine free calcium unbound to protein. Blood chloride and bicarbonate levels may show renal tubular acidosis. Increased blood uric acid levels may indicate gout as the cause.

How it's treated
Because 90% of renal calculi are smaller than 5 mm in diameter, treatment usually consists of measures to promote their natural passage. Along with vigorous hydration, such treatment includes antimicrobial therapy (varying with the cultured organism) for infection; analgesics, such as meperidine and ketorolac tromethamine, for pain; and diuretics to prevent urinary stasis and further calculus formation (thiazide diuretics decrease calcium excretion into the urine, which reduces calculus formation).

Prophylaxis to prevent calculus formation includes a low-calcium diet for absorptive hypercalciuria, parathyroidectomy for hyperparathyroidism, allopurinol for uric acid calculi, and daily administration of ascorbic acid by mouth to acidify the urine.

A calculus that's too large for natural passage may require surgical removal, percutaneous ultrasonic lithotripsy and ESWL, or chemolysis.

What to do

• Strain all urine through gauze or a urine strainer and save the solid material recovered for analysis.
• Promote sufficient intake of fluids to maintain a urine output of 3 to 4 L/day (urine should be very dilute and colorless). If the patient can't drink the required amount of fluid, he can receive supplemental I.V. fluids. Record intake and output and daily weight to assess fluid status and renal function.
• If the patient requires surgery, reassure him by supplementing and reinforcing what the surgeon has told him about the procedure. Explain preoperative and postoperative care.
• Evaluate the patient. A successfully treated and counseled patient is free from pain, has recovered the calculus, and exhibits no signs of complications. He's prepared to follow dietary and medical regimens, if necessary. He verbalizes a good understanding of his illness and the diagnostic procedures. (See *Renal calculi teaching tips*.)

Education edge

Renal calculi teaching tips

• Before discharge, teach the patient and his family the importance of following the prescribed dietary and medication regimens to prevent recurrence of calculi.
• Encourage increased fluid intake.
• Tell the patient to immediately report signs and symptoms of acute obstruction (such as pain and inability to void).

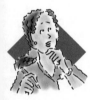

Quick quiz

1. Glomerular filtration is the process of:
   A. filtering the blood that flows through the kidney's blood vessels, or glomeruli.
   B. removing renal calculi from the ureters.
   C. measuring creatinine in the blood.
   D. reabsorbing filtered fluid.

Answer: A. Glomerular filtration is the filtering of the blood that flows through the kidney's blood vessels, or glomeruli.

2. The laboratory tests most specific to renal function are:
   A. potassium and sodium measurements.
   B. chloride and bicarbonate measurements.
   C. BUN and creatinine measurements.
   D. blood glucose and ketone measurements.

Answer: C. Although serum creatinine levels indicate renal damage more reliably than BUN levels do, you need both for a complete view of kidney function. Their simultaneous rise is the key to diagnosing kidney disease.

3. Prerenal failure results from:
   A. bilateral obstruction of urine outflow.
   B. conditions that diminish blood flow to the kidneys.
   C. damage to the kidneys themselves.
   D. any preexisting condition that contributed to renal dysfunction.

Answer: B. Prerenal failure is renal failure due to diminished blood flow to the kidneys.

4. A risk factor for developing a lower UTI is:
   A. frequent urination.
   B. elevated potassium level.
   C. urinary catheterization.
   D. ingestion of a large amount of caffeine.

Answer: C. The presence of an indwelling urinary catheter is a risk factor for developing a lower UTI because the catheter provides a pathway for bacteria to enter the bladder.

5. Which of the following factors can contribute to the formation of renal calculi?
   A. Hypocalcemia
   B. Heart failure
   C. Hypothyroidism
   D. Changes in urine pH

Answer: D. Urine that's consistently acidic or alkaline provides a favorable medium for calculus formation.

Scoring

☆☆☆ If you answered all five questions correctly, excellent! There's no obstruction to your passage of knowledge.

☆☆ If you answered three or four questions correctly, wow! You're headed for perfect filtration of information.

☆ If you answered fewer than three questions correctly, don't get spastic! Just review the chapter and try again.

Reproductive system disorders

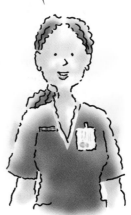

Just the facts

In this chapter, you'll learn:

◆ anatomy and physiology of the female and male reproductive systems

◆ techniques for assessing the reproductive systems

◆ tests to diagnose reproductive disorders

◆ causes, pathophysiology, diagnostic tests, and nursing interventions for common reproductive system disorders.

A look at reproductive disorders

Because of the misinformation and cultural taboos surrounding the reproductive system, reproductive disorders present a special nursing challenge. Problems such as erectile dysfunction, abnormal uterine bleeding, and infertility strike at a patient's deepest sense of self. Besides needing expert health care, each patient requires sensitive counseling and straightforward teaching.

> Cultural taboos can sometimes make discussing reproductive disorders a challenge.

Anatomy and physiology

To meet the patient's needs, you'll need a clear understanding of the female and male reproductive systems.

Female reproductive system

Major female external genitalia include the vulva, which contains the mons pubis, clitoris, labia majora, labia minora, and adjacent structures (Bartholin's glands, Skene's glands, and the urethral meatus).

Major internal genitalia include the vagina, uterus, ovaries, and fallopian tubes. (See *Reviewing the female genitalia.*)

Love those hormones!

Hormonal influences determine the development and function of external and internal female genitalia and affect fertility, childbearing, and the ability to experience sexual pleasure.

Hormones and the menstrual cycle

The hypothalamus, ovaries, and pituitary gland secrete hormones that affect the buildup and shedding of the uterine lining during the menstrual cycle. Ovulation occurs through a network of positive and negative feedback loops that run from the hypothalamus, to the pituitary, to the ovaries, and back to the hypothalamus and pituitary.

The menstrual cycle consists of three phases: menstrual (preovulatory), proliferative (follicular), and luteal (secretory). These phases correspond to the phases of ovarian function. (See *Understanding the menstrual cycle*, page 639.)

Supply exhausted

Cessation of menses usually occurs between ages 40 and 55. Although the pituitary gland still releases follicle-stimulating hormone (FSH) and luteinizing hormone (LH), the body has exhausted the supply of ovarian follicles that respond to these hormones, so menstruation no longer occurs. A woman is considered to have reached menopause after menses are absent for 1 year.

Male reproductive system

The two major organs of the male reproductive system are the penis and testes. This system supplies male sex cells through sperm formation or spermatogenesis and is involved in male sex hormone secretion. (See *Reviewing the male reproductive system*, pages 640 and 641.)

Spermatogenesis

Sperm formation begins when a male reaches puberty and usually continues throughout life. Stimulated by male sex hormones, mature sperm cells are formed continuously within the seminiferous tubules.

(Text continues on page 642.)

A closer look

Reviewing the female genitalia

External and internal structures make up the female genitalia.

External genitalia

The vulva contains the external female genitalia that are visible on inspection. The mons pubis is the cushion of adipose and connective tissue covered by skin and coarse, curly hair in a triangular pattern over the symphysis pubis (the joint formed by union of the pubic bones anteriorly).

The labia majora border the vulva laterally from the mons pubis to the perineum (muscle, fascia, and ligaments between the anus and vulva). The labia minora, two moist lesser mucosal folds, darker pink to red, lie within and alongside the labia majora.

The clitoris is the small, protuberant organ located just beneath the arch of the mons pubis. The clitoris contains erectile tissue, venous cavernous spaces, and specialized sensory corpuscles that are stimulated during coitus.

When the labia are spread, the introitus (vaginal orifice) and the urethral meatus are visible. Less easily visible are the multiple orifices of Skene's glands, mucus-producing glands located on both sides of the urethral opening.

Openings of the two mucus-producing Bartholin's glands are located laterally and posteriorly on either side of the inner vaginal orifice. The hymen, a tissue membrane varying in size and thickness, may completely or partially cover the vaginal orifice. A disrupted hymen appears as remnants of uneven mucosal tissue tags, called *myrtiform caruncles*.

View of external genitalia in lithotomy position

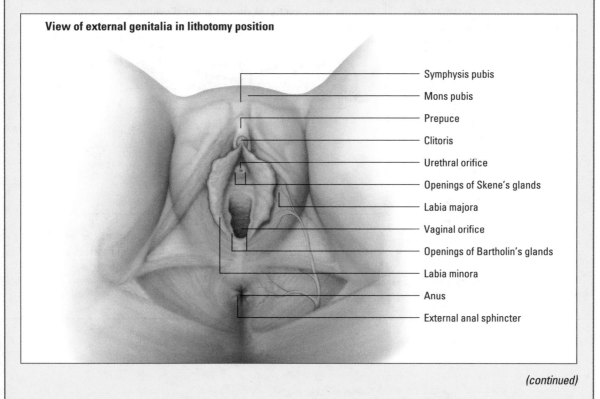

- Symphysis pubis
- Mons pubis
- Prepuce
- Clitoris
- Urethral orifice
- Openings of Skene's glands
- Labia majora
- Vaginal orifice
- Openings of Bartholin's glands
- Labia minora
- Anus
- External anal sphincter

(continued)

Reviewing the female genitalia *(continued)*

Internal genitalia

The vagina, a highly elastic muscular tube, is located between the urethra and the rectum. Between $2^1/_2$″ and $2^3/_4$″ (6.5 to 7 cm) long anteriorly and $3^1/_2$″ (9 cm) long posteriorly, the vagina lies at a 45-degree angle to the long axis of the body.

The uterus, a small, firm, pear-shaped, muscular organ, rests between the bladder and the rectum and usually lies at almost a 90-degree angle to the vagina. However, other locations may be normal. The mucous membrane lining the uterus is called the *endometrium*; the muscular layer, the *myometrium*.

In pregnancy, the elastic, upper uterine portion (the fundus) accommodates most of the growing fetus until term. The uterine neck (isthmus) joins the fundus to the cervix, the uterine part extending into the vagina. The fundus and the isthmus make up the corpus, the main uterine body.

Two fallopian tubes attach to the uterus at the upper angles of the fundus. Usually nonpalpable, these $2^3/_4$″ to $5^1/_2$″ (7 to 14 cm) long, narrow tubes of muscle fibers have fingerlike projections, called *fimbriae*, on the free ends that partially surround the ovaries. Fertilization of the ovum usually occurs in the outer one-third of the fallopian tube.

Palpable, oval, almond-shaped organs measuring $1^1/_4$″ to $1^1/_2$″ (3 to 4 cm) long, $3/_4$″ (2 cm) wide, and $1/_4$″ to

$1/_2$″ (0.5 to 1 cm) thick, the ovaries usually lie near the lateral pelvic walls, a little below the anterosuperior iliac spine.

Lateral view of internal genitalia

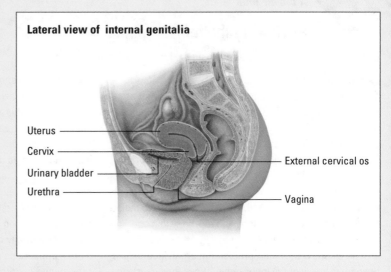

Uterus
Cervix
Urinary bladder
Urethra
External cervical os
Vagina

Anterior cross-sectional view of internal genitalia

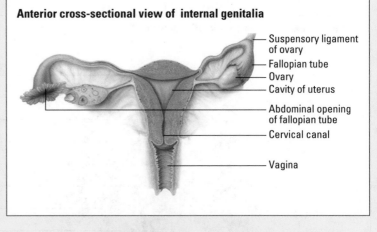

Suspensory ligament of ovary
Fallopian tube
Ovary
Cavity of uterus
Abdominal opening of fallopian tube
Cervical canal
Vagina

Understanding the menstrual cycle

The average menstrual cycle usually occurs over 28 days, although the normal cycle may range from 22 to 34 days. The cycle is regulated by fluctuating hormone levels that, in turn, are regulated by negative and positive feedback mechanisms.

Menstrual (preovulatory) phase

The cycle starts with menstruation (cycle day 1), which usually lasts 5 days. As the cycle begins, low estrogen and progesterone levels in the bloodstream stimulate the hypothalamus to secrete gonadotropin-releasing hormone (GnRH). In turn, this substance stimulates the anterior pituitary to secrete follicle-stimulating hormone (FSH) and luteinizing hormone (LH). When the FSH level rises, LH output increases.

Proliferative (follicular) phase and ovulation

The proliferative phase lasts from days 6 to 14 of the cycle. During this phase, LH and FSH act on the ovarian follicle (mature ovarian cyst containing the ovum), causing estrogen secretion, which in turn stimulates the buildup of the endometrium. Late in the proliferative phase, estrogen levels peak, FSH secretion declines, and LH secretion increases, surging at midcycle (around day 14). Then estrogen production decreases, the follicle matures, and ovulation occurs. Typically, one follicle matures during the ovulatory process and is released from the ovary during each cycle.

Luteal (secretory) phase

During the luteal phase, which lasts about 14 days, FSH and LH levels drop. Estrogen levels decline initially, then increase along with progesterone levels as the corpus luteum (progesterone-producing, yellow structure that develops after the follicle ruptures) begins functioning. During this phase, the endometrium responds to progesterone stimulation by becoming thick and secretory in preparation for implantation of a fertilized ovum.

Between 10 and 12 days after ovulation, the corpus luteum begins to diminish as do estrogen and progesterone levels, until the hormone levels are insufficient to sustain the endometrium in a fully developed secretory state. Then the endometrial lining is shed (menses).

Decreasing estrogen and progesterone levels stimulate the hypothalamus to produce GnRH, and the cycle begins again.

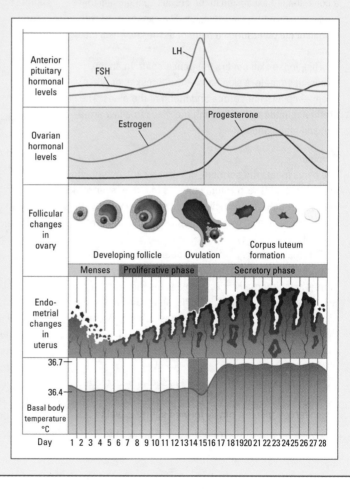

A closer look

Reviewing the male reproductive system

The male reproductive system consists of the penis, the scrotum and its contents, the prostate gland, and the inguinal structures.

Penis

Internally, the cylindrical penile shaft consists of three columns of erectile tissue bound together by heavy fibrous tissue. Two corpora cavernosa form the major part of the penis; on the underside, the corpus spongiosum encases the urethra.

The penile shaft terminates distally in the glans penis, a cone-shaped expansion of the corpus spongiosum that's highly sensitive to sexual stimulus. The expanded lateral margin of the glans forms a ridge of tissue known as the *corona*.

Thin, loose skin covers the penile shaft. In an un-circumcised male, a skin flap — the foreskin, or pre-puce — covers the corona and much of the glans. The urethral meatus opens through the glans to allow urina-tion and ejaculation.

Scrotum

The penis meets the scrotum, or scrotal sac, at the penos-crotal junction. The scrotum consists of a thin layer of skin overlying a tighter, musclelike layer, which in turn overlies the tunica vaginalis, a serous membrane covering the internal scrotal cavity.

Externally, the median raphe (seam of union of the two halves) continues from the penis to superficially bisect the scrotal skin. Internally, a septum divides the scrotum into two sacs, each containing a testis, an epididymis, and a spermatic cord. Each testis measures about 2" (5 cm) long by 1" (2.5 cm) wide and weighs about $1/2$ oz (14 g). The testes contain the seminiferous tubules, where spermato-genesis takes place.

A complex duct system conveys sperm from the tes-tes to the ejaculatory ducts near the bladder. From the seminiferous tubules, newly formed sperm travel to the epididymis — a tubular reservoir for sperm storage and maturation that curves over the posterolateral surface and upper end of the testes.

Mature sperm then move from the epididymis to the vas deferens. This duct begins at the end of the epididymis, passes up through the external inguinal canal, and descends near the bladder fundus, where it enters the ejaculatory duct inside the prostate gland. The vas def-erens is enclosed within the spermatic cord, a compact bundle of vessels, nerves, and muscle fibers.

Prostate gland

Lying under the bladder and surrounding the urethra, the walnut-size (about $1^1/2$" [4 cm] in diameter) prostate gland consists of three lobes — the left and right lateral lobes and the median lobe. The prostate continuously secretes pros-tatic fluid — a thin, milky alkaline fluid. During sexual activ-ity, prostatic fluid adds volume to the semen and enhances sperm motility and possibly fertility by neutralizing the acid-ity of the urethra and of the woman's vagina.

Inguinal structures

The spermatic cord travels from the testis through the inguinal canal, exiting the scrotum through the external inguinal ring and entering the abdominal cavity through the internal inguinal ring. The external inguinal ring is located just above and lateral to the pubic tubercle; the internal ring, about $1/2$" (1 cm) above the midpoint of the inguinal ligament, between the pubic tubercle of the sym-physis pubis and the anterior superior iliac spine.

Between the two rings lies the inguinal canal. Lymph nodes from the penis, scrotal surface, and anus drain into the inguinal lymph nodes. Lymph nodes from the testes drain into the lateral aortic and preaortic lymph nodes in the abdomen.

Male pelvic organs

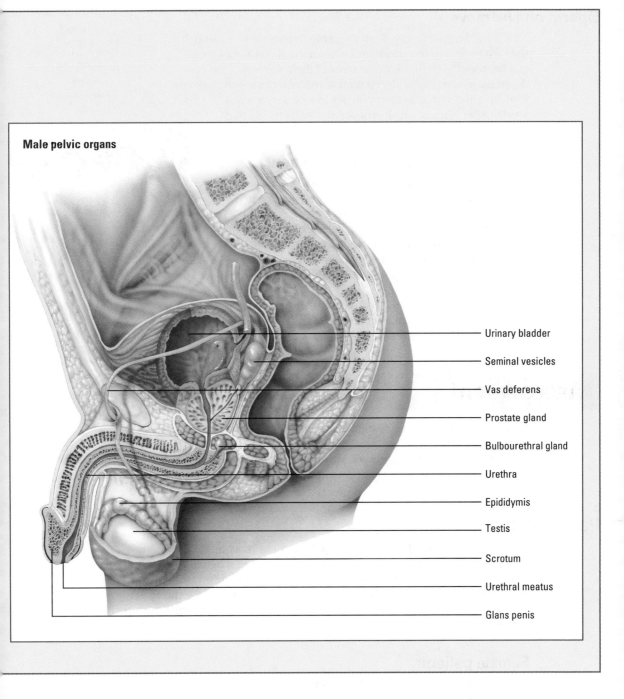

- Urinary bladder
- Seminal vesicles
- Vas deferens
- Prostate gland
- Bulbourethral gland
- Urethra
- Epididymis
- Testis
- Scrotum
- Urethral meatus
- Glans penis

Sperm on the move

Newly mature sperm pass from the seminiferous tubules through the vasa recta into the epididymis. Only a small number of sperm can be stored in the epididymis; most of them move into the vas deferens, where they're stored until sexual stimulation triggers emission. Sperm cells retain their potency in storage for many weeks. After ejaculation, sperm survive for 24 to 72 hours at body temperature.

> I can only survive for 24 to 72 hours, so I gotta get movin'!

Hormones and sexual development

Male sex hormones (androgens) are produced in the testes and the adrenal glands. Leydig's cells are located in the testes between the seminiferous tubules. These cells secrete testosterone, the most significant male sex hormone. They proliferate during puberty and remain abundant throughout life. Testosterone is responsible for the development and maintenance of male sex organs and secondary sex characteristics. It's also required for spermatogenesis.

Male sexuality is also affected by other hormones. Two of these — LH, also known as *interstitial cell-stimulating hormone*, and FSH — directly affect testosterone secretion.

Assessment

Although a reproductive system assessment may be embarrassing for your patient, it's an essential part of an examination. If performed with sensitivity and tact, your assessment may uncover concerns that the patient was previously unwilling to share.

Patient history

First, establish a good rapport to help the patient relax and confide in you. Then begin your assessment by obtaining a detailed reproductive health history. Ask your questions in a comfortable environment that protects the patient's privacy. Leave time for the patient to ask questions about his reproductive organs or sexual activity.

Female patients

Ask the patient about her chief complaint, reproductive history, family history, and social history.

Current illness

Using the PQRST method, help the patient describe her chief complaint, along with any other concerns.

Also ask about the patient's menstrual history. How old was she when she began to menstruate? How long does her period usually last? How often does it occur? Does she have cramps or an unusually heavy or light flow? When was her last period?

Metrorrhagia (bleeding between regular menstrual periods) may be normal in patients taking low-dose oral contraceptives or progesterone; otherwise, it may indicate pathology.

Age 15, period

In girls, menses generally starts about 2 years after breast budding or by age 15. If it hasn't and if no secondary sex characteristics have developed, the patient should be evaluated by a practitioner.

Reproductive history

Ask the patient if she has ever been pregnant. If so, how many times? How many times did she give birth? If she gave birth, did she have a vaginal or cesarean delivery? If indicated, ask the patient about her birth control use.

Family history

Because some reproductive problems tend to be familial, ask about family history. Ask the patient if she or anyone in her family ever had reproductive problems, hypertension, diabetes mellitus (including gestational diabetes mellitus), obesity, heart disease, or gynecologic surgery.

Social history

Ask the patient about her libido and if she's sexually active. If so, ask her when she had sexual relations last and if she has more than one partner. Ask if her sexual partner or partners have any signs or symptoms of infection, such as genital sores, warts, dysuria, or penile or vaginal discharge. If indicated, discuss safe sex practices and prevention of sexually transmitted diseases (STDs).

Male patients

The most common complaints about the male reproductive system are penile discharge, erectile dysfunction, infertility, and scrotal or inguinal masses, pain, and tenderness.

Current illness

Analyze the patient's chief complaint. Also ask him if he's circumcised. If he isn't, can he retract and replace the prepuce easily?

Inquire whether he has any pain or has noticed lumps or ulcers on his penis. These can signal an STD. Does he have scrotal swelling? This can indicate an inguinal hernia, a hematocele, epididymitis, or a testicular tumor. Ask whether he has penile discharge or bleeding.

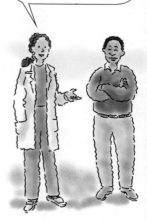

Past problems in other body systems may affect current reproductive function.

Reproductive history

If the patient had reproductive system problems in the past or had problems in other body systems, this may affect his current reproductive function. Be sure to ask these questions:
• Have you fathered any children? If so, how many and how old are they? Have you ever had a problem with infertility? If so, is it a current concern?
• Have you ever been diagnosed with an STD or other infection in the genitourinary tract? If so, what was the specific problem and were there any complications? How long did the problem last? What treatment was provided?
• Do you have a history of undescended testes or an endocrine disorder? Have you ever had mumps? If so, did the disease affect your testes?

Family history

Questions about family health history can provide clues to disorders with known familial tendencies. Ask the patient if anyone in his family has had infertility problems, a hernia, or cancer of the reproductive tract.

Social history

Obtain information about the patient's lifestyle and relationships with others. Ask the patient about his libido, if he's sexually active, and if he has more than one partner. If indicated, ask what precautions he takes to prevent contacting an STD and/or what steps he and his partner take to prevent pregnancy. If he's experiencing sexual difficulty, is it affecting his emotional and social relationships?

Physical examination

Physical assessment of the female patient involves inspection and palpation. You may examine only the external genitalia or perform a complete gynecologic examination, which includes examination of both the external and internal genitalia.

For the male patient, physical assessment involves inspecting and palpating the groin, penis, and scrotum. If the patient is age 50 or over or has a high likelihood of prostate problems, you may also palpate the prostate gland.

Examining the female patient

You may assist a practitioner with a gynecologic assessment or perform the assessment yourself. Before the examination, ask the patient to void to prevent discomfort and inaccurate findings during palpation. Have her disrobe and put on an examination gown. Then perform hand hygiene and put on gloves. Have the patient lie in the supine position, and drape all areas not being examined. Make sure you explain the procedure to her.

Begin by examining the external genitalia; then move to the internal genitalia.

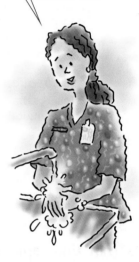

Perform hand hygiene and put on gloves before examining the patient.

Inspecting the external genitalia

If the patient complains of sores or itching, you may only need to inspect her external genitalia to determine the origin of the problem. In any case, uncover the pubic area, and inspect pubic hair for amount and pattern. In younger adult women, it's usually thick and appears on the mons pubis as well as the inner aspects of the upper thighs. Perimenopausal and postmenopausal women typically have thinner pubic hair.

Checking further

Using your index finger and thumb, gently spread the labia majora and look for the labia minora. Both labia should be pink and moist with no lesions.

Check for cervical discharge. Normal discharge varies in color and consistency. It's clear and stretchy before ovulation, white and opaque after ovulation, and usually odorless and nonirritating to the mucosa. No other discharge should be present.

Palpating the external genitalia

Next, spread the labia with one hand and palpate with the other. The labia should feel soft. Note swelling, hardness, or tenderness. If you detect a mass or lesion, palpate it to determine its size, shape, and consistency.

Main squeeze

If you find swelling or tenderness, see if you can palpate Bartholin's glands, which usually aren't palpable. To do this, insert your index finger carefully into the patient's posterior introitus, and place your thumb along the lateral edge of the swollen or tender labium. Gently squeeze the labium. If discharge from the gland results, culture it.

Examining the internal genitalia

As part of a complete gynecologic assessment, obtain a Papanicolaou (Pap) smear after inspecting the cervix. (Obtain the smear before touching the cervix in any manner.) Also obtain other specimens if an abnormal cervical or vaginal discharge indicates infection.

Examining the male patient

Before examining the reproductive system of a male patient, perform hand hygiene and put on gloves. Make the patient as comfortable as possible, and explain what you're doing every step of the way. This helps the patient feel less embarrassed.

Inspection

Inspect the penis, scrotum, and testicles as well as the inguinal and femoral areas.

Penis

First, evaluate the color and integrity of the penile skin. It should be loose and wrinkled over the shaft and taut and smooth over the glans penis. The skin should be pink to light brown in whites, light to dark brown in blacks, and free from scars, lesions, ulcers, or breaks of any kind.

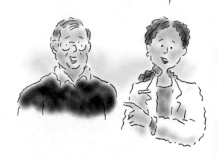

Male patients age 50 and older should also have a prostate examination.

Retract and replace

Ask an uncircumcised patient to retract his prepuce, or foreskin, to expose the glans penis. Inspect the glans for ulcers or lesions. Then ask the patient to replace the foreskin over the glans. He should be able to retract and replace the foreskin easily. Ask him about his cleaning routine.

The urethral meatus, a slitlike opening, is normally located at the tip of the glans. There should be no discharge from it.

Scrotum

First, evaluate the amount, distribution, color, and texture of pubic hair. Hair should cover the symphysis pubis and scrotum.

Scrutinizing scrotal skin

Next, inspect the scrotal skin for lesions, ulcerations, induration (hardness), or reddened areas, and evaluate the scrotal sac for symmetry and size. The scrotal skin should be coarse and more deeply pigmented than the body skin. The left testis usually hangs slightly lower than the right.

Inguinal area

Check the inguinal area for obvious bulges — a sign of hernias. Then ask the patient to bear down as you inspect again. This maneuver increases intra-abdominal pressure, which pushes a herniation downward and makes it more easily visible. Also check for enlarged lymph nodes, a sign of infection.

Palpation

After inspection, palpate the penis and scrotum for structural abnormalities; then palpate the inguinal area for hernias.

Penis

To palpate the penis, gently grasp the shaft between the thumb and first two fingers and palpate along its entire length, noting any indurated, tender, or lumpy areas. The flaccid penis should feel soft and have no nodules.

Scrotum

Like the penis, the scrotum can be palpated using the thumb and first two fingers. Begin by feeling the scrotal skin for nodules, lesions, or ulcers.

Into the sack

Next, palpate the scrotal sac. Typically, the right and left halves of the sac have identical contents and feel the same. You should feel the testes as separate, freely movable oval masses low in the scrotal sac. Their surface should feel smooth and even in contour.

Slight compression of the testes should elicit a dull, aching sensation that radiates to the patient's lower abdomen. This pressure-pain sensation shouldn't occur when the other structures are compressed. No other pain or tenderness should be present.

Posterolateral palpation

Gently palpate the epididymis on the posterolateral surface by grasping each testis between your thumb and forefinger and feeling from the epididymis to the spermatic cord or vas deferens up to the inguinal ring. The epididymis should feel like a ridge of tissue lying vertically on the testicular surface.

The vas deferens should feel like a smooth cord and be freely movable. The arteries, veins, lymph vessels, and nerves, which are located next to the vas deferens, may feel like indefinite threads.

Inguinal area

Palpate the inguinal area for hernias. A hernia will feel like a small bulge or mass.

Diagnostic tests

Diagnostic testing can help you assess reproductive organs and associated structures for abnormalities, detect cancers, or determine the cause of infertility or sexual dysfunction. Diagnostic procedures include endoscopic tests, radiographic and ultrasound studies, and tissue analyses.

Endoscopic tests

Endoscopic tests are invasive procedures that allow examination of internal reproductive structures to assess lesions, cancers, or infections or to perform various therapeutic procedures. Such tests include colposcopy and laparoscopy.

Colposcopy

During colposcopy, the examiner studies the vulva, cervix, and vagina with a colposcope, an instrument that contains a magnifying lens and a light. The areas to be studied are first bathed in white vinegar (5% acetic acid), which causes abnormal areas to turn white.

Coping with a colposcope

Although originally used to screen for cancer, colposcopy is now used to:
• evaluate abnormal cytologic specimens or grossly suspicious lesions
• examine the cervix and vagina to confirm cancer after a positive Pap test result
• monitor patients whose mothers took diethylstilbestrol during pregnancy.

    During the examination, a biopsy may be performed and photographs taken of suspicious lesions using the colposcope and its attachments.

Nursing considerations
• Tell the patient that she doesn't need to restrict food or fluids before the test.
• Explain that the procedure takes 10 to 15 minutes. A biopsy may be performed during the examination and may cause cramping and pain for a short time as well as minimal, easily controlled bleeding.
• Warn the patient to abstain from intercourse after the biopsy and not to insert anything into her vagina (except a tampon) until the practitioner confirms healing of the biopsy site.

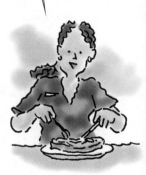

Tell the patient undergoing colposcopy that she doesn't need to worry about restricting food or fluids before the test.

- Instruct the patient to call the practitioner if she begins to bleed more heavily than during a period. She should also call the practitioner if she has signs and symptoms of infection — such as discharge, pain, and fever. Reassure her that abstaining from douching, sexual intercourse, and tub baths will help prevent these complications.

Laparoscopy

Laparoscopy allows a doctor to inspect the organs in the peritoneal cavity by inserting a small fiberoptic telescope (laparoscope) through the anterior abdominal wall.

A scope for all reasons

This test is used to:
- detect abnormalities, such as cysts, adhesions, fibroids, and infection
- determine the cause of pelvic pain
- diagnose endometriosis, ectopic pregnancy, or pelvic inflammatory disease (PID)
- evaluate pelvic masses or the fallopian tubes of infertile patients.
- stage cancer.

Therapeutic uses of this procedure include lysis of adhesions, tubal sterilization, removal of foreign bodies, and fulguration of endometriotic implants.

Nursing considerations

- Instruct the patient to fast after midnight before the test or at least 8 hours before surgery.
- Assure the patient that she'll receive either a local or general anesthetic, and tell her that the procedure will require either an outpatient visit or overnight hospitalization.
- Check the patient's history to make sure she isn't hypersensitive to the anesthetic. Make sure that all laboratory work is completed and results reported before the test.
- During the procedure, check for proper drainage of the urinary catheter, and monitor vital signs and urine output. Report sudden changes immediately — they may indicate complications. After administration of a general anesthetic, check for allergic reactions. Monitor electrolyte and hemoglobin levels and hematocrit as ordered.
- After recovery, help the patient walk as ordered. Instruct her to restrict activity for 2 to 7 days as ordered. Reassure her that some discomfort at the puncture site and in the abdomen, along with shoulder pain (from carbon dioxide pumped into the abdomen during the procedure), is normal and should disappear in 24 to 36 hours. Provide pain medication as ordered.

Radiographic and ultrasound studies

Radiographic and ultrasound studies are tests that use X-rays and high-frequency sound waves to inspect internal reproductive structures.

Hysterosalpingography

Hysterosalpingography allows the doctor to visually inspect the uterine cavity, fallopian tubes, and peritubal area. A contrast medium is injected through a cannula that's inserted through the cervix. Fluoroscopic X-rays are taken as the contrast medium flows through the uterus and the fallopian tubes.

Long name, lotsa uses

This test is usually performed as part of an infertility study to confirm tubal abnormalities, such as adhesions and occlusion, and uterine abnormalities, such as foreign bodies, congenital malformations, and traumatic injuries.

A practitioner may also order this test to evaluate repeated fetal loss or to follow up after surgery, especially uterine unification procedures and tubal reanastomosis.

Nursing considerations

• Warn the patient that she may have moderate cramping, nausea, and dizziness during or after the procedure but that she may receive a mild sedative such as diazepam (Valium) beforehand to relax her. Reassure her that these reactions are transient.
• When monitoring the patient, watch for an allergic reaction to the contrast medium (such as hives, itching, or hypotension) and for signs and symptoms of infection (such as fever, pain, increased pulse rate, malaise, and muscle aches).

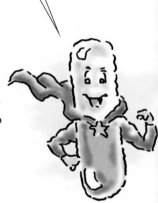

Don't worry about a thing — sedatives can be used to help the patient relax for hysterosalpingography.

Pelvic ultrasonography

During pelvic ultrasonography, a crystal generates high-frequency sound waves that are reflected to a transducer. The transducer then converts sound energy into electrical energy and forms images of the interior pelvic area on an oscilloscope screen. This test is most commonly used to:
• evaluate symptoms that suggest pelvic disease to confirm a tentative diagnosis
• determine fetal viability, position, gestational age, and growth rate during pregnancy.

Nursing considerations

• Reassure the pregnant patient that ultrasonography won't harm the fetus, and provide emotional support during the test.

- Instruct the patient that the test requires a full bladder, so she may have to drink several glasses of water beforehand. A full bladder helps to conduct the sound waves and improves the images of the pelvic organs.
- Explain that a water enema may be necessary to produce a better outline of the large intestine.
- Allow the patient to empty her bladder immediately after the test.

Tissue analysis

Analysis of cervical material may be useful for detecting cancers and infections.

Pap test

A Pap test screens for premalignant and malignant cervical changes in women who have no symptoms or findings suggesting cancer. It's widely used for:
- early detection of cervical cancer
- detection of inflammatory tissue changes that may occur with infections or other cervical diseases
- assessment of the patient's response to chemotherapy and radiation therapy.

Scrape, spread, slide

To perform a Pap test, the practitioner scrapes secretions from the patient's cervix and spreads them on a slide. After the slide is immersed in a fixative, it's sent to the laboratory for cytologic analysis.

Alternatively, the Thin Prep Pap test may be used, in which the collection device is rinsed in a vial of preservative solution and sent to the laboratory.

Paps all around

Recently, the American Congress of Obstetricians and Gynecologists (ACOG) developed new guidelines for Pap tests. These guidelines apply even to women who have been vaccinated against human papillomavirus. ACOG recommends the following schedule:
- Women ages 21 to 30 should have a Pap test every 2 years.
- Women ages 30 to 65 or 70 who have had three consecutive negative test results may undergo screening once every 3 years.
- At age 65 or 70, women who have had no abnormal test results for 10 years may stop testing.

Women with certain risk factors—such as immunosuppression, previous abnormal Pap smears, or a cervical cancer diagnosis—may need more frequent screening. Regardless of age, women who have had a total hysterectomy for noncancerous reasons shouldn't undergo routine cervical cytology testing.

Weighing the evidence

Barriers to Pap testing

Barriers to Pap testing
Even though Papanicolaou (Pap) testing is a vital screening tool, many women choose not to routinely receive a Pap test. To find out why, researchers interviewed high-risk women, examining their knowledge of and attitudes toward Pap testing and cervical cancer.

Clearing up misperceptions
The women told the researchers that they perceived their experiences with pelvic exams and Pap smears negatively. They also incorrectly believed that Pap tests were used to detect sexually transmitted diseases, and they thought that they could avoid cervical cancer without undergoing screening. The researchers concluded that exploring beliefs about Pap testing and perceptions of vulnerability to cervical cancer and providing teaching and counseling could increase Pap testing in high-risk women.

Ackerson, K., et al. (2008). Personal influencing factors associated with pap smear testing and cervical cancer. *Policy, Politics, & Nursing Practice, 9*(1), 50–60.

Nursing considerations
• Explain to the patient that the Pap test allows cervical cells to be studied. Stress the test's importance in detecting cancer at a stage when it commonly produces no symptoms and is still curable. (See *Barriers to Pap testing.*)
• Explain that the test shouldn't be scheduled during menses. The best time is 1 week before or after menses, when there are more cervical cells and less mucus.
• Instruct the patient not to have intercourse for 24 hours before the test and not to douche or insert vaginal medications for 72 hours before the test. These activities can wash away cellular deposits and change the vaginal pH.
• Obtain an accurate patient history, and note any pertinent data on the laboratory request.
• If the patient is anxious, be supportive and tell her that test results should be available within a few days.
• Just before the test, ask the patient to empty her bladder.
• Preserve the slides immediately. A delay in fixing a specimen allows the cells to dry, destroys the effectiveness of the nuclear stain, and makes cytologic interpretation difficult.
• Make sure that you aspirate and scrape the specimen from the cervix. Aspiration of the posterior fornix of the vagina can supplement a cervical specimen but shouldn't replace it.

> The best time to perform a Pap test is 1 week before or after the patient's menses.

• If vaginal or vulval lesions are present, take scrapings directly from the lesion.
• If the patient's uterus is involuted or atrophied from age, use a small pipette, if necessary, to aspirate cells from the squamocolumnar junction and the cervical canal.

Treatments

To provide effective care for the patient with a reproductive disorder, you'll need a working knowledge of current drug therapy, surgery, and related treatments.

All stressed out

Keep in mind that many of these disorders place your patient under enormous social and psychological stress, so your ability to maintain a caring, nonjudgmental attitude will prove especially valuable.

Drug therapy

Drugs are the treatment of choice for many reproductive disorders. For example, estrogens are prescribed for several disorders associated with estrogen deficiency and for inoperable prostatic cancer, breast cancer, and hypogonadism. Gonadotropins are used to treat certain forms of infertility as well as undescended testes in males. Medication in combination with disease management may help men with erectile dysfunction.

Surgery

Women with gynecologic disorders may need surgery. Gynecologic surgeries include dilatation and curettage (D&C), dilatation and evacuation (D&E), and hysterectomy. Such surgery may cause an altered body image. Therefore, you must consistently provide these patients with strong emotional support. Men with erectile dysfunction may benefit from penile prosthesis implantation.

D&C and D&E

During a D&C or D&E — the most common gynecologic procedures — the doctor expands or dilates the cervix to access the endocervix and uterus. In D&C, he uses a curette to scrape endometrial tissue. In D&E, he applies suction to extract the uterine contents.

D&C is used to treat an incomplete abortion, to control abnormal uterine bleeding, and to obtain an endometrial or endocervical tissue specimen for cytologic study. D&E is also a treatment for an incomplete abortion. In addition, it's used for a therapeutic abortion, usually up to 12 weeks' gestation but occasionally as late as 16 weeks'.

Patient preparation

Before the procedure, take these steps:
• Make sure the patient has followed preoperative directions for fasting and has used an enema to empty her colon before admission.
• Remind her that she'll be groggy after the procedure and won't be able to drive. Make sure that she has arranged for help with transportation home.
• Ask the patient to void before you administer preoperative medications, such as meperidine (Demerol) or diazepam (Valium).
• Start I.V. fluids (either dextrose 5% in water or normal saline solution) as ordered to facilitate administration of the anesthetic. The patient may receive monitored sedation, a general anesthetic, a regional paracervical block, or a local anesthetic.

Monitoring and aftercare

After the procedure, take these steps:
• Administer an analgesic as ordered. Expect the patient to have moderate cramping and pelvic and lower back pain. Continuous, sharp abdominal pain that doesn't respond to the analgesic may indicate perforation of the uterus. Report it at once.
• Monitor the patient for hemorrhage and signs of infection such as purulent, foul-smelling vaginal drainage. Also monitor the color and volume of urine (hematuria indicates infection). Report any of these signs immediately.
• Administer fluids as tolerated, and allow food if the patient requests it. Keep the bed's side rails raised, and help the patient walk to the bathroom if she's unsteady on her feet.

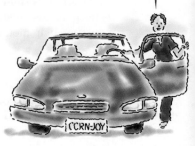

Tell the patient undergoing D&C or D&E that she'll be groggy, so she should arrange for help with transportation home.

Home care instructions

Before the patient is discharged, take these steps:
• Warn the patient to report signs of infection. Tell her not to use tampons or take tub baths until healing is complete because these activities increase the risk of infection.
• Tell her to expect moderate cramps and lower back pain, and to take analgesics as needed. Warn her that she should report unrelenting sharp pain immediately.
• Explain that spotting and discharge may last a week or longer (up to 4 weeks after an abortion procedure). She should report any bright red blood.

• Advise her to follow her practitioner's instructions for scheduling an appointment for a routine checkup.
• Tell the patient to resume activity as tolerated but to follow her practitioner's instructions concerning vigorous exercise and sexual intercourse. These are usually discouraged until 2 weeks after the follow-up visit.
• Advise the patient to seek birth control counseling if needed, and refer her to an appropriate center.

Hysterectomy

A hysterectomy involves removing the uterus. Although it can be performed using a vaginal or an abdominal approach, the abdominal approach allows better visualization of the pelvic organs and a larger operating field.

A different approach

The vaginal approach may be used to repair relaxed pelvic structures, such as cystocele or rectocele, at the same time as hysterectomy. (See *Types of hysterectomy*.)

Patient preparation

The patient will enter the hospital on the day of surgery or 1 day before. Prepare her for surgery by taking these steps:
• Take time to talk to her about what she expects from the surgery and about her menstrual and reproductive status after surgery.
• Review what the surgical approach involves and the extent of the excision.
• If the patient is having an abdominal hysterectomy, tell her that she'll need to:
– douche and have an enema the evening before surgery
– take a shower with an antibacterial soap shortly before surgery
– have an indwelling urinary catheter inserted to keep the bladder empty during surgery and to help prevent urinary retention after surgery
– have a nasogastric (NG) tube or rectal tube inserted if she develops abdominal distention
– expect temporary abdominal cramping and pelvic and lower back pain after the procedure.
• If the patient is scheduled for a vaginal hysterectomy, tell her to expect abdominal cramping afterward. She'll also have a perineal pad in place because moderate amounts of drainage occur postoperatively.
• Inform the patient that after surgery she needs to lie in a supine position or in a low- to mid-Fowler's position.
• Demonstrate the exercises that she'll need to perform to prevent venous stasis.

Types of hysterectomy

Hysterectomy is classified three ways:

☝ A total hysterectomy (panhysterectomy) involves removal of the entire uterus and cervix.

✌ A subtotal hysterectomy removes only a portion of the uterus, leaving the cervical stump intact.

🤟 A radical hysterectomy involves removing all reproductive organs, including the uterus, ovaries, fallopian tubes, and proximal vagina.

A use for each type
Total and subtotal hysterectomies are commonly performed for uterine myomas or endometrial disease. They may also be performed postpartum if the placenta fails to separate from the uterus after a cesarean delivery or if amnionitis is present. A radical hysterectomy is the treatment of choice for uterine, cervical, or ovarian cancer.

Monitoring and aftercare
After the procedure, take these steps:
- If the patient has had a vaginal hysterectomy, change her perineal pad frequently. Provide analgesics to relieve cramps.
- If she has had an abdominal hysterectomy, tell her to remain in a supine position or a low- to mid-Fowler's position. Encourage her to perform the prescribed exercises and to walk early and frequently to prevent venous stasis. Monitor her urine output because retention commonly occurs.
- If abdominal distention develops, relieve it by inserting an NG tube or rectal tube as ordered. Note bowel sounds during routine assessment.

Home care instructions
Before the patient is discharged, take these steps:
- If the patient has had a vaginal hysterectomy, instruct her to report severe cramping, heavy bleeding, or hot flashes (common with oophorectomy) to her practitioner immediately.
- If she has had an abdominal hysterectomy, tell her to avoid heavy lifting, rapid walking, or dancing, which can cause pelvic congestion. Encourage her to walk a little more each day and to avoid sitting for a prolonged period.
- Advise any posthysterectomy patient to eat a high-protein, high-residue diet to avoid constipation, which may increase abdominal pressure. The practitioner may also order increased fluid intake.
- Mention that the practitioner will inform her when she can resume sexual activity (usually 6 weeks after surgery).
- Explain to the patient and her family that abrupt hormonal fluctuations may cause the patient to feel depressed or irritable for a while. She may also have feelings of loss or depression for up to 1 year after the surgery. Encourage family members to respond calmly and with understanding.
- If her ovaries were removed, the patient may receive hormone replacement therapy, which requires monitoring.

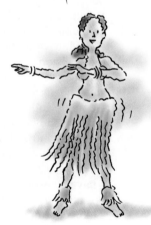

I'm afraid you'll have to avoid dancing after an abdominal hysterectomy...

Penile prosthesis implantation
A penile prosthesis is surgically implanted in the corpora cavernosa of the penis. Prostheses come in two types: those consisting of a pair of semirigid rods and those made of inflatable cylinders. They're used to treat both organic and psychogenic erectile dysfunction.

A semirigid penile prosthesis is especially helpful for the patient with limited hand or finger function because it doesn't require manual dexterity. However, the prosthesis keeps the penis semierect, which may embarrass the patient. Also, some couples complain that the semirigid prosthesis produces an erection that isn't sufficiently stiff to be sexually satisfying.

An inflatable prosthesis provides a more natural erection. The patient controls the erection by squeezing a small pump in the scrotum that releases radiopaque fluid from a reservoir into the implanted cylinders. This device, however, is contraindicated in patients with iodine sensitivity.

Patient preparation

Before implant surgery, take these steps:
- Reinforce the doctor's explanation of the surgery and answer any questions.
- Reassure the patient that the prosthesis won't affect ejaculation or orgasmic pleasure. If the patient experienced either before surgery, he can experience them afterward.
- Recognize that the patient and his partner are likely to be anxious before surgery, so provide emotional support.

Squeaky clean

- Instruct the patient to shower both the evening before and the morning of surgery, using an antimicrobial soap.
- Begin antibiotic therapy if ordered.

Monitoring and aftercare

After surgery, take these steps:
- Apply ice packs to the patient's penis for 24 hours after surgery.
- Empty the surgical drain when it's full, or as ordered, to reduce the risk of infection.
- If the patient has an inflatable prosthesis, tell him to pull the scrotal pump downward to ensure proper alignment.
- With the practitioner's approval, encourage the patient to practice inflating and deflating the prosthesis when the pain subsides. Pumping promotes healing of the tissue sheath around the reservoir and pump.

Home care instructions

Before the patient is discharged, take these steps:
• Tell the patient to wash the incision daily with an antimicrobial soap.
• Caution him to watch for signs of infection and to report them to the practitioner immediately.
• Inform him that scrotal swelling and discoloration may last up to 3 weeks.

Nursing diagnoses

Two nursing diagnoses are commonly used when referring to patients with reproductive disorders. These diagnoses are discussed here, along with appropriate nursing interventions and rationales. See *NANDA-I taxonomy II by domain*, page 936, for the complete list of NANDA diagnoses.

Sexual dysfunction

Related to altered body structure or psychological stress, *Sexual dysfunction* can be applied to such conditions as endometriosis, PID, arousal and orgasmic dysfunction, dyspareunia, vaginismus, impotence, or premature ejaculation.

Expected outcomes

• Patient states understanding of sexual dysfunction related to his current situation.
• Patient discusses concerns with spouse or significant other.
• Patient has resources for postdischarge support, including a sex counselor and other appropriate professional, if necessary.

Nursing interventions and rationales

• Provide a nonthreatening, nonjudgmental atmosphere. This enhances communication and understanding between patient and caregiver.
• Allow the patient to express his feelings openly. This encourages him to ask questions specifically related to his current situation.
• Suggest that the patient discuss concerns with his partner. Sharing concerns helps strengthen relationships.

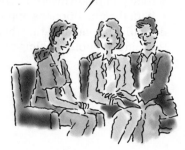

Encourage patients to share their sexuality concerns with their partners.

• Provide support for the patient's partner. Supportive interventions (such as active listening) communicate concern, interest, and acceptance.
• Educate the patient and his spouse or partner about limitations that the patient's physical condition imposes on sexual activity. Understanding these limitations helps the patient avoid complications or injury.
• Suggest referral to a sex counselor or other appropriate professional for future guidance and support.

Ineffective sexuality pattern

Related to illness or medical treatment, *Ineffective sexuality pattern* may be associated with genitourinary or gynecologic disorders or with STDs, such as AIDS, herpes, gonorrhea, and syphilis.

Expected outcomes
• Patient understands diagnosis and treatment.
• Patient communicates with partner concerns regarding change in sexual patterns.

Nursing interventions and rationales
• Plan for uninterrupted time to talk with the patient. This demonstrates your comfort with sexuality issues and reassures the patient that his concerns are acceptable for discussion.
• Provide a nonthreatening, nonjudgmental atmosphere to encourage the patient to express feelings about perceived changes in sexual identity and behaviors. This demonstrates unconditional positive regard for the patient and his concerns.
• Provide the patient and partner with information about the illness and its treatment. Answer questions and clarify any misconceptions. This helps them focus on specific concerns, encourages questions, and avoids misunderstandings.
• Encourage social interaction and communication between the patient and partner. This fosters sharing of concerns and strengthens relationships.
• Offer referral to counselors or support persons, such as a mental health professional, a sex counselor, or an illness-related support group (such as I Can Cope, Reach for Recovery, and the Ostomy Association).

Common reproductive disorders

This section discusses common female and male reproductive disorders, including STDs. For each disorder, you'll find information on causes, assessment findings, diagnostic tests, treatments, nursing interventions, patient teaching, and evaluation criteria.

Endometriosis

In endometriosis, benign endometrial tissue appears outside the lining of the uterine cavity. This ectopic tissue can appear anywhere in the body, but it usually remains in the pelvic area, around the ovaries, fallopian tubes, uterosacral ligaments, and uterovesical peritoneum.

The age of endometriosis

Active endometriosis usually occurs between ages 25 and 35, especially in women who postpone childbearing. Severe symptoms of endometriosis may occur abruptly or develop slowly over many years.

Generally, endometriosis becomes progressively more severe during the menstrual years, and then subsides after menopause. Infertility is the primary complication, although spontaneous abortion may also occur.

Going through stages

A scoring and staging system created by the American Fertility Society quantifies endometrial implants according to size, character, and location.
- Stage I is minimal disease.
- Stage II signifies mild disease.
- Stage III indicates moderate disease.
- Stage IV indicates severe disease.

What causes it

The direct cause is unknown, but having a family member with the disease or having recent surgery that required opening the uterus (such as a cesarean birth) may predispose a woman to endometriosis. Other causes include immune system defects, inflammatory influence, spread through the lymphatic system, or environmental contaminants.

Endometriosis may be in your patient's future if she's between ages 25 and 35 and she has postponed childbearing.

Pathophysiology

Ectopic endometrial tissue responds to estrogen and progesterone with proliferation and secretion. During menstruation, ectopic tissue bleeds and causes inflammation of the surrounding tissues. Inflammation leads to fibrosis, and fibrosis leads to adhesions that produce pain and infertility.

What to look for

Acquired dysmenorrhea is the classic symptom of endometriosis. Pain may be constant. It usually begins 5 to 7 days before menses and lasts for 2 to 3 days.

What a pain

The pain may be in the lower abdomen, vagina, posterior pelvis, and back. It commonly radiates down the legs. Multiple tender nodules occur on uterosacral ligaments or in the rectovaginal system. They enlarge and become more tender during menses. Ovarian enlargement may also be evident on palpation.

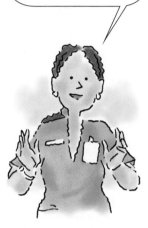

Dysmenorrhea is the classic symptom of endometriosis. Pain usually begins 5 to 7 days before menses and lasts for 2 to 3 days.

Location, location, location

Other signs and symptoms depend on the location of the ectopic tissue:
• appendix and small bowel: nausea and vomiting, which worsen before menses, and abdominal cramps
• bladder: suprapubic pain, dysuria, and hematuria
• cervix, perineum, and vagina: bleeding from endometrial deposits in these areas during menses
• colon and rectovaginal septum: painful bowel movements, rectal bleeding with menses, and pain in the coccyx or sacrum
• cul-de-sac or ovaries: deep-thrust dyspareunia
• ovaries and oviducts: infertility and profuse menses.

What tests tell you

• Laparoscopy may confirm the diagnosis and determine the stage of the disease.
• Barium enema rules out malignant or inflammatory bowel disease.

How it's treated

Treatment varies according to the stage of the disease, the patient's age, and her desire to have children. It includes:
• For young women who want to become pregnant: Conservative therapy includes androgens such as danazol, which produce a temporary remission in stages I and II. Progestins and hormonal contraceptives also relieve symptoms.

• With extensive disease (stages III and IV) or for women who don't want to become pregnant: When ovarian masses are present, they should be removed to rule out cancer. Although this may be accomplished with conservative surgery, the treatment of choice is a total abdominal hysterectomy performed with bilateral salpingo-oophorectomy.

What to do

• Encourage the patient to contact a support group such as the Endometriosis Association for further information and counseling. Remind her to have an annual pelvic examination and Pap test.
• Note whether the patient is free from pain or can at least manage symptoms.
• Check for postoperative complications.
• Explain the possible consequences of delaying surgery if applicable.
• Make sure she understands the importance of frequent gynecologic examinations. (See *Endometriosis teaching tips.*)

Erectile dysfunction

Erectile dysfunction, also known as *impotence*, prevents a man from achieving or maintaining penile erection sufficient to complete intercourse. Two types of impotence exist:

Primary impotence means that the patient has never achieved a sufficient erection.

Secondary impotence (more common and less serious) means that the patient has achieved and maintained erections in the past, even though he can't do so now.

Erectile dysfunction affects men of all ages but is more common and frequent in older men. The prognosis depends on the severity and duration of impotence and on the underlying cause. Transient periods of erectile dysfunction aren't considered dysfunctional and probably occur in 50% of adult males.

What causes it

Eighty percent of cases are believed to have an organic cause, such as arterial insufficiency or, more commonly, venous outflow dysfunction. Other organic causes include alcohol and drug abuse and medications such as amitriptyline, cimetidine (Tagamet), clonidine (Catapres), desipramine (Norpramin), digoxin (Lanoxin), hydralazine, methyldopa, nortriptyline (Aventyl), propranolol (Inderal), thiazide diuretics, and tranylcypromine (Parnate).

Education edge

Endometriosis teaching tips

• Advise the patient to use sanitary napkins instead of tampons if she's an adolescent. This helps prevent retrograde flow in a girl with a narrow vagina or small introitus.
• Warn her that infertility is a possible complication, so if she wants children, she shouldn't postpone childbearing.
• Stress the importance of treatment to prevent or postpone complications, which can include infertility.
• Teach her about strategies to relieve pain, including medications.
• Teach her how to recognize endometrioma rupture and what to do if it occurs.
• Teach her how to relieve dyspareunia and how to recognize and prevent symptoms of anemia.

Twenty percent of cases are believed to be psychogenic in nature, resulting from sexual performance anxiety, low self-esteem, or past failures in sustaining an erection.

Pathophysiology

Inappropriate adrenergic stimulation can cause a lack of autonomic signal or impairment of perfusion. This may interfere with arteriolar dilation and cause premature collapse of the sacs of the corpus cavernosum.

Psychogenic causes may exacerbate emotional problems in a circular pattern, with anxiety causing fear of erectile dysfunction, which in turn causes further emotional problems.

Anticlimax

In arterial insufficiency, there may be inadequate blood flow to the penis. In venous insufficiency, incompetent valves in the veins may cause the blood to exit the penis too quickly and diminish or prevent erection. In addition, pelvic steal syndrome causes increased blood flow to the pelvic muscles, resulting in loss of erection before ejaculation.

What to look for

Begin by assessing the patient's entire health history, including his past and current medications, psychosocial history, and use of alcohol and street drugs. Because the patient's erectile dysfunction won't be obvious to you, you'll need to ask him questions to learn more about it. If he has secondary erectile dysfunction, base your questions on these categories:

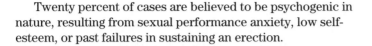 partial: patient can't achieve a full erection

intermittent: patient can sometimes maintain erection with the same partner

selective: patient can maintain erection only with certain partners.

Sorry, but I have to ask

Also ask the patient if he lost erectile function suddenly or gradually. Ask if he ever has an erection upon awakening in the morning. If the cause of his erectile dysfunction is psychogenic, ask if he can still achieve erection through masturbation. Ask how he feels before trying to have intercourse — is he anxious, with sweating and palpitations? Is he totally disinterested in sexual activity?

Also ask the patient if he's depressed. Depression can cause psychogenic impotence and result from both psychogenic and organic impotence.

What tests tell you

Diagnosis can generally be made from the patient's history and physical examination. The following tests can aid in diagnosis:
• Blood tests may help identify underlying causes, such as vascular disease, diabetes, or low testosterone levels.
• Ultrasound imaging and Doppler studies can help identify penile blood flow patterns and problems.

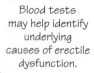

Blood tests may help identify underlying causes of erectile dysfunction.

How it's treated

Treatment includes these measures:
• Sex therapy, largely directed at reducing performance anxiety, may cure psychogenic impotence. Such therapy should include both partners.
• If erectile dysfunction is caused by drug or alcohol abuse, treatment of those specific problems may be the solution.
• Treatment of organic impotence focuses on reversing the cause if possible. If not, psychological counseling may help the couple deal realistically with their situation and explore alternatives for sexual expression.
• Certain patients suffering from organic impotence may benefit from surgically inserted penile implants; those with low testosterone levels, from testosterone replacement therapy.
• Oral erectile dysfunction drugs, such as vardenafil (Levitra), sildenafil (Viagra), and tadalafil (Cialis), help increase blood flow to the penis when it is stimulated, resulting in a harder erection. Other drugs that cause erection, such as alprostadil (Edex), can be injected into the penis or given by penile suppository.
• Vacuum constriction devices can temporarily produce an erection by creating a vacuum that pulls blood into the penis.

What to do

• Help the patient feel comfortable about discussing his sexuality. Assess his sexual health during your initial nursing history. When appropriate, refer him for further evaluation or treatment.
• Help prevent erectile dysfunction by providing information about resuming sexual activity as part of your discharge instructions for any patient with a condition that requires modification of daily activities. Such patients include those with cardiac disease, diabetes, hypertension, or chronic obstructive pulmonary disease, and all postoperative patients.

- Evaluate the patient. He should report achieving and maintaining an erection and express satisfaction with his sexual relationships. (See *Erectile dysfunction teaching tips.*)

PID

PID refers to any acute, subacute, recurrent, or chronic infection of the oviducts and ovaries, with adjacent tissue involvement. It includes inflammation of the cervix (cervicitis), uterus (endometritis), fallopian tubes (salpingitis), and ovaries (oophoritis), which can extend to the connective tissue lying between the broad ligaments (parametritis). (See *Three types of PID*, page 666.)

No time to waste!

Early diagnosis and treatment prevent damage to the reproductive system. Complications of PID include infertility and potentially fatal septicemia, pulmonary emboli, and shock. Untreated PID may be fatal.

What causes it

PID can result from infection with aerobic or anaerobic organisms. About 60% of cases result from overgrowth of one or more of the common bacterial species found in cervical mucus, including staphylococci, streptococci, diphtheroids, chlamydiae, and coliforms such as *Pseudomonas* and *Escherichia coli*.

PID also results from infection with *Neisseria gonorrhoeae*. Finally, multiplication of typically nonpathogenic bacteria in an altered endometrial environment can cause PID. This occurs most commonly during parturition.

PID promoters

These factors increase the patient's chances of developing PID:
- history of STD or bacterial vaginosis
- more than one sexual partner
- conditions, such as uterine infection, or procedures, such as conization or cauterization of the cervix, that alter or destroy cervical mucus, allowing bacteria to ascend into the uterine cavity
- any procedure that risks transfer of contaminated cervical mucus into the endometrial cavity by instrumentation, such as use of a biopsy curet or an irrigation catheter, tubal insufflation, abortion, or pelvic surgery
- infection during or after pregnancy
- an infectious focus within the body, such as drainage from a chronically infected fallopian tube, a pelvic abscess, a ruptured appendix, or diverticulitis of the sigmoid colon.

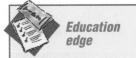

Education edge

Erectile dysfunction teaching tips

- If the patient has had penile implant surgery, tell him to avoid intercourse until the incision site heals, usually in 6 weeks.
- If he has an inflatable prosthesis, provide instructions for its use.
- If he is taking an erectile dysfunction drug, warn him not to take nitrates without first talking to his practitioner.

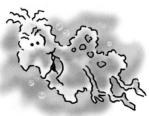

About 60% of PID cases result from overgrowth of common bacterial species.

Three types of PID

Pelvic inflammatory disease (PID) can be classified in three ways, each with its own signs and symptoms and diagnostic findings.

Cause and signs and symptoms	Diagnostic findings
Cervicitis	
• *Acute:* Purulent, foul-smelling vaginal discharge; vulvovaginitis, with itching or burning; red, edematous cervix; cervical bleeding; pelvic discomfort; sexual dysfunction; metrorrhagia; infertility; spontaneous abortion • *Chronic:* Cervical dystocia, laceration or eversion of the cervix, ulcerative vesicular lesion (when cervicitis results from herpes simplex virus type 2)	• Cultures for *Neisseria gonorrhoeae* are positive. • With chronic cervicitis, causative organisms are usually staphylococcus or streptococcus. • Cytologic smears may reveal severe inflammation. • If cervicitis isn't complicated by salpingitis, white blood cell (WBC) count is normal or slightly elevated; erythrocyte sedimentation rate (ESR) is elevated. • With acute cervicitis, cervical palpation reveals tenderness.
Endometritis (usually postpartum or postabortion)	
• *Acute:* Mucopurulent or purulent vaginal discharge oozing from cervix; edematous, hyperemic endometrium, possibly leading to ulceration and necrosis (with virulent organisms); lower abdominal pain and tenderness; fever; rebound pain; abdominal muscle spasm; thrombophlebitis of uterine and pelvic vessels • *Chronic:* Recurring acute episodes (usually from having multiple sexual partners and sexually transmitted infections)	• With severe infection, palpation may reveal boggy uterus. • Uterine and blood samples are positive for causative organism, usually staphylococcus. • WBC count and ESR are elevated.
Salpingo-oophoritis	
• *Acute:* Sudden onset of lower abdominal and pelvic pain, usually after menses; increased vaginal discharge; fever; malaise; lower abdominal pressure and tenderness; tachycardia; pelvic peritonitis • *Chronic:* Recurring acute episodes	• Elevated or normal WBC count. • X-ray may show ileus. • Pelvic examination reveals extreme tenderness. • Smear of cervical or periurethral gland exudate shows gram-negative intracellular diplococci.

Pathophysiology

Various conditions, procedures, or instruments can alter or destroy the cervical mucus, which usually serves as a protective barrier. As a result, bacteria enter the uterine cavity, causing inflammation of various structures.

What to look for

Signs and symptoms vary with the affected area and include:
• profuse, purulent vaginal discharge
• low-grade fever and malaise (especially if *N. gonorrhoeae* is the cause)
• lower abdominal pain
• extreme pain on movement of the cervix or palpation of the adnexa.

What tests tell you

• Gram stain of secretions from the endocervix or cul-de-sac to help identify the infecting organism.
• Culture and sensitivity testing to aid selection of the appropriate antibiotic. Urethral and rectal secretions may also be cultured.
• Ultrasonography to identify an adnexal or uterine mass.
• Culdocentesis to obtain peritoneal fluid or pus for culture and sensitivity testing.

How it's treated

Effective management eradicates the infection, relieves symptoms, and leaves the reproductive system intact. It includes:
• Aggressive therapy with multiple antibiotics beginning immediately after culture specimens are obtained. Therapy can be reevaluated as soon as laboratory results are available (usually after 24 to 48 hours). Infection may become chronic if treated inadequately.
• For PID resulting from gonorrhea: I.V. doxycycline (Vibramycin) and I.V. cefoxitin, followed by doxycycline by mouth (P.O.). Outpatient therapy may consist of I.M. cefoxitin, amoxicillin P.O., or ampicillin P.O. (each with probenecid), followed by doxycycline P.O. A patient with gonorrhea may also require therapy for syphilis.
• Supplemental treatment, including bed rest, analgesics, and I.V. therapy.
• Adequate drainage if a pelvic abscess develops.
• For a ruptured pelvic abscess (a life-threatening complication): Possible total abdominal hysterectomy with bilateral salpingo-oophorectomy.
• Nonsteroidal anti-inflammatory drugs for pain relief (preferred treatment); opioids if necessary.

What to do

• After establishing that the patient has no drug allergies, administer antibiotics and analgesics as ordered.
• Check for elevated temperature.
• Watch for abdominal rigidity and distention, possible signs of developing peritonitis.
• Provide frequent perineal care if vaginal drainage occurs.
• Evaluate the patient. She shouldn't have pain, discharge, fever, or recurring infection. However, many patients experience occasional pain, and up to 25% may become infertile after one episode of PID. (See *PID teaching tips*.)

STDs

STDs are the most common infections in the United States, and chlamydia infection is the most common STD. Morbidity and mortality depend on the type and stage of the disease. Many STDs are easy to treat when detected early.

What causes it

Transmission of the causative organism, which may include bacteria, viruses, protozoans, fungi, or ectoparasites, leads to infection. Patients at high risk include those:

 younger than age 25

 with multiple sexual partners

 with a history of STDs.

Four groups not to join

The incidence of STDs is higher among prostitutes, people having sexual contact with prostitutes, drug abusers, and prison inmates.

Pathophysiology

These contagious diseases are usually transmitted through intimate sexual contact with an infected person. Some are transmitted to an infant during pregnancy or childbirth.

What to look for

The chief signs of STDs are vaginitis, vaginal or penile discharge, epididymitis, lower abdominal pain, pharyngitis, proctitis, and skin or mucous membrane lesions.

Education edge

PID teaching tips

• To prevent recurrence, encourage compliance with treatment, and explain the nature and seriousness of PID.
• Because PID may cause painful intercourse, advise the patient to consult with her practitioner about sexual activity.
• Stress the need for the patient's sexual partner to be examined and treated for infection.
• To prevent infection after minor gynecologic procedures such as dilatation and curettage, tell the patient to immediately report fever, increased vaginal discharge, or pain. After such procedures, instruct her to avoid douching and intercourse for at least 7 days.

The stealthy STD

Many STDs produce no symptoms, especially in women. By the time the STD is detected, the woman may have severe complications, such as PID, infertility, ectopic pregnancy, or chronic pelvic pain.

What tests tell you

The diagnosis of a specific STD is made by physical examination, patient history, and laboratory tests to determine the causative organism.

How it's treated

Treatment is based on the specific causative organism. Treatment guidelines for each STD are available from the Centers for Disease Control and Prevention (CDC). (See *Common sexually transmitted diseases*, pages 670 and 671.)

Recommended resources

The CDC recommends that these resources be available for patients with STDs:
• medical evaluation and treatment facilities for patients with human immunodeficiency virus infection
• hospitalization facilities for patients with complicated STDs, such as PID and disseminated gonococcal infection
• referrals for medical, pediatric, infectious disease, dermatologic, and gynecologic-obstetric services
• family-planning services
• substance abuse treatment programs.

What to do

• Ensure the patient's privacy and confidentiality. Avoid judging the patient's lifestyle and making assumptions about his sexual preference.
• Provide emotional support, and encourage the patient to discuss his feelings. He may be anxious and fearful and may experience altered self-esteem and self-image.
• Evaluate the patient. When assessing treatment outcome, note whether the patient remains asymptomatic without recurrent infections. Make sure the patient understands how to prevent spreading the infection. (See *STD teaching tips*.)

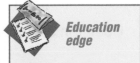

Education edge

STD teaching tips

• Discuss disease transmission, signs and symptoms, the length of the infectious period, infection prevention, and treatment options.
• Explain the health consequences of improper treatment, and emphasize that the patient's partner is also at risk.
• Clarify common misconceptions, and promote understanding of healthful sexual practices.
• Tell the patient to seek immediate treatment if STD symptoms develop.
• Discuss modifications of sexual activity to prevent recurrence: reducing the number of sexual partners, avoiding partners who have multiple partners, and questioning partners about their STD history.
• Talk to the patient about using condoms to prevent transmission of STDs.

Common sexually transmitted diseases

Name and organism	Possible signs and symptoms	Treatment	Special considerations
Chlamydia *Chlamydia* *trachomatis*	• Purulent discharge • *Males:* burning on urination and symptoms of epididymitis • *Females:* usually asymptomatic	Doxycycline (Vibramycin) or azithromycin (Zithromax)	• All sexual contacts must be treated. • Potential complications in females are pelvic inflammatory disease (PID), infertility, and spontaneous abortion; in males, urethritis, epididymitis, and prostatitis. • Patient should take medication as prescribed, follow up in 7 to 10 days, and abstain from sexual activity until treatment is completed.
Genital herpes, herpes simplex Type 2	• *Females:* purulent vaginal discharge • Multiple vesicles on genital area, buttocks, or thighs • Painful dysuria • Fever • Headache • Malaise	Famciclovir (Famvir), valacyclovir (Valtrex), acyclovir (Zovirax), topical anesthetic ointment	• Warm baths and mild analgesics may relieve pain. • Patient should avoid sexual activity during the prodromal stage and during outbreaks until all lesions have dried up. • Many patients have recurrences every 2 to 3 months; local hyperesthesias may occur 24 hours before outbreak of lesions.
Gonorrhea *Neisseria* *gonorrhoeae*	• Purulent discharge • Dysuria • Urinary frequency	Cephalosporins	• All sexual contacts must be treated. • Potential complications in females are PID, sterility, and ectopic pregnancy; in males, prostatitis, urethritis, epididymitis, and sterility. • Patient should take medication as prescribed, follow up in 7 to 10 days, and abstain from sexual activity until treatment is completed.
Human papillomavirus (HPV)	• Pink-gray soft lesions, singularly or in clusters	Podophyllin 10% to 25% to lesions, cryosurgery	• Female patient should receive frequent Papanicolaou tests. • HPV has an 80% chance of recurrence. • HPV is the most common cause of cervical cancer. • The vaccines Gardasil and Cervarix provide protection against HPV and can be given to women ages 9 to 26; Gardasil is also approved for males ages 9 to 26.

Common sexually transmitted diseases (continued)

Name and organism	Possible signs and symptoms	Treatment	Special considerations
Syphilis *Treponema pallidum*	• Chancre on genitalia, mouth, lips, or rectum • Fever • Lymphadenopathy • Positive results for Venereal Disease Research Laboratories test, fluorescent treponemal antibodies test, and rapid plasma reagin test	Penicillin	• Syphilis may be characterized as primary, secondary, or tertiary. • All sexual contacts must be treated. • Patient should take medication as prescribed, follow up in 7 to 10 days, and abstain from sexual activity until treatment is completed.
Trichomoniasis *Trichomonas vaginalis*	• *Males:* urethritis or penile lesions; usually asymptomatic • *Females:* frothy vaginal discharge with erythema and pruritus; may be asymptomatic	Metronidazole (Flagyl)	• All sexual contacts must be treated. • Complications in females include recurrent infections and salpingitis. • Patient should take medication as prescribed, follow up in 7 to 10 days, and abstain from sexual activity until treatment is completed.

Testicular torsion

Testicular torsion is the abnormal twisting of the spermatic cord that results from rotation of a testis or the mesorchium (a fold in the area between the testis and epididymis). It causes strangulation and, if untreated, eventual infarction of the testis.

This condition is almost always unilateral. Although it's most common between ages 12 and 18, it may occur at any age. The prognosis is good with early detection and prompt treatment.

What causes it

Testicular torsion is caused in part by abnormalities inside or outside the tunica vaginalis, the serous membrane covering the internal scrotal cavity.

Twist and shout

Intravaginal torsion is caused by:
• abnormality of the tunica vaginalis and the position of the testis
• incomplete attachment of the testis and spermatic fascia to the scrotal wall, leaving the testis free to rotate around its vascular pedicle.

Extravaginal torsion is caused by:
• loose attachment of the tunica vaginalis to the scrotal lining, causing spermatic cord rotation above the testis
• sudden forceful contraction of the cremaster muscle due to physical exertion or irritation of the muscle.

Pathophysiology

In testicular torsion, the testis rotates on its vascular pedicle and twists the arteries and vein in the spermatic cord. This interrupts blood flow to the testis, resulting in vascular engorgement, ischemia, and scrotal swelling.

What to look for

Torsion produces excruciating pain in the affected testis or iliac fossa. Physical examination reveals tense, tender swelling in the scrotum or inguinal canal and hyperemia of the overlying skin. Scrotal swelling is unrelieved by rest or elevation of the scrotum.

What tests tell you

• Doppler ultrasonography helps distinguish testicular torsion from strangulated hernia, undescended testes, or epididymitis.

How it's treated

If manual reduction is unsuccessful, torsion must be surgically corrected within 6 hours after the onset of symptoms to preserve testicular function (70% salvage rate). Treatment consists of immediate surgical repair by orchiopexy (fixation of a viable testis to the scrotum) or orchiectomy (excision of a nonviable testis).

Without treatment, the testis becomes dysfunctional and necrotic after 12 hours.

What to do

• Before surgery, promote the patient's comfort as much as possible. After surgery, take these steps:
– Administer pain medication as ordered.
– Monitor voiding, and apply an ice bag with a cover to reduce edema.
– Protect the wound from contamination. Otherwise, allow the patient to perform as many normal daily activities as possible.
– Evaluate the patient for pain and postoperative complications. (See *Testicular torsion teaching tips.*)

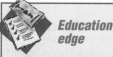

Education edge

Testicular torsion teaching tips

• Explain the surgical procedure and post-operative care to the patient. Even if the testis must be removed, reassure him that his sexual function and fertility should be unaffected.
• Recommend that the patient routinely wear a scrotal support while exercising.

Uterine leiomyomas

Also known as *myomas*, *fibromyomas*, and *fibroids*, uterine leiomyomas are the most common benign tumors in women. They usually occur in the uterine corpus, although they may also appear on the cervix or on the round or broad ligament.

These neoplasms are usually multiple and occur in about 20% of women over age 35. They're three times more common in Blacks than in Whites. They become malignant (leiomyosarcoma) in only 0.1% of patients.

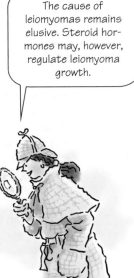

> The cause of leiomyomas remains elusive. Steroid hormones may, however, regulate leiomyoma growth.

Where the leiomyomas are

Leiomyomas are classified three ways, according to location:

- intramural (in the uterine wall)
- submucosal (protruding into the endometrial cavity)
- subserosal (protruding from the serosal surface of the uterus).

In all three cases, the uterine cavity may become larger, increasing the endometrial surface area and causing increased uterine bleeding.

What causes it

The cause of uterine leiomyomas is unknown, but steroid hormones, including estrogen and progesterone, and several growth factors, including epidermal growth factor, have been implicated as regulators of leiomyoma growth.

Pathophysiology

Excessive levels of estrogen and human growth hormone (hGH) probably contribute to uterine leiomyoma formation by stimulating susceptible fibromuscular elements. Large doses of estrogen and the later stages of pregnancy increase tumor size and hGH levels. Conversely, uterine leiomyomas usually shrink or disappear after menopause, when estrogen production decreases.

What to look for

Signs and symptoms of uterine leiomyomas include:
- submucosal hypermenorrhea (cardinal sign) and possibly other forms of abnormal endometrial bleeding, dysmenorrhea, and pain
- with large tumors, a feeling of heaviness in the abdomen, pain, intestinal obstruction, constipation, urinary frequency or urgency, and irregular uterine enlargement.

What tests tell you

- Blood studies showing anemia support the diagnosis.
- D&C or submucosal hysterosalpingography detects submucosal leiomyomas.
- Laparoscopy shows subserous leiomyomas on the uterine surface.

How it's treated

Appropriate intervention depends on the severity of symptoms, the size and location of the tumors, and the patient's age, parity, pregnancy status, desire to have children, and general health. Treatment can include these measures:

- A surgeon may remove small leiomyomas that have caused problems in the past or that appear likely to threaten a future pregnancy. This is the treatment of choice for a young woman who wants to have children.
- Tumors that twist or grow large enough to cause intestinal obstruction require a hysterectomy, with preservation of the ovaries if possible.
- If a pregnant woman has a leiomyomatous uterus no larger than a 6-month normal uterus by the 16th week of pregnancy, surgery is usually unnecessary and the pregnancy outcome is favorable.
- If a pregnant woman has a leiomyomatous uterus the size of a 5-month to 6-month normal uterus by the 9th week of pregnancy, spontaneous abortion will probably occur, especially with a cervical leiomyoma. A hysterectomy may be performed 5 to 6 months after delivery (when involution is complete), with preservation of the ovaries if possible.

What to do

- If your patient develops severe anemia from excessive bleeding, administer iron and blood transfusions as ordered.
- Evaluate the patient for abnormal bleeding or pain and postoperative complications. (See *Uterine leiomyoma teaching tips.*)

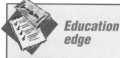

Education edge

Uterine leiomyoma teaching tips

- Tell the patient to report abnormal bleeding or pelvic pain immediately.
- If a hysterectomy or an oophorectomy is indicated, explain the effects of the operation on menstruation, menopause, and sexual activity. Reassure the patient that she won't experience premature menopause if her ovaries are left intact.
- If she must undergo a multiple myomectomy, make sure she understands that pregnancy is still possible.
- If the surgeon must enter the uterine cavity, explain that a cesarean delivery may be necessary.

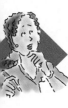

Quick quiz

1. Spermatogenesis is:
    A. the growth and development of sperm into primary spermatocytes.
    B. the division of spermatocytes to form secondary spermatocytes.
    C. the entire process of sperm formation.
    D. the storage of newly developed sperm.

Answer: C. Spermatogenesis refers to the entire process of sperm formation, from the development of primary spermatocytes to the formation of fully functional spermatozoa.

2. Which disorder is characterized by pain in the lower abdomen, vagina, posterior pelvis, and back that lasts for 2 to 3 days and occurs 5 to 7 days before menses?
    A. Ovarian cyst
    B. Endometriosis
    C. PID
    D. Uterine leiomyomas

Answer: B. The classic symptom of endometriosis, acquired dysmenorrhea, may produce the findings listed above.

3. Which statement isn't true about PID?
    A. Risk factors include more than one sexual partner and a history of STD.
    B. Up to 25% of patients may become infertile after one episode of PID.
    C. Untreated PID may be fatal.
    D. The patient's sexual partners don't need to be examined and treated for infection.

Answer: D. It's necessary for the patient's sexual partners to be examined and treated for infection.

4. Which STD is the most common in the United States?
    A. Gonorrhea
    B. Syphilis
    C. Chlamydial infection
    D. Genital herpes

Answer: C. Chlamydial infection is the most common STD in the United States. Transmission usually occurs unknowingly because chlamydia typically produces no symptoms until late in its development.

Scoring

☆☆☆   If you answered all four questions correctly, bravo! You're the diva of reproductive disorders!

☆☆   If you answered three questions correctly, encore! You win the Emmy for excellence in endoscopic tests!

☆   If you answered fewer than three questions correctly, don't worry. A little review and you'll be performing like a star!

Musculoskeletal disorders

![Just the facts]

Just the facts

In this chapter, you'll learn:

♦ anatomy and physiology of the musculoskeletal system

♦ techniques for assessing the musculoskeletal system

♦ tests to diagnose musculoskeletal disorders

♦ causes, pathophysiology, diagnostic tests, and nursing interventions for common musculoskeletal disorders.

A look at musculoskeletal disorders

Be prepared to call on the full range of your nursing skills when providing musculoskeletal care. Why? Because some musculoskeletal problems are subtle and difficult to assess, whereas others are obvious, even traumatic, affecting the patient emotionally as well as physically.

Anatomy and physiology

The three main parts of the musculoskeletal system are the bones, joints, and muscles.

Bones

The 206 bones of the skeleton support the organs and tissues and form the body's framework. The bones also serve as storage sites for minerals and produce blood cells. (See *The skeletal system*, page 678.)

A closer look

The skeletal system

Of the 206 bones in the human skeletal system, 80 form the axial skeleton, or head and trunk, and 126 form the appendicular skeleton, or the extremities. Shown here are the body's major bones.

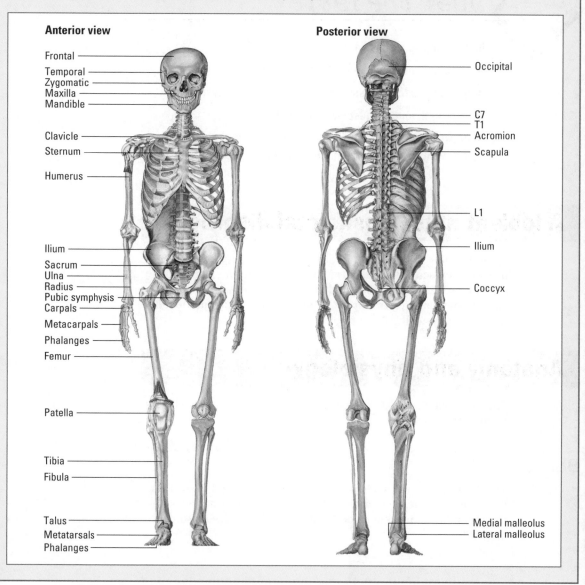

Anterior view

- Frontal
- Temporal
- Zygomatic
- Maxilla
- Mandible
- Clavicle
- Sternum
- Humerus
- Ilium
- Sacrum
- Ulna
- Radius
- Pubic symphysis
- Carpals
- Metacarpals
- Phalanges
- Femur
- Patella
- Tibia
- Fibula
- Talus
- Metatarsals
- Phalanges

Posterior view

- Occipital
- C7
- T1
- Acromion
- Scapula
- L1
- Ilium
- Coccyx
- Medial malleolus
- Lateral malleolus

Bone function

Bones perform anatomic (mechanical) and physiologic functions, including:
- stabilizing and supporting the body
- providing a surface for muscle, ligament, and tendon attachment
- moving through "lever" action when contracted
- producing red blood cells (RBCs) in the bone marrow (hematopoiesis)
- storing mineral salts, including about 99% of the body's calcium
- protecting internal tissues and organs (for example, the 33 vertebrae surrounding and protecting the spinal cord).

Joints

The junction of two or more bones is called a *joint*. Joints stabilize the bones and allow a specific type of movement. There are two types of joints:

✌ nonsynovial

✌ synovial.

In nonsynovial joints, the bones are connected by fibrous tissue or cartilage. They may be immovable, like the sutures in the skull, or slightly movable, like the vertebrae.

Free to be...a synovial joint

Synovial joints move freely. The bones are separate from each other and meet in a cavity filled with synovial fluid, a lubricant. A layer of resilient cartilage covers the surfaces of opposing bones. This cartilage cushions the bones and allows full joint movement by making the surfaces of the bones smooth. (See *Synovial joint*.)

Some popular joints

Synovial joints come in several types, including ball-and-socket joints and hinge joints.

Ball-and-socket joints (found in the shoulders and hips) allow for:

✌ flexion (bending, which decreases the joint angle)

✌ extension (straightening, which increases the joint angle)

✌ adduction (moving toward midline)

✌ abduction (moving away from midline).

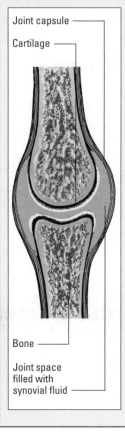

Synovial joint

Typically, bones fit together. Cartilage — a smooth, fibrous tissue — cushions the end of each bone, and synovial fluid fills the joint space. This fluid lubricates the joint and eases movement, much as the brake fluid functions in a car.

Joint capsule

Cartilage

Bone

Joint space filled with synovial fluid

These joints also rotate in their sockets and are assessed by their degree of internal and external rotation.

Hinge joints, such as the knee and elbow, usually move in flexion and extension only.

We've got you surrounded

Synovial joints are surrounded by a fibrous capsule that stabilizes the joint structures. The capsule also surrounds the joint's ligaments (the tough, fibrous bands that join one bone to another).

Muscles

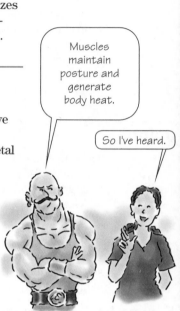

Muscles maintain posture and generate body heat.

So I've heard.

Skeletal muscles are groups of contractile cells or fibers. These fibers contract and produce skeletal movement when they receive a stimulus from the central nervous system (CNS). The CNS is responsible for involuntary and voluntary muscle function. Skeletal muscles also maintain posture and generate body heat.

Tough guy, huh?

Tendons are tough, fibrous portions of muscle that attach the muscles to bone. Bursae — sacs filled with friction-reducing synovial fluid — are located in areas of high friction such as the knee.

Muscle movements

Skeletal muscle allows several types of movement. A muscle's functional name comes from the type of movement it permits. For example, a flexor muscle permits bending (flexion), an abductor muscle permits movement away from a body axis (abduction), and a circumductor muscle allows a circular movement (circumduction).

Assessment

Your sharp assessment skills will help you uncover musculoskeletal abnormalities and evaluate the patient's ability to perform activities of daily living (ADLs). However, because many musculoskeletal injuries are emergencies, you might not have time for a thorough patient history and physical examination.

Patient history

If possible, question the patient about his current illness, past illnesses, medications, and family and social history.

Current illness

Ask the patient about his chief complaint. Patients with joint injuries usually complain of pain, swelling, or stiffness; those with bone fractures have sharp pain when they move the affected area. Muscular injury is commonly accompanied by pain, swelling, and weakness.

Ask the patient if his ability to carry out ADLs is affected. Is pain more intense or has he noticed grating sounds when he moves certain parts of his body? Does he use ice, heat, or other remedies to treat the problem? Is pain worse in the morning?

Past health history

Inquire whether the patient has ever had gout, arthritis, tuberculosis (TB), or cancer, which may have bony metastases. Has he been diagnosed with osteoporosis?

Info on injuries

Ask whether he has had a recent blunt or penetrating trauma. If so, how did it happen? For example, did he suffer knee and hip injuries after being hit by a car, or did he fall from a ladder and land on his coccyx? This information will help guide your assessment and predict hidden trauma.

Also ask the patient whether he uses an assistive device, such as a cane, walker, or brace. If so, watch him use the device to assess how he moves.

Medications

Question the patient about the medications he takes regularly. Many drugs can affect the musculoskeletal system. Corticosteroids, for example, can cause muscle weakness, myopathy, osteoporosis, pathologic fractures, and avascular necrosis of the heads of the femur and humerus.

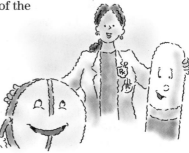

Several drugs affect the musculoskeletal system, so make sure you know what medications your patient is taking.

Family history

Ask the patient if a family member suffers from joint disease. Disorders with a hereditary component include:
• gout
• osteoarthritis of the interphalangeal joints
• spondyloarthropathies (such as ankylosing spondylitis, Reiter's syndrome, psoriatic arthritis, and enteropathic arthritis)
• rheumatoid arthritis.

Social history

Ask the patient about his job, hobbies, and personal habits. Knitting, playing football or tennis, working at a computer, or doing construction work can all cause repetitive stress injuries or injure the musculoskeletal system in other ways. Even carrying a heavy knapsack or purse can cause injury or increase muscle size.

Physical examination

Perform a head-to-toe assessment, simultaneously evaluating the muscle and joint function of each body area. You'll need to observe the patient's posture, gait, and coordination, and inspect and palpate his muscles, joints, and bones.

Inspecting posture, gait, and coordination

Assessment begins the instant you see the patient. Good observation skills enable you to obtain a wealth of information about approximate muscle strength, facial muscle movement, body symmetry, and obvious physical or functional deformities or abnormalities.

Assess the patient's overall body symmetry as he assumes different postures and makes diverse movements. Note marked dissimilarities in side-to-side size, shape, and motion.

Posture

Posture is the attitude, or position, that body parts assume in relation to other body parts and to the external environment. Assessing posture includes inspecting spinal curvature and knee positioning.

Stand by your man (and woman)

To assess spinal curvature, instruct the patient to stand as straight as possible. Then stand at his side, behind his back, and in front of him, in that order, inspecting the spine for alignment and the shoulders, iliac crests, and scapulae for symmetry of position and height. When the patient stands, his thoracic spine should have a convex curvature and his lumbar spine should have a concave curvature.

Next, have the patient bend forward from the waist with his arms relaxed and dangling. Stand behind him and inspect the straightness of his spine, noting flank and thorax position and symmetry.

Other normal findings include:
• a midline spine without lateral curvatures
• a concave lumbar curvature that changes to a convex curvature in the flexed position

• iliac crests, shoulders, and scapulae at the same horizontal level.

Gait
Direct the patient to walk away from you, turn around, and then walk back. Observe his posture, movement (such as pace and length of stride), foot position, coordination, and balance.

Smooth walker
Normal findings when walking include smooth, coordinated movements, the head leading the body when turning, and erect posture with approximately 2″ to 4″ (5 to 10 cm) of space between the feet. Be sure to remain close to an elderly or infirm patient and be ready to help if he should stumble or start to fall.

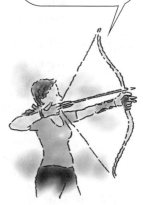

Coordination results from neuromuscular integrity. Just what I need to shoot straight!

Coordination
Evaluate how well a patient's muscles produce movement. Coordination results from neuromuscular integrity; a lack of muscular or nervous system integrity, or both, impairs the ability to make voluntary and productive movements.

You're so fine and gross
Assess gross motor skills by having the patient perform body action involving the muscles and joints in natural directional movements, such as lifting the arm to the side and other range-of-motion (ROM) exercises. Assess fine motor coordination by asking the patient to pick up a small object from a desk or table.

Inspecting and palpating muscles
Expect to perform inspection and palpation simultaneously during the musculoskeletal assessment. You'll evaluate muscle tone, mass, and strength. Palpate the muscles gently, never forcing movement when the patient reports pain or when you feel resistance. Watch the patient's face and body language for signs of discomfort — he may suffer silently.

Tone and mass
Muscle tone is the consistency or tension in the resting muscle. Test it by palpating a muscle at rest and by performing passive ROM exercises. To palpate a muscle at rest, feel from the muscle attachment at the bone to the edge of the muscle. A relaxed muscle should feel soft, pliable, and nontender; a contracted muscle should feel firm.

Check out those muscles

Muscle mass is the size of a muscle. Assessment of muscle mass usually involves measuring the circumference of the thigh, calf, and upper arm. When measuring, mark landmarks with a pen to make sure you're measuring at the same location on each side of the body.

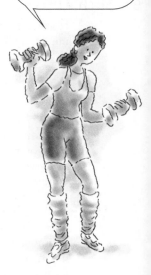

Measuring the circumference of the thigh, calf, and upper arm helps you to assess muscle mass. I'm working to increase my muscle mass!

Strength and joint ROM

Assessing joint ROM tests the joint's function. Assessing muscle strength against resistance tests the function of the muscles surrounding the joint. (See *Testing muscle strength*.)

Inspecting and palpating joints and bones

When evaluating joint and bone characteristics and joint ROM, never force joint movement if you feel resistance or if the patient complains of pain.

Departures from the norm

Deviations include pain, swelling, stiffness, deformities, altered ROM, crepitation (a grating sound or sensation accompanying joint movement), ankylosis (joint fusion or fixation), and contracture (muscle shortening).

Cervical spine

Have the patient sit or stand. Inspect the cervical spine from behind, from the side, and while facing the patient.

Drawing the line

Observe the alignment of the head with the body. The nose should be in line with the midsternum and extend beyond the shoulders when viewed from the side. The head should align with the shoulders. Typically, the seventh cervical and first thoracic vertebrae appear more prominent than the others.

Clavicles

With the patient sitting or standing, inspect and palpate the length of the clavicles, including the sternoclavicular and acromioclavicular joints. Normal findings include firm, smooth, continuous bones.

Scapulae

To inspect and palpate the scapulae, sit directly behind the patient as he sits with his shoulders thrust backward. Usually,

Testing muscle strength

To test the muscle strength of your patient's arm and ankle muscles, use the techniques shown here.

Biceps strength

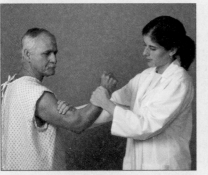

Triceps strength

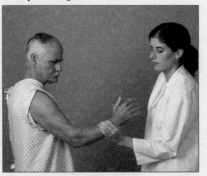

Ankle strength: Plantar flexion

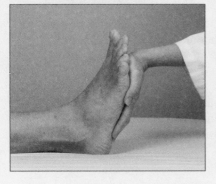

Ankle strength: Dorsiflexion

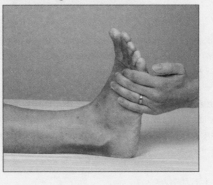

the scapulae are located over thoracic ribs two through seven. Check for an equal distance from the medial scapular edges to the midspinal line.

Ribs

Have the patient remain sitting. After assessing the scapulae, inspect and palpate the anterior, posterior, and lateral surfaces of the ribs. Normal findings include firm, smooth, continuous bones.

Shoulders

With the patient still sitting, palpate the moving joints for crepitus. Inspect the skin overlying the shoulder joints for erythema, masses, or swelling.

Introducing the Ducts, Ad and Ab

Next, palpate the acromioclavicular joint and the area over the greater humeral tuberosity. Ask the patient to stand. Have him hold his arm at his side and then adduct his arm. Next, place your thumb on the anterior portion of the patient's shoulder joint and your fingers on the posterior portion of the shoulder joint. Ask the patient to abduct his arm. Palpate the shoulder joint as he does so.

Stand and rotate

Now stand behind the patient. With your fingertips placed over the greater humeral tuberosity, instruct him to rotate each shoulder internally by moving the corresponding arm behind his back. This allows you to palpate a portion of the musculotendinous rotator cuff as well as the bony structures of the shoulder joint.

Elbows

With the patient sitting or standing, inspect joint contour and skin over each elbow. Palpate the elbows at rest and during movement.

Wrists

With the patient sitting or standing, inspect the wrists for masses, erythema, skeletal deformities, and swelling. Palpate the wrist at rest and during movement by gently grasping it between your thumb and fingers.

Fingers and thumbs

With the patient sitting or standing, inspect the fingers and thumbs of each hand for nodules, erythema, spacing, length, and skeletal deformities. Palpate the fingers and thumbs at rest and during movement.

Thoracic and lumbar spine

In addition to evaluating the curvatures of the thoracic and lumbar spine during the postural assessment, you'll need to palpate the length of the spine for tenderness and vertebral alignment. With the patient standing, check for tenderness, percuss each spinous process (directly over the vertebral column) with the ulnar side of your fist.

Note whether the patient can move with a full ROM while maintaining balance, smoothness, and coordination.

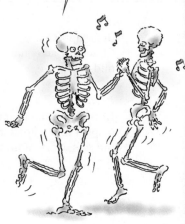

We have all the right moves, along with balance, smoothness, and coordination!

Hips and pelvis

With the patient sitting or standing, inspect and palpate over the bony prominences of the hips and pelvis: iliac crests, symphysis pubis, anterior spine, ischial tuberosities, and greater trochanters. Palpate the hip at rest and during movement.

Knees

Inspect the knees with the patient seated. Palpate the knee at rest and during movement. Inspect and palpate the popliteal spaces behind the knee joint. Knee movements should be smooth.

Ankles and feet

With the patient sitting, inspect and palpate the ankles and feet at rest and during movement.

> With the patient sitting, inspect and palpate her ankles and feet at rest and during movement.

Toes

The patient may be sitting or lying supine for toe assessment. Inspect all toe surfaces. Palpate the toes at rest and during movement.

Diagnostic tests

Diagnostic tests help to confirm the diagnosis and identify the underlying cause of musculoskeletal problems. Common procedures include aspiration tests, endoscopic tests, and radiographic and imaging studies.

Aspiration tests

The doctor may aspirate a specimen from the joint capsule (arthrocentesis) or from the bone marrow to detect various disorders.

Arthrocentesis

Arthrocentesis is a joint puncture that's used to collect fluid for analysis to identify the cause of pain and swelling, to assess for infection, and to distinguish forms of arthritis, such as pseudogout and infectious arthritis. The doctor will probably choose the knee for this procedure, but he may tap synovial fluid from the wrist, ankle, elbow, or first metatarsophalangeal joint.

Telltale findings

In joint infection, for example, synovial fluid looks cloudy and contains more white blood cells (WBCs) and less glucose than normal. When trauma causes bleeding into a joint, synovial fluid contains RBCs. In specific types of arthritis, crystals can confirm the diagnosis — for instance, urate crystals indicate gout.

Doing double duty

Arthrocentesis also has therapeutic value. For example, in symptomatic joint effusion, removing excess synovial fluid relieves pain.

Nursing considerations

• Describe the procedure to the patient. Explain that he'll be asked to assume a certain position, depending on the joint being aspirated, and that he'll need to remain still.
• After the test, the practitioner may ask you to apply ice or cold packs to the joint to reduce pain and swelling.
• If the doctor removed a large amount of fluid, tell the patient that he may need to wear an elastic bandage.
• Advise him not to use the joint excessively for 24 hours after the test to avoid joint pain, swelling, and stiffness.
• Instruct him to report these signs of infection: fever and increased pain, tenderness, swelling, warmth, or redness.

Bone marrow aspiration

In bone marrow aspiration, a doctor removes a small amount of fluid from the bone marrow using a special needle. This procedure can be used to diagnose many abnormalities, including rheumatoid arthritis, TB, amyloidosis, syphilis, bacterial or viral infection, parasitic infestation, tumors, and hematologic problems.

Suck it up

Bone marrow is usually aspirated from the sternum or iliac crests. The site is prepared as for any minor surgical procedure and then is infiltrated with a local anesthetic such as lidocaine. The doctor inserts the marrow needle, with stylet in place, through the cortex into the marrow cavity. Marrow cavity penetration causes the patient to feel a collapsing sensation. Then the doctor removes the stylet, attaches a syringe to the needle hub, and aspirates 0.2 to 0.5 ml of fluid.

Nursing considerations

• Tell the patient that he'll be sedated and that he'll receive a local anesthetic before needle insertion.

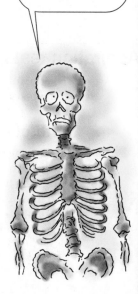

Bone marrow aspiration involves putting a needle where?!

- Explain that the test takes about 10 minutes.
- Warn the patient that he'll feel pressure as the doctor inserts the needle and that aspiration may hurt briefly.
- Watch for signs of infection after the procedure.
- Make sure bleeding stops, particularly if the patient has a clotting disorder.

Endoscopic tests

Endoscopic studies allow direct visualization of joint problems. Arthroscopy is a common endoscopic procedure.

Arthroscopy

Arthroscopy is usually used to evaluate the knee. It helps the doctor assess joint problems, plan surgical approaches, and document pathology.

Needling the knee

After inserting a large-bore needle into the suprapatellar pouch, the surgeon injects sterile saline solution to distend the joint. Then he passes a fiber-optic scope through puncture sites lateral or medial to the tibial plateau, allowing direct visualization. With a large scope, he can remove articular debris and small, loose bodies or repair a torn meniscus.

Nursing considerations

- Tell the patient that he can't eat or drink after midnight before the test.
- Explain that, if ordered, he'll receive a sedative immediately before the test, and that the area around the joint will be prepped.
- If the test will be performed under local anesthesia, check the patient history for hypersensitivity to local anesthetics. Warn the patient that he may feel transient discomfort during injection of the anesthetic.
- Explain that the surgeon will make a small incision and insert the arthroscope into the joint cavity.
- Tell the patient that he'll be allowed to walk as soon as he's fully awake. He'll experience mild soreness and a slight grinding sensation in his knee for 1 to 2 days.
- Instruct him to notify the practitioner if he feels severe or persistent pain or develops a fever with signs of local inflammation.
- Advise against excessive use of the joint for a few days after the test. Tell the patient that he may resume his normal diet.

> Patients should take it easy for a few days after an arthroscopy.

- Ask the surgeon about specific leg exercises, ice application, and dressing changes that are necessary after the procedure and at home.
- Assess the patient for signs of complications, such as infection, hemarthrosis (blood accumulation in the joint), or a synovial cyst.
- Teach the patient proper crutch walking technique if crutches are ordered, and ask him to perform a return demonstration.

Radiographic and imaging studies

Radiographic and imaging studies include bone scans, computed tomography (CT) scans, dual energy X-ray absorptiometry (DEXA), magnetic resonance imaging (MRI), and X-rays.

Bone scan

A bone scan helps detect bony metastasis, benign disease, fractures, avascular necrosis, and infection.

Scintillating study

After I.V. introduction of a radioactive material, such as the radioisotope technetium polyphosphate, the isotope collects in areas of increased bone activity or active bone formation. A scintillation counter detects the gamma rays, indicating abnormal areas of increased uptake (positive findings). The radioisotope has a short half-life and soon passes from the patient's body.

Nursing considerations

- Explain to the patient how this painless test commonly detects bone abnormalities earlier than conventional X-rays.
- Tell him that he can eat and drink as usual before the test.
- Describe how the doctor applies a tourniquet on the patient's arm and then injects a small dose of a radioactive isotope. Assure the patient that the isotope emits less radiation than a standard X-ray machine.
- Explain that after the isotope is injected, there's a 2- to 3-hour waiting period before the scan is done. During this time, the patient must drink four to six glasses of fluid.
- Explain that when it's time for the scan, he'll lie supine on a table within the scanner. The scanner moves back and forth slowly, recording images for about 1 hour. Instruct the patient to lie as still as possible and to expect to assume various positions.

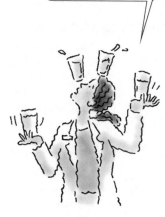

After the isotope is injected for a bone scan, the patient must wait 2 to 3 hours for the scan to be done and drink four to six glasses of fluid. That's a lot of liquid!

CT scan

A CT scan aids diagnosis of bone tumors and other abnormalities. It helps assess questionable cervical or spinal fractures, fracture fragments, bone lesions, and intra-articular loose bodies.

Beam me up, Scotty

Multiple X-ray beams from a computerized body scanner are directed at the body from different angles. The beams pass through the body and strike radiation detectors, producing electrical impulses. A computer then converts these impulses into digital information, which is displayed as a three-dimensional image on a video monitor.

Nursing considerations

• If the patient is scheduled to receive a contrast medium, inform him that he must not eat for 4 hours before the test. Check his records to make sure he isn't hypersensitive to any contrast media. If he is hypersensitive, he may need preprocedure medication.
• Tell the patient that he needs to put on a hospital gown, remove all jewelry, and empty his bladder before the test.
• Instruct him to remain still during the test. Although he'll be alone in the room, assure him that he can communicate with the technician through an intercom system.
• If the patient received a contrast medium by mouth, encourage him to drink plenty of fluids after the test to help flush the contrast medium from his body.

DEXA

DEXA can be used to assess the bone density of the entire body or just the hip or spine. It's used to help diagnose osteoporosis, especially before a fracture occurs. This noninvasive technique involves using a radiography tube to measure bone mineral density and exposes the patient to only minimal radiation.

Alternative approaches

Several other machines can also be used to measure bone density. (See *A bevy of bone density tests*.)

Nursing considerations

• Reassure the patient that this test is painless and noninvasive and usually takes less than 15 minutes.
• Have the patient remove all jewelry from the area that will be examined.

A bevy of bone density tests

These tests measure bone density or mass and are helpful in diagnosing osteoporosis:
• Single energy X-ray absorptiometry measures the wrist or heel.
• Peripheral dual energy X-ray absorptiometry measures the wrist, heel, or finger.
• Single photon absorptiometry measures the wrist.
• Dual photon absorptiometry measures the hip, spine, or total body.
• Radiographic absorptiometry calculates bone density using an X-ray of the hand.

MRI

MRI can show irregularities of the spinal cord and is especially useful for diagnosing disk herniation.

Must be animal magnetism

The MRI scanner uses a powerful magnetic field and radiofrequency energy to produce images based on the hydrogen content of body tissues. The computer processes signals and displays the resulting high-resolution image on a video monitor. The patient can't feel the magnetic fields.

Nursing considerations

• Explain to the patient that he'll be positioned on a narrow bed that slides into a large cylinder housing the MRI magnets.
• Tell him that he'll be asked to put on a hospital gown and to remove all metal objects, including bobby pins, jewelry, watches, eyeglasses, hearing aids, and dental appliances. He should also remove clothes with metal zippers, buckles, or buttons as well as credit, bank, and parking cards, because the scan could erase the magnetic codes. He will also need to remove any medication patches.
• Ask the patient if he has any implanted metal, such as a pacemaker, plate, screws, or an artificial joint. If the patient has implanted metal, an MRI may not be possible.
• Tell the patient he'll hear soft thumping noises during the test. Ask if claustrophobia has ever been a problem for him. If so, sedation may help him tolerate the scan.
• Instruct him to remain still during the test. Although he'll be alone in the room, assure him that he can communicate with the technician through an intercom system.

X-rays

Anteroposterior, posteroanterior, and lateral X-rays allow three-dimensional visualization. They help diagnose:
• traumatic disorders, such as fractures and dislocations
• bone disease, including solitary lesions, multiple focal lesions in one bone, or generalized lesions involving all bones
• joint disease, such as arthritis, infection, degenerative changes, synoviosarcoma, osteochondromatosis, avascular necrosis, slipped femoral epiphysis, and inflamed tendons and bursae around a joint
• masses and calcifications.

X-rays can help diagnose traumatic injuries, bone and joint disease, and masses and calcifications.

If the practitioner needs further clarification of standard X-rays, he may order a CT scan or MRI.

Nursing considerations
- Make sure the patient removes all jewelry from the area to be X-rayed.
- Verify that the X-ray order includes pertinent recent history, such as trauma, and identifies the point tenderness site. It should also include past fractures, dislocations, or surgery involving the affected area.

Treatments

Pain and impaired mobility provide good motivation for obtaining medical care. Consequently, most patients with musculoskeletal problems eagerly seek treatment.

Get up and go again

To restore a patient's mobility, several treatments are used alone or in combination:
- a balanced program of exercise and rest
- a splint, brace, or other device to support a weakened or injured limb or joint
- drug therapy to control pain, inflammation, or muscle spasticity
- nonsurgical treatments, including closed reduction or immobilization
- surgery with subsequent immobilization with a cast, brace, or other device.

Drug therapy

Salicylates are the first line of defense against arthropathies. Other drug therapy includes analgesics, nonsteroidal anti-inflammatory drugs (NSAIDs), corticosteroids, and skeletal muscle relaxants.

Nonsurgical treatments

Some patients with musculoskeletal disorders require nonsurgical treatment. Such treatment may include closed reduction of a fracture or immobilization.

I'm tuned up and ready to mobilize!

Closed reduction

Closed reduction involves external manipulation of fracture fragments or dislocated joints to restore their normal position and alignment. It may be done under local, regional, or general anesthesia or monitored sedation.

Patient preparation

Prepare the patient for reduction by taking these steps:
• If he'll be receiving a general anesthetic, instruct him not to eat after midnight. Tell him he'll receive a sedative before the procedure.
• If appropriate, explain how traction can reduce pain, relieve muscle spasms, and maintain alignment while he awaits the procedure.

Monitoring and aftercare

After the procedure, take these steps:
• Assess for pain and provide pain management, as needed.
• Be prepared to care for a bandage, sling, splint, or cast after the procedure. These devices immobilize the fracture or dislocation.
• Tell the patient that he'll have an X-ray to evaluate the closed reduction.

Home care instructions

Before discharge, take these steps:
• Teach the patient how to apply (if appropriate) and care for the immobilization device. Tell him to regularly check his skin under and around the device for irritation and breakdown.
• Stress the importance of following prescribed exercises.

Immobilization

Immobilization devices are commonly used to maintain proper alignment and limit movement. They also relieve pressure and pain.

Don't move a muscle!

Immobilization devices include:
• plaster and synthetic casts applied after closed or open reduction of fractures or after other severe injuries
• splints to immobilize fractures, dislocations, or subluxations
• slings to support and immobilize an injured arm, wrist, or hand, or to support the weight of a splint or hold dressings in place
• skin or skeletal traction, using a system of weights and pulleys to reduce fractures, treat dislocations, correct deformities, or decrease muscle spasms

- braces to support weakened or deformed joints
- cervical collars to immobilize the cervical spine, decrease muscle spasms, and possibly relieve pain.

Patient preparation

Before the procedure, prepare the patient for immobilization by taking these steps:

- Explain the purpose of the immobilization device. If possible, show the patient the device before application and demonstrate how it works. Reinforce to the patient approximately how long the device will remain in place.
- Explain that he'll have discomfort initially, but reassure him that this will resolve as he becomes accustomed to the device. (See *Comparing traction techniques*, page 696.)

    If the patient is in pain, give analgesics and muscle relaxants as ordered.

I know skeletal traction is beneficial for reducing fractures and other indications, but I feel like a marionette.

Monitoring and aftercare

After the procedure, take these steps:

- Take precautions to help prevent complications of immobility, especially if the patient is in traction or requires long-term bed rest. For example, reposition him frequently to enhance comfort and prevent pressure ulcers.
- As ordered, assist with active or passive ROM exercises to maintain muscle tone and prevent contractures.
- Encourage regular coughing and deep breathing to prevent pulmonary complications.
- Stress adequate fluid intake to prevent urinary stasis and constipation.
- Encourage the bedridden patient to engage in hobbies or other activities to relieve boredom. This also helps maintain the positive mental outlook that's important to recovery.
- Encourage ambulation, if appropriate, and provide assistance as necessary.
- Provide analgesics as ordered. If you're administering opioid analgesics, watch for signs of toxicity or oversedation.
- Provide regular pin care for the patient in skeletal traction to help minimize the risk of infection.

Comparing traction techniques

Traction restricts movement of a patient's affected limb or body part and may confine the patient to bed rest for an extended period. The limb is immobilized by pulling with equal force on each end of the injured area — an equal mix of traction and countertraction. Weights provide the pulling force. Countertraction is produced by using other weights or by positioning the patient's body weight against the traction pull.

Although traction commonly requires confinement to a hospital bed, it does allow the patient limited motion of his affected extremity and permits exercise of his unaffected body parts. Shown here are two types of traction: skin and skeletal.

Skin traction

Skin traction immobilizes a body part intermittently over an extended period through direct application of a pulling force on the patient's skin. The force may be applied using adhesive or nonadhesive traction tape or other skin traction devices, such as a boot, belt, or halter. Adhesive attachment allows more continuous traction, whereas non-adhesive attachment allows easier removal for daily care.

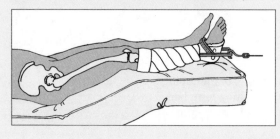

Skeletal traction

Skeletal traction immobilizes a body part for prolonged periods by attaching weighted equipment directly to the patient's bones. This may be accomplished with pins, screws, wires, or tongs.

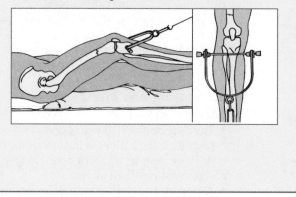

Home care instructions

Before discharge, give the patient these instructions:
• Tell him to promptly report signs of complications, including increased pain, drainage, or swelling in the involved area.
• Stress the need for strict compliance with activity restrictions while the immobilization device is in place.
• If the patient has been given crutches to use with a leg or ankle cast, splint, or knee immobilizer, make sure he understands how to use them. If the patient has a removable device, such as a knee immobilizer, make sure he knows how to apply it correctly.
• Advise the patient to keep scheduled medical appointments to evaluate healing.

Surgery

For some patients with musculoskeletal disorders, surgery can offer a bright alternative to a life of chronic pain and disability. Surgical procedures include amputation, joint replacement, laminectomy and spinal fusion, and open reduction and internal fixation.

Amputation

Perhaps more than any other surgery, amputation can dramatically change a patient's life. Your role includes providing support and detailed instruction in postoperative care.

Patient preparation

Prepare the patient for amputation by taking these steps:
• Before surgery, reinforce the surgeon's explanation of the procedure and contact the surgeon if the patient requires additional information.
• Support the patient as he confronts all of the issues surrounding loss of a limb.

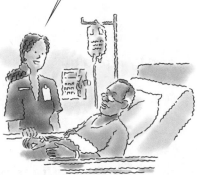

Support the patient as he confronts all of the issues surrounding loss of a limb.

Monitoring and aftercare

After the procedure, take these steps:
• Be prepared to care for the cast or elastic wrap that the surgeon applies around the stump. This helps control swelling, minimize pain, and mold the stump so that it fits comfortably into a prosthesis.
• As appropriate, instruct the patient to report drainage through the cast, warmth, tenderness, or a foul smell.
• Warn the patient that the cast may slip off as swelling subsides. If so, he should immediately wrap the stump or slip on a custom-fitted elastic stump shrinker.

Home care instructions

Before discharge, give the patient these instructions:
• Emphasize that proper home care of the stump can speed healing. Tell the patient to inspect the stump carefully each day, using a mirror. He should call the practitioner if the incision is open, red or swollen, warm, painful to touch, or seeping drainage. Teach him to clean the stump daily with mild soap and water; then rinse and dry it thoroughly.
• Instruct the patient to rub the stump with alcohol daily to toughen the skin. Because alcohol may cause irritation in some patients, warn him to watch for and report this. Teach him not to apply powder or lotion because this may soften or irritate the skin.
• Teach him to massage the stump toward the suture line to mobilize the scar and prevent its adherence to bone.

- Advise him to avoid exposing the skin around the stump to excessive perspiration, which can be irritating. He may need to change his elastic bandages or stump socks during the day to avoid this.
- As stump muscles adjust to amputation, tell the patient he may have twitching, spasms, or phantom limb pain. (See *Predictive factors for phantom limb pain.*) Heat (for example, a hot bath, heating pad, or warm compress), massage, or gentle pressure can decrease these symptoms. If the stump is sensitive to touch, tell the patient to rub it with a dry washcloth for 4 minutes three times per day.
- Stress the importance of performing prescribed exercises to help minimize complications, maintain muscle strength and tone, prevent contractures, and promote independence.
- Stress the importance of positioning to prevent contractures.
- To prepare the stump for a prosthesis, teach progressive resistance maneuvers. First, the patient should push his stump gently against a soft pillow. Have him progress to pushing it against a firm pillow, a padded chair, and finally, a hard chair.

Joint replacement

Total or partial replacement of a joint with a synthetic prosthesis restores mobility and stability, relieves pain, and increases the patient's sense of independence and self-worth.

A pretty hip joint

Recent improvements in surgical techniques and prosthetic devices have made joint replacement a common treatment of

---

Weighing the evidence

Predictive factors for phantom limb pain

Many amputees experience phantom limb pain. Several studies have looked at the severity of the pain and how long it lasts, but results have sometimes conflicted. To determine the prevalence of phantom limb pain over time and the factors associated with increased pain, researchers studied over 130 amputees. They found that, for patients who had undergone lower limb amputation, pain was greatest after 6 months; for upper limb amputees, pain was greatest after 1½ years. They also found that pain decreased over time for both groups, and women and upper limb amputees were more likely to experience phantom pain.

Bosmans, J.C., et al. (2010). Factors associated with phantom limb pain: A 3½ year prospective study. *Clinical Rehabilitation*, 24(5), 444–453.

severe chronic arthritis, degenerative joint disorders, and extensive joint trauma. Many joints can be replaced with prostheses, with hip and knee replacements being the most common.

Patient preparation

Before the procedure, take these steps:
• Tell the patient that because of the complexity of joint replacement, he'll start having extensive tests and studies long before the day of surgery.
• Discuss postoperative recovery with the patient and his family. Explain that his activity will be limited after surgery and that he'll soon begin an exercise program to maintain joint mobility.
• As appropriate, show him ROM exercises. If he's having a total knee replacement, demonstrate the continuous passive motion (CPM) device he'll use during recovery.
• Point out that surgery may not relieve his pain immediately. Reassure him that pain will diminish dramatically after edema subsides and that analgesics will be available as needed.

Monitoring and aftercare

After surgery, help the patient follow activity limitations. When he's in bed, turn him regularly for the prescribed period while maintaining the affected joint in proper alignment. If traction is used, periodically check the weights and other equipment.

Assess the patient's level of pain and provide analgesics, as ordered. If you're administering opioid analgesics, be alert for signs of toxicity or oversedation.

After surgery, assess the patient's level of pain and provide analgesics, as ordered.

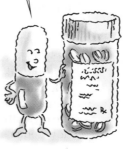

Dangerous globules

During recovery, take these steps:
• Monitor for complications of joint replacement, particularly hypovolemic shock from blood loss during surgery. Also watch for signs of fat embolism. This potentially fatal complication is caused by release of fat molecules in response to increased intermedullary canal pressure from the prosthesis. The fat globules then combine with platelets to form emboli, which may occlude vessels that supply the brain, lungs, kidneys, or other organs. Symptoms typically occur within 24 to 72 hours but may occur up to a week after injury.
• Inspect the incision frequently for signs of infection. Change the dressing as necessary, maintaining strict sterile technique. Periodically assess neurovascular and motor status distal to the joint replacement site.

- Immediately report abnormalities or complications, such as a dislocated total hip replacement. Signs and symptoms of this are sudden, severe pain, shortening, or internal or external rotation of the involved leg.
- Reposition the patient often to enhance comfort and prevent pressure ulcers.
- Encourage coughing and deep breathing to prevent pulmonary complications.
- Stress adequate fluid intake to avert urinary stasis and constipation.
- Have the patient begin exercising the affected joint, as ordered, perhaps even on the day of surgery. The practitioner may prescribe CPM (using a machine or a system of suspended ropes and pulleys) or a series of active or passive ROM exercises.
- Before the patient with a knee or hip replacement is discharged, make sure that he has a walker and knows how to use it.

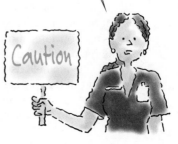

Sudden, severe pain is a symptom of a dislocated total hip replacement. Report it immediately!

Home care instructions

Before discharge, assess whether the patient needs home health care and take these steps:
- Reinforce the practitioner's and physical therapist's instructions for an exercise regimen. Remind the patient to closely adhere to the prescribed schedule and not to rush rehabilitation, no matter how good he feels.
- Review prescribed activity limitations.
- Instruct the patient on the importance of taking anti-inflammatory medication for pain relief and to speed the healing process.
- If the patient has undergone hip replacement, instruct him to keep his hips abducted and not to cross his legs when sitting. This helps reduce the risk of dislocating the prosthesis. Also tell him to avoid flexing his hips more than 90 degrees when rising from a bed or chair. Encourage him to sit in chairs with high arms and a firm seat and to sleep only on a firm mattress.
- Caution the patient to promptly report signs of infection, such as persistent fever and increased pain, tenderness, and stiffness in the joint and surrounding area. Remind him that infection may still develop several months after joint replacement.
- Tell the patient to report a sudden increase of pain, which may indicate dislodgment of the prosthesis.

Laminectomy and spinal fusion

In laminectomy, the surgeon removes one or more of the bony laminae that cover the vertebrae. This procedure has two main uses:

To relieve pressure on the spinal cord or spinal nerve roots resulting from a herniated disk (most common)

To treat compression fracture or dislocation of vertebrae or a spinal cord tumor.

Nothin' confusin' about fusion

After removing the lamina, the surgeon may stabilize the spine by performing spinal fusion using bone chip grafts between vertebral spaces.

Spinal fusion may also be done without a laminectomy in patients whose vertebrae are seriously weakened by trauma or disease. Usually, spinal fusion is done only when more conservative treatments — such as prolonged bed rest, traction, physical therapy, or a back brace — prove ineffective. (See *Alternatives to laminectomy*.)

Alternatives to laminectomy

Percutaneous automated diskectomy and chemonucleolysis are alternatives to laminectomy, the traditional surgical treatment of a herniated disk.

Percutaneous automated diskectomy

In percutaneous automated diskectomy, the surgeon uses a suction technique and X-ray visualization to remove only the disk portion that is causing pain. Depending on the patient's and surgeon's preference, this procedure can be done under local or general anesthesia and on an inpatient or outpatient basis.

Because the procedure causes little muscle trauma, it produces minimal pain. The patient should be on bed rest for the first few days and then gradually resume activities over the next 2 months. A mild analgesic or anti-inflammatory is usually sufficient for pain control.

Chemonucleolysis

Chemonucleolysis involves injection of the drug chymopapain (Chymodiactin) or collagenase to destroy the disk. Usually performed with radiographic visualization, it eliminates the need for surgery.

Chemonucleolysis isn't without risks, however. Disk space narrowing after chemonucleolysis, leading to irreversible osteoarthritis-like changes, is a potential complication.

Nursing care after chemonucleolysis involves monitoring the patient for changes in neurologic status, such as worsened back pain and decreased sensation below the injection site. This may suggest bleeding into the disk space (most common) or an antigenic reaction to the drug.

Patient preparation

Before laminectomy and spinal fusion, take these steps:
• Discuss postoperative recovery and rehabilitation. Point out that surgery won't relieve back pain immediately and that pain may even worsen after the operation. Explain that relief will come only after chronic nerve irritation and swelling subside, which may take several weeks. Reassure him that analgesics and muscle relaxants will be available during recovery.
• Tell the patient that he'll return from surgery with a dressing over the incision and that his activity will be limited postoperatively for a period of time.
• Explain that he'll be turned often to prevent pressure ulcers and pulmonary complications. Show him the logrolling method of turning, and explain that he'll use this method later to get in and out of bed by himself.
• Just before surgery, perform a baseline assessment of motor function and sensation in the patient's lower trunk, legs, and feet. Carefully document the results for comparison with postoperative findings.

Monitoring and aftercare

After the procedure, take these steps:
• Position the patient as ordered by the practitioner for the prescribed period of time.
• When he can assume a side-lying position, make sure he keeps his spine straight with his knees flexed.
• Inspect the dressing frequently for bleeding or cerebrospinal fluid (CSF) leakage, and report either immediately. The practitioner will probably perform the initial dressing change, and you may be asked to perform subsequent changes.
• Assess motor and neurologic function in the patient's trunk and lower extremities, and compare the results with baseline findings. Also evaluate circulation in the patient's legs and feet and report any abnormalities. Give analgesics and muscle relaxants as ordered.
• Every 2 to 4 hours, assess urine output and auscultate for the return of bowel sounds. If the patient doesn't void within 8 to 12 hours after surgery, notify the practitioner and prepare to insert a urinary catheter to relieve retention. If the patient can void normally, assist him in getting on and off a bedpan while maintaining proper alignment.

Home care instructions

Before discharge, take these steps:
• Teach the patient and his caregiver proper incision care measures. Tell them to check the incision site often for signs of infection — such as increased pain and tenderness, redness, swelling, and changes in the amount and character of drainage — and to report any signs immediately.
• Make sure the patient understands the importance of resuming activity gradually after surgery. As ordered, instruct him to start with short walks and to slowly progress to longer distances.
• Review with the patient any prescribed exercises, such as pelvic tilts, leg raises, and toe pointing. Advise him to rest frequently and avoid overexertion.

Get up, stand up

• Review any prescribed activity restrictions. Usually, the practitioner will prohibit sitting for prolonged periods, lifting heavy objects, bending over, and climbing long flights of stairs. He may also impose other restrictions, depending on the patient's condition.
• Teach the patient proper body mechanics to lessen strain and pressure on his spine.
• Instruct the patient to sleep only on a firm mattress. If necessary, advise him to purchase a new one or to insert a bed board between his mattress and box spring.

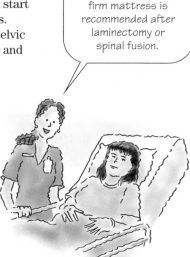

Sleeping on a firm mattress is recommended after laminectomy or spinal fusion.

Open reduction and internal fixation

During open reduction, the surgeon restores the normal position and alignment of fracture fragments or dislocated joints. He then inserts internal fixation devices — such as pins, screws, wires, nails, rods, or plates — to maintain alignment until healing can occur.

Patient preparation

Before the procedure, take these steps:
• Because this procedure requires general or regional anesthesia, instruct the patient not to eat after midnight the night before.
• Tell the patient that he'll likely receive a sedative and antibiotics before going to the operating room.

Monitoring and aftercare

After the procedure, take these steps:
• Describe to the patient the bulk dressing and surgical drain that he'll have in place for several days postoperatively.

• Tell him that he may need a cast or splint for support when the drain is removed and swelling subsides.

Home care instructions

Before discharge, assess whether the patient needs home health care and give the patient these instructions:

• Teach him how to care for the device, if appropriate. Tell him to check his skin regularly under and around the device, if possible, for irritation and breakdown. Also instruct him to watch for signs of incisional infection (redness, swelling, drainage, and foul odor from the site).

• Advise him to follow the practitioner's orders about exercising and placing weight on the affected joint. (See *Reviewing internal fixation devices.*)

Reviewing internal fixation devices

Fractures can be stabilized with various internal devices: pins, nails, rods, or screwplates. Choice of a specific device depends on the location, type, and configuration of the fracture.

For instance, in trochanteric or subtrochanteric fractures, the surgeon may use a hip pin or nail (with or without plate) or a screwplate. Because weight bearing imposes great stresses on this area, the patient requires strong control of both proximal and distal bone fragments.

A pin or plate with extra nails stabilizes the fracture by impacting the bone ends at the fracture site.

In an uncomplicated fracture of the femoral shaft, the surgeon may use an intramedullary rod. This device permits early ambulation with partial weight bearing.

In an upper extremity fracture, the surgeon may use a plate, rod, or nail. Most radius and ulna fractures may be fixed with plates, whereas humerus fractures may be fixed with rods.

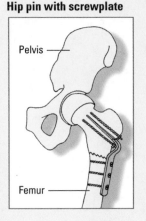

Hip pin with screwplate

Pelvis

Femur

Intramedullary rod

Femur

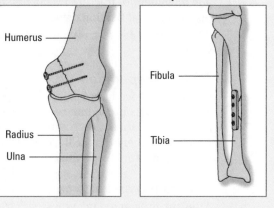

Pins in humerus

Humerus

Radius

Ulna

Screwplate in tibia

Fibula

Tibia

Nursing diagnoses

Several nursing diagnoses are used for patients with musculo-skeletal disorders. Common ones appear in this section, along with appropriate nursing interventions and rationales. See *NANDA-I taxonomy II by domain*, page 936, for the complete list of NANDA diagnoses.

Activity intolerance

Related to impaired physical mobility, *Activity intolerance* may be associated with pain or edema. Alternatively, the patient's activity may be severely restricted by such conditions as fractures requiring skeletal traction, rheumatoid arthritis, vertebral fractures, neurogenic arthropathy, Paget's disease, muscular dystrophy, and other disorders.

Expected outcomes
- Patient reports factors that decrease his activity tolerance.
- Patient progresses to his highest level of possible activity.

Nursing interventions and rationales
- Perform active or passive ROM exercises to all extremities every 2 to 4 hours to foster muscle strength and tone, maintain joint mobility, and prevent contractures.
- Turn and reposition the patient every 2 hours to prevent skin breakdown and improve breathing. Establish a turning schedule for the dependent patient. Post a schedule at the patient's bedside and monitor frequency.
- Maintain proper body alignment at all times to avoid contractures and maintain optimal musculoskeletal balance and physiologic function.
- Encourage active exercise. Provide a trapeze or other assistive device whenever possible. Such devices simplify moving and turning for many patients and allow them to strengthen some upper-body muscles.
- Teach isometric exercises to allow the patient to maintain or increase muscle tone and joint mobility.
- Have the patient perform self-care activities. Begin slowly and increase daily, as tolerated. These activities help the patient regain his health.

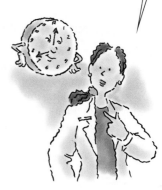

Turn and reposition the patient every 2 hours to prevent skin breakdown and improve breathing.

You can do it!

• Provide emotional support and encouragement to help improve patient self-esteem and provide the motivation to perform ADLs.
• Involve the patient in care-related planning and decision making to improve compliance.
• Monitor physiologic responses to increased activity level, including respirations, heart rate and rhythm, and blood pressure to ensure that they return to normal within a few minutes after exercising.
• Teach caregivers to assist the patient with self-care activities in a way that maximizes the patient's potential. This encourages caregivers to participate in patient care and to support patient independence. Place needed objects within reach to encourage independence.
• Explain the importance of following the prescribed medical and physical therapy regimens. As the patient's understanding of his condition improves, his compliance increases.

Deficient knowledge

Deficient knowledge is related to a lack of information about management and control of disease. Your patient's understanding of his condition will directly affect his ability to cope and his recovery.

Expected outcomes

• Patient reports an increase in knowledge regarding disease.
• Patient demonstrates ability to perform new skill related to his lifestyle.

Nursing interventions and rationales

• Assess the patient's level of understanding of the disease, its course, and its management. This helps you formulate an appropriate teaching plan. Provide a quiet environment, conducive to teaching and learning.
• Provide information at a pace and in a form appropriate for the patient to enhance his understanding and retention of information.
• Identify the patient's learning style. Then select teaching strategies — such as discussion, demonstration, role-playing, and visual materials — that are appropriate to his style. This makes your teaching more effective.
• Identify and teach the skills the patient must incorporate into his daily lifestyle. Ask for a return demonstration of each new skill to help him gain confidence.

- Have the patient incorporate learned skills into his daily routine during hospitalization. This allows him to practice them and receive feedback.
- Provide the patient with the names and telephone numbers of resource people or organizations to provide continuity of care and follow-up after discharge.

Impaired physical mobility

Impaired physical mobility is related to many musculoskeletal disorders involving joint inflammation as well as to fractures, bone disorders, and other disorders that cause decreased mobility.

Expected outcomes

- Patient demonstrates safety measures while increasing mobility.
- Patient reports an increase or optimum mobility.
- Patient describes ways to increase physical mobility.

Nursing interventions and rationales

- Instruct the patient in ROM exercises (active and passive) to increase strength.
- Teach him how to use adaptive aids for mobility so that he can do as much as possible for himself.
- Encourage increased mobility for short durations several times per day to increase strength and confidence.
- Provide emotional support and encouragement to help improve the patient's self-esteem and provide motivation.
- Teach the patient how to walk and transfer from a wheelchair safely to prevent falls or accidents.

Common musculoskeletal disorders

This section discusses musculoskeletal disorders. For each disorder you'll find information on causes, assessment findings, diagnostic tests, treatments, nursing interventions, and patient teaching.

Make sure you have the proper support when using a computer. Strenuous use of the hands can aggravate carpal tunnel syndrome.

Carpal tunnel syndrome

Carpal tunnel syndrome is the most common nerve entrapment syndrome. It results from compression of the median nerve at the wrist, within the carpal tunnel (formed by the carpal bones and the transverse carpal ligament).

The median nerve, along with blood vessels and flexor tendons, passes through this tunnel to the fingers and thumb.

Definitely a hands-on disorder

Carpal tunnel syndrome usually occurs in women between ages 30 and 60 and poses a serious occupational health problem. Assembly-line workers, packers, and people who repeatedly use poorly designed tools are most likely to develop this disorder. Any strenuous use of the hands aggravates this condition.

What causes it

The cause of carpal tunnel syndrome is unknown, but damage to the median nerve may result from:
• repetitive wrist motions involving excessive flexion or extension
• dislocation
• acute sprain.

Pathophysiology

The median nerve controls motions in the forearm, wrist, and hand and supplies sensation to the index, middle, and ring fingers. Compression of the median nerve results in sensory and motor changes in the median distribution of the hand.

What to look for

Signs and symptoms of carpal tunnel syndrome include weakness, pain, burning, numbness, or tingling in one or both hands. This paresthesia affects the thumb, forefinger, middle finger, and one-half of the fourth finger.

A surplus of signs and symptoms

Other indications include decreased sensation to light touch or pinpricks in the affected fingers; an inability to clench the hand into a fist; nail atrophy; dry, shiny skin; and pain, possibly spreading to the forearm and, in severe cases, as far as the shoulder.

What tests tell you

• Diagnosis of carpal tunnel syndrome is based on these characteristic tests and findings:
– Tinel's sign: Tingling occurs over the median nerve on light percussion.
– Phalen's maneuver: Carpal tunnel syndrome symptoms occur when the patient holds his forearms vertically and allows both hands to drop into complete flexion at the wrists for 1 minute.

– Compression test: Blood pressure cuff inflated above systolic pressure on the forearm for 1 to 2 minutes provokes pain and paresthesia along the distribution of the median nerve.

– Electromyography: A median nerve motor conduction delay of more than 5 milliseconds suggests carpal tunnel syndrome.

How it's treated

Conservative treatment includes resting the hands by splinting the wrists in neutral extension for 1 to 2 weeks. If a definite link has been established between the patient's occupation and carpal tunnel syndrome, he may have to seek other work. Effective treatment may also require correction of an underlying disorder.

Free at last!

When conservative treatment fails, the only alternative is surgical decompression of the nerve by sectioning the entire transverse carpal tunnel ligament. Neurolysis (freeing of the nerve fibers) may also be necessary.

What to do

• Administer mild analgesics as needed. Encourage the patient to use his hands as much as possible; however, if the dominant hand is impaired, you may have to help with eating and bathing.

• After surgery, monitor vital signs, and regularly check the color, sensation, and motion of the affected hand. Suggest occupational counseling for the patient who has to change jobs because of carpal tunnel syndrome.

• Evaluate the patient. Following successful interventions (such as splinting and surgery), muscle strength and normal ROM in the affected hand and wrist should progressively return. The patient should be free from pain or paresthesia in the affected hand. (See *Carpal tunnel syndrome teaching tips.*)

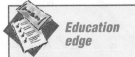

Education edge

Carpal tunnel syndrome teaching tips

• Teach the patient how to apply a splint. Warn him not to make it too tight.

• Show him how to remove the splint and how to perform gentle range-of-motion exercises. Advise him to do these exercises daily.

• Recommend that, after discharge, the patient exercise his hands occasionally in warm water. If his arm is in a sling, tell him to remove the sling several times per day to exercise his elbow and shoulder.

Herniated intervertebral disk

A herniated disk occurs when all or part of the nucleus pulposus (the soft, gelatinous, central portion of an intervertebral disk) forces through the weakened or torn anulus fibrosus (outer ring).

Impingement is irritating

The extruded disk may impinge on spinal nerve roots as they exit from the spinal canal or on the spinal cord itself, resulting in back pain and other signs of nerve root irritation. Most herniation occurs in the lumbar and lumbosacral regions.

A closer look

What happens when a disk herniates?

The spinal column is made of vertebrae that are separated by cartilage called *disks*. Within each disk is a soft, gelatinous center that acts as a cushion during vertebral movement. When severe trauma, strain, or intervertebral joint degeneration occurs, the outer fibrous ring can weaken or tear, the pulpy nucleus can be forced through, and the extruded disk can impinge on the spinal nerve root or spinal column.

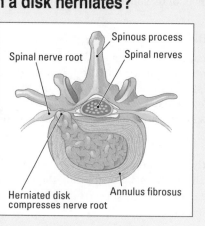

What causes it

Herniated intervertebral disk has two causes:

- Trauma or strain
- Degenerative disk disease.

Pathophysiology

The ligament and posterior capsule of the disk are usually torn, allowing the nucleus pulposus to extrude, compressing the nerve root. Occasionally, the injury tears the entire disk loose, causing protrusion onto the nerve root or compression of the spinal cord. Large amounts of extruded nucleus pulposus or complete disk herniation of the capsule and nucleus pulposus may compress the spinal cord. (See *What happens when a disk herniates?*)

What to look for

The overriding symptom of lumbar herniated disk is severe lower back pain that radiates to the buttocks, legs, and feet (usually unilaterally). The pain intensifies with Valsalva's maneuver, coughing, sneezing, or bending.

The patient may also experience motor and sensory loss in the area innervated by the compressed spinal nerve root and, in later stages, weakness and atrophy of leg muscles.

What tests tell you

Although the straight-leg-raising test and Lasègue's test are perhaps the best tests to determine herniated disk, other tests are used as well:

• Straight-leg-raising test: The patient lies supine while the examiner places one hand on the ilium (to stabilize the pelvis) and the other hand under the ankle. Then the examiner slowly raises the patient's leg. This test is positive only if the patient complains of sciatic (posterior leg) pain and not lower back pain.

• Lasègue's test: The patient lies supine while the examiner flexes his thigh and knee to a 90-degree angle. Resistance and pain as well as absent or decreased ankle or knee deep tendon reflexes indicate spinal root compression.

• Myelography, CT scan, and MRI: These tests provide the most specific diagnostic information, showing spinal compression caused by the herniated disk. CT scan and MRI have, for the most part, replaced myelography.

X out the X-rays

Although X-ray is essential to rule out other abnormalities, it isn't a good diagnostic tool for herniated intervertebral disk. Marked disk herniation can be present despite a normal X-ray.

How it's treated

Initially, conservative treatment consists of several days of bed rest (possibly with pelvic traction), heat applications, and an exercise program.

Medications that mend

Drug therapy includes aspirin to reduce inflammation and edema at the injury site and (rarely) corticosteroids for the same purpose. The patient may also benefit from muscle relaxants, especially diazepam (Valium) or the analgesic hydrocodone with acetaminophen (Vicodin).

Calling the disk doctor

If neurologic impairment progresses rapidly, or a herniated disk fails to respond to conservative treatment, surgery may be necessary:

• Laminectomy, the most common procedure, involves excision of a portion of the lamina and removal of the protruding disk.

• Spinal fusion may be necessary to overcome segmental instability if laminectomy doesn't alleviate pain and disability. Laminectomy and spinal fusion may be performed concurrently to stabilize the spine.

• Chemonucleolysis — injection of the enzyme chymopapain into the herniated disk to dissolve the nucleus pulposus — is a possible alternative to laminectomy. However, this procedure isn't as popular as it once was because it has been found to be less effective than other treatments and may cause severe allergic reaction or nerve damage.

• Microdiskectomy can be used to remove fragments of nucleus pulposus. This form of microsurgery is becoming more popular.

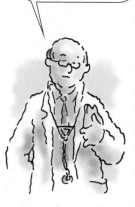

Microdiskectomy is being used more and more for herniated disks.

What to do

• During conservative treatment, watch for a deterioration in neurologic status (especially during the first 24 hours after admission). This may indicate an urgent need for surgery.

• Use antiembolism stockings or a sequential pressure device (stockings) as prescribed, and encourage the patient to move his legs as allowed. Provide high-topped sneakers to prevent footdrop.

• Work closely with the physical therapy department to ensure a consistent regimen of leg- and back-strengthening exercises.

• Give plenty of fluids to prevent renal stasis and constipation and remind the patient to cough, deep-breathe, and use an incentive spirometer to help prevent pulmonary complications.

• Provide good skin care.

Rollin', rollin', rollin'

• After laminectomy, diskectomy, or spinal fusion, enforce activity limitations as ordered. Monitor vital signs and check for bowel sounds and abdominal distention. Use a logrolling technique to turn the patient.

• If a closed drainage system is in use, check the tubing frequently for kinks and a secure vacuum. Empty the Hemovac at the end of each shift as ordered, and record the amount and color of drainage. Report colorless moisture on dressings (possible CSF leakage) or excessive drainage immediately. Observe the neurovascular status of the legs, including color, motion, temperature, and sensation.

• Administer analgesics as ordered, especially 30 minutes before initial attempts at sitting or walking. Assist the patient during his first attempt to walk. Provide a straight-backed chair for limited sitting.

• Before chemonucleolysis, make sure the patient isn't allergic to meat tenderizers (chymopapain is a similar substance). Such an allergy contraindicates the use of this enzyme, which can produce severe anaphylaxis in a sensitive patient.

• After chemonucleolysis, enforce activity limitations as ordered. Administer analgesics and apply heat as needed. Urge the patient to cough and breathe deeply. Assist with special exercises, and tell the patient to continue these exercises after discharge.
• Provide emotional support. Try to raise the patient's spirits during periods of frustration and depression. Assure him of his progress and offer encouragement.
• Evaluate the patient's response to treatment. Look for absence of pain, ability to maintain adequate mobility, and ability to perform ADLs. The patient should also express an understanding of his treatments and any adjustments he must make in his lifestyle. (See *Herniated intervertebral disk teaching tips*.)

Gout

In gout, urate deposits lead to painfully arthritic joints. It can strike any joint but occurs most commonly in the feet and legs. Primary gout usually occurs in men age 30 and older and in postmenopausal women. Secondary gout occurs in the elderly.

All about gout

Gout follows an intermittent course and commonly leaves patients symptom-free for years between attacks. It can lead to chronic disability or incapacitation and, rarely, severe hypertension and progressive renal disease. Prognosis is good with treatment.

What causes it

Although the cause of primary gout remains unknown, it appears to be linked to a genetic defect in purine metabolism, which causes hyperuricemia (overproduction of uric acid), retention of uric acid, or both.

Secondary gout develops during the course of other diseases, such as obesity, diabetes mellitus, hypertension, polycythemia, leukemia, myeloma, sickle cell anemia, and renal disease. It can also follow drug therapy, especially after hydrochlorothiazide or pyrazinamide.

Pathophysiology

In gout, increased concentration of uric acid leads to tophi (urate deposits) in joints or tissues. These crystals trigger an immune response, causing local necrosis or fibrosis.

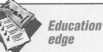

Education edge

Herniated intervertebral disk teaching tips

• Teach the patient who has undergone spinal fusion how to wear a brace if ordered.
• Teach proper body mechanics when lifting: bending at the knees and hips (never at the waist), and standing straight.
• Advise the patient to lie down when tired. He should sleep on his side (never on his abdomen) or in a semi-Fowler's position, using an extra-firm mattress or a bed board to reduce tension on his spine.
• Advise the patient to maintain proper weight to avoid lordosis caused by obesity.
• Warn the patient who must take a muscle relaxant of possible adverse effects. Advise him to avoid activities that require alertness until he has built up a tolerance to the drug's sedative effects.

What to look for

Gout develops in four stages:

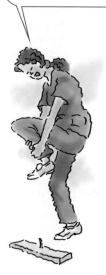

- asymptomatic
- acute
- intercritical
- chronic.

In asymptomatic gout, serum urate levels rise but produce no symptoms. As the disease progresses, it may cause hypertension or nephrolithiasis with severe back pain.

You can't flout gout

The first acute attack strikes suddenly and peaks quickly. Although it usually involves only one joint or a few joints, it's extremely painful. Affected joints appear hot, tender, inflamed, dusky red, or cyanotic.

The metatarsophalangeal joint of the great toe usually becomes inflamed first (podagra), and then the instep, ankle, heel, knee, or wrist joints. Sometimes a low-grade fever is present. Mild acute attacks typically subside quickly but tend to recur at irregular intervals. Severe attacks may persist for days or weeks.

A gap between attacks

Intercritical periods are the symptom-free intervals between gout attacks. Most patients have a second attack within 6 months to 2 years, but in some people, the second attack is delayed for 5 to 10 years.

Delayed attacks are more common in those who are untreated and tend to be longer and more severe than initial attacks. Such attacks are also polyarticular, invariably affecting joints in the feet and legs, and are sometimes accompanied by fever.

Persistent and painful

Eventually, chronic polyarticular gout sets in. This final, unremitting stage of the disease — also called chronic or tophaceous gout — is marked by persistent painful polyarthritis, with large, subcutaneous tophi in cartilage, synovial membranes, tendons, and soft tissue.

Tophi form in the fingers, hands, knees, feet, ulnar sides of the forearms, helix of the ear, Achilles tendons, and, rarely, in internal organs, such as the kidneys and myocardium. The skin over the tophus may ulcerate and release a chalky, white exudate or pus. Chronic inflammation and tophaceous deposits precipitate secondary joint degeneration, with eventual erosions, deformity, and disability.

Kidney involvement, with associated tubular damage, leads to chronic renal dysfunction. Hypertension and albuminuria occur in some patients and urolithiasis is common.

Nothing fake about the symptoms

Pseudogout also causes abrupt joint pain and swelling but results from an accumulation of calcium pyrophosphate in periarticular joint structures.

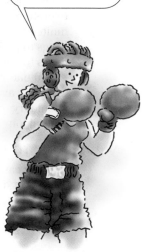

In chronic gout, X-rays show a punched-out look when urate acids replace bony structures.

What tests tell you

• Urate monohydrate crystals in synovial fluid taken from an inflamed joint or tophus establish the diagnosis. Arthrocentesis (aspiration of synovial fluid) or aspiration of tophaceous material reveals needlelike intracellular crystals of sodium urate.
• Although hyperuricemia isn't specifically diagnostic of gout, tests reveal above-normal serum uric acid levels. Uric acid levels are usually higher in secondary gout than in primary gout.
• Initially, X-ray examinations are normal. However, in chronic gout, X-rays show a punched-out look when urate acids replace bony structures. As the disorder destroys cartilage, the joint space narrows and degenerative changes become evident. Outward displacement of the overhanging margin from the bone contour characterizes gout.

How it's treated

Management goals are to terminate an acute attack, reduce hyperuricemia, and prevent recurrence, complications, and calculi formation. Treatment of the patient with acute gout consists of bed rest; immobilization and protection of inflamed, painful joints; and local application of heat or cold.

A medley of meds

Analgesics, such as acetaminophen (Tylenol) or ibuprofen (Motrin), relieve the pain associated with mild attacks. Acute inflammation requires concomitant treatment with oral colchicine (Colcrys) at the first sign of a gout flare.

Indomethacin (Indocin) in therapeutic doses may be used instead but are less specific. Resistant inflammation may require corticosteroids or I.V. drip or I.M. corticotropin or joint aspiration and an intra-articular corticosteroid injection.

Down with serum uric acid!

Treatment of chronic gout aims to decrease serum uric acid levels. The doctor may order a continuing maintenance dosage of allopurinol to suppress uric acid formation or control uric acid levels and prevent further attacks. However, use this powerful drug cautiously in a patient with renal failure. Colchicine prevents recurrent acute attacks until uric acid returns to its normal level, but the drug doesn't affect the acid level.

Uricosuric agents — such as probenecid — promote uric acid excretion and inhibit accumulation of uric acid, but their value is limited in a patient with renal impairment. Don't administer these drugs to patients with calculi. Encourage patients taking these drugs to maintain adequate fluid intake to prevent complications.

Adjunctive therapy emphasizes a few dietary restrictions, primarily avoiding alcohol and high-purine foods. Obese patients should try to lose weight because obesity puts additional stress on painful joints.

Say good-bye to tophi

In some cases, surgery may be necessary to improve joint function or correct deformities. Tophi must be excised and drained if they become infected or ulcerated. They can also be excised to prevent ulceration, improve the patient's appearance, or make it easier for him to wear shoes or gloves.

What to do

• Encourage bed rest, but use a bed cradle to keep covers off extremely sensitive, inflamed joints.
• Give pain medication as needed, especially during acute attacks. Administer anti-inflammatory medication and other drugs as ordered. Watch for adverse effects. Be alert for GI disturbances with colchicine.
• Apply hot or cold packs to inflamed joints.
• Unless contraindicated, urge the patient to drink plenty of fluids (up to 2 qt [2 L] per day) to prevent calculi formation. When forcing fluids, record intake and output accurately. Be sure to monitor serum uric acid levels regularly. Alkalinize urine with sodium bicarbonate or another agent if ordered.
• Watch for acute gout attacks that may occur 24 to 96 hours after surgery. Even minor surgery can precipitate an attack. Before and after surgery, administer colchicine as ordered to help prevent gout attacks.

• Evaluate the patient. When assessing response to treatment, note whether the patient's pain is relieved or controlled. Also note whether he's complying with drug therapy and dietary restrictions to maintain normal serum urate levels and avoid recurrence of acute episodes. (See *Gout teaching tips*.)

Osteoarthritis

Osteoarthritis is the most common form of arthritis. Symptoms usually begin in middle age and may progress with age. A thorough physical examination confirms typical symptoms, and lack of systemic symptoms rules out an inflammatory joint disorder such as rheumatoid arthritis.

Disability depends on the site and severity of involvement and can range from minor limitation of the fingers to severe disability in people with hip or knee involvement. The rate of progression varies, and joints may remain stable for years in an early stage of deterioration.

What causes it

The cause of osteoarthritis is unknown. Primary osteoarthritis, a normal part of aging, results from many things, including metabolic, genetic, chemical, and mechanical factors.

Fateful event

Secondary osteoarthritis usually follows an identifiable predisposing event, most commonly trauma, congenital deformity, or another disease such as Paget's disease. It leads to degenerative changes.

Pathophysiology

This chronic condition causes deterioration of the joint cartilage and reactive new bone formation at the margins and subchondral areas. Degeneration results from a breakdown of chondrocytes, most commonly in the hips and knees. Cartilage flakes irritate the synovial lining, and the cartilage lining becomes fibrotic, causing limited joint movement. Synovial fluid leaks into bone defects, causing cysts.

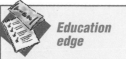

Education edge

Gout teaching tips

• Make sure the patient understands the importance of checking serum uric acid levels.
• Warn him to avoid high-purine foods, such as anchovies, liver, sardines, lentils, and alcoholic beverages, which raise the urate level.
• Explain the principles of a gradual weight reduction diet to obese patients. Such a diet features foods containing moderate amounts of protein and little fat.
• Advise the patient receiving allopurinol (Alloprim), probenecid, and other drugs to report adverse effects. Warn the patient taking probenecid to avoid aspirin or any other salicylate. Their combined effect causes urate retention.
• Inform the patient that long-term colchicine therapy is essential for the first 3 to 6 months of treatment with uricosuric drugs or allopurinol.

What to look for

The severity of these signs and symptoms increases with poor posture, obesity, and occupational stress:
- joint pain (the most common symptom) that occurs particularly after exercise or weight bearing and is usually relieved by rest
- stiffness in the morning and after exercise that's usually relieved by rest
- achiness during changes in weather
- "grating" of the joint during motion
- limited movement.

Irreparable damage

In addition, osteoarthritis of the interphalangeal joints causes irreversible changes in the distal joints (Heberden's nodes) and proximal joints (Bouchard's nodes). Nodes may be painless at first but eventually become red, swollen, and tender, causing numbness and loss of dexterity. (See *Signs of osteoarthritis.*)

> Well, your posture's good and you certainly aren't obese. Could occupational stress be causing your joint pain?

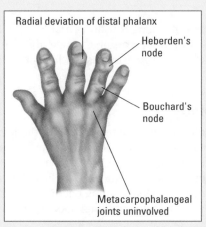

Signs of osteoarthritis

Two easily recognizable signs of osteoarthritis are Heberden's nodes and Bouchard's nodes.

Heberden's nodes
Heberden's nodes appear on the dorsolateral aspect of the distal interphalangeal joints. These bony and cartilaginous enlargements are usually hard and painless. They typically occur in middle-aged and elderly patients with osteoarthritis.

Bouchard's nodes
Bouchard's nodes are similar to Heberden's nodes but are less common and appear on the proximal interphalangeal joints.

Radial deviation of distal phalanx

Heberden's node

Bouchard's node

Metacarpophalangeal joints uninvolved

What tests tell you

• X-rays of the affected joint may show narrowing of the joint space or margins, cystlike bony deposits in the joint space and margins, joint deformity from degeneration or articular damage, and bony growths at weight-bearing areas (such as the hips and knees).
• MRI shows the affected joint, adjacent bones, and disease progression.
• Synovial fluid analysis rules out inflammatory arthritis.

How it's treated

Most measures are palliative. Medications for relief of pain and joint inflammation include aspirin (or other nonopioid analgesics), indomethacin, ketorolac, ibuprofen and, in some cases, intra-articular injections of corticosteroids. Such injections may delay the development of nodes in the hands.

Stabilizing influences

Effective treatment also reduces joint stress by supporting or stabilizing the joint with crutches, braces, a cane, a walker, a cervical collar, or traction. Other supportive measures include massage, moist heat, paraffin dips for hands, protective techniques for preventing undue stress on the joints, adequate rest (particularly after activity), and, occasionally, exercise when the knees are affected.

Surgery for severe cases

Patients who have severe osteoarthritis with disability or uncontrollable pain may undergo one or more of these surgical procedures:
• arthroplasty (partial or total): replacement of a deteriorated joint with a prosthetic appliance
• arthrodesis: surgical fusion of bones, which is used primarily in the spine (laminectomy)
• osteoplasty: scraping of deteriorated bone from a joint
• osteotomy: excision of bone to change alignment and relieve stress.

What to do

• Promote adequate rest, particularly after activity. Plan rest periods during the day, and provide for adequate sleep at night. Moderation is the key; so teach the patient to pace daily activities.
• Assist with physical therapy and encourage the patient to perform gentle ROM exercises. Provide emotional support and

reassurance to help the patient cope with limited mobility. Explain that osteoarthritis isn't a systemic disease.

• Other specific nursing measures depend on the affected joint:

– For the hand, apply hot soaks and paraffin dips as ordered to relieve pain.

– For the lumbar or sacral spine, recommend a firm mattress or bed board to decrease morning pain.

– For the cervical spine, check the cervical collar for constriction; watch for redness with prolonged use.

– For the hip, use moist heat pads to relieve pain, and administer antispasmodic drugs, as ordered. Assist with ROM and strengthening exercises, making sure that the patient gets the proper rest afterward.

– For the knee, twice daily, assist with prescribed ROM exercises, exercises to maintain muscle tone, and progressive resistance exercises to increase muscle strength. Provide elastic supports or braces if needed.

• Check crutches, braces, cane, or walker for proper fit, and teach the patient how to use them correctly. For example, the patient with unilateral joint involvement should use an orthopedic appliance (such as a cane or walker) on the unaffected side. Advise the use of cushions when sitting and suggest an elevated toilet seat.

• Evaluate the patient. Assess whether compliance with the exercise regimen slows down the debilitating effects of osteoarthritis. The patient should maintain or improve his ability to perform ADLs. He should also be able to obtain and use appropriate assistive devices. Note whether he understands and makes use of pain control interventions for involved joints. (See *Osteoarthritis teaching tips*.)

Osteomyelitis

A pyogenic bone infection, osteomyelitis may be chronic or acute. The infection causes tissue necrosis, breakdown of bone structure, and decalcification. Although it commonly remains localized, osteomyelitis can spread through the bone to the marrow, cortex, and periosteum.

In acute osteomyelitis, bacteria or fungi are either carried through the blood from another infectious site or enter the bone through the skin after surgery or trauma. With prompt treatment, the prognosis is good.

Chronic osteomyelitis, which is rare, is characterized by multiple draining sinus tracts and metastatic lesions. More prevalent in adults, it carries a poor prognosis.

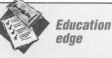

Education edge

Osteoarthritis teaching tips

• Tell the patient to plan for adequate rest during the day, after exertion, and at night.

• Warn him to avoid overexertion. He should also stand and walk correctly and be especially careful when stooping or picking up objects.

• Caution him to take his medication exactly as prescribed and to report adverse effects.

• Advise him to wear well-fitting, supportive shoes.

• Tell him to install safety devices at home such as bathroom handrails.

• Remind him to perform range-of-motion exercises as gently as possible.

• Urge him to maintain proper body weight to lessen joint stress.

• Tell him to discuss any alternative therapy with his practitioner before starting it.

What causes it

Causes of osteomyelitis include:
- traumatic injury
- acute infection originating elsewhere in the body
- organisms, such as *Staphylococcus aureus* (most common), *Streptococcus pyogenes*, *Pneumococcus*, *Pseudomonas aeruginosa*, *Escherichia coli*, and *Proteus vulgaris*
- fungi or viruses.

The rest of the risks

Other risk factors include:
- diabetes
- hemodialysis
- I.V. drug use
- any condition that decreases blood supply to the bone.

Pathophysiology

Organisms settle in a hematoma or weakened area and spread directly to the bone. Pus is produced and pressure builds within the rigid medullary cavity. Then pus is forced through the haversian canals. A subperiosteal abscess forms, depriving the bone of its blood supply. Necrosis results and new bone formation is stimulated. Dead bone detaches and exits through an abscess or the sinuses.

What to look for

Usually, the clinical signs for chronic and acute osteomyelitis are similar. However, chronic infection can persist intermittently for years, flaring up spontaneously after minor trauma. Sometimes the only sign of chronic infection is persistent drainage of pus from an old pocket in a sinus tract. Acute osteomyelitis usually has a rapid onset.

Three sure signals

Local signs and symptoms include:
- sudden pain in the affected bone
- tenderness, heat, and swelling over the affected area
- restricted movement.

What tests tell you

- WBC shows leukocytosis, and the patient has an elevated erythrocyte sedimentation rate (ESR).
- Blood culture results enable the practitioner to identify the causative organisms.

• X-rays may not show bone involvement until the disease has been active for some time, usually 2 to 3 weeks. Bone scans may enable the practitioner to detect infection early.

How it's treated

To prevent further bone damage, interventions against acute osteomyelitis may begin before definitive diagnosis. Measures include:
• administration of large doses of I.V. antibiotics after blood cultures are taken (usually a penicillinase-resistant penicillin, such as nafcillin or oxacillin)
• early surgical drainage to relieve pressure buildup and formation of sequestrum (dead bone fragments that separate from sound bone during necrosis)
• immobilization of the affected bone by plaster cast, traction, or bed rest
• supportive treatment, such as analgesics and I.V. fluids.

Attacking an abscess

If an abscess forms, treatment includes incision and drainage, followed by a culture of the drainage matter. Antibiotic therapy to control infection includes administration of systemic antibiotics, intracavitary instillation of antibiotics through closed-system continuous irrigation with low intermittent suction, limited irrigation with a closed drainage system with suction, and local application of packed, wet, antibiotic-soaked dressings.

If an infected artificial joint is the cause, it's usually removed. Antibiotic therapy is given for 2 to 3 weeks before surgery.

Bad to the bone

Besides antibiotic and immobilization therapy, patients with chronic osteomyelitis usually need surgery to remove dead bone and promote drainage. Even after surgery, the prognosis remains poor. The patient usually feels great pain and requires prolonged hospitalization. Therapy-resistant chronic osteomyelitis in an arm or leg may necessitate amputation.

What to do

Your major concerns are to control infection, protect the bone from injury, and offer meticulous supportive care. To help meet these needs, follow these guidelines:
• Use strict sterile technique when changing dressings and irrigating wounds. If the patient is in skeletal traction for compound fractures, cover insertion points of pin tracks with small, dry

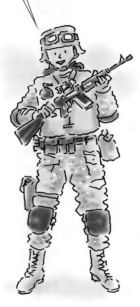

Stand guard against infection. Protect the bone from injury at all costs!

dressings, and tell him not to touch the skin around the pins and wires.
• Administer I.V. fluids to maintain adequate hydration as needed. Provide a diet high in protein and vitamin C.
• Assess vital signs every 4 hours. Assess wound appearance and new pain sites, which may indicate secondary infection, daily.
• Carefully monitor suctioning equipment. Don't let containers of instilled solution become empty — this allows air into the system. Monitor the amount of solution instilled and suctioned.
• Support the affected limb with firm pillows. Keep the limb level with the body, and don't let it sag. Provide good skin care. Turn the patient gently every 2 hours, and watch for signs of developing pressure ulcers.
• Provide good cast care. Support the cast with firm pillows, and "petal" the edges with pieces of adhesive tape or moleskin to smooth roughness. Check circulation and drainage every 4 hours for the first 24 hours postoperatively. Promptly report excessive drainage or signs of neurovascular deficits.
• Protect the patient from mishaps, such as jerky movements and falls that may threaten bone integrity. Report sudden pain, crepitus, or deformity immediately. Watch for sudden malposition of the limb, which may indicate fracture.
• Evaluate the patient. Note whether he sustained any neurovascular deficit secondary to treatment. He should achieve pain relief or pain control. New areas of pain, possibly indicating secondary infection, shouldn't appear.
• Also assess whether the patient pursues meaningful, satisfying activities that avoid the risk of fracture. Is he following therapeutic interventions? If so, look for normal body temperature, absence of pain and edema, and full ROM. (See *Osteomyelitis teaching tips*.)

Education edge

Osteomyelitis teaching tips

• Before discharge, counsel him on how to protect and clean his wound.
• Teach him how to recognize signs of recurring infection, such as increased body temperature, redness, localized heat, and swelling.
• Stress the need for follow-up examinations.
• Urge the patient to seek prompt treatment for possible sources of recurrence, such as blisters, boils, sties, and impetigo.

Osteoporosis

In osteoporosis, bones lose calcium and phosphate salts and become abnormally vulnerable to fracture. Osteoporosis may be primary or secondary to an underlying disease.

Primarily postmenopausal

Primary osteoporosis most commonly develops in postmenopausal women, although men may also develop osteoporosis. It's called *postmenopausal osteoporosis* if it occurs in women ages 50 to 75 and *senile osteoporosis* if it occurs between ages 70 and 85. Risk factors include inadequate intake or absorption of calcium, estrogen deficiency, and sedentary lifestyle.

Osteoporosis primarily affects the weight-bearing vertebrae, ribs, femurs, and wrist bones. Vertebral and wrist fractures are common.

What causes it

The cause of primary osteoporosis remains unknown. Secondary osteoporosis may result from:
• prolonged therapy with steroids, aluminum-containing antacids, heparin, anticonvulsants, or thyroid preparations
• total immobility or disuse of a bone (as with hemiplegia).

Osteoporosis is also linked to alcohol abuse, malnutrition, malabsorption, scurvy, lactose intolerance, hyperthyroidism, osteogenesis imperfecta, and Sudeck's atrophy (localized to hands and feet, with recurring attacks).

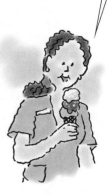

Osteoporosis is linked to several conditions, including lactose intolerance. Fortunately, I tolerate lactose just fine!

Pathophysiology

In osteoporosis, the rate of bone resorption accelerates as the rate of bone formation decelerates. Decreased bone mass results, and bones become porous and brittle.

What to look for

Although osteoporosis develops insidiously, the disease is usually discovered suddenly. An elderly person typically becomes aware of the disorder when he bends to lift something, hears a snapping sound, and then feels a sudden pain in the lower back. Any movement or jarring aggravates the backache.

Other ominous signs

Other signs and symptoms include:
• pain in the lower back that radiates around the trunk
• deformity
• kyphosis (humpback)
• loss of height
• a markedly aged appearance.

What tests tell you

• X-rays show typical degeneration in the lower thoracic and lumbar vertebrae. The vertebral bodies may appear flattened, with varying degrees of collapse and wedging, and may look denser than normal. Loss of bone mineral becomes evident in later stages.
• CT scan accurately assesses spinal bone loss.
• Bone scans show injured or diseased areas.

• Serum calcium, phosphorus, and alkaline phosphatase levels are within normal limits, but parathyroid hormone levels may be elevated.

How it's treated

The patient receives symptomatic treatment aimed at preventing additional fractures and controlling pain. Measures may include:
• a physical therapy program emphasizing gentle exercise and activity
• estrogen to decrease the rate of bone resorption and calcium and vitamin D to support normal bone metabolism (However, drug therapy merely arrests osteoporosis; it doesn't cure it.)
• a bisphosphonate, such as alendronate (Fosamax) or iban-dronate (Boniva), which slows bone resorption but does not decrease bone formation
• a back brace to support weakened vertebrae
• surgery to correct pathologic fractures of the femur by open reduction and internal fixation. Colles' fracture, a fracture of the radius where it joins the wrist, requires reduction followed by plaster-cast immobilization for 4 to 10 weeks.

An *ounce of prevention*

Adequate intake of dietary calcium and regular weight-bearing exercise may reduce a person's chances of developing senile osteoporosis. Although hormone therapy may offer some preventive benefit, it also has risks and adverse effects.

Secondary osteoporosis can be prevented through effective treatment of the underlying disease and by judicious use of steroid therapy, early mobilization after surgery or trauma, decreased alcohol consumption, careful observation for signs of malabsorption, and prompt treatment of hyperthyroidism.

What to do

Your care plan should focus on the patient's fragility, stressing careful positioning, ambulation, prescribed exercises, and injury prevention strategies. Take these steps:
• Check the patient's skin daily for redness, warmth, and new sites of pain, which may indicate new fractures.
• Encourage activity by helping the patient walk several times daily. As appropriate, perform passive ROM exercises, or encourage the patient to perform active exercises. Make sure the patient regularly attends scheduled physical therapy sessions.
• Provide a balanced diet high in nutrients that support skeletal metabolism, such as vitamin D, calcium, and protein.
• Administer analgesics as needed. Apply heat to relieve pain.

• If the patient is prescribed a bisphosphonate to increase bone density, stress the importance of remaining upright for at least 30 minutes after taking the medication to prevent damage to the esophagus.
• Evaluate the patient. Assess whether adherence to the prescribed regimen of medication, exercise, and dietary intake of calcium, vitamin D, and protein is preventing progression of the disease. Note whether the patient demonstrates good body mechanics and if she can identify and subsequently avoid activities that increase the risk of fracture. (See *Osteoporosis teaching tips*.)

Paget's disease

Paget's disease is a slowly progressive metabolic bone disease. It usually localizes in one or several areas of the skeleton (most commonly the lower torso), although occasionally, widely distributed skeletal deformity occurs. Paget's disease can be fatal, particularly if associated with heart failure (widespread disease creates a continuous need for high cardiac output), bone sarcoma, or giant cell tumors.

What causes it

The cause remains unknown, but one theory holds that early viral infection (possibly with mumps virus) causes a dormant skeletal infection that erupts many years later as Paget's disease. The disease also tends to run in families.

Pathophysiology

In the initial phase of Paget's disease (osteoclastic phase), excessive bone resorption occurs. The second phase (osteoblastic phase) involves excessive abnormal bone formation. Affected bones enlarge and soften, and the new bone structure is chaotic, fragile, and weak.

What to look for

Although Paget's disease produces no symptoms in the early stages, it eventually produces severe, persistent pain that intensifies with weight bearing and may impair movement. Characteristic cranial enlargement occurs over frontal and occipital areas (hat size may increase). Headaches also occur with skull involvement. Bony infringement on cranial nerves may impair hearing and visual acuity.

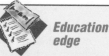

Education edge

Osteoporosis teaching tips

• Thoroughly explain osteoporosis to the patient and her family. They may feel the fractures could have been prevented if they were more careful.
• Before discharge, make sure the patient and her family understand the drug regimen.
• Tell the patient to report new pain sites immediately, no matter how slight the pain.
• Advise her to sleep on a firm mattress and to avoid excessive bed rest.
• If she has a back brace, make sure she knows how to wear it. Teach her good body mechanics.
• If a female patient is taking estrogen, emphasize the need for routine gynecologic checkups, including Papinocolaou tests and mammographys. Tell her to report abnormal vaginal bleeding. Instruct her in the proper technique for breast self-examination and instruct her to perform one monthly.

Other signs may include kyphosis, barrel-shaped chest, and asymmetrical bowing of the tibia and femur. The pagetic sites may be warm and tender, with slow and incomplete healing of fractures. The patient may walk with a waddling gait and have increased susceptibility to pathologic fractures.

What tests tell you

• X-rays may show increased bone expansion and density before overt symptoms develop.
• A bone scan (more sensitive than an X-ray) clearly shows early pagetic lesions. Radioisotope concentrates in areas of active disease.
• A bone biopsy reveals the characteristic mosaic pattern.
• Blood tests reveal anemia and elevated serum alkaline phosphatase levels. Routine biochemical screens, which include serum alkaline phosphatase, make early diagnosis more common.
• A 24-hour urine test shows an elevated hydroxyproline level. (Hydroxyproline is an amino acid excreted by the kidneys and is an index of osteoclastic hyperactivity.)

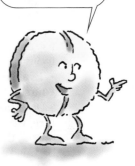

Drug therapy is the main treatment in Paget's disease.

How it's treated

Drug therapy is the primary intervention. It includes the hormone calcitonin, given subcutaneously or I.M.; etidronate (Didronel), taken by mouth; and plicamycin (Mithracin), a cytotoxic antibiotic.

Retarding resorption and reducing levels

Calcitonin and etidronate retard bone resorption and reduce serum alkaline phosphatase levels and urinary hydroxyproline secretion. Although calcitonin requires long-term maintenance therapy, improvement is noticeable after the first few weeks of treatment. Etidronate produces improvement in 1 to 3 months.

Plicamycin decreases calcium, urinary hydroxyproline, and serum alkaline phosphatase levels. This medication produces remission of symptoms within 2 weeks and biochemical improvement in 1 to 2 months. However, it may destroy platelets or compromise renal function.

Surgery still looms

Self-administration of calcitonin and etidronate helps patients with Paget's disease lead near-normal lives. Nevertheless, these patients may need surgery to reduce or prevent pathologic fractures, correct secondary deformities, and relieve neurologic impairment.

To decrease the risk of excessive bleeding from hypervascular bone, drug therapy with calcitonin and etidronate or plicamycin must precede surgery. Joint replacement is difficult if bonding material (methyl methacrylate) is used because it doesn't set properly on pagetic bone.

Other treatment is supportive and varies according to symptoms. Aspirin, indomethacin, or ibuprofen usually controls pain.

What to do

• To evaluate the effectiveness of analgesics, assess the patient's level of pain daily. Watch for new areas of pain or restricted movement, which may indicate new fracture sites. Also watch for sensory or motor disturbances, such as difficulty hearing, seeing, or walking.
• Monitor serum calcium and alkaline phosphatase levels.
• Monitor intake and output. Encourage adequate fluid intake to minimize renal calculi formation.
• If the patient is on prolonged bed rest, prevent pressure ulcers by providing good skin care. Reposition the patient frequently and use a flotation mattress. Provide high-topped sneakers to prevent footdrop.
• Evaluate the patient and assess the success of therapy by asking yourself these questions:
– Does the patient avoid activities that increase the risk of fracture, while at the same time maintaining ROM?
– Does the patient have neurologic deficits, such as footdrop, because of progression of the disease or interventions?
– Does the patient demonstrate effective coping skills for dealing with his illness?
– Has adherence to the prescribed medication and dietary regimens prevented progression of the disease? (See *Paget's disease teaching tips*.)

Rheumatoid arthritis

Rheumatoid arthritis (RA) is a chronic, systemic inflammatory disease that primarily attacks peripheral joints and surrounding muscles, tendons, ligaments, and blood vessels. Spontaneous remissions and unpredictable exacerbations mark the course of the disease. Potentially crippling, RA usually requires lifelong treatment and sometimes surgery.

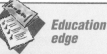

Education edge

Paget's disease teaching tips

• Demonstrate how to inject calcitonin and rotate injection sites. Advise that adverse effects may occur, although they are usually mild.
• Warn him to use analgesics as prescribed.
• Tell the patient receiving etidronate (Didronel) to take the medication with fruit juice 2 hours before or 2 hours after meals, as milk and high-calcium fluids impair absorption, and to divide dosage to minimize adverse effects.
• Tell the patient receiving plicamycin (Mithracin) to watch for signs of infection, easy bruising, bleeding, and temperature elevation and to report for regular follow-up tests.
• Teach him how to pace activities, use assistive devices, and follow a recommended exercise program. Suggest a firm mattress or a bed board to minimize spinal deformities. Advise him to remove small obstacles at home.

From intermittent to incessant

In most patients, the disease **follows** an intermittent course and allows normal activity. However, 10% of patients suffer total disability from severe articular deformity and associated extra-articular symptoms, or both. Prognosis **worsens** with the development of nodules, vasculitis, and high **titers of rheumatoid factor (RF)**.

What causes it

RA is currently believed to have **an** autoimmune basis, although the cause remains unknown.

Pathophysiology

Cartilage damage resulting **from inflammation** triggers further immune responses, including **complement activation**. Complement, in turn, attracts polymorphonuclear leukocytes and stimulates the release of inflammatory mediators, which exacerbates joint destruction.

What to look for

Initial symptoms may include **fatigue**, malaise, anorexia, persistent low-grade fever, weight **loss,** and lymphadenopathy. The patient may also experience **vague** articular symptoms.

Sooner and later

Later, the patient may develop **joint pain**, tenderness, warmth, and swelling. Usually, joint **symptoms occur** bilaterally and symmetrically. Other symptoms may **include morning** stiffness; paresthesia in the hands and feet; and stiff, **weak,** or painful muscles. The patient may also develop **rheumatoid** nodules — subcutaneous, round or oval, nontender **masses,** usually on pressure areas such as the elbow.

Advanced signs include **joint deformities** and diminished joint function. (See *Joint deformities.*)

What tests tell you

In early stages, X-rays show **bone demineralization** and soft-tissue swelling. Later, they help **determine** the extent of cartilage and bone destruction, erosion, **subluxations**, and deformities and show the characteristic **pattern of these** abnormalities. Other tests and findings include:

Joint deformities

In advanced rheumatoid arthritis, marked **edema** and congestion cause spindle-shaped interphalangeal joints and **severe** flexion deformities.

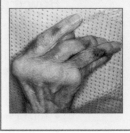

• Positive RF test occurs in 75% to 80% of patients (as indicated by a titer of 1:160 or higher).
• Synovial fluid analysis usually shows increased volume and turbidity but decreased viscosity and complement (C3 and C4) levels, with WBC count possibly exceeding 10,000/μl.
• Serum globulins are elevated.
• ESR is elevated.
• Complete blood count shows moderate anemia and slight leukocytosis.

How it's treated

Salicylates, particularly aspirin, provide the mainstay of RA therapy because they decrease inflammation and relieve joint pain. Other useful medications include:
• NSAIDs, such as indomethacin, ketorolac, and ibuprofen
• antimalarials, such as chloroquine and hydroxychloroquine (Plaquenil)
• tumor necrosis factor inhibitors, such as etanercept (Embrel)
• penicillamine (Depen)
• corticosteroids, such as prednisone
• immunosuppressants, such as methotrexate (Trexall), cyclophosphamide (Cytoxan), and azathioprine (Imuran).

Sleep well, eat right, and rest often

Supportive measures include 8 to 10 hours of sleep every night, adequate nutrition, frequent rest periods between daily activities, and splinting to rest inflamed joints. A physical therapy program, including ROM exercises and carefully individualized therapeutic exercises, forestalls loss of joint function.

Application of heat relaxes muscles and relieves pain. Moist heat, such as hot soaks, paraffin baths, and whirlpools, usually works best for patients with chronic disease. Ice packs are effective during acute episodes.

Advanced disease may require synovectomy, joint reconstruction, or total joint arthroplasty.

What to do

• Assess all joints carefully. Look for deformities, contractures, immobility, and inability to perform ADLs.
• Monitor vital signs and note weight changes, sensory disturbances, and level of pain. Administer analgesics as ordered and watch for adverse effects.

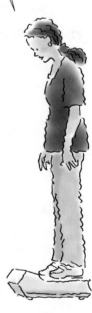

Monitor weight in a patient with RA. Obesity can put more stress on joints.

• Give meticulous skin care. Use lotion or cleansing oil, not soap, for dry skin.
• Explain all diagnostic tests and procedures. Tell the patient to expect multiple blood samples to allow firm diagnosis and accurate monitoring of therapy.

The benefits of bubble baths

• Monitor the duration, not the intensity, of morning stiffness because duration more accurately reflects the severity of the disease. Encourage the patient to take hot showers or baths at bedtime or in the morning to reduce the need for pain medication.
• Apply splints carefully. Observe for pressure ulcers if the patient is in traction or wearing splints.
• Explain the nature of RA. Make sure the patient and his family understand that RA is a chronic disease that requires major lifestyle changes.
• Encourage a balanced diet, but make sure the patient understands that special diets won't cure RA. Stress the need for weight control because obesity adds further stress to joints.
• Urge the patient to perform ADLs, such as dressing and feeding himself. Supply easy-to-open cartons, lightweight cups, and unpackaged silverware.

Can we talk?

• Provide emotional support. Encourage the patient to discuss his fears about dependency, sexuality, body image, and self-esteem. Refer the patient to an appropriate social service agency as needed.
• If appropriate, discuss sexual aids, such as alternative positions, pain medication, and moist heat to increase mobility.
• Before discharge, make sure the patient knows how and when to take his prescribed medication and how to recognize adverse effects such as GI bleeding from salicylate therapy.
• Evaluate the patient. When assessing his response to therapy, note whether compliance with exercise and dietary regimen slows progression of debilitating effects. Has he maintained or improved his ability to perform ADLs? Does he use effective pain control measures? Does he use appropriate assistive devices? (See *RA teaching tips*.)

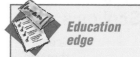

Education edge

RA teaching tips

• Teach the patient how to stand, walk, and sit upright. Tell him to sit in chairs with high seats and armrests. Suggest an elevated toilet seat.
• Instruct the patient to pace daily activities, resting for 5 to 10 minutes out of each hour and alternating sitting and standing tasks.
• Instruct the patient to sleep on his back on a firm mattress and avoid placing a pillow under his knees, which encourages flexion deformity.
• Enlist the aid of the occupational therapist to teach the patient how to simplify activities and protect arthritic joints.
• Suggest dressing aids — such as a shoehorn with a long handle, a reacher, elastic shoelaces, a zipper pull, and a buttonhook — and helpful household items, such as easy-to-open drawers, a handheld shower nozzle, and grab bars.

Scoliosis

Scoliosis — a lateral curvature of the spine — may occur in the thoracic, lumbar, or thoracolumbar spinal segment. The curve may be convex to the right (more common in thoracic curves) or to the left (more common in lumbar curves). Rotation of the vertebral column around its axis occurs and may cause rib cage deformity.

There are two types of scoliosis: functional (postural) and structural. Both types are commonly associated with kyphosis and lordosis.

What causes it

Functional scoliosis isn't a fixed deformity of the vertebral column. It results from poor posture or a discrepancy in leg lengths.

Three sorts of structural scoliosis

Structural scoliosis involves deformity of the vertebral bodies. It can be one of three types:
• Congenital scoliosis is usually related to a congenital defect, such as wedge vertebrae, fused ribs or vertebrae, or hemivertebrae.
• Paralytic, or musculoskeletal, scoliosis develops several months after asymmetrical paralysis of the trunk muscles from polio, cerebral palsy, or muscular dystrophy.
• Idiopathic scoliosis, the most common form, may be transmitted as an autosomal dominant or multifactorial trait. It appears in a previously straight spine during the growing years.

Pathophysiology

In scoliosis, the vertebrae rotate, forming the convex part of the curve. The rotation causes rib prominence along the thoracic spine and waistline asymmetry in the lumbar spine.

What to look for

The most common curve in functional or structural scoliosis arises in the thoracic segment, with convexity to the right. This curve results in compensatory curves (S curves) in the cervical segment above and the lumbar segment below, both with convexity to the left. These curves develop to maintain body balance and mark the deformity.

When the disease becomes well established, backache, fatigue, and dyspnea may occur.

Testing for scoliosis

When assessing the patient for an abnormal spinal curve, use this screening test for scoliosis. Have the patient remove her shirt and stand as straight as she can with her back to you. Instruct her to distribute her weight evenly on each foot. While the patient does this, observe both sides of her back from neck to buttocks. Look for these signs:

• uneven shoulder height and shoulder blade prominence
• unequal distance between the arms and the body
• asymmetrical waistline
• uneven hip height
• a sideways lean.

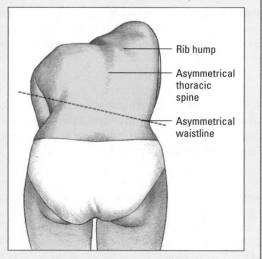

Rib hump

Asymmetrical thoracic spine

Asymmetrical waistline

   With the patient's back still facing you, ask the patient to do the "forward-bend" test. In this test, she places her palms together and slowly bends forward, keeping her head down. Look for these signs:
• asymmetrical thoracic spine or prominent rib cage (rib hump) on either side
• asymmetrical waistline.

Unequal and asymmetrical

Physical examination reveals unequal shoulder heights, elbow levels, and heights of the iliac crests. Muscles on the convex side of the curve may be rounded, whereas those on the concave side are flattened, producing asymmetry of paraspinal muscles. (See *Testing for scoliosis*.)

What tests tell you

• Anterior, posterior, and lateral spinal X-rays, taken with the patient standing upright and bending, confirm scoliosis and determine the degree of curvature and flexibility of the spine.
• Bone growth studies may help determine skeletal maturity.

How it's treated

The severity of the deformity and potential spine growth determine appropriate treatment. Interventions include close observation, exercise, a brace (for example, a Milwaukee brace), surgery, or a combination of these. To be most effective, treatment should begin early, when spinal deformity is still subtle.

Mild curve

A mild curve (less than 25 degrees) can be monitored by X-rays and an examination every 3 months. An exercise program may strengthen torso muscles and prevent curve progression. A heel lift may help.

Moderate curve

A curve of 25 degrees to 40 degrees requires spinal exercises and a brace. Alternatively, the patient may undergo transcutaneous electrical nerve stimulation. A brace halts progression in most patients but doesn't reverse established curvature.

Dangerous curve

A curve of 40 degrees or more requires surgery (spinal fusion, usually with instrumentation) because a lateral curve progresses at the rate of 1 degree per year even after skeletal maturity. Preoperative preparation may include Cotrel-Dubousset segmental instrumentation for 7 to 10 days.

Postoperative care commonly requires immobilization in a localizer cast (Risser jacket) for 3 to 6 months. Periodic checkups follow for several months to monitor stability of the correction.

What to do

• If the patient needs traction or a cast before surgery, check the skin around the cast edge daily. Keep the cast clean and dry and the edges of the cast "petaled" (padded).

Under your skin

• Warn the patient not to insert anything or let anything get under the cast and to immediately report cracks in the cast, pain, burning, skin breakdown, numbness, or odor. Watch for skin breakdown and signs of cast syndrome (such as nausea, abdominal pressure, and vague abdominal pain).
• Evaluate the patient. Make sure that she doesn't develop a neurovascular deficit or loss of skin integrity because of bracing, traction, or surgery. Can she maintain an activity level normal for her age and developmental level?
• Evaluate the results of surgery, if appropriate. Is pain absent or controlled? Are breath sounds, skin color and turgor, elimination patterns, and arterial blood gas levels normal? Are shoulders and hips aligned horizontally? (See *Scoliosis teaching tips.*)

Education edge

Scoliosis teaching tips

For a patient with a brace
• Tell the patient to wear the brace 23 hours per day and to remove it only for bathing and exercise. Recommend that she lie down and rest several times per day until she gets used to the brace.
• To prevent skin breakdown, advise the patient not to use lotions, ointments, or powders on areas where the brace contacts the skin. Instead, she should use rubbing alcohol or compound benzoin tincture to toughen the skin. Tell her to keep the skin dry and clean and to wear a snug T-shirt under the brace.
• Instruct the patient to turn her whole body, not just her head, when looking to the side.

For a patient with a cast or in traction
If the patient needs traction or a cast before surgery, explain these procedures to her and her family. Remember that application of a body cast can be traumatic because it's done on a special frame and the patient's head and face are covered throughout the procedure.

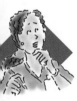

Quick quiz

1.   If your patient can't move his right arm away from his side, you document this as impaired:
    A. supination.
    B. abduction.
    C. eversion.
    D adduction.

Answer: B. Abduction is the ability to move a limb away from the midline.

2.   What's a positive sign of carpal tunnel syndrome?
    A. Trousseau's sign
    B. Phalen's sign
    C. Tzanck test
    D. Tinel's sign

Answer: D. Tinel's sign, a complaint of tingling over the median nerve on light percussion, is a positive sign of carpal tunnel syndrome.

3.   Irreversible changes in the distal joints of the fingers caused by osteoarthritis are known as:
   A. Bouchard's nodes.
   B. lymph nodes.
   C. Heberden's nodes
   D. supraclavicular nodes.

Answer: C. Heberden's nodes are the result of changes in the distal joints of the fingers.

4.   Osteoporosis is characterized by:
   A. crystal deposition and brittleness.
   B. brittleness and swelling of the joints.
   C. porosity and brittleness.
   D. joint stiffness and deformity.

Answer: C. Osteoporosis is a metabolic bone disorder in which bone loses calcium and phosphate and becomes porous, brittle, and abnormally vulnerable to fractures.

5.   Which medication is used to treat RA?
   A. Aspirin
   B. Acetominophen (Tylenol)
   C. Calcitonin
   D. Etidronate (Didronel)

Answer: A. Salicylates, particularly aspirin, provide the mainstay of RA therapy because they decrease inflammation and relieve joint pain.

Scoring

☆☆☆ If you answered all five questions correctly, way to go! You're a bred in the bone musculoskeletal maven!

 ☆☆ If you answered four questions correctly, impressive! Make no bones about it, you have a mastery of musculoskeletal matters!

  ☆ If you answered fewer than three questions correctly, don't become unhinged! Just bone up a bit, and you'll be playing ball and socket with the big boys soon.

16

Hematologic and lymphatic disorders

Just the facts

In this chapter, you'll learn:

♦ anatomy and physiology of the hematologic system

♦ techniques for assessing the hematologic system

♦ causes, pathophysiology, diagnostic tests, and interventions for common hematologic and lymphatic disorders.

A look at hematologic and lymphatic disorders

Because the hematologic system affects every body system, caring for a patient with a hematologic disorder can be especially challenging. For example, a patient's dyspnea may lead you to suspect a respiratory or cardiovascular condition — when his primary problem is anemia.

To help ensure accurate diagnosis and effective care, you'll need to obtain an especially thorough history and physical assessment. With astute, sensitive care founded on a firm understanding of hematologic basics, you can help patients survive these disorders. Even when the prognosis is poor, you can help patients make the necessary adjustments to maintain an optimal quality of life.

Anatomy and physiology

The hematologic system consists of blood — the major body fluid tissue — and the bone marrow, which manufactures new blood cells in a process called *hematopoiesis*. Blood delivers oxygen and nutrients to all tissues, removes wastes, and performs many other tasks. (See *Mapping out blood cell formation*, pages 738.)

A closer look

Mapping out blood cell formation

Blood cells form and develop in the bone marrow by a process called *hematopoiesis*. This chart breaks down the process from the time the myeloid and lymphoid stem cells are "born" from the pluripotent stem cell until they each reach "adulthood" as fully formed cells — erythrocytes, granulocytes (eosinophils, basophils, neutrophils), agranulocytes (monocytes, B-lymphocytes, T-lymphocytes), or platelets.

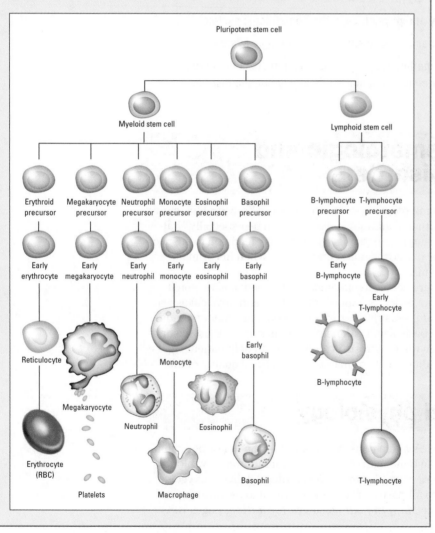

Blood

Blood consists of various formed elements, or blood cells, suspended in a fluid called *plasma*. Formed elements of the blood include:
- red blood cells (RBCs), or erythrocytes
- platelets (thrombocytes)
- white blood cells (WBCs), or leukocytes.

Turf talk

RBCs and platelets function entirely within blood vessels. WBCs, in contrast, act mainly in the tissues outside the blood vessels.

Red blood cells

RBCs transport oxygen and carbon dioxide to and from body tissues. They contain hemoglobin (Hb), the oxygen-carrying substance that gives blood its red color. The RBC surface carries antigens (substances that trigger formation of antibodies that interact specifically with that antigen). These antigens determine a person's blood group, or blood type.

Out with the old...

Constant circulation wears out RBCs, which have an average life span of 120 days. The spleen sequesters, or isolates, the old, worn-out RBCs, removing them from circulation. This process requires the body to manufacture billions of new cells daily to maintain RBCs at normal levels.

... in with the new

The bone marrow releases RBCs into the circulation in an immature form called *reticulocytes*, which mature into RBCs in about 1 day. The rate of reticulocyte release usually equals the rate of old RBC removal. When RBC depletion occurs — for example, with hemorrhage — the bone marrow increases reticulocyte production to maintain normal RBC levels.

Blood groups

Blood falls into one of four types:
- In type A blood, the A antigen appears on RBCs.
- In type B blood, the B antigen appears.
- Type AB blood contains both the A and B antigens.
- Type O blood has neither the A antigen nor the B antigen.

Blood from any of these types may also contain the Rhesus (Rh) factor antigen. Blood with the Rh antigen is Rh-positive; blood without it is Rh-negative.

Antagonistic actions

Plasma may contain antibodies (immunoglobulins) that interact with these antigens, causing the cells to agglutinate (clump together). However, plasma can't contain antibodies to its own cell antigen, or it would destroy itself. Thus, type A blood has A antigen but no anti-A antibodies, although it does have anti-B antibodies.

This principle is important for blood transfusions: The donor's blood type must be compatible with the recipient's. Otherwise, the transfusion may be fatal. That's why precise blood typing and crossmatching (mixing and observing for agglutination of donor cells) are essential.

You think you might be type B but you're not sure? We need to know that to find out if we're compatible!

Platelets

Platelets are small, colorless, disk-shaped, cytoplasmic fragments split from very large bone marrow cells called *megakaryocytes*. Their life span is approximately 10 days.

Platelets perform three vital functions:
• They initiate contraction of damaged blood vessels to minimize blood loss.
• They form hemostatic plugs in injured blood vessels to help stop bleeding.
• Along with plasma, they provide materials that accelerate blood clot formulation, or coagulation.

White blood cells

Five types of WBCs (neutrophils, eosinophils, basophils, monocytes, and lymphocytes) participate in the body's defense and immune systems. WBCs are classified as granulocytes or agranulocytes based on:
• shape of the nucleus (the sphere that contains the genetic codes for maintaining and reproducing that cell)
• presence or absence of granules (small particles) in the cytoplasm (all of the cell's contents excluding the nucleus)
• affinity for laboratory stains or dyes.

Granulocytes

Granulocytes contain a single multilobed nucleus and prominent cytoplasmic granules. Types of granulocytes include neutrophils, eosinophils, and basophils.

Polly wants a shorter name

Collectively, these cells are called *polymorphonuclear leukocytes*. However, each cell type exhibits different properties, and each is activated by different stimuli.

Neutrophils

Neutrophils, the most abundant type of granulocyte, account for 48% to 77% of circulating WBCs. Like granulocytes, neutrophils are phagocytic.

Neutrophils leave the bloodstream by passing through intact capillary walls into surrounding tissues — a process called *diapedesis*. Then they migrate to and accumulate at infection sites.

Eating the enemy

Neutrophils are phagocytes — cells that engulf, ingest, and digest waste material, harmful microorganisms, and other foreign bodies. Consequently, they serve as the body's first line of cellular defense against foreign organisms.

Strike up the bands

Worn-out neutrophils form the main component of pus. Bone marrow produces their replacements — immature neutrophils called *bands*. In response to infection, the bone marrow must produce many immature cells and release them into the circulation, which elevates the band count.

Eosinophils

Eosinophils account for only 0.3% to 7% of circulating WBCs. These granulocytes also migrate from the bloodstream by diapedesis, but do so in response to an allergic reaction. Eosinophils accumulate in loose connective tissue, where they take part in ingesting antigen-antibody complexes.

Basophils

Basophils usually account for less than 2% of circulating WBCs. These cells have little or no phagocytic ability. However, their cytoplasmic granules secrete histamine (a vasodilator) in response to certain inflammatory and immune stimuli. This action causes an increase in vascular permeability and eases fluid passage from capillaries into body tissues.

Agranulocytes

WBCs in this category — monocytes and lymphocytes — lack specific cytoplasmic granules and have nuclei without lobes.

Monocytes

Monocytes, the largest of the WBCs, constitute only 0.6% to 10% of WBCs in circulation. Like neutrophils, monocytes are phagocytic and diapedetic. Outside the bloodstream, they enlarge and mature, becoming tissue macrophages (also called *histiocytes*).

Protection from infection

As macrophages, monocytes may roam freely through the body when stimulated by inflammation. Usually, however, they remain immobile, populating most organs and tissues.

Collectively, monocytes are components of the mononuclear phagocyte system (MPS), formerly called the reticuloendothelial system. The MPS defends against infection and disposes of cell breakdown products.

Fluid finders

Macrophages concentrate in structures that filter large amounts of body fluid — such as the liver, spleen, and lymph nodes — where they defend against invading organisms.

Macrophages are efficient phagocytes of bacteria, cellular debris (including worn-out neutrophils), and necrotic (dead) tissue. When mobilized at an infection site, they engulf and destroy cellular remnants and promote wound healing.

Lymphocytes

Lymphocytes, the smallest of the WBCs and the second most numerous (16% to 43%), derive from stem cells in the bone marrow. They exist in two types:
• T lymphocytes, which directly attack an infected cell
• B lymphocytes, which produce antibodies against specific antigens.

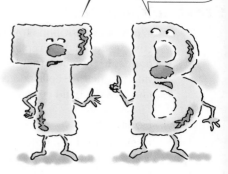

T cells attack infections directly. But B cells, like my buddy here, produce antibodies that do the dirty work for them.

It's easier that way!

Assessment

Many signs and symptoms of hematologic disorders are nonspecific. However, certain ones are more specific and can help you focus on possible disorders. These include:
• abnormal bleeding
• bone and joint pain
• exertional dyspnea
• shortness of breath
• ecchymoses (bruising)
• fatigue and weakness
• fever

- lymphadenopathy (enlarged lymph nodes)
- petechiae (tiny purplish spots caused by minute hemorrhages).

If your patient has one of these more specific signs or symptoms, turn your attention to assessing his hematologic system.

History

Start your assessment by taking a thorough patient history. To increase the patient's cooperation, develop a trusting relationship with him.

Current health status

Ask the patient why he's seeking medical help. Document his response in his own words. Keep in mind that signs and symptoms of hematologic problems can appear in any body system, so patient complaints may be nonspecific — such as lack of energy, light-headedness, or nosebleeds.

Picking out patterns

Nonspecific complaints aren't diagnostic in themselves. However, when considered in the context of a complete patient history, they may establish a pattern that suggests a hematologic disorder.

Previous health status

Ask about the patient's medical history, which may provide clues to his present condition. Stay alert for disorders (such as acute leukemia, Hodgkin's disease, or sarcoma) that necessitated aggressive immunosuppressant or radiation therapies.

If your patient was hospitalized, ask why. Could a previous surgical intervention, such as a splenectomy, be causing a medical problem?

Has the patient received blood products? If so, note when and how many he received to help assess his risk of harboring an infection transmitted by transfusion.

Finally, document all the medications he's taking — prescription and over-the-counter. Some medications interfere with various components of the hematologic system.

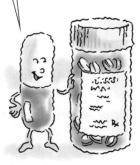

Document all the medications your patient takes, including over-the-counter preparations.

Family history

Ask about deceased family members, recording the cause of death and their ages at death. Note hereditary hematologic disorders, such as hemophilia, von Willebrand's disease, and sickle cell anemia. Plot these disorders on a family genogram to determine the inheritance risk.

Social history

Ask your patient about:
• alcohol intake, diet, sexual habits, and possible drug abuse, which can impair hematologic function
• exposure to such hazardous substances as benzene or Agent Orange, which can cause bone marrow dysfunction (especially leukemia).

Physical examination

Because a hematologic disorder can involve almost every body system, be sure to conduct a complete physical examination.

A seemly sequence

When assessing the abdomen, be sure to inspect first, then auscultate, percuss, and palpate. Palpating or percussing the abdomen before you auscultate it can change the character of bowel sounds and lead to an inaccurate assessment.

Inspection

Focus your inspection on the areas most relevant to a hematologic disorder — the skin, mucous membranes, fingernails, eyes, lymph nodes, liver, and spleen.

Skin and mucous membranes

Skin color directly reflects body fluid composition. Observe for pallor, cyanosis, and jaundice. Because normal skin color can vary widely among individuals, ask the patient if his present skin tone is normal.

Inspect the patient's face, conjunctivae, hands, and feet for plethora (a ruddy color) — a symptom of polycythemia (a disorder marked by excess RBCs). Also look for erythema (redness) of the skin, which may indicate local inflammation or fever.

Not-so-mellow yellow

Next, assess the skin and mucous membranes for jaundice. Be sure to observe the patient in natural light rather than incandescent light, which can mask a yellowish tinge. With a dark-skinned patient, inspect the buccal mucosa, palms, and soles for a yellowish tinge. In a patient with edema, examine the inner forearm for jaundice.

Purplish purpuric patches

If you suspect a blood-clotting abnormality, check the skin for purpuric lesions — purplish spots or patches that vary in size and usually result from thrombocytopenia. With dark-skinned

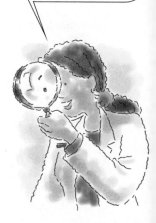

Check your patient's skin for jaundice. If he's dark-skinned, look for a yellowish tinge to the palms, soles, and buccal mucosa.

patients, check the oral mucosa or conjunctivae for petechiae or ecchymoses (bruising).

Anemic indicators

Check the skin for dryness and coarseness, which may indicate iron deficiency anemia.

Mucous membrane appraisal

Finally, inspect the patient's mucous membranes, especially the gingivae (gums). Look for bleeding, redness, swelling, and ulcers.

Fingernails

Inspect the patient's fingernails for longitudinal striations, koilonychia (spoon nail), platyonychia (abnormally broad or flat nails), and nail clubbing (enlargement).

Eyes

Examine the patient's eyes for yellowish sclerae and for retinal hemorrhages and exudates.

Lymph nodes, liver, and spleen

Inspect the abdominal area for enlargement, distention, and asymmetry. Liver and spleen enlargement may result from congestion caused by blood cell overproduction (as in polycythemia or leukemia) or excessive blood cell destruction (as in hemolytic anemia).

Abdominal auscultation

With the patient lying down, auscultate the abdomen before palpation and percussion to avoid altering bowel sounds. Listen for loud, high-pitched tinkling sounds, which herald the early stages of intestinal obstruction.

Finding friction

Next, auscultate the liver and spleen. Listen carefully over both organs for friction rubs — grating sounds that fluctuate with respiration. These sounds usually indicate inflammation of the organ's peritoneal covering.

Percussion of the liver and spleen

To determine liver and spleen size (and possibly detect tumors), percuss all four abdominal quadrants and compare your findings. The normal liver sounds dull.

Establish the organ's approximate size by percussing for its upper and lower borders at the midclavicular line. To determine medial extension, percuss to the midsternal landmark.

Percussing the spleen for sound and size

Percuss the lowest intercostal space in the left anterior axillary line; percussion notes should be tympanic. Ask the patient to take a deep breath, then percuss this area again. If the spleen is normal in size, the area will remain tympanic. If the tympanic percussion note changes on inspiration to dullness, the spleen is probably enlarged.

To estimate spleen size, outline the spleen's edges by percussing in several directions from areas of tympany to areas of dullness.

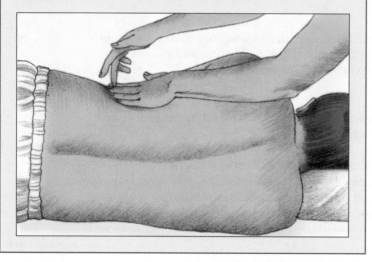

How dull can it get?

Like the liver, the normal spleen sounds dull. Percuss it from the midaxillary toward the midline. The average-sized spleen lies near the eighth, ninth, or tenth intercostal space. You might want to mark liver and spleen borders with a pen for later reference during palpation of these organs. (See *Percussing the spleen for sound and size.*)

Palpation of the lymph nodes, liver, and spleen

Palpate the patient's neck, axillary, epitrochlear, and inguinal lymph nodes. Using your finger pads, move the skin over each area.

As you palpate each node, note its location, size, tenderness, texture (hard, soft, or firm), and fixation (whether it's movable or fixed). For each node group, note the symmetry.

Liver look-over

Accurate liver palpation is difficult and can depend on the patient's size, present comfort level, and whether fluid is present.

If necessary, repeat the procedure, checking your hand position and the pressure you exert.

Quadruple scrutiny

Lightly palpate all four abdominal quadrants to distinguish tender sites and muscle guarding. Deeper palpation helps delineate abdominal organs and masses.

Be sure to palpate tender areas last. Avoid continued palpation if a tumor is suspected.

Diagnostic tests

Diagnostic tests allow direct analysis of the blood, its formed elements, and the bone marrow. Such tests include agglutination tests, coagulation screening tests, and bone marrow aspiration and biopsy.

Agglutination tests

Agglutination tests evaluate the ability of the blood's formed elements to react to foreign substances by clumping together. They include ABO blood typing, crossmatching, and Rh blood typing. (See *Blood and plasma transfusion compatibility*, page 748.)

ABO blood typing

ABO blood typing classifies blood into A, B, AB, or O groups according to the presence of major antigens A and B on RBC surfaces, and according to serum antibodies anti-A and anti-B.

Go forward, then reverse

To prevent a lethal transfusion reaction, both forward and reverse blood typing are required. In *forward* typing, a blood sample is mixed with serum containing anti-A antibodies; another sample is then mixed with serum that contains anti-B antibodies. Clotting patterns are observed and recorded.

In *reverse* typing, the blood sample is mixed with type A and type B blood, and clotting patterns are observed and recorded.

Nursing considerations

• Before the patient receives a transfusion, compare current and past ABO typing and crossmatching to detect mistaken identification and help prevent transfusion reactions. Remember — if the recipient's blood type is A, he may receive type A or O blood. If his blood type is B, he may receive type B or O blood. If his blood

Blood and plasma transfusion compatibility

For a blood or plasma transfusion to be safe, the patient's and donor's blood types must be compatible. The chart below allows you to determine compatibility. Keep in mind that, before transfusing begins, the blood product *must* be crossmatched to fully establish donor-recipient compatibility.

Blood product compatibility chart

Recipient blood type	Compatible whole blood type	Compatible RBC type	Compatible plasma type (Rh match not needed)
O Rh+	O Rh+, O Rh-	O Rh+, O Rh-	O, A, B, AB
O Rh-	O Rh-	O Rh-	O, A, B, AB
A Rh+	A Rh+, A Rh-	A Rh+, A Rh-, O Rh+, O Rh-	A, AB
A Rh-	A Rh-	A Rh-, O Rh-	A, AB
B Rh+	B Rh+, B Rh-	B Rh+, B Rh-, O Rh+, O Rh-	B, AB
B Rh-	B Rh-	B Rh-, O Rh-	B, AB
AB Rh+	AB Rh+, AB Rh-	AB Rh+, AB Rh-, A Rh+, A Rh-, B Rh+, B Rh-, O Rh+, O Rh-	AB
AB Rh-	AB Rh-	AB Rh-, A Rh-, B Rh-, O Rh-	AB

type is AB, he may receive type A, B, AB, or O blood. If his blood type is O, he may receive *only* type O blood.

• Note that recent administration of dextran or I.V. contrast media causes cells to aggregate similarly to agglutination. If the patient received blood during the past 3 months, antibodies to the donor blood may have developed and lingered, interfering with compatibility testing.

Crossmatching

Crossmatching establishes whether donor and recipient blood are compatible and serves as the final check for such compatibility. Lack of agglutination indicates compatibility between donor and recipient blood, which means the blood transfusion can proceed.

Crossmatching in a crisis

Blood is always crossmatched before transfusion, except in extreme emergencies. A complete crossmatch may take 45 minutes to 2 hours, so an incomplete (10-minute) crossmatch may be acceptable in an emergency.

An emergency transfusion must proceed with special awareness of the complications that may result from incomplete typing and crossmatching. After crossmatching, compatible units of blood are labeled and a compatibility record is completed.

Nursing considerations
• If more than 48 hours have elapsed since the previous transfusion, previously crossmatched donor blood must be crossmatched with a new recipient blood sample to detect newly acquired incompatibilities before transfusion.

Verifying protocols
• If the recipient hasn't received the transfusion, donor blood need not be crossmatched again for 72 hours. Check facility transfusion protocols.
• If the patient is scheduled for surgery and has received blood during the previous 3 months, his blood must be crossmatched again to detect recently acquired incompatibilities.

Rh blood typing

The Rh system classifies blood by the presence or absence of the $Rh_o(D)$ antigen on the surface of RBCs. This test is used to establish blood type according to the Rh system to determine if the donor and recipient are compatible before transfusion.

Get right with Rh

Classified as Rh-positive, Rh-negative, or Rh-positive D^u, donor blood may be transfused only if it's compatible with the recipient's blood. (D^u is an $Rh_o[D]$ variant.)

Nursing considerations
Encourage the patient to carry a blood group identification card in his wallet to protect him in an emergency. Most laboratories will provide such a card on request.

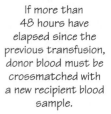

Don't even think about giving a transfusion until ABO typing and crossmatching have been done!

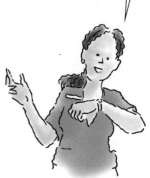

If more than 48 hours have elapsed since the previous transfusion, donor blood must be crossmatched with a new recipient blood sample.

Coagulation screening tests

Coagulation screening tests help detect bleeding disorders and specific coagulation defects. Commonly ordered coagulation tests include partial thromboplastin time (PTT), bleeding time, plasma thrombin time, and prothrombin time (PT). (See *Common coagulation tests.*)

Nursing considerations

- Perform a clean venipuncture. Blood contaminated with tissue thromboplastin causes misleading test results.
- Place the blood sample on ice immediately after obtaining it to preserve its labile factors.
- Allow no more than 4 hours between blood sampling and coagulation testing. Allow only 2 hours between blood centrifugation and coagulation testing; after being centrifuged, RBCs lose their buffering effect on the plasma.

Common coagulation tests

Commonly ordered coagulation tests include partial thromboplastin time (PTT), bleeding time, plasma thrombin time, and prothrombin time (PT).

Partial thromboplastin time
The PTT test evaluates all intrinsic pathway clotting factors (except factors VII and XIII) by measuring the time needed for a fibrin clot to form after calcium and phospholipid emulsion is added to a plasma sample. PTT relies on the activator kaolin to shorten clotting time.

Bleeding time
The bleeding time test measures bleeding duration after a standard skin incision. Bleeding time depends on blood vessel wall elasticity, platelet count, and ability to form a hemostatic plug. The test should involve

two separate punctures, and the results should be averaged.

Plasma thrombin time
Also known as the *thrombin clotting time test*, the plasma thrombin time test measures how quickly a clot forms after a standard amount of bovine thrombin is added to a platelet-poor plasma sample from the patient and to a normal plasma control sample.

Quick but questionable
Because thrombin rapidly converts fibrinogen to a fibrin clot, this test provides a rapid but imprecise estimate of plasma fibrinogen levels.

Prothrombin time
The PT test determines the time needed for a fibrin clot to form in a citrated plasma sample after calcium ion and tissue thromboplastin (factor III) are added. It then compares this time with the fibrin clotting time in a control plasma sample.

Profiting from prothrombin time
This test indirectly measures prothrombin (factor II) and serves as an excellent screening method in evaluating prothrombin, fibrinogen, and extrinsic coagulation factors V, VII, and X. It's the test of choice for monitoring oral anticoagulant therapy.

Biopsy

Biopsy procedures involve removing a small tissue sample for further testing. Bone marrow aspiration is an important test for evaluating the blood's formed elements.

Bone marrow aspiration and needle biopsy

Because most hematopoiesis occurs in the bone marrow, histologic and hematologic bone marrow examination yields valuable diagnostic information about blood disorders. Bone marrow aspiration and needle biopsy provide the material for this examination.

Doubling the diagnostic odds

Aspiration biopsy removes a fluid specimen containing bone marrow cells in suspension. Needle biopsy removes a marrow core containing cells but no fluid. Using both methods provides the best possible marrow specimens.

Bone marrow biopsy helps:
• diagnose aplastic, hypoplastic, and vitamin B_{12} deficiency anemias; granulomas; leukemias; lymphomas; myelofibrosis; and thrombocytopenia
• evaluate primary and metastatic tumors
• determine infection causes
• stage such diseases as Hodgkin's disease
• evaluate chemotherapy effectiveness
• monitor myelosuppression.

Hematologic analysis, including the WBC differential and myeloid-erythroid ratio, can suggest various disorders.

Nursing considerations
• When preparing your patient, explain that the test provides a bone marrow specimen for microscopic examination. Inform him that he need not restrict food or fluids beforehand. Explain who will perform the biopsy, that it usually takes only 5 to 10 minutes, and that results usually are available in 1 day. Inform him that more than one bone marrow specimen may be necessary and that before the biopsy, he'll need to give a blood sample for laboratory testing.
• Check the patient's history for hypersensitivity to the local anesthetic, and make sure the patient's medical record includes a signed consent form.
• After checking with the person who will perform the procedure, tell the patient which bone will serve as the biopsy site (usually the posterior iliac crest). Inform him that he'll receive a local anesthetic but will feel pressure with biopsy needle insertion and a brief pulling pain with marrow removal. (See *Bone marrow aspiration and biopsy sites*, page 752.)

Before bone marrow aspiration, tell the patient that more than one bone marrow specimen may be needed.

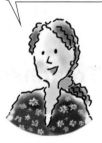

Bone marrow aspiration and biopsy sites

These drawings show the most common sites for bone marrow aspiration and biopsy. These sites are used because the involved bone structures are relatively accessible and rich in marrow cavities.

Posterior superior iliac crest

The posterior superior iliac crest is the preferred site because no vital organs or vessels are nearby. With the patient lying in a prone or lateral position with one leg flexed, the doctor or nurse anesthetizes the bone and inserts the needle several centimeters lateral to the iliosacral junction. Directed downward, the needle enters the bone plane crest and is advanced toward the anterior interior spine. In some cases, the needle enters a few centimeters below the crest at a right angle to the bone surface.

Spinous process

The spinous process is preferred if multiple punctures are necessary or if marrow is absent at other sites. The patient sits on the edge of the bed, leaning over the bedside stand. The doctor selects the spinous process of the third or fourth lumbar vertebrae and inserts the needle at the crest or slightly to one side, advancing it in the direction of the bone plane.

Sternum

The sternum involves the greatest risk but provides the best access. The patient is placed in a supine position on a firm bed or an examination table, with a small pillow beneath his shoulders to raise his chest and lower his head. The doctor secures the needle guard 3 to 4 mm from the tip of the needle to avoid accidentally puncturing the heart or a major vessel. Then he inserts the needle at the midline of the sternum at the second intercostal space.

Posterior
superior
iliac
crest

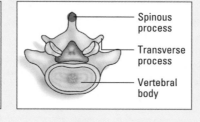

Spinous
process

Transverse
process

Vertebral
body

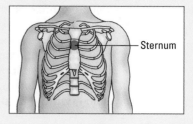

Sternum

- As ordered, administer a mild sedative 1 hour before the test.
- After the procedure, check the biopsy site for bleeding and inflammation. Observe the patient for signs of hemorrhage and infection — rapid pulse rate, low blood pressure, and fever. Change the dressing over the biopsy site every 24 hours to reduce the risk of infection.

Treatments

Treatments for hematologic and lymphatic disorders include drug therapy, transfusions, and surgery.

Drug therapy

Drugs used to treat hematologic and lymphatic disorders include:
• hematinics, which fight anemia by increasing the amount of Hb in the blood
• anticoagulants and heparin antagonists, which impede blood clotting
• hemostatics, which arrest blood flow or reduce capillary bleeding
• blood derivatives, which replace blood loss caused by diseases or surgical procedures
• thrombolytic enzymes, which treat thrombotic disorders
• vitamins, which correct deficiencies of vitamins (such as vitamin B_{12}).

Transfusions

Transfusion procedures allow administration of a wide range of blood products. Here are some examples:
• RBC transfusions revive oxygen-starved tissues.
• Leukocyte transfusions combat infections beyond the reach of antibiotics.
• Transfusions of clotting factors, plasma, and platelets help patients with hemophilia live virtually normal lives.

RBC replacement

A patient with severe anemia or acute bleeding that drug or nutritional therapy can't correct may require transfusion of either whole blood or packed RBCs. A whole blood transfusion replenishes both the volume and oxygen-carrying capacity of the circulatory system by increasing the mass of RBCs.

A paucity of plasma

In contrast, transfusion of packed RBCs—the most common type of transfusion—restores only the oxygen-carrying capacity of the circulatory system because 80% of the plasma has been removed before transfusion. Packed RBCs may also undergo a special washing process to remove WBCs and platelets, decreasing the chance of a reaction in patients who were previously sensitized to transfusions.

Patient preparation
• Become familiar with your facility's policies and procedures for administering blood products.
• Explain the procedure to the patient, and make sure the patient's medical record contains a written physician's order and a signed consent form for the transfusion.

- Verify that the patient has an appropriate, patent peripheral or central venous access site for administration.

Some assembly required

- Assemble the necessary equipment, including a standard blood administration set with an appropriate filter. If needed, flush the venous access with normal saline. Only normal saline may be infused through the same tubing as blood components.
- Obtain the patient's baseline vital signs, and collect the blood from the blood bank. If the blood isn't going to be transfused, it must be returned to the blood bank within 30 minutes.
- Inspect the blood product for abnormal color, cloudiness, clots, and excess air. Match the blood to the written order.
- Verify the patient's identity, using a two-person verification process or a one-person verification process accompanied by automated identification technology (such as bar coding), according to your facility's policy. Involve the patient in the process if possible. Don't start the infusion if you find any discrepancies, and notify the blood bank immediately.

Monitoring and aftercare

- Begin the infusion, check the patient's vital signs, and monitor the patient carefully throughout the transfusion, according to your facility's policy. Keep in mind that many transfusion reactions occur within the first 15 minutes of starting a transfusion. (See *Guide to immediate transfusion reactions.*)
- Complete RBC transfusions within 4 hours. If the patient needs multiple units, change the administration tubing after every second unit to help prevent infection.
- If the patient develops an adverse reaction, stop the transfusion at once and notify the physician according to facility policy. Keep the vein open with normal saline, obtain vital signs, and begin appropriate nursing interventions.

Factor replacement

I.V. infusion of deficient clotting factors is a major part of treatment of coagulation disorders. Factor replacement typically corrects clotting factor deficiencies, thereby stopping or preventing hemorrhage. The blood product used depends on the specific disorder being treated.

Cold comfort

Fresh frozen plasma, for instance, helps treat clotting disorders whose causes aren't known, clotting factor deficiencies resulting from hepatic disease or blood dilution, consumed clotting factors secondary to disseminated intravascular coagulation (DIC), and

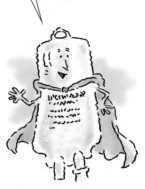

Fresh frozen plasma may be given to treat clotting factor deficiencies caused by liver disease, blood dilution, DIC, and certain other conditions.

Guide to immediate transfusion reactions

Any patient receiving a transfusion of blood or blood products is at risk for a transfusion reaction. An immediate reaction may occur during the transfusion itself or several hours after the transfusion. The chart below describes immediate reactions.

Reaction	Causes	Signs and symptoms	Nursing interventions
Acute hemolytic	Administration of incompatible blood	Chest pain, dyspnea, facial flushing, fever, chills, hypotension, flank pain, bloody oozing at the infusion or surgical incision site, nausea, tachycardia	• Monitor the patient carefully, especially during the first 15 minutes of any transfusion. If you see signs of a reaction, stop the transfusion immediately. • Administer I.V. fluids, oxygen, epinephrine, and a vasopressor, as ordered. • Observe the patient for signs of coagulopathy.
Bacterial contamination	Contamination of blood product	Chills, fever, vomiting, abdominal cramping, diarrhea, shock	• Provide broad-spectrum antibiotics, as prescribed. • Monitor the patient for fever for several hours after completion of the transfusion. • Obtain blood cultures from a site other than the I.V. infusion site. • Keep all blood bags and tubing and send them to the blood bank.
Febrile nonhemolytic	Bacterial lipopolysaccharides Antileukocyte recipient antibodies directed against donor white blood cells	Fever within 2 hours of transfusion, chills, rigors, headache, palpitation, cough, tachycardia	• Relieve symptoms with an antipyretic. • If the patient requires further transfusions, consider using a leukocyte removal filter.
Transfusion-related acute lung injury	Granulocyte antibodies in the donor or recipient that cause complement and histamine release	Severe respiratory distress within 6 hours of transfusion, fever, chills, cyanosis, hypotension	• Stop the transfusion immediately. • Provide oxygen as needed. • Monitor pulse oximetry. • Prepare for intubation and ventilatory support and hemodynamic monitoring.
Allergic reaction	Allergen in donor blood	Urticaria, fever, nausea, vomiting, anaphylaxis (facial swelling, laryngeal edema, respiratory distress) in extreme cases	• Stop the transfusion and administer antihistamine, corticosteroid, or epinephrine, as ordered. • Prepare for intubation and respiratory support if the patient develops anaphylaxis.

(continued)

Guide to immediate transfusion reactions (continued)

Reaction	Causes	Signs and symptoms	Nursing interventions
Transfusion-associated circulatory overload	Rapid infusion of blood Excessive volume of transfusion	Chest tightness, chills, dyspnea, tachypnea, hypoxemia, hypertension, jugular vein distention that occurs 2 to 6 hours after transfusion	• Monitor intake and output, breath sounds, and blood pressure. • Administer diuretics as needed. • Watch elderly patients and those with a history of cardiac disease carefully because they are at higher risk.
Hypocalcemia	Rapid infusion of citrate-treated blood resulting in the citrate binding to calcium	Arrhythmias, hypotension, muscle cramps, nausea and vomiting, seizures, prolonged QT interval	• Administer I.V. calcium gluconate as ordered. • Monitor the patient's electrocardiogram for arrhythmias or a prolonged QT interval. • Monitor patients with an elevated potassium level closely because they're at greater risk for hypocalcemia.

deficiencies of clotting factors (such as factor V) for which no specific replacement product exists.

For cryin' out loud

Administration of cryoprecipitate, which forms when fresh frozen plasma thaws slowly, helps treat von Willebrand's disease, fibrinogen deficiencies, and factor XIII deficiencies.

Eight is really great

Factor VIII (antihemophilic factor) concentrate is the long-term treatment of choice for hemophilia A because it contains a less variable amount of factor VIII than cryoprecipitate. It's given I.V. to hemophiliac patients who have sustained injuries. It is also used to treat von Willebrand's disease.

Pooled assets

Prothrombin complex — which contains factors II, VII, IX, and X — is used to treat hemophilia B, severe liver disease, and acquired deficiencies of the factors it contains. However, it carries a high risk of transmitting hepatitis because it's collected from large pools of donors.

Patient preparation

• Become familiar with your facility's policies and procedures for administering blood products.
• Explain the procedure to the patient.

- Assemble the necessary equipment: a standard blood administration set for giving fresh frozen plasma or prothrombin complex, a component syringe or drip set for giving cryoprecipitate, a plastic syringe for I.V. injection of factor VIII, or a plastic syringe and infusion set for I.V. infusion.
- Obtain the plasma fraction from the blood bank or pharmacy. Check the expiration date, and carefully inspect the plasma fraction for cloudiness and turbidity. If you'll be transfusing fresh frozen plasma, administer it within 4 hours because it doesn't contain preservatives.
- Take the patient's vital signs. If an I.V. line isn't in place, perform venipuncture and infuse normal saline solution at a keep-vein-open rate.

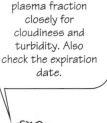

Inspect the plasma fraction closely for cloudiness and turbidity. Also check the expiration date.

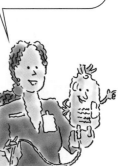

Monitoring and aftercare

- During and after administration of clotting factors, monitor the patient for signs and symptoms of anaphylaxis, other allergic reactions, and fluid overload.
- Monitor for fever, bleeding, and increased pain or swelling at the transfusion site.
- Closely monitor the patient's PTT.
- Alert the practitioner if adverse reactions occur or if you suspect bleeding.
- Follow your facility's protocol for monitoring vital signs.
- Instruct the patient and his family on proper care and use of the patient's vascular access device.

Home care instructions

The patient or his family can administer factor replacement therapy at home. If home therapy is ordered, cover these topics:
- Demonstrate correct infusion techniques to the patient and his family.
- Tell them to keep factor replacement and infusion equipment readily available and to start treatment immediately if the patient experiences bleeding.
- Teach them to watch for signs and symptoms of anaphylaxis, allergic reactions, and fluid overload. Instruct them to call the doctor immediately if such reactions occur.

Surgery

Surgical removal of the spleen is sometimes done to treat various hematologic disorders.

Splenectomy

The spleen may be removed to reduce the rate of RBC and platelet destruction or to stage Hodgkin's disease. It's also done as an emergency procedure to stop hemorrhage after traumatic splenic rupture.

Look Ma, no spleen

Splenectomy is the treatment of choice for such diseases as hereditary spherocytosis and chronic idiopathic thrombocytopenic purpura in patients who don't respond to steroids or danazol therapy. Besides bleeding and infection, splenectomy can cause other complications, such as pneumonia and atelectasis.

Infection alert

Keep in mind that the spleen's location close to the diaphragm and the need for a high abdominal incision restrict lung expansion after surgery. Also, splenectomy patients — especially children — are vulnerable to infection because of the spleen's role in the immune response.

> You can lead a normal life without your spleen, but you'll need to take extra precautions against infection.

Patient preparation

• Explain to the patient that splenectomy involves removal of the spleen under general anesthesia. Inform him that he can lead a normal life without the spleen, although he'll be more prone to infection.
• Obtain the results of blood studies, including coagulation tests and complete blood count (CBC), and report them to the practitioner.
• If ordered, transfuse blood to correct anemia or hemorrhagic loss. Similarly, give vitamin K to correct clotting factor deficiencies. Give pneumonia vaccine as ordered.
• Take the patient's vital signs and perform a baseline respiratory assessment. Note signs and symptoms of respiratory tract infection, such as fever, chills, crackles, rhonchi, and cough. Notify the practitioner if you suspect such infection; he may delay surgery.
• Teach the patient coughing and deep-breathing techniques to help prevent postoperative pulmonary complications.

Monitoring and aftercare

• During the early postoperative period, check closely (especially if the patient has a bleeding disorder) for bleeding from the wound or drain and for signs of internal bleeding, such as hematuria (bloody urine) or hematochezia (bloody feces).
• Know that leukocytosis (an increased WBC count) and thrombocytosis (an increased platelet count) follow splenectomy and may persist for years. Because thrombocytosis may predispose the patient to thromboembolism, help him exercise and walk as soon as possible after surgery. Encourage him to perform coughing and deep-breathing exercises to reduce the risk of pulmonary complications.

• Watch for signs and symptoms of infection, such as fever and sore throat, and monitor the results of hematologic studies. If infection develops, give an antibiotic as prescribed.

Home care instructions
• Inform the patient that he's at increased risk for infection, and urge him to report signs and symptoms of infection promptly.
• Teach him measures to help prevent infection, such as getting the pneumococcal pneumonia vaccine.

Nursing diagnoses

When caring for patients with hematologic disorders, you'll typically use several nursing diagnoses. These diagnoses appear here, along with appropriate nursing interventions and rationales. See *NANDA-I taxonomy II by domain*, page 936, for the complete list of NANDA diagnoses.

Fatigue

Related to anemia caused by decreased hematocrit (HCT) and Hb, *Fatigue* may be associated with sickle cell anemia, pernicious anemia, folic acid and iron deficiency anemias, aplastic or hypoplastic anemias, thalassemias, leukemia, and sideroblastic anemias.

Expected outcomes
• Patient demonstrates that he's adequately rested by being able to participate in routine daily activities.
• Patient identifies measures to prevent or modify fatigue.
• Patient states that he has increased energy.

Nursing interventions and rationales
• Help the patient avoid unnecessary activity — for example, avoid scheduling two energy-draining procedures on the same day. Consult an occupational therapist for practical suggestions in modifying the home and work environments. Using energy-conserving techniques avoids overexertion and potential for exhaustion.
• Help the patient conserve energy through rest, planning, and setting priorities, to prevent or alleviate fatigue.

Divide and conquer
• Alternate activities with periods of rest. Encourage the patient to engage in activities that he can complete in short periods or divide into several segments. Regular rest periods help decrease fatigue and increase stamina.

• Discuss the effects of fatigue on daily living and personal goals. Explore with the patient the relationship between fatigue and his disorder, to enhance his ability to cope.

• Structure the patient's environment to encourage compliance with the treatment regimen. For example, devise a daily schedule based on his needs and desires.

• Encourage the patient to eat foods rich in iron and minerals, unless contraindicated, to help prevent anemia and demineralization.

• Provide small, frequent feedings to conserve the patient's energy and encourage optimal nutrition.

• Establish a regular sleeping pattern. Getting 8 to 10 hours of sleep nightly helps reduce fatigue.

• Avoid highly emotional situations, which worsen fatigue. Encourage the patient to explore feelings and emotions with a supportive counselor, clergy, or other professional to help cope with illness.

Memory jogger

Think **BEEP** to remember the signs of minor bleeding:

Bleeding gums

Ecchymoses (bruises)

Epistaxis (nosebleed)

Petechiae (tiny purplish spots).

Ineffective tissue perfusion

Related to inadequate blood volume or HCT, *Ineffective tissue perfusion* may be associated with hemophilia, thrombocytopenia, various purpuras, DIC, and von Willebrand's disease.

Expected outcomes
• Patient's vital signs are within baseline values.
• Patient's pulse oximetry value is within normal limits.

Nursing interventions and rationales
• Monitor the patient's vital signs every 4 hours. Assess for signs and symptoms of both *minor* bleeding (such as bleeding gums, ecchymoses, epistaxis [nosebleed], and petechiae) and *serious* bleeding (such as changed mental status, headache, hematemesis [vomiting of blood], hemoptysis [coughing up of blood], hypotension, melena [black, tarry stools], orthostatic changes, and tachycardia). Detecting bleeding early helps control complications.
• Take steps to prevent bleeding. Avoid invasive measures, such as injections, rectal enemas or suppositories, and urinary catheterization. Avoid giving aspirin or aspirin-containing products if possible. Shave the patient with an electric razor only. Give oral care with a soft toothbrush. These measures prevent complications by maintaining skin integrity.

If your patient has bleeding problems, don't perform invasive measures, such as giving injections, enemas, or suppositories.

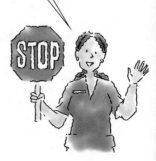

Common hematologic disorders

This section discusses common hematologic disorders, from anemias (such as aplastic anemia and sickle cell anemia) to hemorrhagic disorders (such as hemophilia and thrombocytopenia).

Aplastic anemia

Aplastic, or hypoplastic, anemia results from injury to or destruction of stem cells in the bone marrow or the bone marrow matrix, causing pancytopenia (deficiency of RBCs, WBCs, and platelets) and bone marrow hypoplasia (underdevelopment).

Alarming mortality

Although commonly used interchangeably with other terms for bone marrow failure, aplastic anemia properly refers to pancytopenia resulting from decreased functional capacity of a hypoplastic, fatty bone marrow. Aplastic anemia with severe pancytopenia carries a mortality of 80% to 90%. Death may result from bleeding or infection.

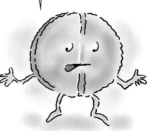

Adverse drug reactions are among the many possible causes of aplastic anemia.

What causes it

Aplastic anemia may result from:
- adverse drug reactions
- exposure to toxic agents, such as benzene and chloramphenicol
- radiation
- immunologic factors
- severe disease, especially hepatitis
- preleukemia and neoplastic infiltration of bone marrow
- congenital abnormalities
- induced changes in fetal development (suspected as a cause when no consistent genetic history of aplastic anemia exists).

Pathophysiology

Aplastic anemia usually develops when damaged or destroyed stem cells inhibit RBC production. Less commonly, it arises when damaged bone marrow microvasculature creates an unfavorable environment for cell growth and maturation.

What to look for

Clinical features of aplastic anemia vary with the severity of pancytopenia. They commonly develop gradually, and may include:
- pallor, ecchymoses, and petechiae
- retinal hemorrhages

- weakness and fatigue
- alterations in level of consciousness
- bibasilar crackles
- tachycardia
- gallop murmur
- fever
- oral and rectal ulcers
- sore throat
- nausea.

What tests tell you

- RBC tests usually show RBCs of normal size, shape, and color, although larger-than-normal RBCs and RBCs of varying size may be present. Total RBC count is 1 million/µl or less.
- Absolute reticulocyte count is very low.
- Serum iron level is elevated (unless bleeding occurs), but total iron-binding capacity is normal or slightly reduced. Hemosiderin (a blood protein) is present, and tissue iron storage is visible microscopically.
- Platelet and WBC counts fall. A lower platelet count is reflected in abnormal coagulation tests (bleeding time).

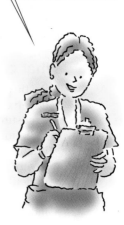

In aplastic anemia, absolute reticulocyte count, platelet count, and WBC count fall below normal.

Tapped out

- Bone marrow biopsies taken from several sites may yield a "dry tap" or show severely hypocellular or aplastic marrow, with a varying amount of fat, fibrous tissue, or gelatinous replacement; absence of tagged iron and megakaryocytes; and depression of RBC elements.

How it's treated

Effective treatment must eliminate identifiable causes of anemia and provide vigorous supportive measures, such as packed RBC, platelet, and human leukocyte antigen (HLA)-matched leukocyte transfusions. Even then, recovery may take months.

Bone marrow transplantation is the preferred treatment of anemia stemming from severe aplasia and for patients needing constant RBC transfusions.

Patients with low WBC counts may need interventions to avoid infection. They may receive antibiotics, but prophylactic use encourages resistant strains of organisms. Patients with low Hb levels may need oxygen therapy and blood transfusion.

Stimulate, suppress, or complement

Other treatments for aplastic anemia include:
- bone marrow-stimulating agents, such as androgens (controversial)
- immunosuppressants (if the patient doesn't respond to other therapies)

- colony-stimulating factors, which encourage growth of specific cellular components in patients who have had chemotherapy or radiation therapy; agents include granulocyte colony-stimulating factor, granulocyte-macrophage colony-stimulating factor, and erythropoietic stimulating factor
- alternative and complementary therapies to treat associated fatigue.

What to do

- If the patient's platelet count is below 20,000/μl, take steps to prevent hemorrhage. For instance, avoid I.M. injections; suggest that the patient use an electric razor and a soft toothbrush; give humidifying oxygen, if ordered, to prevent drying of mucous membranes (dry mucosa may bleed); and promote regular bowel movements through stool softeners and a proper diet. Also, apply pressure to venipuncture sites until bleeding stops. Detect bleeding early by checking for blood in the urine and stools and assessing the skin for petechiae.
- Help prevent infection by performing hand hygiene thoroughly before entering the patient's room, making sure the patient eats a nutritious diet high in vitamins and proteins to boost his resistance, and encouraging meticulous mouth and perianal care. Make sure routine throat, urine, and blood cultures are done regularly to check for infection.

Keep an eye on it

- Watch for life-threatening hemorrhage, infection, adverse drug reactions, and transfusion reaction.
- Schedule frequent rest periods for a patient with a low Hb level.
- Administer oxygen therapy as needed and ordered.
- If blood transfusions are given, assess for transfusion reaction by checking the patient's temperature and monitoring him for rash, hives, itching, back pain, restlessness, and shaking chills.
- To prevent aplastic anemia, monitor blood drug levels carefully if the patient is receiving a drug that could cause anemia.
- Evaluate the patient. He should experience fewer infections, his blood cell counts should return to normal, he should breathe easily, and he should no longer experience trauma-induced hemorrhagic episodes. He and his family should demonstrate knowledge of energy-saving strategies. (See *Aplastic anemia teaching tips.*)

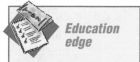
Education edge

Aplastic anemia teaching tips

- Reassure and support the patient and his family by teaching them about aplastic anemia and its treatment, particularly if the patient has recurring acute episodes.
- Teach the patient how to recognize signs and symptoms of infection, and tell him to report these immediately.
- If the patient doesn't require hospitalization, encourage him to continue his normal lifestyle with appropriate restrictions (such as regular rest periods) until remission occurs.

Disseminated intravascular coagulation

DIC is a grave blood coagulation disorder that occurs as a complication of conditions that accelerate clotting. It causes small blood vessel occlusion, organ necrosis, depletion of circulating clotting factors and platelets, and activation of the fibrinolytic (blood-clot promoting) system.

The case of the consumed clotting factors

These processes, in turn, can provoke severe hemorrhage as clotting factors are consumed. Clotting in the microcirculation usually affects the kidneys and extremities, but also may occur in the brain, lungs, pituitary and adrenal glands, and GI mucosa.

Although usually acute, DIC may be chronic in cancer patients. Prognosis depends on early detection and treatment, hemorrhage severity, and treatment of the underlying disease.

> In DIC, small blood vessel occlusion is one in a series of events leading to severe hemorrhaging.

What causes it

DIC can result from:
• infection, such as gram-negative or gram-positive septicemia; viral, fungal, or rickettsial infection; or protozoal infection (falciparum malaria)
• obstetric complications, such as abruptio placentae, amniotic fluid embolism, or retained dead fetus
• neoplastic disease, such as acute leukemia or metastatic carcinoma
• tissue necrosis from extensive burns or trauma, brain tissue destruction, transplant rejection, or hepatic necrosis.

Other possible causes of DIC include cardiac arrest, heatstroke, shock, poisonous snakebite, cirrhosis, fat embolism, incompatible blood transfusions, intraoperative cardiopulmonary bypass, giant hemangioma (a benign vascular tumor), severe venous thrombosis, and purpura fulminans (a severe, rapidly fatal form of nonthrombocytopenic purpura).

Pathophysiology

DIC arises when one of the predisposing conditions listed above activates the coagulation system. Excess fibrin forms (triggered by the action of thrombin, an enzyme) and becomes trapped in the microvasculature along with platelets, causing clots.

Horrific hemorrhaging

Blood flow to the tissues then decreases, resulting in acidemia, blood stasis, and tissue hypoxia. These conditions may lead to organ failure. Both fibrinolysis (fibrin dissolution) and antithrombotic mechanisms induce anticoagulation. Platelets and clotting factors are consumed, and massive hemorrhage may ensue. (See *Deciphering DIC*.)

What to look for

Abnormal bleeding, without a history of a serious hemorrhagic disorder, can signal DIC. Signs of such bleeding include:
• cutaneous oozing
• petechiae

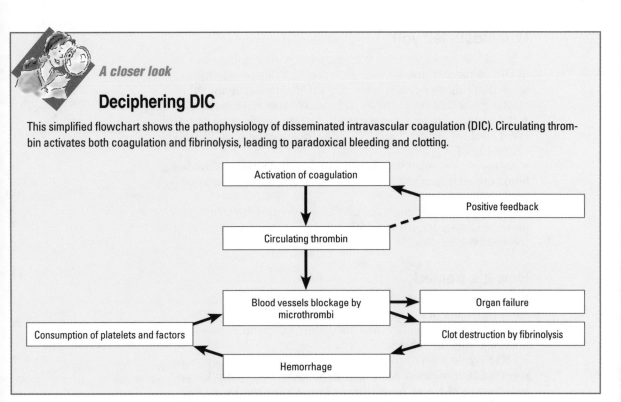

A closer look

Deciphering DIC

This simplified flowchart shows the pathophysiology of disseminated intravascular coagulation (DIC). Circulating thrombin activates both coagulation and fibrinolysis, leading to paradoxical bleeding and clotting.

- ecchymoses
- hematomas
- bleeding from sites of surgical or invasive procedures (such as incisions and I.V. sites)
- GI tract bleeding.

Assessment add-ons

Also, assess the patient for acrocyanosis (symmetrical cyanosis) and acute tubular necrosis (damage to renal tubule cells, leading to renal failure).

Related symptoms and other possible effects of DIC include:
- nausea and vomiting
- dyspnea
- oliguria (reduced urine output)
- seizures
- coma
- shock
- severe muscle, back, and abdominal pain
- failure of major organ systems.

What tests tell you

• Initial laboratory findings that support a tentative diagnosis of DIC include PT greater than 15 seconds, PTT exceeding 60 seconds, fibrinogen levels below 150 mg/dl, platelet count below 100,000/µl, and fibrin degradation products above 100 mcg/ml.
• Supportive data may include positive fibrin monomers, diminished levels of factors V and VIII, RBC fragmentation, and Hb level below 10 g/dl.
• Assessment of renal status shows urine output below 30 ml/hour, blood urea nitrogen level above 25 mg/dl, and serum creatinine level above 1.3 mg/dl.

Additional diagnostic measures may be done to determine the underlying disorder, because other disorders may cause many of the same test results.

How it's treated

Effective treatment of DIC requires prompt recognition and adequate treatment of the underlying disorder. Treatment may be supportive (for example, when the underlying disorder is self-limiting) or highly specific.

If the patient isn't actively bleeding, supportive care alone may reverse DIC. But active bleeding may necessitate heparin I.V. and transfusions of blood, fresh frozen plasma, platelets, or packed RBCs to support hemostasis.

Dissension over heparin

Heparin therapy is controversial. It may be used early in DIC to prevent microclotting or as a last resort in an actively bleeding patient. In thrombosis, heparin therapy is usually mandatory. In most cases, it's given with transfusion therapy.

What to do

• Focus patient care on early recognition of the primary signs and symptoms of abnormal bleeding, prompt treatment of the underlying disorder, and prevention of further bleeding.
• To prevent clots from dislodging, don't scrub bleeding areas.
• Use pressure, cold compresses, and topical hemostatic agents to control bleeding.
• Protect the patient from injury. Enforce complete bed rest during bleeding episodes. If the patient is agitated, pad the side rails.
• Check all I.V. and venipuncture sites frequently.
• Apply pressure to injection sites for at least 10 minutes.
• Monitor fluid intake and output hourly in patients with acute DIC, especially when giving blood products. Watch for transfusion reactions and indications of fluid overload.

• To measure the amount of blood lost, weigh dressings and linens and record drainage.
• Weigh the patient daily, particularly if there's renal involvement.
• Check the patient for headache, and assess neurologic status periodically.
• Watch for GI and genitourinary tract bleeding. To detect intra-abdominal bleeding, measure the patient's abdominal girth at least every 4 hours and monitor closely for signs and symptoms of shock. Monitor the results of serial blood studies (especially HCT, Hb levels, and coagulation times).
• Evaluate the patient. With successful treatment, he should be free from bleeding, and tests should show his coagulation parameters and renal status within normal limits. (See *DIC teaching tips*.)

Hemophilia

Hemophilia is a hereditary bleeding disorder that results from lack of specific clotting factors. It occurs in two main forms:
• Hemophilia A (classic hemophilia), seen in more than 80% of hemophilia cases, results from deficiency of factor VIII.
• Hemophilia B (Christmas disease), which accounts for roughly 15% of hemophilia cases, results from deficiency of factor IX.

A prettier picture

Treatment advances have greatly improved prognosis, and many hemophiliacs have normal life spans. Surgery can be done safely under a hematologist's guidance at special hemophilia treatment centers.

What causes it

Hemophilia A and B are inherited as X-linked recessive traits. This means female carriers have a 50% chance of transmitting the gene to each son or daughter. Daughters who receive the gene are carriers; sons who receive it are born with hemophilia.

Nonfunctional factors?

Although traditionally seen as a deficiency of clotting factors, recent evidence suggests that hemophilia may result from non-functioning factors VIII and IX.

Pathophysiology

Hemophilia produces abnormal bleeding. Depending on the degree of factor deficiency, the bleeding may be mild, moderate, or severe. Overall prognosis is best in patients with mild hemophilia, which doesn't cause spontaneous bleeding or joint deformities.

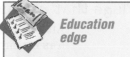

Education edge

DIC teaching tips

• Explain applicable diagnostic tests and procedures to the patient. Allow time for questions.
• Inform the family of the patient's progress. Prepare them for his appearance, including the possibility of I.V. lines, nasogastric tubes, bruises, and dried blood.
• Provide emotional support. As needed, enlist the aid of a social worker, chaplain, and other health care team members in providing such support.

Plugs that preclude clots

After a platelet plug forms at a bleeding site, lack of clotting factors impairs formation of a stable fibrin clot. Delayed bleeding is more common than immediate hemorrhage.

What to look for

Signs and symptoms vary with the severity of hemophilia.
• With *mild* hemophilia, bleeding doesn't occur spontaneously or after minor trauma. However, major trauma or surgery typically causes prolonged bleeding.
• With *moderate* hemophilia, spontaneous bleeding occurs occasionally. Surgery or trauma causes excessive bleeding.
• With *severe* hemophilia, bleeding occurs spontaneously and may be severe even with minor trauma, leading to large subcutaneous and deep I.M. hematomas.

Bleeding and deformity

Bleeding into joints and muscles also may occur and causes pain, swelling, extreme tenderness and, possibly, permanent deformity.

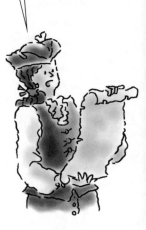

Hear ye, hear ye! These test results show that the patient's factor levels are 4% of normal. That means he has moderate hemophilia.

What tests tell you

Characteristic findings in patients with hemophilia A include:
• factor VIII assay 0% to 30% of normal
• prolonged PTT
• normal platelet count and function, bleeding time, and PT.
   Characteristic findings in patients with hemophilia B include:
• deficient factor IX assay
• baseline coagulation results similar to those in hemophilia A, except with normal factor VIII levels.

Three degrees of deficiency

With either hemophilia A or B, the degree of factor deficiency determines the severity of the illness:
• mild hemophilia: factor levels 5% to 40% of normal
• moderate hemophilia: factor levels 1% to 5% of normal
• severe hemophilia: factor levels less than 1% of normal.

How it's treated

Although hemophilia isn't curable, treatment can prevent crippling deformities and prolong life expectancy. Correct treatment quickly stops bleeding by increasing plasma levels of deficient clotting factors. This helps prevent disabling deformities that result from repeated bleeding into muscles and joints.

Treatment includes:
• For hemophilia A, cryoprecipitated antihemophilic factor (AHF), lyophilized AHF, or both are given in doses large enough to raise clotting factor levels above 25% of normal to support normal hemostasis. Before surgery, AHF is given to raise clotting factors to hemostatic levels. Levels are then kept within a normal range until the wound has healed. Fresh frozen plasma also can be given.

Multiple risks

• Inhibitors to factor VIII develop after multiple transfusions in 10% to 20% of patients with severe hemophilia, causing resistance to factor VIII infusions. Desmopressin (DDAVP) may be given to stimulate release of stored factor VIII, raising the blood level of this factor. In hemophilia B, administering factor IX concentrate during bleeding episodes increases factor IX levels.
• A patient who undergoes surgery needs careful management by a hematologist experienced in caring for hemophiliacs. The deficient factor must be replaced before and after surgery (possibly even minor surgery such as dental extractions). Aminocaproic acid (Amicar) is commonly used for oral bleeding, to inhibit the active fibrinolytic system in the oral mucosa. Human immunodeficiency virus screening reduces the risk of acquired immunodeficiency syndrome from transfusion.

What to do

• During bleeding episodes, administer the deficient clotting factor or plasma as ordered. The body uses up AHF in 48 to 72 hours, so repeat the infusion, as ordered, until bleeding stops.
• Apply cold compresses or ice bags, and elevate the injured part.
• To prevent recurrent bleeding, restrict the patient's activity for 48 hours after bleeding is under control.
• If bleeding into a joint occurs, immediately elevate the affected joint.
• Control pain with an analgesic, such as acetaminophen (Tylenol), codeine, or meperidine (Demerol) as ordered.
• Know that aspirin and aspirin-containing medications are contraindicated because they decrease platelet adherence and may worsen bleeding.
• Avoid I.M. injections because of possible hematoma formation at the injection site.
• After bleeding episodes and surgery, watch closely for signs and symptoms of further bleeding, such as increased pain and swelling, fever, or indications of shock. Closely monitor PTT.
• To restore mobility in an affected joint, begin range-of-motion exercises, if ordered, at least 48 hours after bleeding is controlled. Tell the patient to avoid bearing weight on the joint until bleeding stops and swelling subsides.

• Evaluate the patient. He should be free from bleeding; he should understand how to minimize bleeding risks and know what to do if bleeding occurs. (See *Hemophilia teaching tips*.)

Sickle cell anemia

A type of congenital hemolytic anemia (shortened RBC survival and inability of bone marrow to compensate for decreased RBC life span), sickle cell anemia occurs mainly in African-Americans. It results from a defective Hb molecule (HbS), which causes RBCs to roughen and become sickle shaped and more fragile.

Renegade RBCs

The abnormal RBCs impair circulation, resulting in chronic ill health, periodic crises, long-term complications, and premature death.

What causes it

Sickle cell anemia may stem from homozygous inheritance of the HbS–producing gene, which causes the amino acid valine to replace glutamic acid in the Hb beta chain. (See *Understanding sickle cell trait.*)

Pathophysiology

Blood vessel obstruction by rigid, tangled RBCs causes tissue oxygen starvation and possible necrosis. These conditions, in turn,

Hemophilia teaching tips

• Teach the parents of a child with hemophilia which precautions they must take to prevent bleeding episodes as well as proper procedures for managing these episodes when they occur.
• Refer new patients to a hemophilia treatment center for evaluation. The center can develop a treatment and management plan for the patient's primary care practitioner and serve as a resource for medical personnel, dentists, or others involved in the patient's care.

Understanding sickle cell trait

Sickle cell trait is a relatively benign condition that results from heterozygous inheritance of a sickle hemoglobin S (HbS) gene. Like sickle cell anemia, sickle cell trait is most common in African-Americans. However, sickle cell trait *never* progresses to sickle cell anemia.

It's all in the percentages
In people with sickle cell trait (called *sickle cell carriers*), 20% to 40% of the total Hb is HbS; the rest of the Hb is normal. These people rarely experience symptoms, have normal Hb levels and hematocrit, and can have a normal life span.

Genetic risks
Genetic counseling is essential for sickle cell carriers. If two sickle cell carriers have children, each of their children has a 25% chance of inheriting sickle cell anemia.

lead to painful vaso-occlusive crisis, a hallmark of the disease. Bone marrow depression results in aplastic (megaloblastic) crisis.

Crises and their causes

Factors that predispose a patient to sickle cell crisis include deoxygenation (as from pneumonia, hypoxia, or scuba diving), cold exposure, acidosis, and infection.

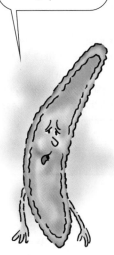

When I get sickled, the patient gets sick. Signs include aching bones, chest pain, fatigue, and dyspnea.

What to look for

Signs and symptoms of sickle cell anemia include:
- aching bones
- cardiomegaly (heart enlargement)
- chest pain
- chronic fatigue
- diastolic and systolic murmurs or tachycardia
- exertional or unexplained dyspnea
- hepatomegaly (liver enlargement) or jaundice
- increased susceptibility to infection
- ischemic leg ulcers (especially on the ankles)
- joint swelling
- pallor.

Crisis components

During a painful vaso-occlusive crisis, the patient may experience:
- severe abdominal, thoracic, muscular, or bone pain
- low-grade fever
- possible increased jaundice and dark urine
- diminished spleen size in chronic disease. (See *Caring for a patient in sickle cell crisis*, page 772.)

What tests tell you

- Stained blood smear showing sickle-shaped RBCs and Hb electrophoresis showing HbS confirm the diagnosis.
- CBC shows low RBC and elevated WBC and platelet counts. Hb levels may be low or normal.
- Erythrocyte sedimentation rate and RBC survival time are decreased; serum iron levels and reticulocyte counts are increased.

How it's treated

Although sickle cell anemia can't be cured, treatment can ease symptoms and prevent painful crises. Treatment includes:
- Polyvalent pneumococcal and *Haemophilus influenzae* B vaccinations; anti-infectives, such as low-dose oral penicillin; and

What do I do?

Caring for a patient in sickle cell crisis

Suspect a sickle cell crisis if your patient has these signs and symptoms:
• severe pain
• a temperature over 104.7° F (40.4° C) or a fever of 100.7° F (38.2° C) lasting at least 2 days
• pale lips, tongue, palms, or nailbeds
• lethargy or listlessness
• difficulty awakening
• irritability.

Taking action
Implement these measures:
• Provide effective pain management, including use of opioid analgesics if needed. Assess the patient's pain frequently. Have him rate the pain on a scale of 0 to 10 (or according to your facility's policy). Give opioid analgesics as prescribed.

• Apply warm compresses to painful areas. Never use cold compresses because they may aggravate the condition.
• Cover the patient with a blanket.
• Give an analgesic-antipyretic, such as aspirin or acetaminophen as ordered.
• Encourage bed rest, and place the patient in a sitting position.
• If dehydration or severe pain occurs, hospitalization may be necessary.

chelating agents, such as deferoxamine (Desferal), help minimize complications.
• Analgesics can relieve the pain of vaso-occlusive crisis. (See *Pain management and sickle cell anemia: When emergency departments don't make the grade.*)
• An iron supplement may be given if folic acid levels are low.
• An antisickling agent may be given. However, the most commonly used agent, sodium cyanate, has many adverse effects.
• During an acute sequestration crisis, treatment may include sedation, analgesia, blood transfusions, oxygen therapy, and large amounts of oral or I.V. fluids.

What to do
• Advise the patient to avoid tight clothing that restricts circulation.
• Emphasize the need for prompt treatment of infection.
• Evaluate the patient. He should be free from pain and infection. He and his family should understand what steps to take to avoid exacerbating the disease. (See *Sickle cell anemia teaching tips.*)

Thrombocytopenia

The most common hemorrhagic disorder, thrombocytopenia is characterized by a deficiency of circulating platelets. Because platelets play a vital role in blood clotting, this disorder seriously threatens hemostasis.

Weighing the evidence

Pain management and sickle cell anemia: When emergency departments don't make the grade

When patients with sickle cell anemia seek treatment at an emergency department (ED), how quickly do they receive treatment for pain, and how effective is that treatment? Researchers looked at ED pain management for 155 sickle cell anemia patients to answer those questions. They found that, on average, patients waited 74 minutes for initial analgesia and that they perceived their pain relief at discharge as lower than documented pain relief scores. The data showed that not only did patients experience significant delays in receiving initial analgesia, they were still in more pain than they considered desirable at discharge. Such findings can help spur EDs to devise strategies to improve pain control for sickle cell patients.

Tanabe, P., et al. (2010). Adult emergency department patients with sickle cell pain crisis: A learning collaborative model to improve analgesic management. *Academic Emergency Medicine, 17*(4), 399–407.

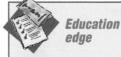

Education edge

Sickle cell anemia teaching tips

• Instruct the patient to avoid strenuous exercise, vasoconstricting medications, cold temperatures, unpressurized aircraft, high altitudes, and conditions that provoke hypoxia.
• Stress meticulous wound care, good oral hygiene, regular dental and eye checkups, and a balanced diet as safeguards against infection.
• Advise to maintain a high fluid intake to prevent dehydration.
• Recommend that family members be screened to determine if they're heterozygous carriers of the sickle cell trait.
• Warn a female patient that both pregnancy and oral contraceptives can pose risks for her. Refer her to a gynecologist for birth control counseling.
• Inform a male patient that he may experience sudden, painful episodes of priapism (abnormal errection of the penis).

Predicting recovery

Drug-induced thrombocytopenia carries an excellent prognosis if the causative drug is withdrawn; recovery may be immediate. Otherwise, prognosis depends on the patient's response to treatment of the underlying cause.

What causes it

Thrombocytopenia may be congenital or acquired (more common). In either case, it usually results from:
• decreased or defective platelet production in the bone marrow
• increased platelet destruction outside the marrow, caused by an underlying disorder (such as cirrhosis of the liver, DIC, or severe infection)
• sequestration (as in hypothermia or increased RBC destruction in the spleen) or platelet loss.

An acquired affliction

Acquired thrombocytopenia may result from such drugs as nonsteroidal anti-inflammatory agents, sulfonamides, histamine blockers, heparin, alkylating agents, or antibiotic chemotherapeutic agents.

Fleeting forms

In children, thrombocytopenia of unknown cause (idiopathic thrombocytopenia) is common. Transient thrombocytopenia may follow a viral infection, such as Epstein-Barr or infectious mononucleosis.

Pathophysiology

In thrombocytopenia, lack of platelets may cause inadequate hemostasis. The four responsible mechanisms include:
• decreased platelet production
• decreased platelet survival
• pooling of blood in the spleen
• intravascular dilution of circulating platelets.

Minding megakaryocytes

Platelet production falls when the number of megakaryocytes decreases or when platelet production becomes dysfunctional.

What to look for

Watch for these signs and symptoms:
• abnormal bleeding (typically of a sudden onset, with skin petechiae or ecchymoses, or bleeding into mucous membranes)
• malaise and fatigue
• general weakness and lethargy
• large, blood-filled bullae (elevations) in the mouth.

What tests tell you

• Coagulation tests show diminished platelet count with prolonged bleeding time.
• Bone marrow studies may reveal increased megakaryocytes and shortened platelet survival.

How it's treated

The underlying cause must be treated. In drug-induced thrombocytopenia, the offending drug is withdrawn.

Outlining the options

Treatment may include:
• splenectomy for hypersplenism
• chemotherapy for acute or chronic leukemia
• steroids, danazol, or I.V. immune globulin for idiopathic thrombocytopenia
• platelet transfusions (to reduce the risk of spontaneous bleeding) if the platelet count falls below 20,000/µl.

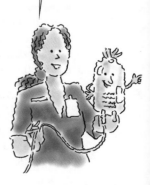

When giving platelet concentrate, remember that platelets are fragile and must be infused quickly.

What to do

• Take every possible precaution against bleeding, including guarding the patient from trauma. Keep the bed side rails up and pad them, if possible. Instruct him to use an electric razor and a soft toothbrush. Avoid all invasive procedures, such as venipuncture or urinary catheterization, if possible. When venipuncture is unavoidable, exert pressure on the puncture site for at least 20 minutes or until bleeding stops.

• Monitor platelet counts daily. Test stools for occult blood, and test urine and vomitus for blood. Watch for signs of bleeding (including petechiae, ecchymoses, surgical or GI bleeding, and menorrhagia).

• When the patient is bleeding, enforce strict bed rest if necessary.

• When giving platelet concentrate, remember that platelets are extremely fragile. Infuse them quickly, using the administration set recommended by the blood bank. During platelet transfusion, monitor the patient for febrile reaction (flushing, chills, fever, headache, tachycardia, and hypertension).

• Be aware that HLA–typed platelets may be ordered when the patient no longer responds to pooled platelets (because of antibody development). WBC–depleted platelets may be ordered to reduce the risk of febrile reactions. A patient with a history of minor reactions may benefit from acetaminophen and diphenhydramine (Benadryl) before the transfusion.

• During steroid therapy, monitor the patient's fluid and electrolyte balance and blood glucose level. Watch for infection, pathologic fractures, and mood changes.

• Evaluate the patient. He should lack signs and symptoms of gross and microscopic bleeding. He and his family should know how to reduce bleeding risks. (See *Thrombocytopenia teaching tips.*)

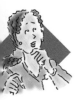

Quick quiz

1. The blood cells that transport oxygen and carbon dioxide to and from body tissues are:
   A. RBCs.
   B. WBCs.
   C. platelets.
   D. granulocytes.

Answer: A. RBCs transport oxygen and carbon dioxide. Because of their biconcave shape, they have the flexibility to travel through blood vessels of different sizes.

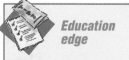

Education edge

Thrombocytopenia teaching tips

• Caution the patient to avoid aspirin in any form as well as other drugs that impair coagulation. Teach him how to recognize aspirin compounds listed on labels of over-the-counter preparations.

• Advise the patient to avoid coughing and straining during defecation. Both can lead to increased intracranial pressure, possibly causing cerebral hemorrhage. Provide a stool softener if necessary.

• If thrombocytopenia is drug-induced, stress the importance of avoiding the offending drug.

• If the patient must receive long-term steroid therapy, teach him to watch for and report cushingoid signs (such as acne, moon face, hirsutism, and edema). Emphasize that steroids must never be stopped suddenly; they must be discontinued gradually.

2. A patient with blood type B can receive a transfusion of:
  A. type A or type O blood.
  B. type B or type O blood.
  C. type AB or type O blood.
  D. type A or type B.

Answer: B. Type B blood contains B antigens and anti-A antibodies, but no anti-B antibodies. Therefore, a patient with type B blood can receive type B or type O blood (which contains neither anti-A nor anti-B antibodies).

3. Which type of anemia results from deficiency of all the blood's formed elements, caused by failure of the bone marrow to generate enough new cells?
  A. Sickle cell anemia
  B. Folic acid deficiency anemia
  C. Aplastic anemia
  D. Iron deficiency anemia

Answer: C. Aplastic anemia usually develops when damaged or destroyed stem cells inhibit RBC production.

4. Which disorder results from a deficiency of circulating platelets?
  A. Hemophilia
  B. Sickle cell anemia
  C. Von Willebrand's disease
  D. Thrombocytopenia

Answer: D. Thrombocytopenia, the most common hemorrhagic disorder, results from a deficiency of circulating platelets.

Scoring

★★★ If you answered all four questions correctly, you're certainly brainy about blood! Whatever your blood type, on this test you're clearly an A+!

★★ If you answered three questions correctly, nice phagocytic footwork! You've obviously ingested and absorbed the bulk of this chapter!

★ If you answered fewer than three questions correctly, your hematologic expertise is a bit anemic. We recommend rereading this chapter for a quick knowledge transfusion.

Immunologic disorders

Just the facts

In this chapter, you'll learn:

♦ anatomy and physiology of the immune system

♦ effects of the immune system on other body systems

♦ techniques for assessing the immune system

♦ causes, pathophysiology, diagnostic tests, and nursing interventions for common immune disorders.

A look at immunologic disorders

A normally functioning immune system guards against the effects of invasion by microorganisms and maintains equilibrium within the body by governing degradation and removal of damaged cells. When the immune system functions abnormally, physiologic effects can be devastating.

Immunologic disorders can result from or cause problems in other systems. This makes accurate assessment and intervention both crucial and challenging.

Besides endangering the patient's health—or even his life—some immunologic disorders pose a serious health risk to caregivers. This is yet another of the many challenges you'll face when caring for a patient with an immunologic disorder.

Anatomy and physiology

The immune system consists of specialized blood cells (lymphocytes and macrophages) and specialized structures, including the lymph nodes, spleen, thymus, bone marrow, tonsils, adenoids, and appendix.

The blood is an important part of this protective system. Although the blood and immune system are distinct entities, they're closely related. Their cells share a common origin in the bone marrow, and the immune system uses the bloodstream to transport its components to the site of an invasion.

Immunity

Immunity refers to the body's capacity to resist invading organisms and toxins, thus preventing tissue and organ damage. The cells and organs of the immune system perform that function. (See *Unraveling the immune system*, pages 780 and 781.)

Scavengers on surveillance

The immune system recognizes, responds to, and eliminates foreign substances (antigens), such as bacteria, fungi, viruses, and parasites. It also preserves the internal environment by scavenging dead or damaged cells and by performing surveillance.

Triple tactics

To perform these functions efficiently, the immune system uses three basic defense strategies:

physical and chemical barriers to infection

inflammatory response

immune response.

Breaking through the barriers

Physical barriers, such as the skin and mucous membranes, prevent most organisms from invading the body. Organisms that penetrate this first barrier simultaneously trigger the inflammatory and immune responses. Both responses involve stem cells—primitive cells in the bone marrow from which all types of blood cells derive.

Types of immunity

In general host defenses, all foreign substances elicit the same response. In contrast, particular microorganisms or molecules activate *specific* immune responses, and initially can involve specialized sets of immune cells. These specific responses are classified as either *humoral* or *cell-mediated* immunity. Lymphocytes (B cells and T cells) produce the responses.

> B and T cells like us play crucial roles in humoral and cell-mediated immunity.

> You can count on us!

Humoral immunity

In the humoral response, an invading antigen causes B cells to divide and differentiate into plasma cells. Each plasma cell, in turn, produces and secretes large amounts of antigen-specific immunoglobulins (Ig) into the bloodstream.

Mind your Igs

Immunoglobulins exist in five types—IgA, IgD, IgE, IgG, and IgM. Each type serves a particular function:
- IgA, IgG, and IgM guard against viral and bacterial invasion.
- IgD acts as an antigen receptor of B cells.
- IgE causes an allergic response.

Thanks for the complement

Indispensable to humoral immunity, the complement system consists of about 25 enzymes that "complement" the work of antibodies by aiding phagocytosis or destroying bacterial cells (through puncture of their cell membranes).

Cell-mediated immunity

Cell-mediated immunity protects the body against bacterial, viral, and fungal infections. It also resists transplanted cells and tumor cells. In the cell-mediated immune response, a type of scavenger cell called a *macrophage* processes the antigen, which is then presented to T cells.

Memory jogger

A stand-up comedian who gets no laughs might say his audience has humoral immunity. But humor is the Latin word for "liquid," and humoral immunity comes from elements in the blood—specifically, antibodies.

Contrast this with cellular immunity, which comes about through the actions of T cells.

Assessment

Accurately assessing the immune system can challenge your skills because immune disorders commonly cause vague symptoms, such as fatigue or dyspnea. Initially, these symptoms may seem to be related to other body systems.

History

Begin your assessment with a thorough history. Because the immune system affects all body functions, be sure to investigate the patient's overall health.

Current health status

Among patients with immunologic disorders, common complaints include fatigue or lack of energy, light-headedness, frequent bruising, and slow wound healing.

(Text continues on page 782.)

Unraveling the immune system

The immune system includes organs and tissues in which *lymphocytes* (a type of white blood cell) predominate as well as cells that circulate in peripheral blood. The central lymphoid organs are the bone marrow and thymus. Peripheral lymphoid organs include the lymph nodes and vessels, spleen, tonsils, adenoids, appendix, and intestinal lymphoid tissue (Peyer's patches).

Bringing up baby cells

The bone marrow and thymus play a role in developing the primary immune system cells—B lymphocytes (B cells) and T lymphocytes (T cells). Both cell types probably originate in the bone marrow.

    B cells may also mature and differentiate from pluripotential stem cells in the bone marrow. T cells mature and differentiate in the thymus, a two-lobed endocrine gland in the upper mediastinum. B and T cells are distributed throughout the tissue of peripheral lymphoid organs, especially the lymph nodes and spleen.

Lymph nodes

Most abundant in the head, neck, axillae, abdomen, pelvis, and groin, lymph nodes are small, oval-shaped structures located along a network of lymph channels. They help remove and destroy antigens (such as toxins, bacteria, and other foreign matter) that circulate in the blood and lymph. Lymph nodes are also a primary source of circulating lymphocytes, which provide specific immune responses.

    Surrounding each lymph node is a fibrous capsule. Bands of connective tissue (trabeculae) from the capsule extend into the node, dividing it into three compartments: superficial cortex, deep cortex, and medulla.

• The *superficial cortex* contains follicles consisting mainly of B cells. During an immune response, the follicles enlarge and develop a germinal area with large proliferating cells.
• The *deep cortex* consists mostly of T cells, as do the areas between follicles.
• The *medulla* contains numerous plasma cells that secrete immunoglobulins (antibodies) during an immune response.

Lymphatic vessels

Afferent lymphatic vessels carry lymph (a colorless fluid consisting mainly of water with dissolved salts and protein) into the node's subcapsular sinus. From here, lymph flows through cortical sinuses and smaller radial

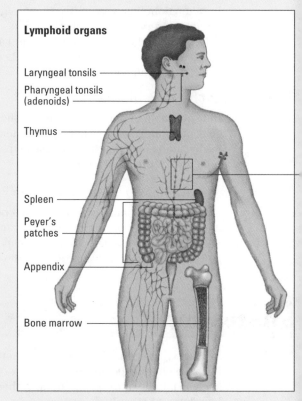

Lymphoid organs

Laryngeal tonsils
Pharyngeal tonsils (adenoids)
Thymus
Spleen
Peyer's patches
Appendix
Bone marrow

medullary sinuses. In the deep cortex and medullary sinuses, phagocytes (cells that engulf, ingest, and digest foreign material) attack the antigen. The antigen may also be trapped in the follicles of the superficial cortex.

Wayfaring lymph

Clean lymph leaves the node through efferent lymphatic vessels at the hilum. These vessels drain into specific lymph node chains that, in turn, drain into large lymph vessels known as trunks, which empty into the subclavian vein of the vascular system. In most parts of the body, lymphatic

Lymphatic and blood capillaries

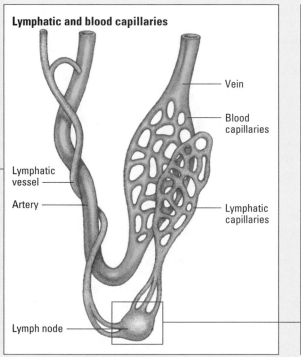

Vein

Blood capillaries

Lymphatic vessel

Artery

Lymphatic capillaries

Lymph node

Lymph node

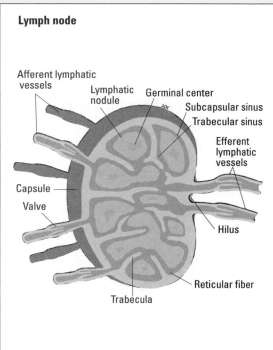

Afferent lymphatic vessels

Lymphatic nodule

Germinal center

Subcapsular sinus

Trabecular sinus

Efferent lymphatic vessels

Capsule

Valve

Hilus

Reticular fiber

Trabecula

vessels and lymphatic capillaries help veins and blood capillaries function by draining body tissues and increasing the return of blood to the heart.

Protecting the center

Lymph usually travels through more than one lymph node because numerous nodes line the lymphatic channels that drain a particular region. For example, axillary nodes filter drainage from the arms, whereas femoral nodes (located in the inguinal region) filter drainage from the legs. This arrangement prevents organisms that enter peripheral body areas from migrating unchallenged to central areas.

Spleen

The spleen is located in the left upper quadrant of the abdomen beneath the diaphragm. It gathers and isolates worn-out red blood cells, foreign materials, and cellular debris. It also stores blood and about 20% to 30% of the body's platelets.

Accessory organs

Other lymphoid tissues—tonsils, adenoids, appendix, thymus, and Peyer's patches (located in the small intestine)—also remove foreign debris in much the same way as lymph nodes do. They're positioned in food and air passages—likely areas of microbial access.

Key queries

Ask these questions to elicit details about your patient's current illness:
- Have you noticed enlarged lymph nodes?
- Have you experienced weakness or joint pain? If so, when did you first notice the problem? Does it affect one side of your body or both sides?
- Have you recently had a rash, abnormal bleeding, or a slow-healing sore?
- Have you experienced vision disturbances, fever, or changes in elimination patterns?
- Have you felt more tired recently? If so, when did it start?

Previous health status

Explore the patient's previous major illnesses, recurrent minor illnesses, accidents or injuries, surgical procedures, and allergies. Ask if he has had a procedure that could affect the immune system, such as a blood transfusion or an organ transplant.

Family and social history

Find out if the patient has a family history of cancer or hematologic or immune disorders. Ask about his home and work environments to help determine if he's being exposed to hazardous chemicals or other agents.

Physical examination

The effects of immune disorders are far-reaching and may materialize in several body systems. Pay special attention to the skin, hair, nails, and mucous membranes.

Inspection

- Observe for pallor, cyanosis (blue-tinged skin), and jaundice. Also check for erythema (redness), indicating a local inflammation, and plethora (a red, florid complexion).
- Evaluate skin integrity. Note signs and symptoms of inflammation or infection, such as redness, swelling, heat, tenderness, poor wound healing, wound drainage, induration (tissue hardening), and lesions.
- Check for rash, and note its distribution.
- Observe hair texture and distribution, noting alopecia (hair loss) on the arms, legs, or head.

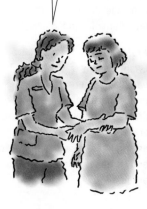

Check the patient's skin for rash, and note its distribution.

- Inspect nails for color, texture, longitudinal striations, onycholysis (separation from the nail bed), and clubbing (enlargement of the fingertips).
- Inspect the oral mucous membranes for fluffy white patches, white plaques, lesions, swollen gums, redness, and bleeding.
- Inspect areas where the patient reports "swollen glands" or "lumps" for color abnormalities and visible lymph node enlargement.
- Observe respiratory rate, rhythm, and energy expenditure related to respiratory effort. Note the position the patient assumes to ease breathing.
- Assess peripheral circulation. Inspect for Raynaud's phenomenon (intermittent arteriolar vasospasm of the fingers or toes and, sometimes, the ears and nose).
- Inspect the anus for inflammation or breaks in the mucosal surface.

Palpation

After inspection, palpate the peripheral pulses, which should be symmetrical and regular. Next, palpate the abdomen, noting enlarged organs and tenderness, and then the joints, checking for swelling, tenderness, and pain.

Noting the nodes

Palpate the superficial lymph nodes in the head and neck and in the axillary, epitrochlear, inguinal, and popliteal areas. If palpation reveals an enlarged node or other abnormalities, note the node's location, size, shape, surface, consistency, symmetry, mobility, color, tenderness, temperature, pulsations, and vascularity. (See *Locating lymph nodes in the head and neck*, page 784.)

Percussion

Next, percuss the anterior, lateral, and posterior thorax, comparing one side with the other. A dull sound indicates consolidation, which may occur with pneumonia. Hyperresonance (increased percussion sounds) may result from trapped air, as from bronchial asthma.

Auscultation

Finally, auscultate over the lungs to check for adventitious (abnormal) sounds. Wheezing suggests asthma or an allergic response. Crackles may signal a respiratory tract infection such as pneumonia.

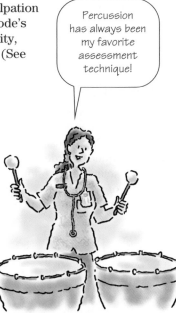

Percussion has always been my favorite assessment technique!

Locating lymph nodes in the head and neck

This illustration shows the location of the lymph nodes in the head and neck.

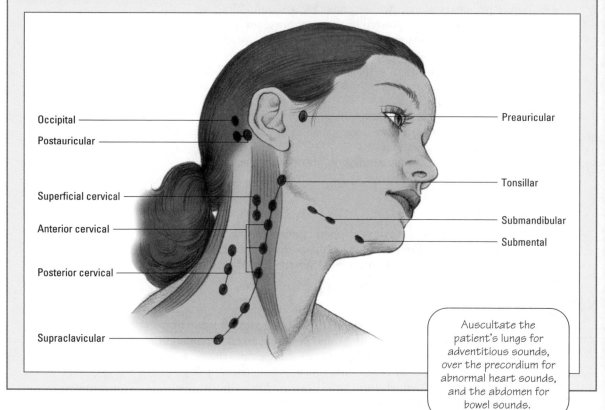

Occipital

Postauricular

Superficial cervical

Anterior cervical

Posterior cervical

Supraclavicular

Preauricular

Tonsillar

Submandibular

Submental

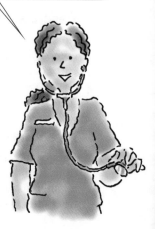

Auscultate the patient's lungs for adventitious sounds, over the precordium for abnormal heart sounds, and the abdomen for bowel sounds.

Sounding it out

Auscultate for heart sounds over the precordium. Normal auscultation reveals only the first and second heart sounds (lub-dub).

Next, auscultate the abdomen for bowel sounds. With autoimmune disorders that cause diarrhea, bowel sounds increase. With scleroderma (skin hardening and thickening, with degeneration of connective tissue) and other autoimmune disorders that cause constipation, bowel sounds decrease.

Diagnostic tests

Two commonly ordered studies to evaluate the immune response are general cellular tests (which help diagnose immunodeficiency disorders) and delayed hypersensitivity skin tests (which evaluate the cell-mediated immune response).

General cellular tests

General cellular tests, such as T- and B-lymphocyte assays, help diagnose primary and secondary immunodeficiency disorders.

T- and B-lymphocyte surface marker assays

Surface marker assays identify specific cells involved in the immune response and examine the balance between the regulatory activities of several interacting cell types—notably, T-helper and T-suppressor cells. These tests use highly specific monoclonal antibodies to define levels of lymphocyte differentiation and to analyze both normal and malignant cells.

Plethora of purposes

The results of T- and B-lymphocyte surface marker assays help to:
• assess immunocompetence in chronic infections
• evaluate immunodeficiencies
• classify lymphocytic leukemia, lymphoma, and immunodeficiency diseases such as acquired immunodeficiency syndrome (AIDS)
• identify immunoregulation associated with autoimmune disorders
• diagnose disorders marked by abnormal numbers and percentages of T-helper cells, T-suppressor cells, and B lymphocytes.

Nursing considerations
• Inform the patient that the test requires a blood sample.
• As ordered, perform a venipuncture. Send the blood sample to the laboratory immediately to ensure viable lymphocytes. The sample must not be refrigerated or frozen. Apply pressure to the venipuncture site until bleeding stops.
• Many patients with T- and B-cell changes have a compromised immune system, so be sure to keep the venipuncture site clean and dry.

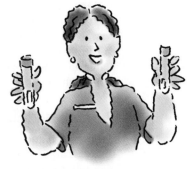

Be sure to send the blood sample to the laboratory immediately. Lymphocytes don't stay viable too long.

Delayed hypersensitivity skin tests

Delayed hypersensitivity skin tests evaluate the cell-mediated immune response. They include intradermal skin tests and scratch and puncture allergy tests.

Intradermal skin tests

For intradermal skin tests, recall antigens (antigens to which the patient may have been previously sensitized) are injected into the superficial skin layer with a needle and syringe or a sterile four-pronged lancet.

TB or not TB?

Tuberculin skin tests (such as the tine or Mantoux) produce a delayed hypersensitivity reaction in patients with active or dormant tuberculosis (TB).

Recalling past antigens

Recall antigen tests for *Candida*, tetanus, and mumps induce depressed or negative delayed hypersensitivity reactions in patients with infections and immunodeficiencies. Recall antigen tests induce positive delayed hypersensitivity reactions in patients who can maintain a nonspecific inflammatory response to the antigen. (See *Administering test antigens.*)

Nursing considerations
• Tell the patient when he can expect a reaction to appear (usually after 2 days). Check his history for hypersensitivity to the test antigens and for previous reactions to a skin test.
• Using alcohol, clean the volar surface (palm side) of the arm, about 2 or 3 fingerbreadths distal to the antecubital space (triangle of the elbow) to protect the wheal from potential infection. You may also clean the area with acetone to remove skin oils that may interfere with test results.
• Make sure the test site you've chosen has adequate subcutaneous tissue and is free from hair and blemishes. Let the skin dry completely before administering the injection to avoid inactivating the antigen.
• Instruct an outpatient to return at the prescribed time to have test results read.

Scratch and puncture allergy tests

Skin scratch and puncture allergy tests evaluate the immune system's ability to respond to known allergens. A tiny amount of allergen is scratched across or lightly pricked into the skin of a

Administering test antigens

This illustration shows the arm of a patient undergoing a recall antigen test, which determines whether he has previously been exposed to certain antigens. A sample panel of four test antigens has been injected into his forearm, and the test site has been marked and labeled for each antigen.

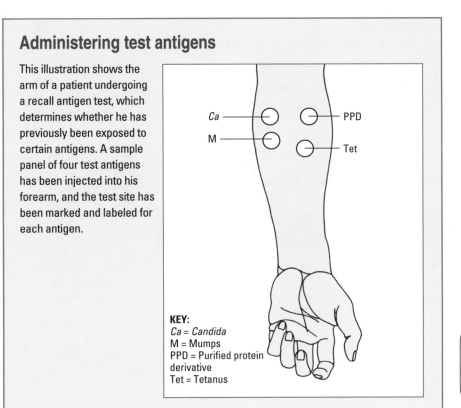

KEY:
Ca = Candida
M = Mumps
PPD = Purified protein derivative
Tet = Tetanus

This scratch and puncture test may tell us which substances you're allergic to.

hairless area, such as the scapula, volar surface of the forearm, or anterior surface of the thigh. If the patient has an allergy, the specific allergens he's allergic to will cause redness and swelling.

Teensy weensy doses

These tests provoke delayed hypersensitivity reactions mediated by T cells. Although minute amounts of test allergens usually can demonstrate an intact immune response, test results may indicate an anergic (diminished or absent) reaction in elderly patients as well as in patients with acute leukemia, Hodgkin's disease, congenital immunodeficiencies, or overwhelming infections.

Scratch and puncture tests are contraindicated in patients with inflammation, skin diseases, or significant immunologic impairment.

Nursing considerations
- Use the volar surface of the arm to perform the test in an adult; use the upper back in a child.
- After 20 minutes, check for a pale, raised, urticarial area around the puncture or scratch site (wheal), surrounded by a reddened area that's generally round (flare). This indicates a positive response, meaning a patient is allergic to the specific allergen tested.
- Record the greatest diameter of the wheal and flare for each allergen.
- Have epinephrine available in case of an anaphylactic reaction.

Treatments

Treatments for immune disorders include drug therapy and bone marrow transplantation. Both may cause additional immunosuppression, so you'll need to take special precautions to maintain strict asepsis and prevent infection and injury.

Epinephrine should be given immediately to a patient who's suffering an acute anaphylactic reaction.

Drug therapy

Many immune disorders are treated with drugs, so you'll need to be familiar with the indications, dosages, and nursing considerations for such drugs as:
- antihistamines, which prevent or relieve allergic reactions
- immunosuppressants, used to combat tissue rejection and help control autoimmune disorders
- corticosteroids, which prevent or suppress the cell-mediated immune response and reduce inflammation
- cytotoxic drugs, which kill immunocompetent cells
- adrenergics, which stimulate the sympathetic nervous system.

Prime drugs

For certain immune disorders, drugs are the primary treatment. For instance, epinephrine is the drug of choice for treating acute anaphylactic reaction. For other immune disorders, drugs are prescribed to treat associated symptoms.

Medication roster

Besides epinephrine, other drugs used to treat immune disorders include:
- azathioprine (Imuran)
- cyclosporine (Sandimmune)

- cytomegalovirus immune globulin (human)
- didanosine (Videx)
- hepatitis B immune globulin, human
- immune globulin
- lamivudine (Epivir)
- $Rh_o(D)$ immune globulin
- stavudine (Zerit)
- zidovudine (Retrovir).

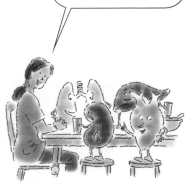

Immunosuppressant therapy can be used to prevent rejection of an organ transplant.

Immunosuppressant therapy

Iatrogenic (treatment-induced) immunodeficiency may be a complicating adverse effect of chemotherapy or other treatment. In some cases, however, it's the goal of therapy—for instance, to suppress immune-mediated tissue damage from an autoimmune disorder or to prevent rejection of an organ transplant. To induce immunodeficiency, a patient may receive various types of immunosuppressant drugs.

Antilymphocyte serum

Antilymphocyte serum is a powerful nonspecific immunosuppressant that destroys circulating lymphocytes. It reduces T-cell number and function, thus suppressing cell-mediated immunity. It has been used effectively to prevent cell-mediated rejection of tissue grafts or transplants.

Antithymocyte globulin

Antithymocyte globulin (ATG) causes specific destruction of T lymphocytes. Usually, it's given immediately before transplantation and continued for some time afterward.

Sickening the serum

Adverse effects of ATG include anaphylaxis and serum sickness. Arising 1 to 2 weeks after ATG injection, serum sickness is marked by fever, malaise, rash, arthralgias and, sometimes, glomerulonephritis or vasculitis.

Corticosteroids

Corticosteroids are adrenocortical hormones used widely to treat immune-mediated disorders because of their potent anti-inflammatory and immunosuppressant effects. They stabilize the vascular membrane, blocking tissue infiltration by neutrophils and monocytes and thus inhibiting inflammation. They also "kidnap" T cells in the bone marrow, causing lymphopenia.

Memory jogger

Searching for a "hook" to use when assessing patients for serum sickness? Just think of the word **FARM.** Each letter stands for a key sign or symptom of serum sickness:

Fever

Arthralgias

Rash

Malaise.

Lymphocyte bounce-back

However, because these drugs aren't toxic to cells, lymphocyte concentration can quickly return to normal within 24 hours after the corticosteroid is withdrawn. Also, corticosteroids seem to inhibit immunoglobulin synthesis and interfere with binding of immunoglobulin to antigen.

Cyclosporine

Cyclosporine selectively suppresses the proliferation and development of T-helper cells, resulting in depressed cell-mediated immunity.

Cytotoxic drugs

Cytotoxic drugs kill immunocompetent cells while they're replicating. Unfortunately, most of these agents aren't selective, which means they interfere with all rapidly proliferating cells. As a result, they cause depletion of lymphocytes and phagocytes and interfere with lymphocyte synthesis and release of immunoglobulins and lymphokines.

Dicey drug therapy

Cyclophosphamide (Cytoxan), a potent cytotoxic drug commonly used as an immunosuppressant, initially depletes B cells, suppressing humoral immunity. Long-term therapy also depletes T cells, suppressing cell-mediated immunity, too. Cyclophosphamide may be given to patients with systemic lupus erythematosus (SLE), Wegener's granulomatosis, or certain autoimmune disorders.

Because it nonselectively destroys rapidly dividing cells, the drug can cause severe bone marrow suppression with abnormally low levels of red blood cells, or RBCs (anemia), neutrophils (neutropenia), or platelets (thrombocytopenia). It may also lead to gonadal suppression, resulting in sterility, alopecia, hemorrhagic cystitis, nausea and vomiting, stomatitis, and an increased risk of lymphoproliferative neoplasm.

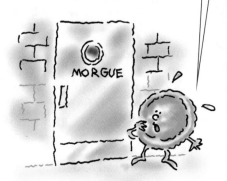

Cyclophosphamide destroys all rapidly dividing cells, including red blood cells. I'm too young to go!

Other immune busters

Other cytotoxic drugs used to suppress the immune system include:
• azathioprine (Azasan), commonly used in kidney transplant
• methotrexate (Trexall), occasionally used in rheumatoid arthritis and other autoimmune disorders.

Bone marrow transplantation

Patients with certain immune disorders may be candidates for bone marrow transplant. This procedure also is being explored as a treatment of certain hematologic disorders and cancers, such as multiple myeloma and some solid tumors.

Bone up on transplantation

In bone marrow transplantation, bone marrow cells are collected from the patient or another donor and then administered to the patient after his diseased bone marrow is destroyed by chemotherapy or total body radiation. The goal is to allow the patient to resume normal blood cell production.

The preferred treatment for aplastic anemia and severe combined immunodeficiency syndrome (SCID), bone marrow transplantation also is used to treat leukemia patients who are at high risk for relapse or who have undergone high-dose chemotherapy and total body radiation therapy.

Patient preparation

Before the procedure, take these steps:
• Inform the patient that bone marrow transplant will deplete his white blood cells (WBCs), putting him at high risk for infection immediately after the procedure. As a safeguard, he'll be placed in reverse isolation for several weeks.
• Prepare him for the pretransplant regimen, which may include cytotoxic chemotherapy and total body radiation. During this regimen, he should expect adverse reactions, such as parotitis (inflammation or infection of the parotid salivary glands), diarrhea, fever, nausea, vomiting, and signs and symptoms of bone marrow depression (such as fever, fatigue, chills, bruising, and bleeding).

Monitoring and aftercare

During and after the procedure, take these steps:
• During the transfusion, monitor the patient's vital signs closely to promptly detect such reactions as fever, dyspnea, and hypotension.
• Assess the patient every 4 hours for signs and symptoms of infection, such as fever and chills.
• Maintain strict asepsis when caring for the patient. Take measures to protect him from injury.

Being a bad host

• Watch for signs of graft-versus-host (GVH) disease, such as dermatitis, hepatitis, hemolytic anemia, and thrombocytopenia. GVH disease usually occurs during the first 90 days after the transplant

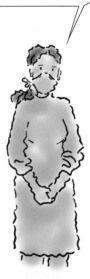

If your patient is in reverse isolation, apply a clean mask every time you enter his room, and make sure visitors do the same.

and may become chronic—or it may cause transplant failure, lymphatic depletion, infection, or death.

Home care instructions

Before discharge, give the patient these instructions:
• Tell the patient to guard against infection. Warn him that he may remain unusually vulnerable to infection for up to 1 year after bone marrow transplantation.
• Urge him to keep regular medical appointments so the practitioner can monitor his progress and detect late complications.

Nursing diagnoses

When caring for patients with immunologic disorders, you'll find that several nursing diagnoses can be used over and over. Commonly used diagnoses appear here, along with appropriate nursing interventions and rationales. See *NANDA-I taxonomy II by domain*, page 936, for the complete list of NANDA diagnoses.

Risk for infection

Related to external or internal factors, *Risk for infection* may be associated with AIDS, SCID, pernicious anemia, and other immune disorders.

Expected outcomes

• Patient remains free from signs and symptoms of infection.
• Patient maintains adequate respiratory function.
• Patient states ways to prevent infection, including proper hand washing and good personal hygiene.

Nursing interventions and rationales

• Practice strict hand hygiene before and after patient contact to avoid spreading pathogens.
• Monitor the patient closely for signs and symptoms of infection, such as fever and chills. Check vital signs every 4 hours. Close monitoring allows for timely intervention.
• Maintain skin and mucous membrane integrity to help prevent infection. Encourage ambulation, and help turn the patient every 2 hours. Don't give an enema or a suppository or take the patient's rectal temperature. Encourage mouth care with sodium bicarbonate and natural saline rinse (1 teaspoonful per 8 oz) to inhibit microbial growth. Perform daily hygiene and oral assessment.

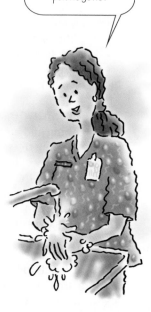

Practice strict hand hygiene before and after patient contact to avoid spreading pathogens.

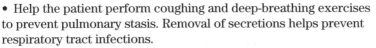

• Help the patient perform coughing and deep-breathing exercises to prevent pulmonary stasis. Removal of secretions helps prevent respiratory tract infections.
• Make sure visitors and staff members with upper respiratory tract infections wear masks when with the patient to protect him from pathogens.
• Teach the patient measures to minimize the risk of infection. Participating in his care encourages his compliance with therapy and lifestyle modifications.

Ineffective coping

Related to perceived or impending personal loss, *Ineffective coping* may be associated with life-threatening immunodeficiency disorders.

Expected outcomes
• Patient identifies mechanisms for coping effectively.
• Patient demonstrates an active role in self-care activities.
• Patient identifies appropriate resources to maximize his status.

Nursing interventions and rationales
• Encourage the patient and his family to discuss past coping mechanisms and their effectiveness. Doing this reinforces successful coping behaviors and fosters a sense of control.
• Urge the patient and his family to participate in care and ongoing decision making, to increase their sense of self-worth and mastery over the current situation and allow the patient to progress at his own pace.
• Refer the patient and his family to appropriate community resources as needed for continued support to restore and maintain psychological equilibrium and prevent future crisis.

Common immunologic disorders

Immunologic disorders range from mild ailments (such as hypersensitivity vasculitis) to life-threatening ones (such as anaphylaxis). Some are congenital, whereas others are acquired.
    Immunologic disorders may result from:
• hyperreactivity, as in allergic rhinitis
• autoimmunity, as in SLE
• immunodeficiency, as in AIDS.

Acquired immunodeficiency syndrome

Marked by progressive weakening of cell-mediated immunity, AIDS increases susceptibility to opportunistic infections and unusual cancers. (See *Opportunistic infections in AIDS*.) Diagnosis comes from careful correlation of the patient's history and clinical features with counts of certain types of T cells.

Time and mortality

The time between probable exposure to the human immunodeficiency virus (HIV, the agent that causes AIDS) and diagnosis of AIDS averages 8 to 10 years. Children seem to have a shorter incubation time, with a mean of 8 months. Worldwide, more than 75% of AIDS patients die within 2 years of diagnosis. Patients may be HIV-positive and asymptomatic for varying periods.

What causes it

AIDS is caused by infection with HIV, a retrovirus present in body fluids, such as blood and semen. Modes of HIV transmission include:
• sexual contact, especially associated with trauma to the rectal or vaginal mucosa

---

Opportunistic infections in AIDS

This table shows some of the complicating infections that may occur in patients with acquired immunodeficiency syndrome (AIDS). Other opportunistic conditions seen in AIDS patients include Kaposi's sarcoma, wasting disease, and AIDS dementia complex.

Microbiological agent	Organism	Condition
Protozoa	*Pneumocystis jiroveci*	*Pneumocystis* pneumonia
	Cryptosporidium	Cryptosporidiosis
	Toxoplasma gondii	Toxoplasmosis
	Histoplasma	Histoplasmosis
Fungi	*Candida albicans*	Candidiasis
	Cryptococcus neoformans	Cryptococcosis
Viruses	Herpes	Herpes simplex 1 and 2
	Cytomegalovirus	Cytomegalovirus retinitis
Bacteria	*Mycobacterium tuberculosis*	Tuberculosis
	M. avium-intracellulare	MAI infection

• transfusion of contaminated blood or blood products
• use of contaminated needles
• placental transmission from an infected mother to a fetus through cervical or blood contact at delivery
• breast milk from an infected woman.

Compromising circumstances

Risk factors for AIDS include:
• sexual contact with someone who has AIDS or is at risk for it
• present or past abuse of I.V. drugs
• transfusion of blood or blood products.

Prenatal and perinatal exposure to AIDS increases the risk of AIDS in infants, as does breast-feeding if the mother has AIDS or is at risk for it.

Pathophysiology

HIV attaches to helper T cells having an antigen called *CD4+* on their surface. CD4+ serves as a receptor for the virus, allowing it to enter the cell. After invading the cell, HIV either replicates, leading to cell death, or the virus becomes latent.

By hook or by crook

HIV infection results in profound pathology—either directly or indirectly. Direct pathologic effects come about through destruction of CD4+ cells, other immune cells, and neuroglial cells. Indirect pathologic consequences occur through the secondary effects of CD4+ T-cell dysfunction and the resulting immunosuppression.

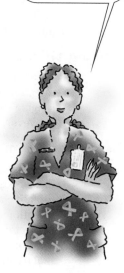

A patient with a history of injectable drug use is at risk for AIDS, which can be transmitted through contaminated needles.

What to look for

After initial exposure, an infected person may have no signs or symptoms—or may have a flulike illness (seroconversion illness) and then remain asymptomatic for years.

Cunning contagion

However, as the syndrome progresses, he may have neurologic signs and symptoms caused by HIV encephalopathy or signs and symptoms of an opportunistic infection or disease, such as *Pneumocystis jiroveci* pneumonia, cytomegalovirus, or cancer. Eventually, repeated opportunistic infections overwhelm his weakened immune defenses, invading every body system.

What tests tell you

• The Centers for Disease Control and Prevention defines AIDS as a CD4+ cell count below 200 cells/μl or when a patient has an opportunistic infection in the setting of HIV infection.

• Enzyme-linked immunosorbent assay and a confirmatory Western blot assay detect HIV antibodies to diagnose HIV infection.
• Levels of circulating HIV ("viral load") are measured regularly to assess the risk of disease progression and the patient's response to therapy.

How it's treated

Although no cure exists for AIDS, signs and symptoms can be managed with treatment. Primary therapy for HIV infection includes four categories of antiretroviral drugs:
• Reverse transcriptase inhibitors include nucleoside and nonnucleoside reverse transcriptase inhibitors. Drugs in this category include abacavir (Ziagen), delavirdine (Rescriptor), didanosine, lamivudine, nevirapine (Viramune), tenofovir (Viread), and zidovudine (Retrovir).
• Protease inhibitors include fosamprenavir (Lexiva), indinavir (Crixivan), ritonavir (Norvir), saquinavir (Invirase), and tipranavir (Aptivus).
• Fusion inhibitors include enfuvirtide (Fuzeon).
• Integrase inhibitors include raltegravir (Isentress).
    Used in various combinations, these drugs are designed to inhibit HIV viral replication.

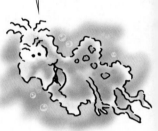

Repeated opportunistic infections eventually overwhelm the weakened immune system of a person with AIDS. We pathogens don't give up easily.

Slowing things down

Treatment with zidovudine effectively slows the progression of HIV infection, decreasing the number of opportunistic infections, prolonging survival, and slowing the progress of associated dementia. However, the drug can cause severe adverse and toxic reactions.

Tweaking the immune system

Other drug therapies used in AIDS include immunomodulatory drugs, designed to boost the weakened immune system, and anti-infective and antineoplastic agents, used to combat opportunistic infections and associated cancers. HIV and AIDS drugs are the subject of a great deal of research. New drugs are constantly being developed, and many studies are under way to determine the optimal treatment regimens.

What to do

• Monitor the patient for fever, noting its pattern.
• Assess for tender, swollen lymph nodes, and check laboratory values regularly.
• Watch for signs and symptoms of infection, such as skin breakdown, cough, sore throat, and diarrhea.
• Watch for signs of oral candida infection (thrush).

- Follow standard precautions as directed by your facility, depending on the patient's disease stage and condition.
- Offer support in coping with the social impact and discouraging prognosis of AIDS.
- Evaluate the patient. After counseling and treatment, he should be able to state the early signs and symptoms of infection, explain how HIV is transmitted, and describe the limitations AIDS may impose on his lifestyle. He also should be able to maintain an optimal nutritional status. (See *AIDS teaching tips*.)

Anaphylaxis

Anaphylaxis is an exaggerated hypersensitivity reaction to a previously encountered antigen. A severe anaphylactic reaction may induce vascular collapse, leading to systemic shock and, in some cases, death.

What causes it

An anaphylactic reaction results from systemic exposure to a sensitizing drug or other antigen, such as:
- penicillin (the most common cause) or other antibiotics
- serums
- vaccines
- allergen extracts
- enzymes
- hormones
- sulfonamides
- local anesthetics
- salicylates
- polysaccharides.

Toxic triggers

Anaphylaxis may also result from diagnostic chemicals (including radiographic contrast media containing iodine), foods, sulfites, insect venom (such as from a bee sting) and, rarely, a ruptured hydatid cyst (a liver cyst containing tapeworm larvae).

Pathophysiology

Here's how an anaphylactic reaction occurs:

On initial exposure to an antigen, the immune system responds by producing IgE antibodies in the lymph nodes. Helper T cells enhance this process.

Antibodies bind to membrane receptors located on mast cells in connective tissues and on basophils.

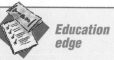

Education edge

AIDS teaching tips

- Explain how acquired immunodeficiency syndrome (AIDS) affects the immune response and makes him susceptible to opportunistic infection. Discuss ways to prevent infection.
- Discuss measures to prevent the spread of AIDS, such as wearing a condom during vaginal or anal intercourse, not sharing needles or syringes, and not donating blood, body organs or tissue, or sperm.
- Discuss contraceptive measures with a female patient. Explain that a mother can transmit AIDS to her fetus during pregnancy and to an infant through her breast milk.
- Teach the patient about your facility's infection-control policies and how they're implemented.

The next time the person encounters this antigen, the IgE antibodies, or cross-linked IgE receptors, recognize it as foreign and activate the release of powerful chemical mediators.

What to look for

An anaphylactic reaction usually produces sudden distress within seconds or minutes after exposure to an allergen. (A delayed or persistent reaction may occur up to 24 hours later.) Severity of signs and symptoms depends on the original sensitizing dose of antigen, amount and distribution of antibodies, and the antigen's entry route and dose.

Right out of the gate...

Initial signs and symptoms of anaphylaxis include:
- a feeling of impending doom or fright
- weakness
- sweating
- sneezing
- pruritus (itching)
- urticaria (an itchy skin eruption causing wheals) and angioedema (acute swelling of the face, neck, lips, larynx, hands, feet, genitalia, or internal organs)
- cardiovascular changes, such as hypotension, shock, and arrhythmias
- respiratory signs and symptoms, including swelling of the nasal mucosa, profuse runny nose, nasal congestion, sudden sneezing attacks, and hoarseness, stridor, and dyspnea (early signs of acute respiratory failure)
- GI and genitourinary signs and symptoms (severe stomach cramps, nausea, diarrhea, and urinary urgency and incontinence).

How it's treated

Anaphylaxis is always an emergency. It requires an immediate injection of epinephrine 1:1,000 aqueous solution, repeated every 5 to 20 minutes as necessary.

Epi to the rescue

In the early stages of anaphylaxis, when the patient still has normal blood pressure and is conscious, give epinephrine I.M. or subcutaneously. Massage the injection site to help the drug move into circulation faster.

With severe reactions, when the patient has lost consciousness and is hypotensive, give epinephrine I.V.

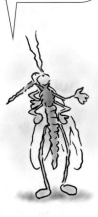

Chemicals, foods, sulfites, and insect venom can trigger anaphylaxis.

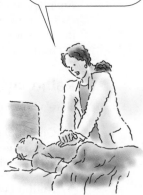

If your anaphylactic patient goes into cardiac arrest, start CPR immediately.

What to do

• Maintain a patent airway. Observe the patient for early signs of laryngeal edema (stridor, hoarseness, and dyspnea), which typically necessitate endotracheal intubation or a tracheotomy and oxygen therapy. If he's in cardiac arrest, begin cardiopulmonary resuscitation (CPR) at once.

• Watch for hypotension and shock, and maintain circulatory volume with volume expanders (plasma, saline solution, and albumin), as needed and ordered.

• After the initial emergency, give other medications as ordered: epinephrine solution or suspension subcutaneously, corticosteroids and diphenhydramine I.V. for long-term management, and aminophylline I.V. over 10 to 20 minutes for bronchospasm. Keep in mind that rapid aminophylline (Truphylline) infusion may cause or aggravate severe hypotension.

• If a patient must receive a drug to which he's allergic, help prevent a severe reaction by making sure he's carefully desensitized beforehand with gradually increasing doses of the antigen or advance steroid administration.

• Evaluate the patient. On recovery, his blood pressure should be within normal limits and his respirations should be regular and unlabored. (See *Anaphylaxis teaching tips.*)

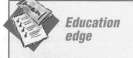

Education edge

Anaphylaxis teaching tips

• To prevent anaphylaxis, teach the patient to avoid exposure to known allergens. If he has a food or drug allergy, tell him to avoid the offending food or drug in all its forms. If he's allergic to insect bites or stings, tell him to avoid open fields and wooded areas during the insect season and to carry an anaphylaxis kit (containing epinephrine, antihistamine, and tourniquet) when outdoors.

• Advise the patient to wear medical identification jewelry identifying his allergy or allergies.

Asthma

A chronic reactive airway disorder, asthma causes episodic, reversible airway restriction with bronchospasm, increased mucus secretion, and mucosal edema. Although this common condition can strike at any age, children under age 10 account for 50% of the cases.

From within or without

Asthma can be intrinsic or extrinsic. Extrinsic asthma results from sensitivity to specific external allergens. In intrinsic asthma, the symptoms aren't associated with an allergic reaction, and the immune system isn't involved in the reaction.

All in the family?

About one-third of all asthmatics share the condition with at least one member of their immediate family, and roughly three-fourths of children with two asthmatic parents also have asthma.

What causes it

Extrinsic asthma follows exposure to pollen, animal dander, house dust or mold, pillows containing feathers or a silky material called kapok, food additives containing sulfites, or other sensitizing substances. Intrinsic asthma may be triggered by irritants, anxiety, fatigue, endocrine changes, temperature and humidity changes, or viruses.

Cataloging causes

Other causes of asthma include aspirin, various nonsteroidal anti-inflammatory drugs (NSAIDs, such as indomethacin [Indocin] and mefenamic acid [Ponstel]), tartrazine (a yellow food dye), exercise, and occupational exposure to an allergenic factor (such as platinum).

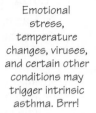

Emotional stress, temperature changes, viruses, and certain other conditions may trigger intrinsic asthma. Brrr!

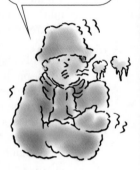

Pathophysiology

In asthma, tracheal and bronchial linings overreact to various stimuli, causing episodic smooth-muscle spasms that severely narrow the airways. Mucosal edema and thickened secretions further block the airways.

There's inflation...and then there's hyperinflation

During an asthma attack, expiratory airflow decreases, trapping gas in the airways and causing alveoli to hyperinflate. Atelectasis (lung tissue collapse) may occur in some lung regions. Increased airway resistance leads to labored breathing.

What to look for

Usually, extrinsic asthma is accompanied by signs and symptoms of atopy (IgE-mediated allergy), such as eczema and allergic rhinitis. It commonly follows a severe respiratory tract infection, especially in adults.

Drama and distress

An acute asthma attack may begin dramatically, with simultaneous onset of severe multiple symptoms. Sometimes, however, onset is slow, with gradually increasing respiratory distress. Asthma that causes cyanosis, confusion, and lethargy indicates the onset of life-threatening status asthmaticus and respiratory failure.

Signs and symptoms of asthma include:
- sudden dyspnea, wheezing, and tightness in the chest
- coughing that produces thick, clear, or yellow sputum
- tachypnea and use of accessory respiratory muscles.

Other findings may include a rapid pulse, profuse perspiration, hyperresonant lung fields, and diminished breath sounds.

What tests tell you

• Pulmonary function studies reveal signs of obstructive airway disease (decreased flow rates and forced expiratory volume in 1 second), low-normal or diminished vital capacity, and increased total lung and residual capacity.
• Arterial blood gas analysis reveals reduced partial pressure of oxygen and partial pressure of arterial carbon dioxide ($Paco_2$). With severe asthma, $Paco_2$ may be normal or elevated, indicating severe bronchial obstruction.
• A chest X-ray may show lung hyperinflation, with areas of local atelectasis.
• Skin testing for specific allergens may be necessary if the patient lacks a history of allergy.
• Inhalation bronchial challenge testing evaluates the significance of allergens identified by skin testing.

> If your patient has asthma, a chest X-ray may show hyperinflated lungs with areas of atelectasis.

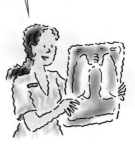

How it's treated

Treatment usually is tailored to each patient and focuses on identifying and avoiding precipitating factors, such as allergens or irritants. Usually, such stimuli can't be removed entirely. Although desensitization to specific antigens may be helpful, it's rarely totally effective or persistent.

Drug therapy usually includes a bronchodilator and proves more effective when begun soon after symptom onset. Other drugs used to treat asthma may include:
• rapid-acting epinephrine
• terbutaline
• long-acting beta agonists (Serevent) or short-acting beta agonists (Maxair)
• theophylline and oral preparations containing theophylline
• oral sympathomimetics
• oral or inhaled corticosteroids
• cromolyn (Intal) to help prevent release of the chemical mediators (histamine and leukotrienes) that cause bronchoconstriction
• leukotriene receptor modifiers (Singulair) to help block inflammatory reactions in the lungs.

What to do

• During an acute asthma attack, take appropriate measures to maintain respiratory function and relieve bronchoconstriction, while allowing mucus plug expulsion.
• If the attack was caused by exertion, have the patient sit down, rest, and sip warm water.

Tempering the terror

- Severe breathing difficulty is terrifying. Reassure the patient that you'll help him. Place him in semi-Fowler's position, encourage diaphragmatic breathing, and urge him to relax as much as possible.
- Know that status asthmaticus unrelieved by epinephrine is a medical emergency. Severe hypoxemia may require endotracheal intubation and mechanical ventilation.
- Administer drugs and I.V. fluids as ordered.
- Evaluate the patient. With successful treatment, his respirations should be regular and unlabored, and he should exhibit signs of adequate gas exchange, such as absence of cyanosis and confusion. Also, the patient and his family should be able to identify predisposing factors and state measures to eliminate them. (See *Asthma teaching tips*.)

Systemic lupus erythematosus

A chronic inflammatory disorder of the connective tissue, SLE affects multiple organ systems (as well as the skin) and can be fatal. It's marked by recurring remissions and exacerbations, which are especially common during the spring and summer.

SLE strikes eight times as many women as men, increasing to 15 times as many during childbearing years. SLE occurs worldwide, and is most prevalent among Asians and blacks.

Prognosis: Mixed

The prognosis improves with early detection and treatment but is poor for patients who develop cardiovascular, renal, or neurologic complications or severe bacterial infections.

About 1 out of 20 patients with discoid lupus erythematosus, another form of lupus erythematosus, later develops SLE.

What causes it

The cause of SLE remains a mystery, but evidence points to interrelated immunologic abnormalities and environmental, hormonal, and genetic factors as possible causes.

A grab bag of causes

Factors that may increase the risk of SLE exacerbation include:
- genetic predisposition
- stress
- streptococcal or viral infections
- exposure to sunlight or ultraviolet light
- immunization

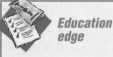

Education edge

Asthma teaching tips

- Help the patient identify asthma triggers. Explain how these triggers cause bronchospasm, airway edema, and mucus production.
- Explain how to recognize and prevent respiratory tract infection.
- Teach the patient how to control an asthma attack.
- Discuss prescribed drugs and how to use them. Teach the patient how to use an oral inhaler. Explain that he should keep his nebulizer handy at all times. Caution him to take no more than two or three inhalations every 4 hours. If he needs the nebulizer more frequently, advise him to call the practitioner. Explain that nebulizer overuse can weaken his response and diminish the drug's therapeutic effect. Warn him that extended overuse can lead to cardiac arrest and death.
- Tell the patient about asthma support groups such as the American Lung Association.

- pregnancy
- abnormal estrogen metabolism.

Medications that increase the risk of SLE include procainamide, hydralazine, anticonvulsants and, less commonly, penicillins, sulfa drugs, and hormonal contraceptives.

Pathophysiology

Autoimmunity is thought to be the prime mechanism associated with SLE. The body produces antibodies against components of its own cells, resulting in immune complex disease. Patients with SLE may produce antibodies against various tissue components (such as RBCs, neutrophils, platelets, lymphocytes) or virtually any organ or tissue in the body.

What to look for

Characteristic findings in SLE include facial erythema (butterfly rash), nonerosive arthritis, and photosensitivity. (See *Recognizing butterfly rash.*)

> One of the characteristic findings in SLE is a classic butterfly rash.

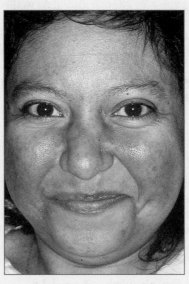

Recognizing butterfly rash

In the classic butterfly rash of systemic lupus erythematosus, lesions appear on the cheeks and the bridge of the nose, creating a characteristic butterfly pattern. The rash may vary in severity from malar erythema (redness of the cheeks) to discoid lesions (plaques).

A rash of reactions

The patient may also experience discoid rash (an itchy, scaly, or flaky round or oval rash most common on the face, scalp, neck and chest after sun exposure), oral or nasopharyngeal ulcers, pleuritis, pericarditis, seizures, patchy alopecia, and even psychoses.

The patient also commonly has some combination of these systemic signs and symptoms: aching, malaise, fatigue, low-grade or spiking fever, chills, anorexia, weight loss, lymph node enlargement, abdominal pain, nausea and vomiting, diarrhea or constipation, Raynaud's phenomenon, and irregular menses or amenorrhea.

> Sun exposure may trigger an itchy discoid rash on the face of a patient with SLE.

What tests tell you

- For most patients with active disease, antinuclear antibody, anti-DNA, and lupus erythematosus cell tests are the most specific SLE tests.
- Complete blood count with differential may show anemia and decreased WBC counts. Platelet count may also be decreased.
- Erythrocyte sedimentation rate may be elevated.
- Serum electrophoresis may show hypergammaglobulinemia (an excess of gamma globulins in the blood).
- Urine studies may show urinary RBCs and WBCs, urine casts and sediment, and significant urine protein loss (more than 3.5 g/24 hours).
- Blood studies showing decreased serum complement (C3 and C4) levels indicate active disease.
- A chest X-ray may show pleurisy or lupus pneumonitis (lung inflammation).

How it's treated

Patients with mild disease need little or no medication. Aspirin and other NSAIDs may control arthritis symptoms.

Skin lesions require topical treatment. For acute lesions, corticosteroid creams are recommended. Refractory skin lesions are treated with intralesional corticosteroids or antimalarial drugs, such as hydroxychloroquine (Plaquenil) and chloroquine (Aralen).

Systemic symptoms? Stick with steroids

Corticosteroids remain the treatment of choice for systemic symptoms of SLE, acute generalized exacerbations, and serious disease related to vital organ systems (such as pleuritis, pericarditis, lupus nephritis, vasculitis, and central nervous system involvement).

What to do

- Watch for such signs and symptoms as joint pain or stiffness, weakness, fever, fatigue, and chills, and provide comfort measures for the patient.
- Observe the patient for dyspnea, chest pain, and edema of the arms and legs.
- Note the size, type, and location of skin lesions.
- Check the urine for blood.
- Inspect the scalp for hair loss, and check skin and mucous membranes for petechiae (tiny purplish spots indicating minute hemorrhages), bleeding, ulcers, pallor, and bruising.
- Provide a balanced diet. A patient with renal involvement may require a low-sodium, low-protein diet.
- Apply heat packs to relieve joint pain and stiffness. Encourage regular exercise to maintain full range of motion and prevent contractures.
- Monitor vital signs, fluid intake and output, weight, and laboratory findings.
- Evaluate the patient. With successful therapy, she should be free from pain and stiffness and her vital signs should be within normal limits. (See *SLE teaching tips*.)

> A patient with SLE should eat a balanced diet. If she has renal involvement, instruct her to limit sodium and protein intake.

Education edge

SLE teaching tips

- Tell the patient to avoid crowds and people who might be contagious to minimize the risk of infection.
- Review range-of-motion exercises and body alignment techniques to help minimize joint pain.
- Tell the patient to call her practitioner if she develops a fever, cough, or rash or if chest, abdominal, muscle, or joint pain becomes worse.
- Stress the importance of eating a balanced diet.
- Emphasize the importance of keeping follow-up appointments.
- Tell the patient to wear protective clothing and to use sunscreen when she goes outside to help minimize skin flare-ups.
- Make sure she understands and can maintain her medication regimen.
- Tell her to talk with her practitioner before trying to become pregnant.

Quick quiz

1. If a patient who's allergic to peanut butter eats peanut butter cookies, which antigen-specific immunoglobulin will his body produce?

    A. IgA
    B. IgD
    C. IgE
    D. IgG

Answer: C. IgE is responsible for allergic reactions.

2. The most common anaphylaxis-causing agent is:

    A. shellfish.
    B. contrast dye.
    C. bee venom.
    D. penicillin.

Answer: D. Penicillin is the most common anaphylaxis-causing antigen because of its systemic effects on the body.

3. Asthma is most strongly associated with:

    A. a family history of asthma.
    B. a history of anaphylactic reactions.
    C. high blood pressure.
    D. a history of frequent upper respiratory infections.

Answer: A. About one-third of asthmatics share the condition with at least one member of their immediate family, and three-fourths of children with two asthmatic parents also have asthma.

4. In most cases, the treatment of choice for SLE is:

    A. antibiotics.
    B. antifungals.
    C. corticosteroids.
    D. cyclosporine.

Answer: C. Corticosteroids are the treatment of choice for systemic symptoms of SLE.

Scoring

★★★   If you answered all four questions correctly, we're impressed! Your top score has earned you immunity from having to reread this chapter!

★★   If you answered three questions correctly, well done! Your knowledge of the immune system is a far cry from deficient!

★   If you answered fewer than three questions correctly, don't break out in hives! Just read this chapter again to improve your anergic performance!

Skin disorders

In this chapter, you'll learn:
♦ anatomy and physiology of the skin and its appendages
♦ techniques for assessing the skin and its appendages
♦ causes, pathophysiology, diagnostic tests, and nursing interventions for common skin disorders.

A look at skin disorders

As the body's main protective system, the skin's various functions include sensory perception, regulation of temperature, prevention of water and electrolyte loss, and excretion. Nursing care for skin disorders requires careful examination and observation, prevention of infection, and hands-on treatment regimens, such as topical application of medication and wound debridement.

Anatomy and physiology

The skin (integument) covers the body's internal structures and protects them from the external world. The skin has two distinct layers:
• The *epidermis*, or outer layer, is made up of squamous epithelial tissue, which itself contains several layers—the stratum corneum, stratum lucidum, stratum spinosum, and stratum basale.
• The *dermis*, the deeper second layer, consists of connective tissue and an extracellular material called *matrix*, which contributes to the skin's strength and pliability. The dermis contains and supports the blood vessels, lymphatic vessels, nerves, and sweat and sebaceous glands and serves as the site of wound healing and infection control. Beneath the dermis lies the subcutaneous tissue. (See *Skin: The inside story*, page 808.)

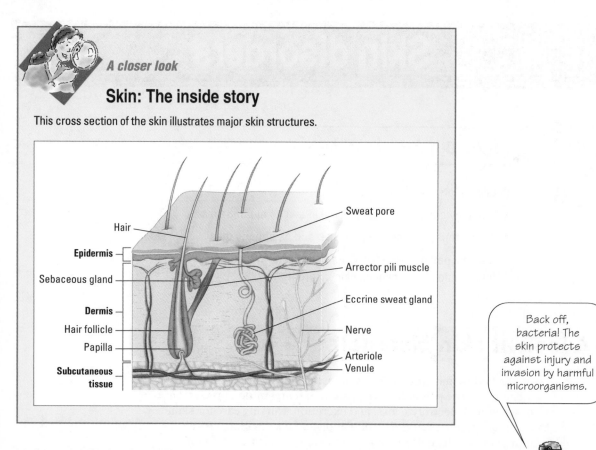

A closer look

Skin: The inside story

This cross section of the skin illustrates major skin structures.

Back off, bacteria! The skin protects against injury and invasion by harmful microorganisms.

Value-added appendages

Numerous epidermal appendages occur throughout the skin. They include the hair, nails, sebaceous glands, and sweat glands. The two types of sweat glands are the *apocrine* glands (found in the axillae and groin near hair follicles) and the *eccrine* glands (located over most of the body except the lips).

Skin functions

The skin performs many functions, including:
- protecting the tissues from trauma and bacteria
- preventing loss of water and electrolytes from the body
- allowing temperature, pain, touch, and pressure sensation
- regulating body temperature through sweat production and evaporation

- synthesizing vitamin D
- promoting wound repair by intensifying normal cell replacement mechanisms.

Assessment

Skin disorders may involve or stem from disorders that originate in other body systems. During your assessment, be sure to investigate even minor symptoms and systemic complaints.

History

Begin the assessment by taking a thorough history. With a skin disorder, expect the patient to report such problems as changes in the skin's appearance, pruritus (itching), pain, or drainage from lesions.

Current health status

Ask these questions to elicit information about the patient's chief complaint:
- How long have you had this problem? When did it begin? Have you had it before?
- What does the problem area look like, including its shape, size, color, location, character, and distribution?
- Is the area painful? Tender? Numb? Warm?
- Does anything seem to trigger the problem (such as stress, menstruation, or sunlight exposure)? Does anything make it worse? Does anything relieve it?
- Have you had recent contact with detergents, chemicals, or plants?
- Did you recently change soaps or skin care products?
- Have you tried using anything to make the condition feel better, such as compresses, lotions, or over-the-counter preparations?

Previous health status

Ask whether the patient has ever had a similar skin condition. (Some skin disorders, such as psoriasis, can recur.) Find out if he has ever had an allergic reaction to medication, food, or other substances (such as cosmetics). Past and present allergies—including those caused by cutaneous, ingested, or inhaled allergens—may predispose a patient to other skin disorders.

Also find out if the patient has a history of diabetes mellitus, vascular problems, or immunodeficiency.

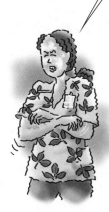

A patient with a skin disorder is likely to complain of problems such as pain, drainage from lesions, and — ooh! — itching.

Family history

Some skin disorders, such as atopic dermatitis, acne, and psoriasis, tend to run in families. Contagious skin problems, such as scabies, may be transmitted by family members. Ask the patient if anyone in his family has had a skin problem. If so, what was it and when did it occur?

Allergies may also run in families. Find out if any family members have allergies. If so, what are they and how have they been treated?

Social history

Obtain relevant information about the patient's lifestyle, including occupation, travel, diet, hobbies, smoking, alcohol and drug use, sun exposure, stress, and sexual contact.

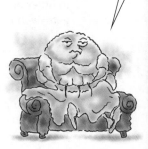

Scabies and other contagious skin problems can pass from one family member to another. I've settled in here quite comfortably, thank you.

Physical examination

Start by observing the overall appearance of the patient's skin to identify areas that need further assessment. Then inspect and palpate the skin one area at a time, focusing on color, texture, turgor, moisture, and temperature. Be sure to check for and note skin lesions.

Color

Look for localized areas of ecchymosis (bruising), cyanosis, pallor, and erythema (redness). Check for color uniformity and for areas with darker or lighter pigmentation than the rest of the patient's body. Remember that color changes may vary depending on skin pigmentation.

Texture and turgor

Inspect and palpate the skin's texture, noting its thickness and mobility. It should look smooth and be intact.

Turgor on trial

Assess turgor by gently grasping and pulling up a fold of skin, releasing it, and observing how quickly it returns to normal shape. Normal skin will resume its flat shape immediately.

Moisture

Observe the skin's moisture content. The skin should be relatively dry, with a minimal amount of perspiration. Skin-fold areas also should be fairly dry.

Temperature

Palpate for skin temperature by using the back (dorsal surface) of your fingers or hands, which are most sensitive to temperature perception. The skin should feel warm to cool, and areas should feel the same when compared bilaterally.

Lesions

Whenever you see a skin lesion, evaluate it to determine its origin. Start by classifying it as primary or secondary. A *primary* lesion is a change in the skin's color or texture that can stem from environmental factors, allergic reactions, or infectious diseases, or may even be present from birth. (See *Identifying primary skin lesions*.)

Collateral *damage*

Secondary lesions result from changes to primary lesions due to natural progression or from external factors, such as trauma or manipulation.
• Measure and record the lesion's size, shape or configuration, color, degree of elevation or depression, pedunculation (connection to the skin by a stem or stalk), and texture.
• Evaluate the lesion's odor, color, consistency, and amount of exudate.
• Assess the lesion's distribution pattern, including the extent and pattern of involvement. Note the location of the lesion or lesions,

> Use the backs of your fingers or hands when palpating skin temperature. They're more sensitive to temperature perception.

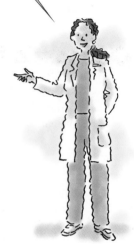

Identifying primary skin lesions

Are you having trouble identifying your patient's skin lesion? Here's a quick look at three common lesions. Remember to keep a centimeter ruler handy so you can measure lesion size accurately.

Macule
Flat circumscribed area of altered skin color; generally less than 1 cm. Examples: freckle, flat nevus

Papule
Raised, circumscribed, solid area; generally less than 1 cm. Examples: elevated nevus, wart

Vesicle
Circumscribed, elevated lesion; contains serous fluid; less than 1 cm. Example: early chickenpox

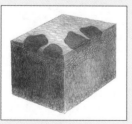
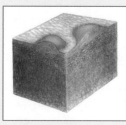
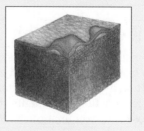

such as on a specific dermatome (cutaneous areas of peripheral nerve innervation), on flexor or extensor surfaces, in skin folds, on clothing or jewelry lines, or on palms or soles—or whether lesions appear randomly.
• Accurately describe the arrangement of lesions to help determine their cause. Is each lesion discrete? Are the lesions grouped? Do they merge together? Are they diffuse? Linear? Annular (ring shaped)? Arciform (curved or arced)? Do the lesions revolve around a fixed point (gyrate)?

Diagnostic tests

Several studies can help differentiate among integumentary disorders. They include the patch test, potassium hydroxide (KOH) preparation, skin biopsy, and the Tzanck test.

Patch test

The patch test identifies the cause of allergic contact sensitization. Indicated in patients with suspected allergies or allergies from an unknown cause, this test uses a sample of common allergens, or antigens, to determine if one or more will produce a positive reaction. If the doctor suspects a particular causative agent, he may test it for a positive reaction.

Nursing considerations
• If the patient has an acute inflammation, postpone the patch test until the inflammation subsides because a patch test may worsen it.
• Apply the patch to normal, hairless skin on the back or on the inner surface of the forearm.
• Instruct the patient to leave the patch in place for 48 hours—but to remove it immediately if pain, itching, or irritation develops.
• Check findings after removing the patch, and then recheck 48 hours later for a delayed reaction.

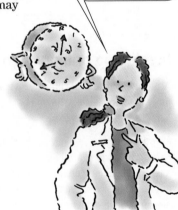

Wait another 48 hours after your initial inspection to check your patient's patch test results for a delayed reaction.

Potassium hydroxide preparation

KOH preparation helps identify fungal skin infections. It involves scraping scales from the skin, mixing them with a few drops of 10% to 25% KOH on a glass slide, and then lightly heating the slide. Skin cells lyse, leaving fungal elements (hyphae and spores) visible on microscopic examination.

Nursing considerations

• Gently scrape the border of a rash or skin lesion with a sterile scalpel blade to obtain a specimen. After scraping, inspect the area for bleeding and apply light pressure, if necessary.
• Tell the patient that the KOH preparation may identify a fungal infection—but because the test may be inconclusive, he should comply with treatment until fungal culture results are known.

Skin biopsy

During a skin biopsy, a small piece of tissue from a suspected malignancy or other skin lesion is excised. One of three techniques—excision, shave, or punch—may be used to secure the specimen.
• An *excision* biopsy removes a small lesion in its entirety. This technique is indicated for rapidly expanding lesions; sclerotic, bullous, or atrophic lesions; and examination of the border of a lesion and surrounding normal skin.
• A *shave* biopsy cuts the lesion above the skin line, leaving the lower dermal layers intact.
• A *punch* biopsy removes an oval core from the center of a lesion.

Nursing considerations

• Explain to the patient that he'll first receive a local anesthetic.
• After the procedure, apply pressure to the biopsy site to stop bleeding, if necessary, and apply a dressing.
• After the biopsy specimen is obtained, place it in a container with 10% formaldehyde solution.
• If the patient has sutures, instruct him to keep the area clean and as dry as possible. Tell him when the sutures will be removed.
• If the patient has adhesive strips, instruct him to leave them in place for 14 to 21 days.

Tzanck test

In the Tzanck test, vesicular fluid or exudate from an ulcer is smeared on a glass slide and stained with Papanicolaou's, Wright's, Giemsa, or methylene blue stain. Herpesvirus is confirmed if microscopic examination of the slide reveals multinucleated giant cells, intranuclear inclusions, and ballooning degeneration.

Nursing considerations

• To obtain a specimen for staining, unroof an intact vesicle and, using a sterile scalpel blade, scrape the base of the lesion to obtain fluid and skin cells. Apply the specimen to a glass slide, allow it to air dry, and then stain.

Memory jogger

Did you know that the practitioner uses ESP to perform a skin biopsy? No, that doesn't mean he uses extrasensory perception. ESP simply refers to the three different techniques—Excision, Shave, or Punch— used to secure a skin biopsy specimen.

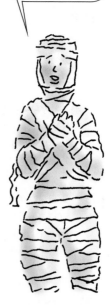

OK, so I'm exaggerating a little. But after a skin biopsy, you may need to apply a pressure dressing to the site.

• Always wear gloves while obtaining the specimen because herpesvirus is transmissible.

Treatments

Usually, treatment for skin disorders involves hands-on care. Most medications are applied topically. Surgery is usually performed with only a local anesthetic, and monitoring depends less on laboratory tests than on simple observation.

Drug therapy

Categories of drugs used to treat skin disorders include:
• anti-infectives, such as acyclovir (Zovirax), bacitracin, clotrimazole (Lotrimin AF), lindane, and mupirocin
• astringents, such as aluminum acetate and calcium acetate
• topical corticosteroids, such as hydrocortisone (Cortaid) and triamcinolone (Kenalog)
• demulcents, emollients, and protectants, such as calamine, oatmeal, and para-aminobenzoic acid
• keratolytics, such as podophyllum and salicylic acid
• miscellaneous agents, such as acitretin (Soriatane), isotretinoin (Sotret), topical minoxidil (Rogaine), selenium sulfide, and tretinoin (Retin-A).

Surgery

Surgical techniques used to treat skin disorders include cryosurgery, laser surgery, Mohs' micrographic surgery, and skin grafting.

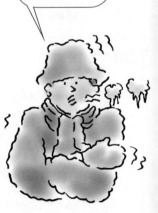

Brrrr! With cryosurgery, extreme cold is applied to the skin to cause tissue destruction.

Cryosurgery

Cryosurgery is a common procedure in which extreme cold is applied to the skin to induce tissue destruction. Cryosurgery causes epidermal-dermal separation above the basement membranes, helping to prevent scarring after reepithelialization.

Simple to sophisticated

The procedure can be performed quite simply, using nothing more than a cotton-tipped applicator dipped in liquid nitrogen and applied to the skin, or it may involve a complex cryosurgical unit.

Patient preparation

Before the procedure, take these steps:
• Ask the patient if he has any allergies or hypersensitivities, especially to iodine or cold.
• Tell him he'll initially feel cold, followed by a burning sensation, during the procedure.

Monitoring and aftercare

After the procedure, take these steps:
• After cryosurgery, clean the area gently with a cotton-tipped applicator soaked in hydrogen peroxide.
• If necessary, apply an ice bag to relieve swelling and give the patient an analgesic, as ordered, to relieve pain.

Home care instructions

Before discharge, give the patient these instructions:
• Tell the patient that he should expect pain, redness, and swelling, and that a blister will form within 24 hours of treatment. The blister may be large, and it may bleed. Usually, it flattens within a few days and sloughs off in 2 to 3 weeks. Serous exudation may follow during the first week, and a crust or a dry scab may develop.

Don't touch!

• To promote healing and prevent infection, warn the patient not to touch the blister. Tell him that if the blister becomes uncomfortable or interferes with daily activities, he should call the practitioner, who can decompress it with a sterile blade or pin.
• Tell the patient to clean the area gently with soap and water, alcohol, or a cotton-tipped applicator soaked in an anti-infective agent, as ordered.
• To prevent hyperpigmentation, instruct him to cover the wound with a loose dressing when he's outdoors. After the wound heals, he should apply a sunblock over the area.

Laser surgery

Laser surgery uses the intense, highly focused light of a laser beam to treat dermatologic lesions. Performed on an outpatient basis, laser surgery spares normal tissue, promotes faster healing, and helps prevent postsurgical infection.

Patient preparation

Before the procedure, take these steps:
• If the surgical suite has windows, keep shades or blinds closed. Cover reflective surfaces and remove flammable materials.

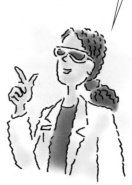

During laser surgery, everyone in the room—patient included—must wear goggles to protect their eyes.

• Make sure everyone in the room, including the patient, is wearing safety goggles, because reflection of the laser beam may damage the eyes.

Monitoring and aftercare

After the procedure, apply direct pressure over any bleeding wound for 20 minutes. Initial wound care varies with the procedure.

Home care instructions

Before discharge, give the patient these instructions:
• Tell the patient to dress the wound daily. Permit him to take showers, but advise him not to immerse the wound site in water.
• If bleeding occurs, instruct the patient to apply direct pressure on the site with clean gauze or a washcloth for 20 minutes. If pressure doesn't control the bleeding, he should call the doctor immediately.
• To avoid pigmentation changes, caution the patient to protect the wound from sun exposure.

Mohs' micrographic surgery

Mohs' micrographic surgery involves serial excision and histologic analysis of cancerous or suspected cancerous tissues. By allowing step-by-step tumor excision, Mohs' surgery minimizes the size of the scar (important if the treatment is done on the face) and helps prevent recurrence by removing all malignant tissue. This surgery is especially effective in basal cell carcinomas.

Support for scarring

Mohs' surgery has two common complications: bleeding and facial scarring. Bleeding is easily controlled with direct pressure. The potentially devastating psychological effects of a large facial scar or defect are harder to treat and require considerable emotional support.

Patient preparation

Before the procedure, take these steps:
• Make sure the patient understands that the procedure usually takes many hours, most of which will be spent waiting for histologic results.
• Explain that the doctor will use electrocauterization to control bleeding and that a grounding plate will be affixed to the patient's leg or arm to complete the circuit between the cautery pencil and generator. Warn him to expect a burning odor.

Monitoring and aftercare

After the procedure, take these steps:
• Assess the patient's level of pain, and provide an analgesic, as ordered.

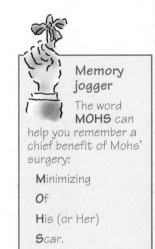

Tell the patient he can take showers, but he shouldn't immerse the wound site in water.

Memory jogger

The word **MOHS** can help you remember a chief benefit of Mohs' surgery:

Minimizing

Of

His (or Her)

Scar.

- Periodically check for excessive bleeding. If it occurs, remove the dressing and apply pressure over the site for 20 minutes.

Home care instructions

Before discharge, give the patient these instructions:
- Tell the patient to leave the dressing in place for 24 hours and to change the dressing daily afterward.
- If he experiences frank bleeding, advise him to reinforce the bandage and apply direct pressure to the wound for 20 minutes, using clean gauze or a clean washcloth. If this measure doesn't control bleeding, he should call the practitioner.
- Instruct the patient to report signs or symptoms of infection.
- Advise him to refrain from alcohol, aspirin, and excessive exercise for 48 hours to prevent bleeding and promote healing.
- Recommend acetaminophen (Tylenol) for discomfort.

Skin grafting

Skin grafting covers defects caused by burns, trauma, and surgery. This procedure is indicated:
- to repair surgical defects when primary closure isn't possible or desirable
- to cover areas denuded of skin.
  Grafting may be done using a general or local anesthetic. It can be performed on an outpatient basis for small facial or neck defects.

Getting graphic about grafts

Types of skin grafts include:
- split-thickness grafts, which consist of the epidermis and a small portion of dermis
- full-thickness grafts, which include all of the dermis as well as the epidermis
- composite grafts, which also include underlying tissues, such as muscle, cartilage, or bone.

Patient preparation

Before the procedure, take these steps:
- Because successful skin grafting begins with a good graft, preserve potential donor sites by providing meticulous skin care.
- Assess the recipient site. The graft's survival depends on close contact with the underlying tissue. Ideally, the recipient site should consist of healthy granulation tissue free from eschar (a dry crust or thick scab appearing after a burn), debris, or the products of infection.

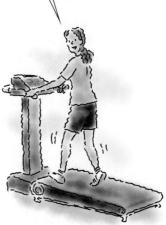

After the procedure, advise the patient to refrain from excessive exercise for 48 hours to prevent bleeding and promote healing. This treadmill can wait for a couple of days!

Monitoring and aftercare

After the procedure, your primary role is to ensure graft survival.
• Position the patient so that his graft site is protected. If possible, keep the graft area elevated and immobilized.
• Modify your nursing care to protect the graft. For example, never use a blood pressure cuff over a graft site.

Keep it clean

• Use sterile technique when changing the dressing, and work gently to avoid dislodging the graft.
• Keep the donor site clean, dry, and protected.

Home care instructions

Before discharge, give the patient these instructions:
• Advise the patient not to disturb the dressings on the graft or donor sites for any reason. If they need to be changed, instruct him to call the practitioner.
• If grafting was done as an outpatient procedure, stress that the graft site must be immobilized to promote proper healing.
• After the graft has healed, instruct the patient to apply an emollient cream to the site several times daily to keep the skin pliable and aid scar maturation.
• Because sun exposure can affect graft pigmentation, advise the patient to limit his time in the sun and to use a sunblock on all grafted areas.
• Explain that when scar maturation is complete, the practitioner may use other plastic surgery techniques to improve graft appearance.

Debridement

Debridement may involve mechanical, chemical, or surgical techniques to remove necrotic tissue from a wound. Although debridement can be extremely painful, it's necessary to prevent infection and promote healing of burns and skin ulcers.

Mechanical debridement

Mechanical debridement consists of wet-to-dry dressings, irrigation, hydrotherapy, and bedside debridement.
• Wet-to-dry dressings are appropriate for partially healed wounds with only slight amounts of necrotic tissue and minimal drainage.
• Irrigation of a wound with an antiseptic solution cleans tissues and removes cell debris and excess drainage.
• Hydrotherapy (commonly called "tubbing" or "tanking") involves immersing the patient in a tank of warm water, which

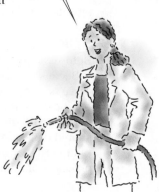

Irrigation provides mechanical debridement. The antiseptic solution cleans tissues and removes cell debris.

is agitated intermittently. Hydrotherapy is often performed on burn patients.
• Bedside debridement of a burn wound involves careful prying and cutting of loosened eschar with forceps and scissors to separate it from viable tissue beneath. One of the most painful types of debridement, it may be the only practical way to remove necrotic tissue from a severely burned patient.

Chemical debridement

In chemical debridement, topical debriders are used to absorb exudate and particulate debris. These agents also absorb bacteria, thus reducing the risk of infection.

Surgical debridement

Surgical debridement is done under general or regional anesthesia. It provides the fastest and most complete debridement, but it's usually reserved for burn patients or those with extremely deep or large ulcers. It's commonly performed with skin grafting.

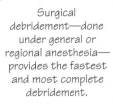

Surgical debridement—done under general or regional anesthesia—provides the fastest and most complete debridement.

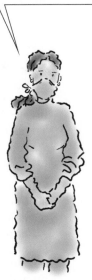

Patient preparation
Before the procedure, take these steps:
• Explain the type of debridement the patient will undergo. Reassure him that he'll receive an analgesic if needed.
• If ordered, give analgesics 20 minutes before the procedure.

Monitoring and aftercare
After the procedure, take these steps:
• Assess the patient's pain, and provide analgesics, as ordered.
• During dressing changes, note the amount of granulation tissue, necrotic debris, and drainage. Watch for signs of wound infection.
• If the patient's arm or leg was debrided, keep it elevated to promote venous return—especially if the patient has a stasis ulcer.

Home care instructions
Before discharge, take these steps:
• Teach the patient how to perform dressing changes if appropriate.
• Instruct him to watch for and report signs or symptoms of infection or poor healing.

Nursing diagnoses

When caring for patients with skin disorders, you'll find that several nursing diagnoses are applicable to many situations. These nursing diagnoses appear here, along with appropriate nursing interventions and rationales. See *NANDA-I taxonomy II by domain*, page 936, for the complete list of NANDA diagnoses.

Impaired skin integrity

Related to illness, *Impaired skin integrity* can be associated with infection, immobility, excessive moisture, trauma, advanced age, and impaired blood flow.

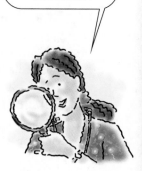

Inspect the patient's skin daily, particularly noting changes in status. Early detection prevents or minimizes skin breakdown.

Expected outcomes

• Patient verbalizes and demonstrates an understanding of all procedures and skin care regimens to prevent further tissue breakdown.
• Patient verbalizes feelings about his skin condition.

Nursing interventions and rationales

• Inspect the patient's skin daily and document findings, particularly noting any change in status. Early detection prevents or minimizes skin breakdown.
• Perform the prescribed treatment regimen for the patient's skin condition; monitor progress. Report favorable and adverse responses to treatment so the current regimen can be maintained or modified as needed.

Hygiene help

• Assist the patient with general hygiene and comfort measures as needed to promote comfort and a general sense of well-being.
• Promote mobility, and establish a pressure ulcer prevention routine if indicated.
• Apply a bed cradle to protect lesions from bed covers.
• Encourage the patient to express his feelings about his skin condition. This helps to allay anxiety and develop coping skills.
• Discuss precipitating factors if known. If the patient has a skin allergy to food, explain dietary restrictions to help reduce the occurrence and severity of skin reactions.
• Teach the patient about his skin care regimen to ensure compliance.

Risk for infection

Related to impaired skin integrity, *Risk for infection* may also apply to any condition that impairs the skin's ability to guard against invasion by microorganisms.

Expected outcomes

- Patient remains free from additional infections.
- Patient maintains normal temperature and laboratory values.

Nursing interventions and rationales

- Minimize the patient's risk of infection through proper hand washing and by using standard precautions when providing direct care.

Fever fears

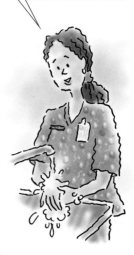

Instruct the patient to wash his hands before and after meals and after using the bathroom, bed pan, or urinal.

- Take the patient's temperature at least every 4 hours. Report elevations immediately. Sustained postoperative fever may signal the onset of pulmonary complications, wound infection or dehiscence (premature splitting open of the wound layers), or urinary tract infection.
- Monitor white blood cell (WBC) count as ordered. Report elevations or depressions. An elevated WBC count indicates infection.
- Inspect skin lesions for erythema, warmth, or purulent drainage to detect secondary infection.
- Culture urine, respiratory secretions, wound drainage, or blood according to your facility's policy and the practitioner's orders. This procedure identifies pathogens and guides antibiotic therapy.
- Instruct the patient to wash his hands before and after meals and after using the bathroom, bedpan, or urinal.
- Ensure adequate nutritional intake. Offer high-protein supplements, unless contraindicated, to aid healing, stabilize weight, and improve muscle tone and mass.
- Teach the patient about good hand-washing technique, factors that increase his infection risk, and signs and symptoms of infection. Doing this helps him participate in care and modify his lifestyle to maintain optimal health.

Common skin disorders

This section covers common skin disorders and includes information on their causes, assessment findings, diagnostic tests, treatment, nursing interventions, patient teaching, and evaluation criteria.

Cellulitis

A diffuse inflammation of the dermis and subcutaneous tissue, cellulitis commonly appears around a skin break—usually a fresh wound or small puncture site. With timely treatment, prognosis is usually good.

What causes it

Cellulitis usually results from an infection by group A beta-hemolytic streptococci or *Staphylococcus aureus*. It may also stem from infection by other organisms.

Pathophysiology

A break in skin integrity almost always precedes infection. As the offending organism invades the compromised area, it overwhelms the defensive cells (such as neutrophils, eosinophils, basophils, and mast cells) that usually contain and localize the inflammation. As cellulitis progresses, the organism invades tissue around the initial wound site.

What to look for

Signs and symptoms of cellulitis include:
• a tender, warm, erythematous, swollen area, which is usually well demarcated
• a warm, red, tender streak following the course of a lymphatic vessel
• fever and chills.

What tests tell you

• Although diagnosis usually can be made from the clinical presentation, the doctor may order a Gram stain and culture of skin tissue.
• If the patient is acutely ill, blood cultures may be taken.

How it's treated

Preventing widespread skin destruction requires I.V. or oral antibiotic therapy depending on the severity of the infection.

If gangrene occurs, the patient must undergo surgical debridement and incision and drainage of surrounding tissue.

What to do

• Monitor the patient's vital signs (especially temperature) every 4 hours.
• Assess the patient every 4 hours for an increase in the size of the affected area or worsening of pain.
• Administer an antibiotic, an analgesic, and warm compresses, as ordered.
• Evaluate the patient. He should show signs of resolution of erythema, pain, and warmth and improved skin integrity. (See *Cellulitis teaching tips.*)

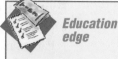

Education edge

Cellulitis teaching tips

• Emphasize the importance of complying with treatment to prevent relapse.
• Teach the patient how to apply warm compresses.
• Advise him to elevate the affected limb to reduce swelling.
• Tell him to limit activity until his condition improves.

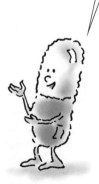

To treat cellulitis, the practitioner will order antibiotics.

Cutaneous ulcers

Cutaneous ulcers are localized areas of cellular necrosis that arise from areas of poor tissue oxygenation. The ulcers may be superficial or deep (originating in underlying tissue). Ulcers that arise from deep tissues typically go undetected until they penetrate the skin.

What causes them

The three most common cutaneous ulcers include *pressure ulcers*, caused by pressure; *arterial ulcers*, which result from chronic arterial insufficiency that stems from peripheral arterial disease; and *venous ulcers*, the result of venous insufficiency. Less common causes of cutaneous ulcers include infection, lymphedema, vasculitis, malignancy, adverse medication reactions, and ulcerating skin diseases such as pyoderma gangrenosum.

A roll call of risk factors

Conditions that increase the risk of developing pressure ulcers include:
• altered mobility
• inadequate nutrition (leading to weight loss with reduction of subcutaneous tissue and muscle bulk)
• breakdown in skin or subcutaneous tissue (from edema or incontinence).

Other predisposing factors for pressure ulcers are infection, trauma, pathologic conditions, and obesity.

Conditions that increase the risk of developing arterial ulcers include:
• damage to arteries from atherosclerosis, hypertension, diabetes, smoking, trauma, or irradiation
• inflammatory vasculitis disorders, such as thromboangiitis obliterans, polyarteritis nodosa, and hypersensitivity arteritis
• vasospastic disorders such as Raynaud's phenomenon
• congenital anomalies of the arterial system such as coarctation of the aorta.

Several conditions increase the risk of developing venous ulcers:
• In inherited or acquired venous valve disorders, valves are absent or don't work properly. Incompetent venous valves allow blood to leak backwards through the valve cusps instead of moving towards the heart.
• In deep vein thrombosis, clots obstruct the veins and damage the venous valves. Such obstructions can lead to postphlebitic syndrome, characterized by chronic edema and ulcers that don't heal well.

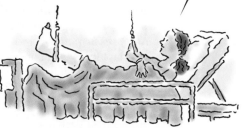

Altered mobility—such as being in traction—increases the risk of developing pressure ulcers.

824

- Conditions such as edema from heart failure, abdominal surgery, obesity, and lymphedema can cause vein compression and impair venous outflow.

Pathophysiology

Pressure ulcers are caused by pressure that interrupts normal circulatory function. Intensity and duration of the pressure determine ulcer severity. Pressure exerted over an area for a moderate length of time (1 to 2 hours) produces tissue ischemia and increased capillary pressure, leading to edema, inflammation, cellular necrosis, and ulceration.

The fallout from faulty flow

In arterial ulcers, damage to the artery walls can lead to blockages, aneurysms, and microvascular changes. Impaired blood flow decreases the oxygen delivered to the tissue, which results in necrosis and ulcers.

In venous ulcers, blood flow towards the heart is impaired, causing high pressures within the veins. This venous hypertension causes local tissue inflammation, resulting in skin changes, tissue anoxia, necrosis, and ulcers.

What to look for

Pressure ulcers commonly develop over bony prominences. Early features of superficial lesions include shiny, erythematous changes over the compressed area, caused by localized vasodilation when pressure is relieved, and superficial erythema progressing to small blisters or erosions. As the lesion progresses, it may develop ulceration and necrosis.

Gauging the stage

On admission, every patient with pressure ulcers should receive a complete skin assessment, including pressure ulcer staging and an assessment for the risk of developing new pressure ulcers. Such assessments should be ongoing, at regular intervals and any time the patient's condition changes, according to the facility's policy. Early detection of skin changes associated with pressure ulcer development plays a key role in preventing pressure ulcers. (See *Staging pressure ulcers.*)

Arterial ulcers often occur in areas of increased focal pressure, such as the tips of the toes, metatarsal heads, and lateral malleolus. These ulcers are commonly dry and can cause signs and symptoms of ischemia in

Experts recommend staging pressure ulcers at their onset and at least every week thereafter.

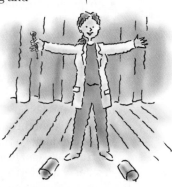

Staging pressure ulcers

The classification system developed by the National Pressure Ulcer Advisory Panel (NPUAP) is the most widely used system for staging pressure ulcers. NPUAP's system includes six categories, including two recently redefined stages for deep tissue injury and unstageable ulcers.

Suspected deep tissue injury

Deep tissue injury is characterized by a purple or maroon localized area of intact skin or a blood-filled blister caused by damage of underlying soft tissue from pressure or shear. The injury may be preceded by tissue that's painful, firm, mushy, boggy, or warm or cool compared to adjacent tissue. It may be difficult to detect in individuals with dark skin tones.

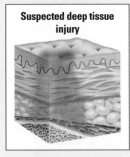

Suspected deep tissue injury

Stage I

The skin is intact with non-blanchable redness over a localized area (typically over a bony prominence). Darkly pigmented skin may not visiblly blanch, but its color may differ from the surrounding area. Compare the suspected area to an adjacent area or to the same region on the other side of the body. Stage I ulcers exhibit differences in skin temperature, tissue consistency, and sensation.

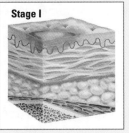

Stage I

Stage II

Partial-thickness loss of the dermis presents as a shallow, open ulcer with a red-pink wound bed without slough. It may also present as an intact or open serum-filled blister.

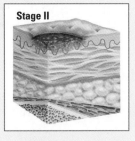

Stage II

Stage III

Full-thickness loss is present and subcutaneous fat may be visible, but bone, tendon, and muscle aren't exposed. Slough may be present but doesn't obscure the depth of tissue loss. Undermining and tunneling may be present.

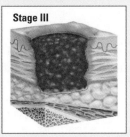

Stage III

Stage IV

Full-thickness loss occurs with exposed bone, tendon, and muscle. Slough or eschar may be present on some parts of the wound bed. Undermining and tunneling are common.

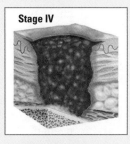

Stage IV

Unstageable ulcer

An unstageable ulcer is characterized by full-thickness tissue loss in which the ulcer base in the wound bed is covered with slough (yellow, tan, gray, green, or brown), eschar (tan, brown, or black), or both. Until enough eschar or slough is removed to expose the wound base, the true depth, and therefore stage, can't be determined.

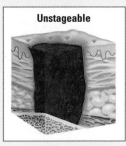

Unstageable

the affected limb, such as limb pain, pallor, decreased pulses, coolness, nail changes, and hair loss.

Venous ulcers most commonly occur just above the medial ankle and are typically superficial and moist. The skin may appear brawny and brown from fibrotic changes, and the patient may have chronic edema and varicosities.

What tests tell you

Wound culture and sensitivity testing of ulcer exudate identify infecting organisms and help determine whether an antibiotic is needed.

How they're treated

Treatment is similar for many types of cutaneous ulcers. Treatment begins by addressing any underlying disease process and maximizing blood flow to improve tissue oxygenation. Open lesions are cleaned with normal saline solution. Dressings, if needed, should be porous and taped lightly to healthy skin. Composite dressings (such as Coverderm and Tegaderm) are appropriate for wounds with minimal to heavy drainage, necrotic tissue, or healthy granulation tissue. Debridement of necrotic tissue may be necessary to promote healing.

What to do

• Clean the skin with warm water and a mild cleaning agent; then apply moisturizer if indicated. Raise the head of the bed to 30 degrees to prevent shearing pressure. Protect the wound from further trauma.
• Turn and reposition the patient every 1 to 2 hours unless contraindicated. For at-risk patients, use a pressure-relieving mattress.
• Ensure adequate dietary intake of protein and calories.
• Use pressure-reduction devices and control excess moisture.
• Evaluate the wound-healing process. With successful treatment, the ulcer should reepithelialize. The patient and caregivers should take adequate measures to prevent recurrence of cutaneous ulcers. (See *Cutaneous ulcer teaching tips*.)

Herpes zoster

Also called *shingles*, herpes zoster is an acute unilateral and segmental inflammation of certain nerve roots. Usually appearing in adults over age 40, herpes zoster causes localized vesicular skin lesions confined to a dermatome (an area of the skin innervated by sensory fibers from a single spinal nerve).

Education edge

Cutaneous ulcer teaching tips

• Advise the patient to eat a diet with adequate calories, protein, and vitamins and to quit smoking.
• Teach a patient with venous ulcers to avoid prolonged standing, to elevate the legs above heart level to promote venous return, and to wear antiembolism stockings during the day.
• Emphasize the importance of changing positions regularly. Teach the patient and his family how to change the patient's position correctly.
• Teach the patient how to inspect and care for his skin. Advise him to treat dry skin with moisturizers after bathing.
• Caution the patient to avoid rubbing his skin, which can damage capillaries.
• If the patient is confined to a chair or uses a wheelchair, advise him to shift his weight every 30 minutes to promote blood flow to compressed tissues.

No gain from this pain

Severe neuralgic pain occurs in peripheral areas fed by the nerves arising in the inflamed ganglia.

What causes it

Herpes zoster results from the varicella-zoster virus, a herpesvirus that also causes chickenpox. Roughly 20% of people who have had chickenpox eventually get herpes zoster.

It isn't known what causes the virus to reactivate in healthy people. Perhaps a temporary weakness in immunity allows it to multiply and travel along nerve fibers toward the skin.

Pathophysiology

Herpes zoster erupts when the varicella-zoster virus reactivates after dormancy in the cerebral ganglia (extramedullary ganglia of the cranial nerves) or the ganglia of posterior nerve roots. The virus may multiply as it reactivates, and antibodies remaining from the initial infection may try to neutralize it.

Neutralizing neurons

If antibodies don't effectively neutralize the virus, it continues to multiply in the ganglia, destroys neurons, and spreads down the sensory nerves to the skin.

What to look for

Onset of herpes zoster is characterized by fever and malaise. Within 2 to 4 days, severe deep pain, pruritus, and paresthesia (burning, itching, prickling, or tingling sensations) or hyperesthesia (increased sensitivity to touch) develop—usually on the trunk and occasionally on the arms and legs. Pain may be continuous or intermittent.

Unilateral attack

Small, red, nodular skin lesions then usually erupt over the painful areas and spread unilaterally around the thorax or vertically over the arms or legs. They quickly become vesicles, or blisters, filled with clear fluid or pus. About 10 days after they appear, the vesicles dry and form scabs. (See *Zooming in on herpes zoster.*)

What tests tell you

• The dermatomic distribution of lesions is usually sufficient to confirm the diagnosis.
• A Tzanck test of vesicular fluid and infected tissue shows eosinophilic intranuclear inclusions and varicella virus.

> ## Zooming in on herpes zoster
>
> The classic vesicles of herpes zoster, shown here, have erupted along a peripheral nerve in the torso.
>
>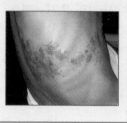

• In unusual cases, a Tzanck smear, biopsy, and viral culture may be needed to confirm the diagnosis.

How it's treated

Relief of itching and neuralgic pain may require calamine lotion or another topical antipruritic and pain medication. If bacteria have infected ruptured vesicles, treatment includes a systemic antibiotic.

Potent potions

Trigeminal zoster with corneal involvement calls for instillation of an antiviral agent. To help the patient cope with the intractable pain of postherpetic neuralgia, the doctor may order analgesics, a systemic corticosteroid to reduce inflammation, or a tranquilizer, sedative, or tricyclic antidepressant with a phenothiazine.

Acyclovir or another antiviral is used to stop progression of the skin rash and prevent visceral complications.

An ounce of prevention

A vaccine called Zostavax can help prevent herpes zoster in those age 60 and up. However, Zostavax won't cure herpes zoster once it occurs, and patients who have already had herpes zoster shouldn't receive the vaccine.

What to do

• Promote patient comfort.
• Administer medications as ordered.
• If lesions are severe and widespread, apply a wet dressing. If vesicles rupture, apply a cold compress as ordered.
• Watch an immunosuppressed patient closely for signs and symptoms of dissemination (such as generalized lesions) and central nervous system infection (such as headache, weakness, fever, and stiff neck).
• Evaluate the patient. With successful treatment, he should show resolution of all skin lesions, although extensive lesions may produce scars. Determine whether he has postherpetic neuralgia. (See *Herpes zoster teaching tips.*)

Education edge

Herpes zoster teaching tips

• Focus on helping the patient with herpes zoster minimize pain and prevent infection spread.
• Instruct him to avoid touching the lesions.
• To decrease the pain of oral lesions, advise him to use a soft toothbrush, eat a soft diet, and use saline solution mouthwash.
• Provide diversionary activities to take his mind off the pain and pruritus.
• Caution the patient to avoid contact with people who haven't had chickenpox until his eruption has resolved.

Psoriasis

A chronic disorder, psoriasis is a noncontagious inflammatory skin disease marked by reddish papules (solid elevations) and plaques covered with silvery scales. The condition takes a recurrent course, with remissions and exacerbations. Psoriatic lesions vary widely in severity and distribution. The disorder occurs in about 1% of the North American population, with usual onset between ages 25 and 30.

What causes it

The tendency to develop psoriasis may be genetically determined. Researchers have found a significantly higher-than-normal incidence of human leukocyte antigen (HLA) in patients with psoriasis, suggesting a possible autoimmune deficiency.

Pathophysiology

Psoriatic skin cells have a shortened maturation time as they migrate from the basal membrane to the surface or stratum corneum.

Plaque attack

As a result, the stratum corneum develops thick, scaly plaques (the chief sign of psoriasis).

What to look for

Small, erythematous papules usually are the initial sign of psoriasis. These lesions enlarge or merge to form red, elevated plaques with silver scales. Most commonly, they're symmetrical and seen on the scalp, face, chest, elbows, knees, back, buttocks, and genitalia.

Other features of psoriasis include pruritus, nail pitting, and joint stiffness (psoriatic arthritis).

What tests tell you

- Skin biopsy helps rule out other disorders.
- The serum uric acid level may be elevated.
- In early-onset familial psoriasis, tests typically show the presence of the HLA known as Cw6, B13, and Bw57.

How it's treated

Interventions for psoriasis vary because no permanent cure exists. All treatments are merely palliative.

Lukewarm baths and application of occlusive ointment bases (petroleum jelly or preparations containing urea) or salicylic acid preparations may soften and remove psoriatic scales. Steroid creams are the mainstay of therapy.

> Lukewarm baths and occlusive ointment bases or salicylic acid preparations may soften and remove psoriatic scales.

A sunny suggestion

To slow rapid cell proliferation, the practitioner may recommend exposure to ultraviolet light (wavelength B [UVB] or natural sunlight) to the point of minimal redness.

Advice on anthralin

Anthralin, combined with a paste mixture, may be used for well-defined plaques. However, this drug must not be applied to unaffected areas because it may cause inflammation. Anthralin irritates and stains the skin. It also stains clothing and household items such as the bathtub.

Tar? Sounds bizarre

For a patient with severe chronic psoriasis, the Goeckerman treatment—which combines tar application and UVB treatments—may help achieve remission and clear the skin.

The Ingram technique, a variation of the Goeckerman treatment, uses anthralin instead of tar. Psoralen plus ultraviolet A (PUVA) therapy combines methoxsalen (a psoralen derivative) with exposure to ultraviolet A light. Methotrexate may help severe, refractory psoriasis.

Oatmeal, emollients, and aspirin

Low-dosage antihistamines, oatmeal baths, emollients (perhaps with phenol and menthol), and open wet dressings may relieve pruritus.

Aspirin and local heat alleviate the pain of psoriatic arthritis; severe cases may require NSAIDs such as indomethacin.

For scalp psoriasis, therapy usually consists of a tar shampoo, followed by application of a steroid lotion while the hair is still wet.

Severe disease may require systemic treatment with drugs such as methotrexate (Trexall), cyclosporine (Gengraf), etanercept (Enbrel), or infliximab (Remicade).

Not much for nails

No effective treatment exists for psoriasis of the nails. However, the nails usually improve as skin lesions improve.

What to do

• Monitor for adverse reactions to therapy. The patient may develop allergic reactions to anthralin, atrophy and acne from steroids, and burning, itching, nausea, and skin cancer from PUVA. Methotrexate may cause liver or bone marrow toxicity.
• Evaluate the patient. With successful treatment, skin eruptions should be under control; he should be able to demonstrate proper skin care. Note whether he keeps follow-up appointments required to monitor for adverse reactions to therapy. (See *Psoriasis teaching tips*.)

Education edge

Psoriasis teaching tips

• Teach the patient how to apply prescribed creams and lotions.
• Tell the patient using the Goeckerman treatment to apply tar with a downward motion to avoid rubbing it into the follicles.
• Instruct him to apply anthralin to psoriatic plaques only. Advise him to wear gloves because anthralin stains the skin. After application, he may dust himself with powder to prevent anthralin from rubbing off on his clothes. Warn him never to put an occlusive dressing over anthralin. Suggest using mineral oil, then soap and water, to remove anthralin. Caution him to avoid scrubbing his skin vigorously.
• Tell him that flare-ups are commonly related to specific environmental and systemic factors.
• Inform the patient undergoing psoralen plus ultraviolet A therapy that treatment may cause burning, itching, nausea, and skin cancer.

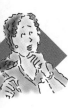

Quick quiz

1. Functions of the skin include:
   A. protection, regulation of temperature, prevention of water and electrolyte loss, and excretion.
   B. sensory perception, immunity, and blood pressure regulation.
   C. regulation of temperature, blood pressure, and respirations; protection; and immunity.
   D. vitamin C synthesis, sensory perception, and immunity.

Answer: A. The skin's many functions include protection, sensory perception, temperature regulation, prevention of water and electrolyte loss, vitamin synthesis, and excretion.

2. Which nursing diagnosis is most likely to be applicable to a patient with a skin disorder?
   A. *Risk for imbalanced nutrition: More than body requirements*
   B. *Ineffective tissue perfusion*
   C. *Risk for infection*
   D. *Impaired physical mobility*

Answer: C. *Risk for infection* applies to any condition that impairs the skin's ability to protect the body from microorganisms.

3. Wet-to-dry dressings, irrigation, hydrotherapy, and bedside debridement are components of which type of debridement?
   A. Surgical
   B. Chemical
   C. Prophylactic
   D. Mechanical

Answer: D. Mechanical debridement uses wet-to-dry dressings, irrigation, hydrotherapy, and bedside debridement.

4. Your patient complains of an itchy rash. On inspection, you note red, scaly, silvery patches on her back. Which disorder can cause these findings?
   A. Scabies
   B. Cellulitis
   C. Psoriasis
   D. Herpes zoster

Answer: C. Psoriasis is characterized by red, elevated plaques with silvery scales.

Scoring

☆☆☆ If you answered all four questions correctly, excellent! Your integumentary intelligence quotient has hit the uppermost stratum!

☆☆ If you answered three questions correctly, kudos! You've added several layers to your comprehension of cutaneous matters!

☆ If you answered fewer than three questions correctly, don't over-work your sweat glands! Just settle into a nice therapeutic bath and review this chapter until it really gets under your skin!

Cancer care

Just the facts

In this chapter, you'll learn:

♦ epidemiology and pathophysiology of cancer

♦ techniques for assessing, diagnosing, and treating specific cancers

♦ causes, diagnostic tests, and nursing interventions for patients with cancer.

A look at cancer care

Cancer is an umbrella term for a group of disorders in which abnormal cells grow, multiply uncontrollably, and have the ability to invade other tissues and metastasize. Abnormal tissue masses are called solid tumors and may be benign or malignant (cancerous).

Cancer causes more than 560,000 deaths in the United States annually, making it the second-leading killer after cardiovascular disease. The American Cancer Society (ACS) estimates that half of all men and one-third of all women currently living in the United States will eventually develop some form of cancer.

Pathophysiology

In many cases, the exact cause of cancer remains unknown. However, specific factors have been implicated in some types of cancer. They include:
• chemical carcinogens
• ultraviolet (UV) light exposure
• hereditary predisposition
• viruses
• gender.

Where there's smoke...

Smoking can cause lung cancer and has been strongly implicated in cancers of the mouth, throat, bladder, kidney, and several other organs. Although not everyone who smokes will get cancer, smoking increases the cancer risk. Similarly, high alcohol intake and smokeless (chewing) tobacco increase the risk of oral cancers.

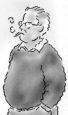

Not everyone who smokes will get cancer, but it increases the risk. I strongly suggest you put that out.

Genetic mutation

Smoking and other risk factors can affect the cell's genetic material, interfering with normal gene replication before cell division (mitosis) takes place. Such interference can increase the likelihood of a mutation—an abnormal change in some portion of the cell's gene complement. (See *Reviewing cancer risk factors.*)

Genetic mutation may result from aging; exposure to chemicals, radiation, or hormones; and other factors. Over time, numerous gene mutations may occur in a cell, permitting it to divide and grow in a way that eventually leads to cancer.

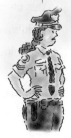

Uncontrolled growth

Cancer cells first develop from a genetic mutation in a single cell. (See *Cancer cell characteristics.*) This cell grows without the control that characterizes normal cell growth. Also, it fails to mature into the type of normal cell from which it originated.

Uncontrolled localized growth follows. Unlike normal cells, cancer cells keep growing and multiplying even after lost cells have been replaced.

Metastasis

In addition to this uncontrolled localized growth, cancer cells may spread from their origin site in a process called *metastasis.* Cancer cells metastasize in three ways:
- by circulation through the bloodstream and lymphatic system
- by accidental transplantation during surgery or other invasive procedures
- by spreading to adjacent organs and tissues.

Cancer classifications

Cancer is classified by the tissues or blood cells in which it originates. Most cancers derive from epithelial tissues and are called *carcinomas.*

Cancer cell characteristics

Cancer cells are characterized by uncontrolled cellular growth and development. Typically, these cells:
- vary in size and shape
- aren't encapsulated
- undergo abnormal mitosis
- function abnormally
- don't resemble their cells of origin
- produce substances rarely associated with the original cell or tissue
- can spread to other sites.

Reviewing cancer risk factors

Although cancer can strike anyone, adults and children alike, its incidence rises with age. Many other factors, internal and external, contribute to an individual's predisposition to cancer. Here are some examples.

Internal risk factors

Internal risk factors include age, gender, race, and genetic, immunologic, and psychological factors.

Age

Age of exposure to carcinogens may increase the cancer risk. Fetuses, infants, and children are at greater risk because they're still developing. Blistering sunburns in children under age 12 may predispose them to skin cancer.

Researchers are examining the effects of low electromagnetic fields, as in electric blankets or high-voltage power lines, on children.

Gender

Overall, women have a lower cancer incidence than men and higher survival rates. In females, breast, lung, colon, and uterine cancers are the most common. In males, lung, colon, and bladder cancers predominate.

Race

Cancer incidence and mortality are higher in blacks, possibly due to economic, social, and environmental factors that may delay prompt detection and increase exposure risk to industrial carcinogens.

Genetic factors

Certain cancers tend to run in families. For example, women who have first-degree relatives (mothers or sisters) with breast cancer are at greater risk than the general population.

Immunologic factors

According to the immune surveillance theory, antigenic differences between normal and cancerous cells may help the body eliminate malignant cells. Thus, immunosuppression may increase susceptibility to cancer.

Psychological factors

Emotional stress may increase a person's cancer risk by leading to poor health habits (such as frequent smoking), by depressing the immune system, or by leading him to ignore early warning signs.

External risk factors

External risk factors include exposure to chemical carcinogens or radiation, viruses, diet, tobacco and alcohol use, and chemotherapeutic drugs.

Chemical carcinogens

Occupational exposure to chemical carcinogens, such as those used in nickel refining or in the asbestos industry, is an important external risk factor.

Chemical carcinogens typically cause cancer in a two-step process—initiation and promotion.
* *Initiation* involves exposure to the carcinogen. This irreversible step converts normal cells into latent tumor cells.
* In *promotion*, repeated exposure to the same or some other substance stimulates the latent cells to become actively neoplastic.

Radiation

Ionizing radiation of all kinds (from X-rays to nuclear radiation) are carcinogenic, although their potencies vary.

Fair-skinned people have a higher risk for skin cancer from ultraviolet radiation. Skin cancer develops on exposed extremities, and its incidence correlates with the amount of exposure.

Viruses

Some human viruses have carcinogenic potential. The Epstein-Barr virus, for example, has been linked to lymphoma and nasopharyngeal carcinoma, and human papilloma virus can cause cervical cancer.

Deoxyribonucleic acid viruses (such as herpes simplex virus type 2) have been associated with uterine cervical cancer. Ribonucleic acid viruses are linked to breast cancer in mice.

Diet

Certain foods may supply carcinogens (or precarcinogens), affect carcinogen formation, or modify other carcinogens' effect. Diet has been implicated in colon cancer, which may result from low fiber intake and excessive fat consumption.

(continued)

Reviewing cancer risk factors (continued)

Liver tumors are linked to food additives, such as nitrates (commonly used in smoked and processed meat) and alfatoxin (a fungus that grows on stored grains, nuts, and other foodstuffs).

Tobacco use
Lung cancer is the leading cause of cancer deaths in both men and women. Cigarette smoking accounts for about 30% of all cancers and is implicated in cancers of the mouth, pharynx, larynx, esophagus, pancreas, cervix, and bladder. Pipe smoking and chewing tobacco are linked to oral cancer.

Studies show increased cancer risks associated with inhalation of secondhand smoke by nonsmokers (particularly children).

Alcohol use
Alcohol may act synergistically with tobacco. Smokers who drink heavily run an increased risk of head, neck, and esophageal cancers. Heavy beer consumption may increase the risk of colorectal cancer through an unknown mechanism.

Chemotherapeutic drugs
Some chemotherapeutic drugs may be directly carcinogenic or may enhance neoplastic development by suppressing the immune system.

By altering the body's normal endocrine balance, hormones may contribute to (rather than directly stimulate) neoplastic development—especially in endocrine-sensitive organs, such as the breast or prostate. The risk of secondary cancers from these agents must be weighed carefully against their benefits.

Other cancers arise from these tissues and cells:
- glandular tissues (adenocarcinomas)
- connective, muscle, and bone tissues (sarcomas)
- brain and spinal cord tissues (gliomas)
- pigmented cells (melanomas)
- plasma cells (myelomas)
- lymphatic tissue (lymphomas)
- leukocytes (leukemia)
- erythrocytes (erythroleukemia).

Cancers

This section discusses the most prevalent cancers of each body system. For each disorder, you'll find information on causes, assessment findings, diagnostic tests, treatment, nursing interventions, patient teaching, and evaluation criteria.

Acute leukemia

In acute leukemia, cancerous white blood cell (WBC) precursors called *blasts* proliferate in the bone marrow or lymph tissue and then accumulate in peripheral blood, bone marrow, and body tissues. Untreated, acute leukemia invariably leads to death, usually from complications of leukemic cell infiltration of bone marrow or vital organs.

Acute leukemia ranks 15th as a cause of cancer-related deaths among people of all ages. With treatment, prognosis varies. Among children, acute leukemia is the most common cancer.

Classifying acute leukemia

The most common forms of acute leukemia are:
• acute lymphoblastic leukemia (ALL), marked by abnormal growth of lymphocyte precursors (lymphoblasts)
• acute myelogenous leukemia (AML), characterized by rapid accumulation of myeloid precursors (myeloblasts)
• acute monocytic leukemia, or Schilling's type, which involves a marked increase in monocyte precursors (monoblasts).

Other leukemia variants include acute myelomonocytic leukemia and acute erythroleukemia.

Survival stats

The 5-year relative survival rate for leukemia is over 50%. The survival rate depends on the type of leukemia, age at diagnosis, gender, and race.

What causes it

The cause of acute leukemia is unknown. According to some experts, risk factors include:
• a combination of viruses
• genetic and immunologic factors
• exposure to radiation and certain chemicals.

Pathophysiology

The pathogenesis of acute leukemia isn't clearly understood. Immature, nonfunctioning WBCs appear to accumulate first in the tissue where they originate (lymphocytes in lymph tissue, granulocytes in bone marrow). These immature WBCs then spill into the bloodstream and infiltrate other tissues. Eventually, they cause organ malfunction from encroachment or hemorrhage.

What to look for

Typical clinical features of acute leukemia include:
• fever and infection
• abnormal bleeding, easy bruising, and petechiae

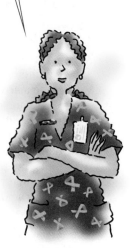

The 5-year relative survival rate for leukemia is over 50%, although the specific rate depends on the type of leukemia and a patient's age at diagnosis, gender, and race.

- fatigue and weight loss
- bone pain
- enlarged lymph nodes.

Be less specific...

Nonspecific signs and symptoms include low-grade fever, pallor, and weakness and lassitude that may persist for months before other signs and symptoms arise.

As the disease progresses, the patient may develop dyspnea, fatigue, malaise, tachycardia, palpitations, systolic ejection murmur, and abdominal or bone pain. In meningeal leukemia, early symptoms typically include confusion, lethargy, and headache.

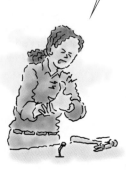

Some common signs of acute leukemia include abnormal bleeding, petechiae, and easy bruising. Don't forget to look for nonspecific signs, too.

What tests tell you

- Bone marrow biopsy is performed in a patient with typical clinical findings but whose aspirate is dry or free from leukemic cells. Bone marrow aspiration typically shows proliferation of immature WBCs and confirms the diagnosis.
- WBC differential determines cell type.
- Complete blood count (CBC) shows decreased levels of hemoglobin (anemia), platelets (thrombocytopenia), and neutrophils (neutropenia).
- Lumbar puncture detects meningeal involvement.
- Uric acid measurement may be done to detect hyperuricemia.

How it's treated

Systemic chemotherapy aims to eradicate leukemic cells and induce remission, restoring normal bone marrow function. Chemotherapy varies with the specific leukemia:
- For meningeal leukemia, treatment includes intrathecal instillation of methotrexate (Trexall) or cytarabine (Cytosar-U), along with cranial radiation.
- For ALL, treatment consists of vincristine and prednisone (Deltasone) with intrathecal methotrexate or cytarabine; I.V. asparaginase (Elspar), daunorubicin (DaunoXome), and doxorubicin; and maintenance with mercaptopurine (Purinethol) and methotrexate.
- For AML, treatment consists of a combination of I.V. daunorubicin or doxorubicin, cytarabine, and oral thioguanine. If these agents fail to induce remission, the patient may receive a combination of cyclophosphamide (Cytoxan), vincristine, prednisone, or methotrexate; high-dose cytarabine alone or with other drugs; amsacrine; mitoxantrone (Novantrone); or maintenance with additional chemotherapy.

Other treatments

Treatment may also include antibiotics, antifungals, and antivirals (given along with granulocyte injections to control infection and platelet transfusions to prevent bleeding). Red blood cell (RBC) transfusions may be given to prevent anemia. For some patients, bone marrow transplantation is an option.

What to do

• Control infection by placing the patient in a private room and imposing reverse isolation, if necessary. (Benefits of reverse isolation are controversial.) Coordinate care so the patient doesn't come in contact with staff members who also care for patients with infections or infectious diseases. Avoid using indwelling catheters and giving intramuscular injections, which can pave the way for infection. Screen staff members and visitors for contagious diseases. Watch for and report signs and symptoms of infection.

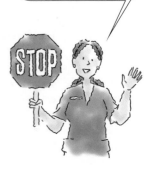

If your patient is being treated for leukemia, don't give aspirin, take rectal temperatures, or perform digital rectal exams.

Fending off fever

• Monitor the patient's vital signs every 2 to 4 hours. A temperature over 101° F (38.3° C) accompanied by a decreased WBC count calls for prompt antibiotic therapy.
• Watch for bleeding. If it occurs, apply ice compresses and pressure, and elevate the affected extremity. Avoid giving aspirin and aspirin-containing drugs. Also avoid taking rectal temperatures, giving rectal suppositories, and performing digital rectal examinations (DRE).

Supine for safety

• Watch for signs and symptoms of meningeal leukemia. If these occur, provide care after intrathecal chemotherapy. After instillation, place the patient in the Trendelenburg position for 30 minutes. Give plenty of fluids, and keep him supine for 4 to 6 hours. Check the lumbar puncture site often for bleeding.
• If the patient has received cranial radiation, teach him about potential adverse effects, and try to minimize them.
• Take steps to prevent hyperuricemia—a possible result of rapid chemotherapy-induced leukemic cell lysis. Give the patient about 2 qt (2 L) of fluids daily, and administer acetazolamide (Diamox), sodium bicarbonate tablets, and allopurinol (Zyloprim), as ordered. Check urine pH often—it should be above 7.5. Watch for rash and other hypersensitivity reactions to allopurinol.
• Control mouth ulcers by checking often for obvious ulcers and gum swelling and by providing frequent mouth care and saline solution rinses.

Weighing the evidence

Life after cancer: Families feel it, too

Although a growing body of research looks at the impact of cancer on the quality of life of patients, less is known about the effects of a cancer diagnosis on family caregivers. To find out more about family members' experiences, researchers surveyed 1,635 caregivers of cancer survivors 2 years after the cancer diagnosis, assessing their mental and physical health as well as their psychological adjustment and spirituality. They found that overall, caregivers reported normal levels of quality of life, along with an increased awareness of spirituality. Significant predictors of quality of life included the caregiver's age and income, and the care recipient's mental and physical well-being.

Care for the caregivers

The researchers found that younger, lower-income caregivers providing care to relatives with poor mental and physical functioning often needed spiritual and psychological support. In contrast, older caregivers were more likely to need support to reduce the physical burden of caregiving. The bottom line? It's not just the patient who needs care; family caregivers need resources and support, too.

Kim, Y., & Spillers, R. L. (2010). Quality of life of family caregivers at 2 years after a relative's cancer diagnosis. *Psychooncology, 19*(4), 431–440.

- Check the rectal area daily for induration, swelling, erythema, skin discoloration, and drainage.
- Minimize stress by providing a calm, quiet atmosphere that promotes rest and relaxation.
- Provide psychological support by establishing a trusting relationship with the patient. Allow him and his family to express their anger, anxiety, and depression. Encourage them to participate in patient care as much as possible. Refer them to a local chapter of the Leukemia Society of America. (See *Life afer cancer: Families feel it, too*.)
- For a patient with terminal disease that resists chemotherapy, provide supportive care directed at promoting comfort; managing pain, fever, and bleeding; and offering emotional support. Provide the opportunity for spiritual counseling if appropriate. Discuss the option of home or hospice care.

• Evaluate the patient. He and his family should understand the rationale for treatment and potential complications of chemotherapy. They should also know how to recognize signs and symptoms of infection and understand that they must notify the practitioner if these occur. They should be able to discuss treatment options and verbalize concerns about a poor prognosis. (See *Acute leukemia teaching tips*.)

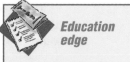

Education edge

Acute leukemia teaching tips

• If your patient has leukemia, teach him and his family the signs and symptoms of infection (such as fever, chills, cough, and sore throat) and abnormal bleeding (such as bruising and small purplish spots, or petechiae, caused by tiny hemorrhages). Also teach them how to stop bleeding, such as by applying pressure or ice.
• Instruct the patient to use a soft-bristle toothbrush and to avoid hot, spicy foods and alcohol-based commercial mouthwashes.

Breast cancer

Breast cancer is the most common cancer among females in the United States and the second-leading cause of cancer deaths in women ages 35 to 54. Breast cancer also occurs in men, although it's rare.

Thanks to earlier diagnosis and expanded treatment options, the 5-year survival rate for patients with localized breast cancer has improved from 78% in 1940 to 92% today.

Surviving in situ

For noninvasive cancer in situ (confined to the origin site without invading neighboring tissue), the survival rate is near 100%. If the cancer has spread regionally, the survival rate is 71%. With distant metastasis, it falls to 20%.

What causes it

Although the exact cause of breast cancer is unknown, certain risk factors exist. Primary risk factors include:
• gender (more than 90% of breast cancers occur in women)
• age (risk increases after age 50)
• personal history of the disease (15% of women develop breast cancer in the opposite breast)
• family history of the disease (women who have a first-degree relative with breast cancer have a twofold to threefold increased risk).

Secondary risk factors

Secondary risk factors for breast cancer include:
• never having given birth
• giving birth to a first child after age 30
• prolonged hormonal stimulation (menarche before age 12 and menopause after age 50)
• atypical hyperplasia (abnormal cell multiplication) on a previous breast biopsy
• exposure to excessive ionizing radiation (as in Hodgkin disease treatment)
• history of endometrial, ovarian, or colon cancer.

The discovery of specific genes linked to breast cancer, called *BRCA1* and *BRCA2*, indicates that the disease can be inherited. Someone who inherits either gene has roughly an 80% lifetime chance of developing breast cancer.

Pathophysiology

Breast cancer is more commonly found in the left breast than the right. It's also more common in the upper outer quadrant. (See *Breast tumor sites.*)

Growth rates vary. Theoretically, slow-growing breast cancer may take up to 8 years to become palpable at 1 cm in size.

Spread pattern

Breast cancer spreads via the lymphatic system and bloodstream, through the right side of the heart to the lungs, and may spread to the other breast, chest wall, liver, bone, and brain.

What to look for

Signs and symptoms of breast cancer include:
- painless lump or mass in the breast
- changes in breast symmetry or size
- changes in breast skin, such as dimpling (called *peau d'orange*), edema, or ulcers
- changes in nipples; for instance, itching, burning, erosion, retraction, or discharge
- skin temperature changes (a warm, hot, or pink area).

If you detect any of these changes, suspect cancer in a nonlactating woman past childbearing age until proven otherwise. Investigate spontaneous discharge of any kind in a non–breast-feeding, nonlactating woman.

Signs and symptoms of metastasis

Metastatic disease may cause shoulder, hip, or pelvic pain; cough; anorexia; persistent dizziness; or enlarged axillary or supraclavicular lymph nodes.

What tests tell you

- Detection of a breast lump or tumor on breast self-examination, clinical breast examination, or mammography suggests breast cancer. (See *Breast cancer screening recommendations.*)

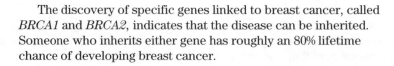

Memory jogger

ASH is an easy way to remember the primary risk factors for breast cancer:

Age: The risk increases after age 50.

Sex: About 90% of breast cancers are found in women.

History: A personal or family history of breast cancer increases the risk for the disease.

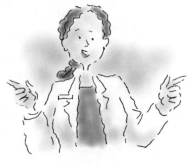

Breast cancer more commonly affects the left breast than the right and is more common in the upper outer quadrant.

Breast tumor sites

This illustration shows the location and frequency of breast cancer. The upper outer quadrant is the most common breast cancer site.

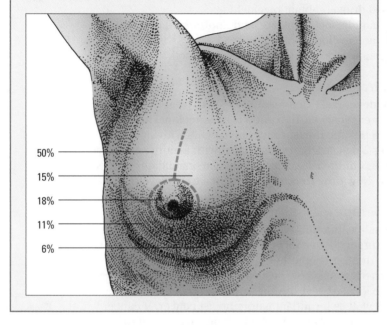

50% —
15% —
18% —
11% —
6% —

Breast cancer screening recommendations

These recommendations from the American Cancer Society focus on early detection of breast cancer to improve survival rates:

• Women age 40 and older should have yearly mammograms.
• Women age 40 and older should have a clinical breast examination every year. Women ages 20 to 39 should have such examinations every 3 years.
• Women at high risk should undergo magnetic resonance imaging and mammography every year.

• Diagnosis hinges on biopsy and pathologic evaluation of the suspicious tissue. The staging workup may include chest X-rays as well as liver and bone scans.
• A hormonal receptor assay of tumor tissue obtained by biopsy can determine whether the tumor's growth is stimulated by estrogen (estrogen-dependent) or progesterone (progesterone-dependent). Such determination guides therapeutic decisions.

How it's treated

Treatment may include one or any combination of the following options.

Chemotherapy

Chemotherapy for breast cancer may involve various cytotoxic drug combinations. In patients with axillary lymph node involvement but no evidence of distant metastasis, chemotherapy may be adjuvant (used after the primary tumor has been removed) or neoadjuvant (used as a preliminary therapy preceding a necessary second treatment modality).

Breast cancer staging may warrant chest X-rays and liver and bone scans.

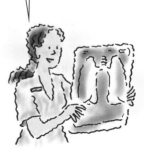

If metastasis has occurred, chemotherapy may be done as primary therapy based on such factors as the patient's premenopausal or postmenopausal status.

Chemo combos

Commonly used drug combinations include:
- cyclophosphamide, methotrexate, and fluorouracil (Adrucil)
- doxorubicin and cyclophosphamide
- cyclophosphamide, doxorubicin, and fluorouracil.

Other drug treatments

Paclitaxel and docetaxel (Taxotere) are used to treat recurrent or metastatic breast cancer. Herceptin is a monoclonal antibody used to treat metastatic breast cancer in patients with an overexpression of Her-2/neu, a protein associated with a more aggressive tumor. About 30% of breast cancer patients are candidates for herceptin therapy. New drug treatments continue to be developed.

Radiation therapy

Primary external-beam radiation therapy typically begins 2 to 4 weeks after surgery, when incisions have healed. It may be given before, during, or after chemotherapy.

Radiation therapy may also be used as adjunctive therapy for tumors that are located near the chest wall or are locally advanced or recurrent as well as for inflammatory breast cancer. If cancer has spread to the bone, radiation therapy may be targeted to specific bone sites to reduce pain.

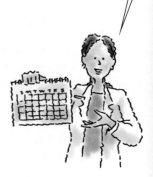

Primary radiation therapy typically begins 2 to 4 weeks after surgery, when incisions have healed.

Surgery

Lumpectomy, or tumor excision, usually is the initial surgery. It also provides biopsy material to determine tumor cell type.

Typically, lumpectomy is performed on an outpatient basis. For some patients—especially those with small tumors and no evidence of axillary node involvement—it's the only surgery required. However, lumpectomy is commonly combined with radiation therapy.

Lumpectomy is performed in two stages. First, the surgeon removes the lump and confirms malignancy. Then he discusses treatment options with the patient.

Other operation options

Other surgical procedures for breast cancer include:
- lumpectomy with sentinel node biopsy or axillary lymph node dissection, which removes the tumor and axillary lymph nodes while leaving the breast intact

- simple mastectomy, which removes the breast but not axillary lymph nodes or pectoral muscles
- modified radical mastectomy, which removes the breast and axillary nodes
- radical mastectomy (rare), which removes the breast, pectoralis major and minor muscles, and axillary nodes.

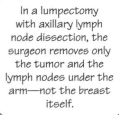

In a lumpectomy with axillary lymph node dissection, the surgeon removes only the tumor and the lymph nodes under the arm—not the breast itself.

Rebuilding the breast

Postmastectomy reconstructive surgery can create a breast mound if the patient desires it, which may help her to cope with changes in her body image.

Other methods

Other breast cancer treatments may include:
- estrogen, progesterone, or androgen therapy
- antiandrogen therapy with aminoglutethimide
- antiestrogen therapy.

Antiestrogen therapy involves administration of tamoxifen, a drug with few adverse effects that inhibits deoxyribonucleic acid synthesis. In postmenopausal women, aromatase inhibitors such as anastrozole (Arimidex) effectively combat estrogen-dependent tumors.

What to do

- Obtain a patient history. Assess the patient's feelings and knowledge about her diagnosis, and determine her expectations.
- Explain treatment options at the patient's level of understanding.
- Evaluate the patient. With effective treatment, she should recover uneventfully from surgery, radiation, chemotherapy, or other treatments. She should perform appropriate exercises and understand postoperative safety precautions for the affected arm. Also, she should correctly demonstrate breast self-examination. (See *Breast cancer teaching tips*.)

Cervical cancer

The third most common cancer of the female reproductive system (after uterine and ovarian cancer), cervical cancer may be preinvasive or invasive. With early detection and proper treatment, the preinvasive form has a high cure rate.

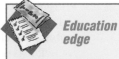

Education edge

Breast cancer teaching tips

- To promote early diagnosis and treatment of breast cancer, teach female patients the importance of mammography and appropriate follow-up care.
- Postoperatively, instruct the patient to continue these practices to detect new breast lesions.

Unwelcome invasion

If untreated (and depending on the exact cancer form), the disease may progress to become invasive. Invasive cervical cancer causes 4,000 deaths annually in the United States. Rare before age 20, it usually occurs between ages 30 and 50.

What causes it

The cause of cervical cancer is unknown. However, the most important risk factor is infection by human papillomavirus (HPV). HPV is responsible for about 70% of cervical cancer cases. HPV recombinant vaccine (Gardasil or Cervarix) is recommended for women and girls ages 9 to 26 to protect against cervical cancer.

Other risk factors include:
- chlamydia infection
- immunosuppression
- poor diet and obesity
- early pregnancy and multiple pregnancies
- cigarette smoking.

Pathophysiology

Preinvasive cervical cancer ranges from minimal cervical dysplasia, in which the lower third of the epithelium contains abnormal cells, to carcinoma in situ, which involves the full thickness of epithelium.

No basement bargains

In invasive cancer, cancer cells penetrate the basement membrane and may spread directly to adjacent pelvic structures or to distant sites via the lymph system.

What to look for

Preinvasive cervical cancer is asymptomatic. Abnormal vaginal bleeding, persistent vaginal discharge, and postcoital pain and bleeding may signal early invasive disease.

Advanced disease may cause pelvic pain or vaginal leakage of urine and feces from a fistula, along with anorexia, weight loss, and fatigue.

What tests tell you

• A Papanicolaou (Pap) test can detect cervical cancer before symptoms arise. The ACS recommends annual Pap tests starting about 3 years after the initiation of sexual intercourse but no later than age 21. Women ages 30 to 70 with three or more consecutive satisfactory examinations with normal findings should have a

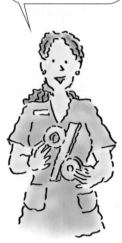

The percentages for surviving preinvasive cervical cancer are high, with the cure rate approaching 100%.

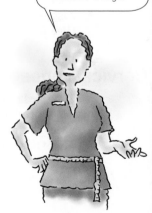

Effective treatment for cervical cancer is tailored to the cancer stage.

Pap test every 2 to 3 years. For women age 70 and older with three or more consecutive satisfactory examinations and no abnormal Pap tests in the past 10 years, screening may stop.

• The HPV DNA test is recommended to detect HPV in women older than age 30 who have had abnormal Pap tests.

• Colposcopy (examination of the vaginal and cervical epithelium using a colposcope) can reveal the presence and extent of pre-clinical lesions.

• Biopsy and histologic examination confirm the diagnosis.

• Additional studies, such as lymphangiography, cystography, and scans, can detect metastasis.

How it's treated

Effective treatment is tailored to the cancer stage. Preinvasive lesions may warrant total excisional biopsy, cryosurgery, laser destruction of the tumor, conization (removal of a cone-shaped section of the cervix) with frequent Pap test follow-up or, rarely, hysterectomy. Invasive squamous cancer may require radical hysterectomy and radiation therapy (internal, external, or both).

What to do

• Provide comprehensive patient teaching and emotional and psychological support.

• If the patient will receive internal radiation, determine if the radioactive source will be inserted while she's in the operating room (preloaded) or at the bedside (afterloaded). Remember that safety precautions—time, distance, and shielding—must start as soon as the radioactive source is in place. Tell the patient she'll require a private room.

• Check the patient's vital signs every 4 hours. Watch for skin reactions, vaginal bleeding, abdominal discomfort, and evidence of dehydration.

Within arm's reach

• Make sure she can reach everything she needs without stretching or straining. Assist her in range-of-motion arm exercises; be aware that leg exercises and other body movements could dislodge the radiation source.

• Organize the time you spend with the patient to minimize your radiation exposure. Inform visitors of safety precautions, and hang a sign listing these precautions on the patient's door.

• Evaluate the patient. When assessing her response to treatment, note how well she tolerates the therapy. She should understand that it won't impair her ability to have sex. She should also understand the importance of complying with the treatment regimen. (See *Cervical cancer teaching tips.*)

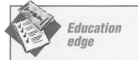

Education edge

Cervical cancer teaching tips

• If your patient with cervical cancer undergoes excisional biopsy, cryosurgery, or laser therapy, tell her to expect discharge or spotting for about 1 week. Advise her not to douche, use tampons, or have sexual intercourse during this time.

• Explain that outpatient radiation therapy (if needed) continues for 4 to 6 weeks.

• Tell the patient she may be hospitalized for a 2- to 3-day course of internal radiation treatment if necessary.

• Because radiation therapy may make her more susceptible to infection by lowering her white blood cell count, instruct her to avoid people with obvious infections during therapy.

• Reassure the patient that cervical cancer and its treatment need not adversely affect sexual function.

Colorectal cancer

Colorectal cancer is the third most common cause of cancer deaths in the United States. It affects men and women equally.

Nearly all colorectal cancers are adenocarcinomas. About 50% are rectosigmoid lesions that adhere closely to the mucosal surface (called *sessile*). The rest are polyps.

Slow to spread, easier to cure

Because colorectal cancer spreads slowly, it's potentially curable with early diagnosis. The 5-year survival rate for colon and rectal cancers caught in the early stages is 91%. After the cancer spreads regionally, survival drops to 70%.

What causes it

The cause of colorectal cancer remains unknown. Studies show, however, that it's prevalent in areas of higher economic development. This suggests it's linked to a high-fat diet.

Other factors that increase the risk for this disease include:
• age over 50
• inflammatory bowel disease
• history of polyps
• inherited tendency toward colon polyps
• sedentary lifestyle and obesity
• heavy alcohol use
• diet high in red meat
• family history of colorectal cancer, especially before age 60.

Pathophysiology

Most lesions of the large bowel are moderately differentiated adenocarcinomas. Tumors tend to grow slowly and remain asymptomatic for long periods.

Stretching the circumference

Tumors in the sigmoid and descending colon grow circumferentially and constrict the intestinal lumen. At diagnosis, tumors in the ascending colon are usually large and palpable on physical examination.

What to look for

Signs and symptoms of colorectal cancer include malaise and fatigue. Other findings result from local obstruction and, in later stages, from direct extension to adjacent organs (such as the bladder, prostate, ureters, vagina, and sacrum) or from distant metastasis (usually to the liver).

Later signs and symptoms include:
- weight loss
- pain
- pallor
- bloody stools
- cachexia (malnutrition, weakness, and emaciation)
- ascites (buildup of serous fluid in the abdominal cavity)
- hepatomegaly (liver enlargement)
- lymphangiectasis (widening of the lymphatic vessels).

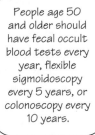

People age 50 and older should have fecal occult blood tests every year, flexible sigmoidoscopy every 5 years, or colonoscopy every 10 years.

What tests tell you

- Only a tumor biopsy can verify colorectal cancer, but other tests help detect it. For women and men age 50 and older, the ACS recommends one of the following tests: fecal occult blood test (FOBT) or fecal immunochemical test (FIT) every year, flexible sigmoidoscopy every 5 years, FOBT or FIT every year plus flexible sigmoidoscopy every 5 years, colonoscopy every 10 years, or double-contrast barium enema every 5 years.
- DRE detects nearly 15% of colorectal cancers. It can be used to detect suspicious rectal and perianal lesions.
- FOBT and FIT detect blood in stools, a warning sign of rectal cancer.
- Proctoscopy or sigmoidoscopy permits visualization of the lower GI tract and can detect up to two-thirds of colorectal cancers.

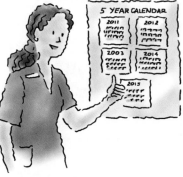

Photographing the evidence

- Colonoscopy allows visual inspection (and photographs) of the colon up to the ileocecal valve. It also provides access for polypectomy and biopsy of suspected lesions.
- MRI uses magnetic fields to obtain detailed images of body structures.
- Carcinoembryonic antigen testing, although not specific or sensitive enough for early diagnosis, helps monitor the patient before and after treatment to detect metastasis or recurrence.

How it's treated

Surgery seeks to remove the cancerous tumor and adjacent tissues as well as lymph nodes that may contain cancer cells. The type of surgery depends on tumor location. (See *Treating colorectal cancer*, page 850.)

Treating colorectal cancer

The most effective treatment for colorectal cancer is surgery to remove the malignant tumor, adjacent tissues, and cancerous lymph nodes. The surgical site depends on tumor location. The illustrations below show the different locations in the colon that may be resected for tumor removal and the different types of possible anastomoses (reattachments).

Postoperative treatment

After surgery, treatment typically includes chemotherapy or radiation therapy. If the cancer has spread to other sites or the patient has residual disease or a recurrent inoperable tumor, chemotherapy is essential.

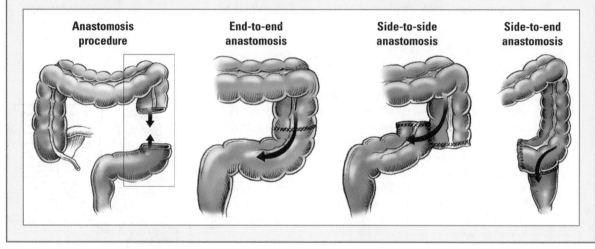

| Anastomosis procedure | End-to-end anastomosis | Side-to-side anastomosis | Side-to-end anastomosis |

Surgical options

- For tumors of the cecum or ascending colon, right hemicolectomy for advanced disease may include resection of the terminal segment of the ileum, cecum, ascending colon, and right half of the transverse colon with corresponding mesentery.
- For tumors of the proximal and middle transverse colon, right colectomy includes transverse colon and mesentery corresponding to midcolonic vessels. Alternatively, the surgeon may perform segmental resection of the transverse colon and associated midcolonic vessels.
- For sigmoid colon tumors, surgery is usually limited to the sigmoid colon and mesentery.
- Upper rectum tumors usually call for anterior or low anterior resection. A newer method using a stapler allows resections much lower than were previously possible.
- For tumors in the lower rectum, abdominoperineal resection and permanent sigmoid colostomy are usually performed.

Better living through chemotherapy

Chemotherapy may be used as adjuvant therapy or for patients with metastasis, residual disease, or recurrent inoperable tumors. Commonly used drugs include:
- 5-fluorouracil, with or without leucovorin
- irinotecan (Camptosar)
- oxaliplatin (Eloxatin)
- capecitabine (Xeloda).

Researchers are developing new therapies that target the genes and proteins that lead to cancer.

Radiation

Radiation therapy may induce tumor regression and may be used before and after surgery.

What to do

- If the patient will have colorectal surgery, monitor his diet and give laxatives, enemas, and antibiotics, as ordered (to clean the bowel and minimize abdominal and perineal cavity contamination during surgery).
- Evaluate the patient. He should verbalize an understanding of the treatment regimen, including ostomy care, and the need for long-term follow-up. (See *Colorectal cancer teaching tips.*)

Hodgkin disease

Hodgkin disease is a lymphatic cancer marked by painless, progressive enlargement of the lymph nodes, spleen, and other lymphoid tissue. Left untreated, it follows a variable but progressive and ultimately fatal course.

Promising odds

However, recent advances in therapy make Hodgkin disease potentially curable, even in advanced stages. Appropriate treatment yields long-term survival in about 85% of patients.

What causes it

The exact cause of Hodgkin disease is unknown, although indirect evidence suggests it may involve a virus. The disease is most common in young adults.

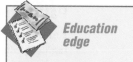

Education edge

Colorectal cancer teaching tips

- If your patient with colorectal cancer will have a colostomy, teach him and his family about the procedure. Consider referring the patient to an enterostomal therapist before surgery.
- Because a history of colorectal cancer increases the risk for other primary cancers, instruct the patient to have close follow-up and screening and to increase his dietary fiber intake.
- Instruct the patient's family about the familial risks of colorectal cancer, and teach them about dietary modifications to reduce their risk. Also teach them how to recognize early signs and symptoms of colorectal cancer.

Pathophysiology

Enlargement of the lymph nodes, spleen, and other lymphoid tissues results from proliferation of lymphocytes, histiocytes, eosinophils, and Reed-Sternberg cells. The latter cells are hall-marks of the disease.

What to look for

Usually, the first sign is painless swelling in a cervical lymph node (or, occasionally, in a lymph node in another area). Other signs and symptoms include pruritus (itching), persistent fever, night sweats, fatigue, weight loss, and malaise.

Late-stage signs and symptoms include facial and neck edema, jaundice, nerve pain, enlarged retroperitoneal lymph nodes, and nodular infiltration of the spleen, liver, and bones.

What tests tell you

• Lymph node biopsy reveals abnormal histologic proliferation, nodular fibrosis, necrosis, and Reed-Sternberg cells. Lymph node biopsy is also used to determine lymph node and organ involvement.
• Blood tests show mild to severe normocytic anemia (anemia with RBCs of normal size); normochromic anemia (marked by normal hemoglobin amounts) in 50% of cases; an elevated, normal, or reduced WBC count; and WBC differential showing any combination of neutrophilia (excessive neutrophil levels), lymphocytopenia (deficient lymphocyte levels), monocytosis (excessive monophil levels), and eosinophilia (excessive eosinophil levels).
• Serum alkaline phosphatase levels may be elevated, indicating liver or bone involvement.
• A staging laparotomy is necessary for patients under age 55 and for those without obvious advanced disease (stages III or IV), lymphocyte predominance histology, or medical contraindications.
• Computed tomography (CT) scans evaluate the extent of the disease.

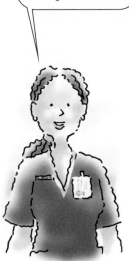

A combination of chemotherapy and radiation therapy is used to treat patients with Hodgkin disease.

How it's treated

Depending on the disease stage, treatment may include chemotherapy, radiation, or both. Choice of therapy depends on careful physical examination, accurate histologic interpretation, and proper clinical staging. Correct treatment prolongs survival and induces an apparent cure in many patients.

A favorable outlook

Patients with favorable prognoses may benefit from a combination of targeted radiation and chemotherapy. Commonly used chemotherapy combinations include:
• doxorubicin, bleomycin, vinblastine, and dacarbazine
• cyclophosphamide, doxorubicin, etoposide, oncovin, bleomycin, procarbazine, and prednisone.

What to do

• Monitor the patient closely for indications of toxicity caused by chemotherapy or radiation. As appropriate, manage symptoms to help prevent the need for a treatment hiatus or reduction.
• Provide emotional support and offer appropriate counseling and reassurance.
• Evaluate the patient. He should understand and comply with the self-care regimen for radiation and chemotherapy. He should know how to recognize adverse effects of treatment and know when to notify the practitioner. He should also be able to control weight loss and remain free from infection. (See *Hodgkin disease teaching tips*.)

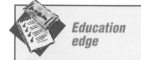

Lung cancer

Although largely preventable, lung cancer is the most common cause of cancer deaths in men and women. It usually develops within the wall or epithelium of the bronchial tree.

Histologic headings

There are two major types of lung cancer:
• Small cell lung cancer—also called oat cell cancer—accounts for 10% to 15% of lung cancers. It usually starts in the bronchi and spreads widely.
• Non–small cell lung cancer accounts for 85% to 90% of lung cancers and includes squamous cell cancers, adenocarcinomas, and large-cell (undifferentiated) carcinomas.

Gloomy forecast

Prognosis varies with cell type and extent of spread at the time of diagnosis. Only 15% of patients with later-stage lung cancer survive 5 years after diagnosis.

What causes it

Tobacco smoking accounts for approximately 90% of lung cancers and is closely associated with all histologic types. Other risk factors include genetic predisposition and exposure to carcinogenic industrial or air pollutants (such as asbestos, uranium, arsenic, nickel, iron oxides, chromium, radioactive dust, and coal dust). Some people without any risk factors develop lung cancer.

Pathophysiology

Lung tumors show bronchial epithelial changes progressing from squamous cell changes or metaplasia (abnormal changes in adult cells) to carcinoma in situ. Tumors originating in the bronchi produce more mucus.

Tumor growth causes partial or complete airway blockage, resulting in collapse of lung lobes distal to the tumor.

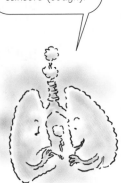

Tobacco smoking (cough) accounts for about 90% (cough) of lung cancers (cough).

Thoracic sprawl

Early metastasis occurs to other thoracic structures, such as the hilar lymph nodes and mediastinum. Distant metastasis may involve the brain, liver, bone, and adrenal glands.

What to look for

Because early-stage lung cancer tends to have a gradual onset, the disease is usually well developed by the time it's diagnosed.

With small cell cancer and squamous cancers, late-stage respiratory findings include smoker's cough, hoarseness, wheezing, dyspnea, hemoptysis (expectoration of blood), and chest pain. With non–small cell cancer and adenocarcinoma, findings include fever, weakness, weight loss, anorexia, and shoulder pain.

Hormonal disharmony

Sometimes, lung cancer causes hormone-related changes, including:
• gynecomastia, or breast enlargement in males (with non–small cell cancer)
• bone and joint pain (with non–small cell cancer and adenocarcinoma)
• signs or symptoms of Cushing's syndrome, such as central obesity, round face, supraclavicular fat pads, muscle atrophy, edema, and emotional changes (with small cell cancer)
• signs or symptoms of carcinoid syndrome, such as flushing, diarrhea, cramps, skin lesions, labored breathing, and palpitations (with small cell cancer)
• signs or symptoms of hypercalcemia, such as muscle pain and weakness.

Spreading signs

If lung cancer spreads, signs and symptoms vary. With bronchial obstruction, metastatic signs and symptoms include hemoptysis, atelectasis (lung tissue collapse), pneumonitis (lung inflammation), and dyspnea.

With recurrent nerve invasion, findings may include vocal cord paralysis. With chest wall invasion, the patient may have piercing chest pain, increasing dyspnea, and severe shoulder pain radiating down the arm. With local lymphatic spread, expect cough, hemoptysis, stridor (a harsh sound on expiration), and pleural effusion.

What tests tell you

• A chest X-ray usually shows an advanced lesion, but can detect a lesion up to 2 years before symptoms appear. It also defines tumor size and location.
• Bronchoscopy can locate the tumor site. Bronchoscopic washings provide material for cytologic and histologic examination. Using a flexible fiberoptic bronchoscope increases test effectiveness.
• Needle biopsy uses biplane fluoroscopic visual control to detect peripheral tumors, allowing firm diagnosis in 80% of patients.
• Tissue biopsy of accessible metastatic sites includes supraclavicular and mediastinal node and pleural biopsy.
• Thoracentesis (removal of fluid from the chest cavity) allows chemical and cytologic examination of pleural fluid.
• Tests to detect metastasis include bone scan (a positive scan may lead to bone marrow biopsy; bone marrow biopsy is also recommended for patients with small cell cancer); CT scan of the brain; liver function studies; and gallium scan (noninvasive nuclear scan) of the liver, spleen, and bone.

A chest X-ray can detect a lung tumor up to 2 years before symptoms appear.

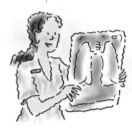

How it's treated

Treatment involves combinations of surgery, radiation, and chemotherapy. Although treatment may improve prognosis and prolong survival, it's largely palliative because most cancers are diagnosed at an advanced disease stage.

Surgery

Surgery is the main treatment for non–small cell cancer—unless the tumor is nonresectable or other conditions (such as cardiac disease) rule out surgery. Surgery may involve partial removal of a lung (as in wedge resection and lobectomy) or total lung removal (as in pneumonectomy and radical pneumonectomy).

Radiation therapy

Preoperative radiation therapy may reduce tumor bulk to allow surgical resection, but its value is questionable. Radiation therapy is generally recommended for early-stage (stage I and stage II) lesions if surgery is contraindicated and as an adjunct to surgery (either preoperatively or postoperatively).

Prophylactic cranial irradiation may be used to prevent or slow brain metastasis in small cell lung cancer. Some patients undergo radiation to control cancer-related symptoms or to prolong their functional lives.

Chemotherapy

Chemotherapy for small cell lung cancer uses a combination of drugs such as:
- cisplatin (Platinol) and etoposide
- carboplatin and etoposide
- cisplatin and irinotecan (Camptosar).

For non–small cell cancers, cisplatin, carboplatin, paclitaxel (Abraxane), and docetaxel (Taxotere) are among the drugs used.

Other treatments

Other possible treatment methods include radiofrequency ablation, photodynamic therapy, and laser therapy.

What to do

- Provide comprehensive supportive care and patient teaching to minimize complications and promote recovery from surgery, radiation, or chemotherapy.
- Evaluate the patient. He should experience an uneventful recovery from surgery, radiation, or chemotherapy. He and his family should verbalize an understanding of risk factors and alter their smoking behavior as appropriate. The patient should follow the treatment regimen and understand the need for good pulmonary hygiene and follow-up. He should also recognize signs and symptoms of respiratory tract infection and understand the need to report these immediately. (See *Lung cancer teaching tips*.)

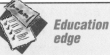

Education edge

Lung cancer teaching tips

- Before discharge, teach the patient with lung cancer how to use home oxygen therapy. Make sure the patient and his family know the signs and symptoms of respiratory tract infection and the need to report them to the practitioner.
- To help prevent lung cancer, teach high-risk patients to stop smoking. Refer smokers who want to quit to the local branch of the American Cancer Society or American Lung Association. Inform patients that nicotine gum or a nicotine patch and an antidepressant may be prescribed in combination with educational and support groups.
- Encourage patients with recurring or chronic respiratory tract infections and those with chronic lung disease to see the doctor promptly for evaluation if they detect changes in the character of a cough.

Malignant melanoma

The most lethal form of skin cancer, malignant melanoma remains uncommon but is increasing at a rate of about 4% per year. An estimated 68,000 new cases develop each year, with about 8,700 deaths. Peak incidence occurs from ages 45 to 55.

The four types of melanoma are:
- superficial spreading melanoma
- nodular melanoma
- acral-lentiginous melanoma
- lentigo maligna melanoma.

What causes it

The cause of malignant melanoma is unknown. Risk factors include a family tendency, a history of melanoma or dysplastic nevi, excessive sun exposure, a history of severe sunburns, and fair skin.

Ancestral affliction

Most people who develop melanoma have blond or red hair, fair skin, and blue eyes; are prone to sunburn; and are of Celtic or Scandinavian ancestry. Other risk factors are immunosuppressant therapy and psoralen UVA treatment for psoriasis.

Pathophysiology

Melanoma arises from melanocytes (cells that synthesize the pigment melanin). In addition to the skin, melanocytes are less commonly found in the meninges (membranes of the brain and spinal cord), eyes, mouth, and vagina.

When melanoma goes mobile

Melanoma spreads through the lymphatic and vascular systems to the regional lymph nodes, skin, liver, lungs, and central nervous system. Prognosis varies with tumor thickness. Typically, superficial lesions are curable, whereas deeper lesions tend to metastasize and carry a poorer prognosis.

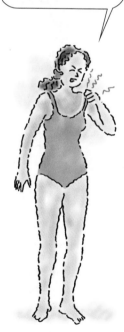

Excessive sun exposure and a history of severe sunburns are risk factors for malignant melanoma. Ouch!

What to look for

Suspect melanoma when any skin lesion or nevus enlarges, changes color, becomes inflamed or sore, itches, ulcerates, bleeds, changes texture, or shows signs of surrounding pigment regression (halo nevus or vitiligo). (See *Recognizing potentially malignant nevi*.)

Superficial spreading melanoma

Features of superficial spreading melanoma, the most common type, include:
- a red, white, and bluish tinge over a brown or black background
- irregular, notched margins
- an irregular surface
- a small, elevated nodule that may ulcerate and bleed
- horizontal growth pattern.

Nodular malignant melanoma

Nodular malignant melanoma usually grows vertically, invades the dermis, and metastasizes early. It commonly appears as a polyp and has uniformly dark discoloration; sometimes, it's grayish, resembling a blackberry. Occasionally, it matches the patient's skin color. Pigment flecks may appear around the lesion's base, which may be inflamed.

Acral-lentiginous melanoma

Acral-lentiginous melanoma occurs mainly on the palms and soles—especially on the tip of a finger or toe or in the nail fold or bed; sometimes, it's seen on mucosal surfaces, such as the vulva or vagina. It appears as an irregular, enlarging black macule and has a prolonged nonvinvasive stage. Although relatively rare, it's the most common melanoma type in nonwhite persons.

Lentigo malignant melanoma

Lentigo malignant melanoma, a relatively rare type, develops over many years from a lentigo maligna (a black or brown, mottled, slowly enlarging lesion with irregular borders) on an exposed skin surface. Usually diagnosed between ages 60 and 70, the lesion looks like a flat, large (2.5 to 6.5 cm) freckle.

A neutral palette

The lesion may be tan, brown, black, white, or slate; and may have scattered black nodules on the surface. Eventually, it may become ulcerated.

Memory jogger

Use the **ABCD** rule to assess a mole's malignant potential:

Asymmetry: Is the mole irregular in shape?

Border: Is its border irregular, notched, or poorly defined?

Color: Does the color vary—for example, between shades of brown, red, white, or black?

Diameter: Is the diameter more than 6 mm?

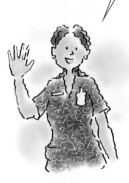

Acral-lentiginous melanoma occurs mainly on the palm of the hand and sole of the foot.

Recognizing potentially malignant nevi

Skin lesions called *nevi* (moles) commonly are pigmented and may be hereditary. They begin to grow in childhood and become more numerous during young adulthood.

Up to 70% of patients with melanoma have a history of a preexisting nevus at the tumor site. Of these, about one-third are congenital; the remainder develop later in life.

Changes in nevi (for example, in color, size, shape, or texture or onset of ulceration, bleeding, or itching) suggest possible malignant transformation. Presence or absence of hair within a nevus has no significance.

Types of nevi include blue nevi, compound nevi, dermal nevi, dysplastic nevi, junctional nevi, and lentigo maligna.

Blue nevi

Blue nevi are flat or slightly elevated lesions from 0.5 to 1 cm in diameter. Twice as common in women as in men, they appear on the head, neck, arms, and back of the hands. Their blue color results from dermal pigment and collagen, which reflect blue light but absorb other wavelengths. They must be excised to rule out pigmented basal cell epithelioma or melanoma or for cosmetic reasons.

Compound nevi

Compound nevi usually are tan to dark brown and slightly raised, although size and color vary. They contain melanocytes in the dermis and epidermis and rarely undergo malignant transformation. Excision may be needed to rule out malignant transformation or for cosmetic reasons.

Dermal nevi

Dermal nevi are elevated lesions from 2 to 10 mm in diameter that vary in color from tan to brown. Typically, they develop in older adults on the upper part of the body. They're generally removed only to rule out malignant transformation.

Dysplastic nevi

Dysplastic nevi usually are more than 5 mm in diameter, with irregularly notched or indistinct borders. Most often, they're tan or brown but sometimes have red, pink, or black pigmentation. No two of these lesions are exactly alike. They occur in great numbers (typically over 100 at a time), rarely singly—most commonly on the back, scalp, chest, and buttocks.

Dysplastic nevi are potentially malignant, especially in patients with a personal or family history of melanoma. Skin biopsy confirms diagnosis; treatment is by surgical excision, followed by regular physical examinations (every 6 months) to detect new lesions or changes in existing lesions.

Junctional nevi

Junctional nevi are flat or slightly raised and light to dark brown, with melanocytes confined to the epidermis. Usually, they appear before age 40. They may change into compound nevi if junctional nevus cells proliferate and penetrate the dermis.

Lentigo maligna

Also called *melanotic freckle* or *Hutchinson's melanotic freckle,* lentigo maligna is a precursor to malignant melanoma. About one-third of them eventually give rise to malignant melanoma.

Typically, they occur in persons over age 40, especially on exposed skin areas such as the face. At first, these lesions are flat tan spots, but they gradually enlarge and darken, developing black speckled areas against their tan or brown background. Removal by simple excision (not electrodessication and curettage) is recommended.

What tests tell you

- A skin biopsy with histologic examination distinguishes malignant melanoma from a benign nevus, seborrheic keratosis, or pigmented basal cell epithelioma. It also determines tumor thickness.
- Chest X-ray aids staging.
- Blood studies may show anemia and an elevated erythrocyte sedimentation rate. With metastasis, these tests may also reveal an abnormal platelet count and abnormal liver function studies.

How it's treated

Wide surgical resection is imperative in treating malignant melanoma. The extent of resection depends on the size and location of the primary lesion. Surgery may include regional lymphadenectomy.

Chemotherapy and biotherapy

Deep primary lesions may merit adjuvant chemotherapy with dacarbazine and nitrosureas carmustine (BCNU) and cisplatin (Platinol). Biotherapy with interferons, interleukin-2, tumor necrosis factor, and vaccine therapy is being studied.

Radiation therapy

Radiation therapy is usually reserved for metastatic disease. It doesn't prolong survival but may reduce tumor size and relieve pain. Prognosis depends on tumor thickness.

What to do

• After surgery, take steps to prevent infection. Check the wound often for excessive drainage, foul odor, redness, and swelling. If surgery involved lymphadenectomy, minimize lymphedema by applying a compression stocking and instruct the patient to keep the extremity elevated.
• During chemotherapy, know which adverse reactions to expect and do what you can to minimize these. For instance, give an antiemetic as ordered to reduce nausea and vomiting.
• For advanced metastatic disease, control and prevent pain by giving an analgesic around the clock. Don't wait until pain begins to initiate pain relief.
• Provide psychological support to help the patient cope with anxiety. Encourage him to express his fears. Answer his questions honestly without destroying hope.
• Evaluate the patient. He should recover uneventfully from surgery. He should also understand risk factors for melanoma and the importance of getting careful treatment follow-up, preventing sun exposure, and performing monthly skin self-examinations. (See *Malignant melanoma teaching tips.*)

Prostate cancer

The most common cancer in men over age 50, prostate cancer is the second-leading cause of cancer deaths among males. Incidence is highest among Blacks and men with blood type A and lowest in Asians. Incidence isn't affected by socioeconomic status or fertility.

Education edge

Malignant melanoma teaching tips

• Inform the patient with malignant melanoma that the donor site for a skin graft may be as painful as (or even more painful than) the tumor excision site itself.
• When preparing the patient for discharge, emphasize the need for close follow-up care to detect recurrences early. Explain that recurrences and melanoma spread (if they occur) are commonly delayed, so follow-up must continue for years.
• Teach the patient how to recognize signs of melanoma recurrence.
• To help prevent malignant melanoma, stress the hazards of exposure to sunlight. Recommend that the patient use sunblock or sunscreen whenever he's outdoors. Teach him and his family to conduct monthly skin self-examinations and to have yearly screenings by a dermatologist.

Testing, testing

Both DRE and serum prostate-specific antigen (PSA) testing are used to screen for prostate cancer. There are limits to screening, however, and the ACS recommends that patients discuss screening with their practitioners.

Prognoses and predictions

When prostate cancer is treated in its localized form, the 5-year survival rate is 84%. After metastasis occurs, the rate drops below 35%. Death typically results from widespread bone metastasis.

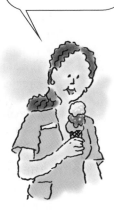

Risk factors for prostate cancer include a diet high in saturated fats. So tell your patient to go light on the ice cream—or skip it entirely!

What causes it

The cause of prostate cancer is unknown. Risk factors may include:
- age over 40
- diet high in saturated fats
- hormonal factors (testosterone may initiate or promote prostate cancer).

Pathophysiology

Prostate cancer grows slowly. When primary lesions spread beyond the prostate, they invade the prostatic capsule and spread along the ejaculatory ducts in the space between the seminal vesicles.

What to look for

Signs and symptoms of prostate cancer appear only in advanced disease stages and may include:
- difficult urination
- urinary dribbling
- urine retention
- unexplained cystitis (urinary bladder inflammation)
- hematuria (blood in the urine), a rare sign
- back or pelvic pain.

    DRE may reveal a hard nodule, which may be felt before other signs and symptoms develop.

What tests tell you

- PSA testing may be used to detect cancer.
- Transrectal prostatic ultrasonography can detect a mass.
- Biopsy confirms the diagnosis.

• Serum acid phosphatase levels are elevated in two-thirds of patients with metastasized prostate cancer. Successful therapy restores a normal enzyme level; a subsequent rise points to cancer recurrence.
• Increased alkaline phosphatase levels and a positive bone scan suggest bone metastasis. However, routine bone X-rays don't always show evidence of metastasis.

How it's treated

Treatment varies with each disease stage, but generally includes:
• radiation
• prostatectomy (prostate removal)
• orchiectomy (removal of one or both testes) to decrease androgen production
• cryoablation (tumor removal by freezing)
• hormone therapy with synthetic estrogen (diethylstilbestrol [DES]) or leuprolide (Lupron) and flutamide (Eulexin).

Radical measures

For localized lesions with no evidence of metastasis, radical prostatectomy (removal of the prostate with its capsule, seminal vesicles, ductus deferens, some pelvic fasciae and, sometimes, pelvic lymph nodes) is usually effective.

Radiation therapy

Radiation therapy is used in the early stages to relieve bone pain from metastatic skeletal involvement, or prophylactically for patients with regional lymph node tumors.

Planting a seed

Alternatively, implantating radioactive seeds (brachytherapy) focuses radiation on the prostate while minimizing exposure of surrounding tissue.

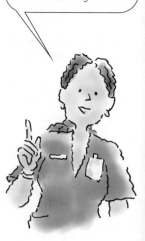

A radioactive seed may be implanted to focus radiation on the prostate while minimizing the effects on surrounding tissue.

Chemotherapy

If hormone or radiation therapy and surgery can't be done or prove ineffective, chemotherapy may be tried. Common combinations include vinblastine, doxorubicin, estramustine (Emcyt), paclitaxel (Abraxane), and vindesine.

What to do

• Provide supportive care if the patient is scheduled for prostatectomy, along with good postoperative care and symptomatic treatment of radiation and postsurgical complications.

• If incontinence or erectile dysfunction follows treatment, the patient and his significant other should be informed about corrective techniques and educational and support groups. Encourage the patient to contact the ACS for information.

• If the patient has received radiation or hormonal therapy, watch for and treat nausea, vomiting, dry skin, and alopecia. Also watch for adverse effects of DES (such as gynecomastia, fluid retention, nausea, and vomiting) and thrombophlebitis (such as pain, tenderness, swelling, warmth, and redness in a calf).

• Evaluate the patient. He should understand the treatment regimen and be aware of adverse reactions that require immediate medical attention (such as thrombophlebitis). He should also express his feelings about potential sexual dysfunction. (See *Prostate cancer teaching tips*.)

Squamous cell carcinoma

Squamous cell carcinoma is an invasive tumor with metastatic potential that arises from squamous cells—thin, flat cells on the outer layer of the skin. The disease commonly develops on sun-damaged areas.

Except for those on the lower lip and the ears, lesions on sun-damaged skin are less likely to metastasize as readily as lesions arising on unexposed skin. With treatment, prognosis is excellent for well-differentiated lesions on sun-damaged areas.

What causes it

Squamous cell carcinoma may result from overexposure to UV rays, radiation, chronic skin irritation and inflammation, ingestion of herbicides containing arsenic, and exposure to local carcinogens (such as tar and oil).

Sunbathing sequelae

Risk factors for squamous cell carcinoma include:
• being white, male, and over age 60
• having an outdoor job
• living in a sunny, warm climate
• premalignant lesions
• such hereditary diseases as xeroderma pigmentosum or albinism
• psoriasis or chronic discoid lupus erythematosus
• smallpox vaccination.

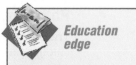

Education edge

Prostate cancer teaching tips

• Explain to the patient the expected after-effects of surgery (such as erectile dysfunction and incontinence) and radiation therapy. Discuss tube placement and dressing changes.

• Teach the patient to perform perineal exercises 1 to 10 times an hour. Have him squeeze his buttocks together, hold this position for a few seconds, and then relax. Encourage him to begin perineal exercises within 24 to 48 hours after surgery.

Pathophysiology

Transformation from a premalignant lesion to squamous cell carcinoma may start with hardening and inflammation of a preexisting lesion. When the disease arises from normal skin, the nodule grows slowly on a firm, hardened base. If untreated, this nodule eventually ulcerates and invades underlying tissues.

What to look for

Physical findings may include lesions on the face, ears, or backs of the hands and forearms as well as on other sun-damaged skin areas. Lesions may be scaly and keratotic (marked by excessive growth of horny skin tissue), with raised, irregular borders.

Powder and crust

In late disease, lesions grow outward from the epithelium, are friable (easily reduced to powder), and tend toward chronic crusting.

What tests tell you

Excisional biopsy of the lesion confirms the diagnosis.

How it's treated

Depending on the lesion, treatment may consist of wide surgical excision or electrodesiccation (destruction by electrical current) followed by curettage (tissue removal). These procedures offer good cosmetic results for smaller lesions.

Radiation therapy is usually used for older or debilitated patients. Mohs' surgery (serial excision and histologic analysis of cancerous tissues) may also be indicated.

What to do

• Disfiguring lesions may be distressing to the patient. Try to accept him as he is, develop strategies to increase his self-esteem, and project a caring relationship.
• Develop a consistent care plan for changing the patient's dressings. A standard routine helps the patient and his family learn how to care for the surgical wound. Keep the wound dry and clean. Try to control odor with balsam of Peru, yogurt flakes, oil of cloves,

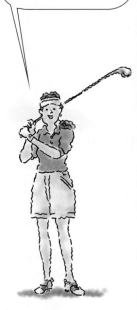

Overexposure to ultraviolet rays, as from sunlight, may lead to squamous cell carcinoma. So don't forget that sunblock when you're outdoors!

or other odor-masking substances (although they're usually ineffective for long-term use). Topical or systemic antibiotics also temporarily control odor and eventually alter the lesion's bacterial flora.

• Evaluate the patient. He should recover from surgery uneventfully. He should also demonstrate an understanding of sun protection methods and the importance of follow-up care. (See *Squamous cell carcinoma teaching tips.*)

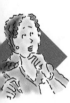

Quick quiz

1.   Reed-Sternberg cells are associated with:
   A.   prostate cancer.
   B.   malignant melanoma.
   C.   Hodgkin disease.
   D.   multiple myeloma.

Answer: C. The diagnosis of Hodgkin disease hinges on the presence of Reed-Sternberg cells.

2.   According to the ACS, how often should a woman have a mammogram?
   A.   Once every 3 years starting at age 21
   B.   Once a year starting at age 35
   C.   Every 5 years starting at age 30
   D.   Once a year starting at age 40

Answer: D. The ACS recommends a yearly mammogram for all women age 40 and older.

3.   One risk factor for prostate cancer is:
   A.   a history of infertility.
   B.   poverty.
   C.   being between ages 15 and 34.
   D.   being older than age 40.

Answer: D. Prostate cancer seldom develops before age 40. Socioeconomic status and infertility don't appear to affect the risk of this cancer.

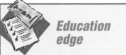

Education edge

Squamous cell carcinoma teaching tips

To help prevent recurrence of squamous cell carcinoma, cover these topics when providing patient teaching:

• Avoid excessive sun exposure.

• Apply sunscreen 30 to 60 minutes before sun exposure. Use a strong sunscreen containing para-aminobenzoic acid, oxybenzone, and zinc oxide.

• Wear protective clothing, such as a hat and long sleeves, when outdoors.

• Use a lipscreen to protect the lips from sun damage.

• Periodically examine the skin for precancerous lesions, which should be removed promptly.

4. The leading cause of cancer death in women is:
    A. breast cancer.
    B. lung cancer.
    C. cervical cancer.
    D. ovarian cancer.

Answer: B. Lung cancer is the second most common cancer among females in the United States (after breast cancer) and is the leading cause of cancer death in women.

Scoring

☆☆☆ If you answered all four questions correctly, congratulations! You've conquered the cancer chapter and are ready to move on with your life.

☆☆ If you answered three questions correctly, pat yourself on the back! Your cancer comprehension is nearly complete.

☆ If you answered fewer than three questions correctly, don't withdraw. Just review the chapter again, and your knowledge deficit is bound to go into remission.

Obesity

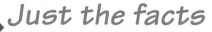
Just the facts

In this chapter, you'll learn:

♦ effects of and complications associated with obesity

♦ causes of overweight and obesity

♦ guidelines for evaluating weight

♦ risk factors associated with obesity

♦ treatments to help ensure successful weight loss.

A look at obesity

The prevalence of obesity in the United States has increased markedly over the past two decades. According to the Centers for Disease Control and Prevention (CDC), approximately one-third of American adults age 20 and older are either overweight or obese. The trend toward obesity has been steadily increasing. Children haven't escaped the trend, with 17% of 2 to 5 year olds 19% of 6 to 11 year olds, and 18% of 12 to 19 year olds overweight.

Taking an awfully big risk

Excess weight substantially increases the risk of diabetes, cardiovascular disease, certain types of cancer, and other diseases, including:
- gynecologic abnormalities
- osteoarthritis
- gallbladder disease
- stress incontinence.

The risk of death from all causes in obese people is 50% to 100% greater than in people of normal weight. In addition, the annual health care cost of obesity is estimated to exceed $140 billion per year.

A morbid thought

In addition to the risk of morbidity from obesity-related diseases, obesity can increase the morbidity of other preexisting disorders.

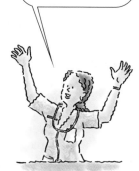

Obesity is a huge problem that can lead to a multitude of other diseases and complications.

Obese patients with existing coronary artery disease (CAD), type 2 diabetes, stroke, and sleep apnea are at high risk for developing disease-related complications that can lead to death.

And if that isn't disturbing enough

Obesity is also associated with complications during surgery, pregnancy, and labor and delivery. A major contributor to preventable deaths, obesity also leads to low self-esteem, negative self-image, hopelessness, and negative social consequences, such as stereotyping, prejudice, social isolation, and discrimination.

> I'm telling you, if you take in that many calories, you'll have to work extra hard to burn them off. Why don't we just skip dessert?

Causes

The basic cause of obesity is an energy imbalance that results when the number of calories taken in exceeds the number of calories used for energy. A recurring imbalance leads to weight gain over time. This imbalance most commonly results from overeating, inactivity, or both.

Risk factors

You may notice that some people who are overweight eat only moderate amounts of food but still gain weight and that some average-weight people overeat but never gain weight. That's because other factors can also influence fat accumulation in the body.

Inheriting grandma's hips...

A family history of obesity increases a person's chance of becoming obese by 25% to 30%. In addition, body fat distribution is influenced by genetics. Families also share diet and lifestyle habits that can contribute to obesity.

...and her remote control

Environment also strongly influences obesity. This includes such lifestyle behaviors as eating habits, diet, and level of physical activity. Americans tend to eat high-fat foods and put taste and convenience ahead of nutrition. Only 22% of Americans achieve the recommended 30 minutes of physical activity each day.

Calorie conundrum

Nutrition also plays an important role in weight gain. Although the type of food makes a difference, consuming too many calories in any form leads to weight gain. High-fat foods are known to be

> An inactive lifestyle can contribute to obesity. Let's get moving!

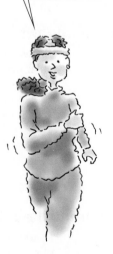

high in calories, but eating too much of low-fat foods can lead to overconsumption, too.

Eating under the influence

Psychological factors can also influence eating habits. Many people eat in response to positive emotions, such as excitement, or to negative emotions, such as boredom, sadness, and anger.

It can get rather complicated

Some illnesses can lead to obesity or a tendency to gain weight. Examples include hypothyroidism, Cushing's syndrome, depression, and certain neurological problems that can lead to overeating. Also, such drugs as steroids, antipsychotics, and some antidepressants can cause weight gain. A practitioner can tell whether underlying medical conditions are causing weight gain or making weight loss difficult.

A few more factors

Sociocultural factors, such as race, gender, income, education, and ethnicity, may also contribute to obesity. For example, males older than age 45 and females who are postmenopausal are at greater risk.

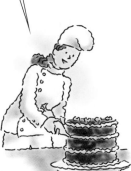

You say you tend to eat when you're excited? Well, you'll have to tone down your excitement because I just finished frosting this!

Evaluating weight

The CDC has developed definitions for what constitutes being overweight and obese. According to the definitions, an adult who has a body mass index (BMI) of between 25 and 29.9 is considered overweight; an adult with a BMI of 30 or higher is considered obese.

A person's BMI usually correlates with the amount of body fat he has. Other methods besides BMI of estimating body fat include waist circumference and skinfold thickness measurements. Once a patient's body fat has been determined, his risk factors for diseases and other conditions can be evaluated.

BMI

BMI is a measurement of weight in relationship to height. It can be calculated using conventional pounds and inches or the metric system (using kilograms and centimeters). (See *Calculating BMI*, page 870.) BMI can also be estimated without doing any calculations. (See *Using a BMI chart*, page 871.)

Calculating BMI

You can use one of the formulas below to calculate your patient's body mass index (BMI).

$$BMI = \left(\frac{\text{weight in pounds}}{\text{height in inches} \times \text{height in inches}}\right) \times 703$$

OR

$$BMI = \left(\frac{\text{weight in kilograms}}{\text{height in centimeters} \times \text{height in centimeters}}\right) \times 10{,}000$$

OR

$$BMI = \left(\frac{\text{weight in kilograms}}{\text{height in meters} \times \text{height in meters}}\right)$$

A little or a lot o' weight

Officially, a person with a BMI of 25 to 29.9 is considered overweight, whereas someone with a BMI of 30 or above is considered obese. Obesity may be further categorized as follows:

- Class I—BMI of 30 to 34.9
- Class II—BMI of 35 to 39.9
- Class III—BMI of 40 or more.

Tipping the scales

Keep in mind that the relationship between body weight and good health is more complicated than simply comparing the number on the scale to a weight range table. In fact, weight range tables aren't appropriate to use with all individuals because not everyone whose weight falls within the "healthy" range is necessarily at a healthy weight. For example, one patient might have more fat and less muscle than what's considered healthy, and another person might have more muscle than fat yet may be fine.

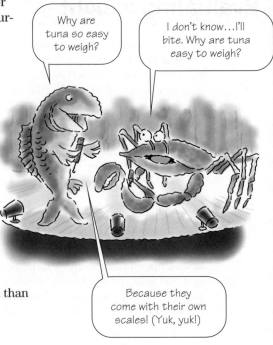

Why are tuna so easy to weigh?

I don't know...I'll bite. Why are tuna easy to weigh?

Because they come with their own scales! (Yuk, yuk!)

Using a BMI chart

Body mass index (BMI) is a relationship of weight to height. The BMI ranges shown here are for adults. They aren't exact ranges for healthy or unhealthy weights; however, they show that health risks increase at higher levels of overweight and obesity. To use this graph, find your patient's weight along the bottom and then go straight up until you come to the line that matches his height. The shaded area indicates whether your patient is healthy, overweight, or obese.

A BMI of 18.5 to 24.9 defines healthy weight.

A BMI of 25 to 29.9 defines overweight.

A BMI 30 or higher defines obesity.

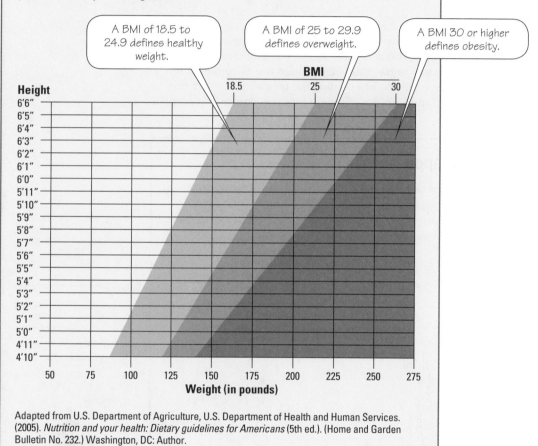

Adapted from U.S. Department of Agriculture, U.S. Department of Health and Human Services. (2005). *Nutrition and your health: Dietary guidelines for Americans* (5th ed.). (Home and Garden Bulletin No. 232.) Washington, DC: Author.

Waist circumference

Where a person's fat is deposited on the body (weight distribution) may be a more important indicator of health problems than how much fat he actually has. People with a high distribution of fat around their waists (apple-shaped) as opposed to their hips and thighs (pear-shaped) are at greater risk for such diseases as type 2 diabetes, dyslipidemia, hypertension, and cardiovascular disease. (See *Pear- or apple-shaped?*)

Middle measure

To evaluate weight distribution, measure waist circumference. Locate the upper hip bone and the top of the iliac crest. Place a measuring tape in a horizontal place around the abdomen at the level of the iliac crest. Before reading the tape measure, ensure that the tape is snug, but doesn't compress the skin, and is parallel

Pear- or apple-shaped?

The illustrations below depict an apple-shaped person and a pear-shaped person. Studies indicate that where excess body fat is deposited may be a more important and reliable indicator of disease risk than degree of total body fat.

Pear-shaped

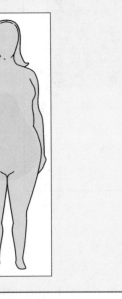

Apple-shaped

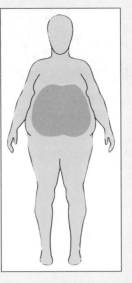

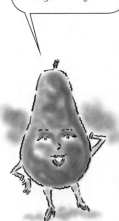

I think my shape is divine, but it might not look so good on you...

to the floor. Measure at the end of expiration. If the measurement is greater than 35″ (89 cm) for women or 40″ (102 cm) for men with a normal BMI, your patient has a greater risk of health problems. If the BMI is 35 or higher, waist measurement is irrelevant because disease risk is already high based on the BMI alone.

Risk factors

Determining how many health risk factors your patient has will further help you assess his need for weight control. The more risk factors present, the more your patient will benefit from weight loss.

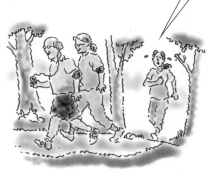

You should ask your patients (puff) how much exercise they get each day—if you can catch up with them! (gasp)

Questions, questions

Ask your patient the following questions to assess his risk factors for obesity:
• Do you smoke? If so, how many packs per day?
• How much exercise do you get each day? Do you have a sedentary lifestyle or job?
• What is your age?
• Are you postmenopausal (for women)?
• Do you have a personal or family history of heart disease?
• Do you have diabetes or an impaired fasting glucose level?
• Do you have high blood pressure or have risk factors for high blood pressure?
• Do you have high low-density lipoprotein (LDL) cholesterol levels or low high-density lipoprotein (HDL) cholesterol levels?
• Are your triglyceride levels elevated?

Complications

Obese patients are more susceptible to certain complications than nonobese patients. The most common complications involve the pulmonary, cardiovascular, GI, and musculoskeletal systems. (See *Complications of obesity*, pages 874 and 875.)

Complications of obesity

Obese patients typically have more complications that affect various body systems. Here are some of the more common complications along with their pathophysiology and related nursing interventions.

System	Pathophysiologic consequences	Potential problems	Nursing interventions
Pulmonary	• Decreased diaphragmatic excursion • Decreased vital capacity • Decreased alveolar ventilation • Decreased compliance • Decreased respiratory drive • Chronic carbon dioxide retention	• Increased respiratory rate • Ventilation-perfusion mismatch • Hypoxemia • Respiratory acidosis • Difficulty weaning from the ventilator • Obstructive sleep apnea • Increased risk of aspiration	• Try noninvasive positive pressure ventilation, such as bilevel positive airway pressure or continuous positive airway pressure. • Be prepared for intubation. • Calculate tidal volume based on ideal weight, not actual weight. • Minimize time the patient spends in a supine position. • Control secretions to maintain airway patency. • Reposition at least every 2 hours.
Cardiovascular	• Left ventricular hypertrophy • Increased total blood volume • Increased stroke volume • Increased cardiac output • Increased cardiac deconditioning	• Right-sided and left-sided heart failure • Hypertension • Myocardial infarction • Stroke • Chronic venous insufficiency • Deep vein thrombosis • Pulmonary embolism	• Encourage mobility as tolerated. • Watch for signs of fluid overload. • Monitor blood pressure. • Administer medications as ordered.
Endocrine	• Increased metabolic requirements • Increased insulin resistance	• Type 2 diabetes • Hyperlipidemia	• Carefully monitor blood glucose levels, especially if the patient is receiving a steroid. • Work with a dietitian to ensure that metabolic needs are met.
Gastrointestinal	• Increased intra-abdominal pressure • Increased gastric volume	• Increased incidence of gastroesophageal reflux disease • Increased risk of aspiration, especially with enteral feedings • Increased constipation • Increased risk of pancreatitis	• Administer medications as ordered. • Keep head of bed at 30 degrees when possible. • Increase fluid and fiber intake. • Monitor amylase and lipase levels. • Be alert for altered pharmacokinetics for some drugs.

Complications of obesity *(continued)*

System	Pathophysiologic consequences	Potential problems	Nursing interventions
Immune	• Impaired immune response • Impaired cell-mediated immunity	• Impaired healing • Increased risk of wound infections • Increased skin breakdown and pressure ulcers • Decreased resistance to infection	• Monitor wounds for early signs of infection. • Reposition the patient at least every 2 hours. • Monitor skin folds for pressure ulcers or skin breakdown. • Work with a dietitian to ensure that metabolic needs are met for proper healing.
Musculoskeletal	• Increased joint trauma • Decreased mobility • Increased atrophy from lack of use • Increased pain with movement	• Osteoarthritis • Rheumatoid arthritis	• Encourage mobilization. • Perform range-of-motion exercises with the patient. • Provide nonpharmacologic pain-relief measures.

Treatment

Treatment of obesity can be long and difficult. No single treatment method or combination of methods is guaranteed to produce weight loss or maintain weight loss in all people. Treatment can be directed using guidelines from the National Heart, Lung and Blood Institute. (See *Treatment algorithm for obesity*, page 876.)

Keep in mind that the road to successful weight loss is long and difficult. Watch out for road blocks and the occasional flat tire along the way.

Diet therapy

Diet, or nutrition, therapy includes instructing patients how to modify their diets to decrease calorie intake.

Calorie culprits

A key element of the current recommendation is a moderated reduction in calories to achieve a slow, progressive weight loss of 1 to 2 lb (0.5 to 1 kg) per week. Calories should be reduced only to the level required to achieve the goal weight.

Weighing the evidence

Treatment algorithm for obesity

This algorithm can help guide your treatment of an obese patient.

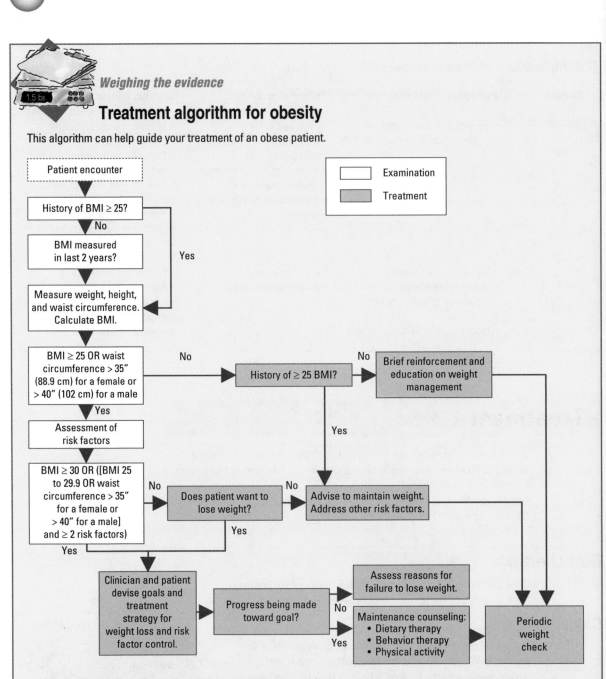

Source: U.S. Department of Health and Human Services, Public Health Service, National Institutes of Health, National Heart, Lung, and Blood Institute. (1988). *Clinical guidelines on the identification, evaluation, and treatment of overweight and obesity in adults: The Evidence Report* (NIH Publication No. 98-4083). Rockville, MD: Author.

Mindful menus

Successful weight reduction is more likely to occur when the patient's food preferences are included in the menu and when dietary education is performed.

Dietary tips of beef

When educating your patient, be sure to:
• cover the energy value of different foods and discuss food components, such as fats, carbohydrates (including dietary fiber), and proteins
• encourage the patient to read nutrition labels
• promote new habits of purchasing, especially low-calorie foods
• instruct on food preparation, especially the need to avoid adding high-calorie ingredients (such as fats and oils) during cooking
• warn against the overconsumption of high-calorie foods
• stress the importance of adequate water intake, reducing portion sizes, and limiting alcohol consumption.

> When educating a patient about weight loss, remember to stress the importance of reducing calories and planning meals that include the foods he likes. In other words, teach him to spend his calorie allowance wisely.

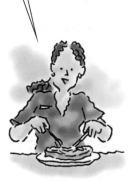

Increased physical activity

Exercise plays a critical role in the loss and maintenance of body weight. Exercise is important for increasing energy expenditure, maintaining or increasing lean body mass, and promoting fat loss. These changes in body composition result in improved body dimensions and, possibly, an increased metabolic rate.

First, talk the talk...

Patients with medical problems, however, commonly have difficulty exercising. Any patient who wishes to start an exercise routine should first discuss it with their practitioner and get approval to start exercising.

> Remember that not all patients can just begin increasing activity on their own. Advise them to discuss exercising with their practitioner first.

...then walk the walk

Daily walking is an attractive form of physical exercise, especially for the obese patient. Advise your patient to begin by walking 10 minutes 3 days per week, and then build up to 30 to 45 minutes of more intense walking at least 5 to 7 days per week. With this regimen, an additional 100 to 200 calories/day can be expended. A moderate amount of physical activity that burns about 250 calories can be achieved in various ways. (See *Burning calories*, page 878.)

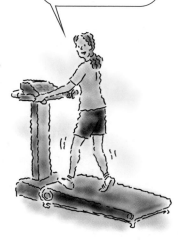

Every little bit helps

Reducing sedentary time, such as time spent watching television, is another way to increase activity. Patients should build

Burning calories

This chart shows the activity and duration needed to burn 150 calories for an average 154-lb (70-kg) adult.

Activity	Intensity	Duration (in minutes)
Volleyball, noncompetitive	Moderate	43
Walking, moderate pace (3 mph, 20 minutes/mile)	Moderate	37
Walking, brisk pace (4 mph, 15 minutes/mile)	Moderate	32
Table tennis	Moderate	32
Raking leaves	Moderate	32
Social dancing	Moderate	29
Lawn mowing (powered push mower)	Moderate	29
Jogging	Hard	18
Field hockey	Hard	16
Running	Very hard	13

physical activities into each day. For example, parking farther than usual from work or shopping and walking up stairs instead of taking elevators are easy ways to increase daily physical activity.

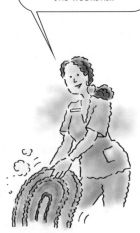

All those little daily chores and extra steps can add up. Think of how many calories you'll burn—and how much cleaner your house will be—by the weekend!

Behavior therapy

Behavior therapy is a useful adjunct to planned decreases in food intake and increases in physical activity. The goal of behavior therapy is to overcome barriers to compliance with eating and activity habits.

Changing for the long haul

The primary assumptions of behavior therapy are listed below. (Remember, long-term weight reduction most likely won't succeed unless new habits are acquired.)

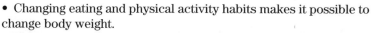

- Changing eating and physical activity habits makes it possible to change body weight.
- Eating and physical activity behaviors are learned and can be modified.
- Environment must be changed to change patterns.

Strategies for success

Various strategies must be used for behavior modification because no single method is superior.

Monitor thyself

- Self-monitoring of eating and physical activity—This strategy involves recording the amount, type, caloric value, and nutrient composition of food eaten and the frequency, intensity, and type of physical activity performed each day. Recording this information allows the patient to gain insight into his behavior.

Cool, calm, and collected

- Stress management—Stress triggers dysfunctional eating habits. Using coping strategies, meditation, relaxation techniques, and exercise can help relieve stress.

Keep the safety on the trigger

- Stimulus control—This strategy involves identifying triggers—stimuli that encourage incidental eating—and taking the necessary steps to limit them; for example, by keeping high-calorie foods out of the house, limiting times and places of eating, and avoiding situations in which overeating occurs.

Alternatives, please

- Problem solving—This includes identifying weight-related problems and planning and implementing alternative behaviors.

Now that's rewarding!

- Contingency management—Rewarding positive changes in behavior, such as increasing exercise or reducing consumption of a specific food, can be an effective strategy.

A mental pat on the back

- Cognitive restructuring—This strategy involves changing self-defeating thoughts and feelings by replacing them with positive thoughts and setting reasonable goals.

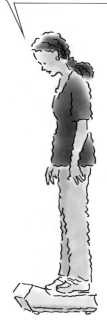

Unfortunately, when trying to lose weight, there's no escaping the dreaded scale. Yikes!

With a little help from friends

- Social support—A strong support system can help provide the emotional support needed to lose weight. Including friends and family in physical activity and diet or joining a support group can be beneficial.

Pharmacotherapy

Drug therapy should be considered if, after 6 months of diet therapy and increased activity, the patient hasn't lost the recommended 1 lb (0.5 kg) per week.

Don't be so modest

Drugs produce a modest weight loss of 4.4 to 22 lb (2 to 10 kg) within the first 6 months and can help maintain the weight loss. However, most studies show a rapid weight gain after the drugs are stopped. When drug therapy is effective and adverse effects are manageable, therapy can be continued long-term; however, no one knows how long drug therapy can safely be maintained.

When the risks are high

Because few long-term studies have been conducted on the safety and effectiveness of weight loss medication, such drugs should be used only by patients who are at an increased medical risk because of their weight. These patients include those with a BMI of 30 or more and those with one of the following disorders:
- hypertension
- dyslipidemia
- CAD
- type 2 diabetes
- sleep apnea.

Weighing the odds of success

Not every patient responds to drug therapy. Tests show that initial responders tend to continue to respond, while nonresponders are less likely to respond even with increases in dosage. Drug therapy should be discontinued if adverse effects are unmanageable or if therapy is ineffective. The decision to add a drug to an obesity treatment program should be made after consideration of all potential risks and benefits and only after all behavioral options have been used.

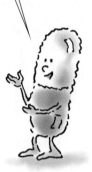

No one knows for sure how long weight-loss medications can be used safely. So, it's best to use them only when patients are at an increased medical risk because of their weight and all other options have been used.

Altering absorption

If the patient is a good candidate for drug therapy, the practitioner may prescribe or recommend orlistat (Xenical by prescription and Alli over the counter). This drug works peripherally to inhibit pancreatic lipase and, therefore, decreases fat absorption in the GI tract. It should be used in conjunction with a reduced-calorie diet with 30% of calories from fat. Adverse reactions include headache, flatus with discharge, fecal urgency, fatty or oily stool, pancreatitis, and abdominal pain. Absorption of fat-soluble vitamins also is decreased.

Other drugs for weight loss are under development.

Weight-loss surgery

Surgery is an option for some patients who are experiencing complications from severe and resistant obesity. It should be considered if the risk of remaining obese is greater than the risk of surgery.

Committed to success

Long-term success of surgery depends on the patient's ability to change behavior and commit to lifelong follow-up. About 70% of patients maintain a weight loss of 50% for 5 years.

Two options

Two types of surgeries are primarily used to promote weight loss: restrictive and malabsorptive-restrictive procedures.

Restrictive procedures

In gastric restriction, also known as *vertical banded gastroplasty* and *adjustable gastric banding*, the size of the stomach is surgically decreased so that a patient feels full after eating a small amount of food.

Tighten it up

In vertical banded gastroplasty, a vertical row of staples is inserted across the patient's stomach, decreasing the stomach's size to 15 to 30 ml. A band decreases the opening from the upper pouch to about 1 cm, which delays gastric emptying. Over time, the pouch can stretch to hold more food. (See *Surgical weight loss procedures*, page 882.)

Surgical weight loss procedures

Two types of surgical procedures promote weight loss: restrictive and combination malabsorptive-restrictive procedures.

Restrictive procedures

Adjustable gastric banding

Vertical banded gastroplasty

Malabsorptive-restrictive procedures

Gastric bypass (Roux-en-Y)

Biliopancreatic diversion with duodenal switch

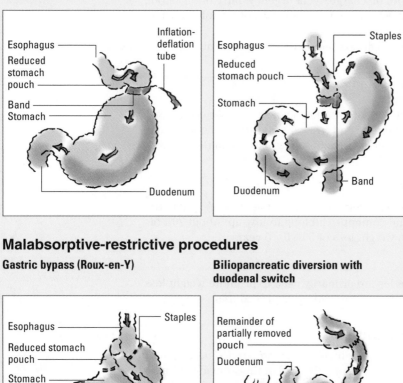

Rubber-banded and ready for action

In adjustable gastric banding, a silicone rubber band is placed around the upper portion of the stomach, creating a small pouch with a narrow opening into the larger portion of the stomach. The band can be inflated or deflated with saline solution through a tube attached to an access port under the skin, allowing the size of the stomach opening to be adjusted. This procedure may be performed laparoscopically.

Complicating the situation

Complications of gastric restriction may include bursting of the staples if too much food or liquid is consumed before the staple line heals and obstruction if food isn't chewed well. Nutritional complications include hypoalbuminemia and vitamin deficiencies as well as nausea and vomiting.

Malabsorptive-restrictive procedures

Malabsorptive-restrictive procedures, which reduce stomach size as well as the number of calories and nutrients the body can absorb, produce better weight loss results than gastric resection.

Get rid of it...quickly!

After surgery, rapid dumping of food from the stomach into the small intestine limits calorie absorption, leading to weight loss. Nausea, diarrhea, and abdominal cramping may occur, but these adverse effects improve over time.

Take the bypass route

Two types of malabsorptive-restrictive procedures are currently being done.
• Gastric bypass—Also known as *Roux-en-Y gastric bypass*, this procedure combines gastric resection with a bypass of the duodenum and the first portion of the jejunum. It's the most commonly performed surgical weight loss procedure and is recommended for long-term weight loss.
• Biliopancreatic diversion—This is a more complicated surgery in which the lower part of the stomach is removed and the remaining pouch is connected to the terminal segment of the small intestine, thus bypassing the duodenum and jejunum. This procedure isn't commonly used because it can lead to nutritional deficiencies. Patients who have undergone biliopancreatic diversion must take fat-soluble vitamin (A, D, E, and K) supplements.

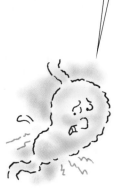

Malabsorptive-restrictive procedures may help with weight loss, but I hate when they give me cramps!

Everything in moderation

In a modified version of the procedure, a larger portion of the stomach and pyloric valve are in place, allowing control of the movement of stomach contents into the duodenum. With this variation, the patient can eat more food than following other procedures.

Nursing considerations

Many of the nursing considerations are the same, regardless of the type of weight loss surgery performed.

Pre-op preparations

- Before surgery, make sure the patient has undergone a complete medical and psychological evaluation. The patient will commonly have extensive nutritional counseling before the procedure also.
- Make sure the patient has signed an appropriate consent form.
- Administer I.V. fluids and total parenteral nutrition (TPN), as ordered.

Post-op care

- If the patient has a nasogastric tube in place after surgery, don't reposition the tube unless ordered by the practitioner.
- Encourage early mobility and coughing and deep-breathing exercises. Remember that obese patients are at higher risk for pulmonary complications.
- Monitor the patient's vital signs, intake and output, and daily weight.
- Administer I.V. fluids, TPN, and electrolyte replacements, as ordered.
- Carefully monitor laboratory values, and be alert for electrolyte disturbances.
- Administer pain medication, as needed.
- Remind the patient of the importance of following his set diet. Advise him that he may need vitamin supplements.
- Inform the patient about possible complications and when to notify the practitioner.

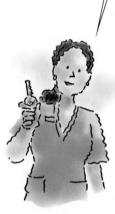

Weight-loss surgery can be a key factor in successfully controlling weight.

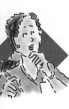

Quick quiz

1. Which of the following changes is a benefit of weight loss?
    A. Lower HDL levels
    B. Higher LDL levels
    C. Increased blood pressure
    D. Reduced risk of diabetes and cardiovascular disease

Answer: D. Benefits of weight loss include higher HDL levels, decreased blood pressure, and a reduced risk of diabetes and cardiovascular disease.

2. A patient with a BMI of 37.9 falls into which BMI class?
    A. Class I
    B. Class II
    C. Class III
    D. Class IV

Answer: B. There are three classes of BMI. Class I is a BMI of 30 to 34.9, Class II is a BMI of 35 to 39.9, and Class III is a BMI of 40 or more.

3. One of the complications of obesity is:
    A. hypertension.
    B. type 1 diabetes.
    C. hypothyroidism.
    D. cancer.

Answer: A. Hypertension is one of the complications of obesity. Obese patients are more likely to have type 2 diabetes, not type 1. Hypothyroidism and cancer aren't known to be complications of obesity.

4. Which type of weight-loss surgery can lead to the most nutritional deficiencies?
    A. Adjustable gastric banding
    B. Biliopancreatic diversion
    C. Vertical banded gastroplasty
    D. Gastric bypass

Answer: B. Biliopancreatic diversion can lead to the most nutritional deficiencies because the patient can no longer absorb fat-soluble vitamins (A, D, E, and K).

Scoring

⭐⭐⭐ If you answered all four questions correctly, terrific! You've taken
a heavy weight off your shoulders by knowing all the right
answers.

⭐⭐ If you answered three questions correctly, well done! Practice a
little cognitive restructuring and turn those negative thoughts
into positive ones.

⭐ If you answered fewer than three questions correctly, don't get
down on yourself and start heading for the cookie jar yet.
Keep in mind the goal is just to do better next time!

21

Gerontologic care

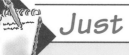

Just the facts

In this chapter, you'll learn:

♦ normal physiologic changes associated with aging

♦ techniques for assessing an older adult

♦ signs and symptoms of common adverse drug effects and interactions

♦ methods to manage urinary incontinence and prevent falls.

A look at gerontologic care

People age 65 and older require health care services more often than any other age-group. Chances are, you'll care for a great many older adults—especially if you practice in California, New York, Florida, Illinois, Texas, Ohio, Pennsylvania, Michigan, or New Jersey, where 52% of people age 65 and older live.

Attitudes about aging are improving among the general public and health care professionals alike. More people have come to view aging as a normal lifelong process that begins at conception and culminates with old age.

The American Nurses Association (ANA) emphasizes holistic care and treatment of elderly patients. Significantly, the ANA now uses the term *gerontologic* rather than *geriatric* to describe the process of providing nursing care for older adults. Not just a matter of semantics, this change acknowledges the need to address not only age-related diseases but also associated physiologic, pathologic, psychological, economic, and sociologic issues.

Demographic trends

The older adult population is growing rapidly and becoming more racially and ethnically diverse, reflecting the demographic changes in the U.S. population. In 2008, 38.9 million people age 65 and older were living in the United States, and the number of older adults is projected to grow to 55 million by 2020.

The old get older

Furthermore, the older adult population of the United States is getting progressively older. In 2006, there were over 5.3 million people age 85 and older.

Gender trends

Older women outnumber older men, and the proportion of women to men increases with age. There are approximately 22.4 million older women, compared with 16.5 million older men.

Health perceptions among the elderly

Contrary to stereotypes, most older adults view their health positively. Even if they have chronic illnesses, four out of five describe their health as good or excellent.

Still, the likelihood of having a chronic illness rises with age. More than 20% of people age 65 and over have at least one chronic condition, and many have multiple chronic conditions.

Implications for nursing

These demographic trends have important implications for health care. For one thing, they show a need for increased long-term care services and more gerontologic nurses, especially in states that have high numbers of elderly people.

Also, as the number of elderly women increases, so does the need for information about women's health across the entire life span.

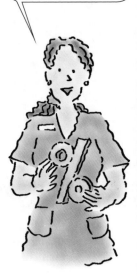

The likelihood of having a chronic illness rises with age, with more than 20% of those age 65 and over having at least one chronic condition.

Normal changes of aging

With aging comes the loss of some body cells and reduced metabolism in others. These changes lead to altered body composition and reductions in certain body functions. For instance, adipose (fatty) tissue stores typically increase with age, whereas lean body mass and bone mineral content diminish.

Aging and its effect on the body

Although the effects of aging vary with the specific tissue or organ, all older adults eventually become more susceptible to fatigue and disease. Here are some of the physiologic changes that occur with aging.

- Gradual loss of subcutaneous fat and elastin causes the skin to wrinkle and sag.
- After about age 50, brain cells decrease at a rate of 1% per year.

- Between ages 30 and 75, the heart's efficiency decreases by about 30%, and the lungs' by about 40%
- Between ages 40 and 90, renal function and bladder size and capacity decrease by as much as 50%.
- The liver's efficiency decreases by 10%.

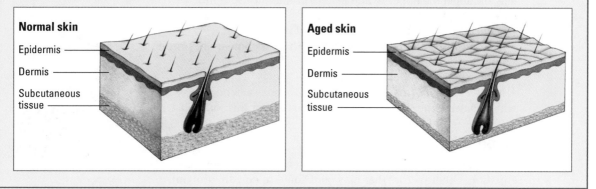

Normal skin
- Epidermis
- Dermis
- Subcutaneous tissue

Aged skin
- Epidermis
- Dermis
- Subcutaneous tissue

Older but not necessarily ill

Although an older person's body tends to work less efficiently than a younger person's, illness doesn't inevitably accompany old age. Certainly, the heart, lungs, kidneys, and other organs are less efficient at age 60 than at age 20, but that doesn't mean aging always leads to the breakdown of body systems.

As a nurse, you must recognize these gradual changes in body function so you can adjust your assessment techniques accordingly. (See *Aging and its effect on the body*.) It's also important to understand how aging increases the risk of developing certain diseases and sustaining certain types of injuries.

Nutritional aspects of aging

Protein, vitamin, and mineral requirements usually remain stable as we age, but caloric needs decrease. Diminished activity may lower daily energy requirements by about 200 calories for men and women between ages 51 and 75, by 400 calories for women older than age 75, and by 500 calories for men older than age 75.

Notes on nutrition

Other physiologic changes that can affect an elderly patient's nutritional status include:
• decreased renal function, which heightens susceptibility to dehydration and renal calculi formation
• loss of calcium and nitrogen (in patients who aren't ambulatory)
• diminished enzyme activity
• reduced pepsin and hydrochloric acid secretion, which may reduce the absorption of calcium and vitamins B_1 and B_2
• decreased salivary flow and a reduced taste sensation, which may diminish the appetite and lead to greater consumption of sweet and spicy foods
• reduced gastric motility and intestinal peristalsis
• thinning of tooth enamel, causing teeth to become more brittle
• decreased biting force
• diminished gag reflex
• limited mobility (in persons with certain health conditions), which may hamper the ability to prepare food or feed oneself.

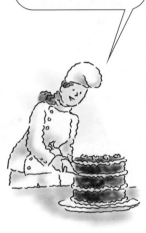

Some older adults eat more sweet or spicy foods because taste sensation diminishes with age.

GI problems

Reduced intestinal motility may lead to such GI disorders as constipation. Other factors that may contribute to constipation in older adults include:
• nutritionally inadequate diets that are high in soft, refined foods and low in dietary fiber
• physical inactivity
• emotional stress
• use of certain medications
• inadequate fluid intake due to decreased thirst perception.

Laxative overload

Some older adults abuse laxatives, resulting in rapid transport of food through the GI tract. This, in turn, decreases digestion and absorption.

Socioeconomic and psychological factors

Socioeconomic and psychological factors that can affect an older person's nutritional status include:
• loneliness
• perceived decline in his importance to the family
• susceptibility to nutritional misinformation
• lack of money to buy nutritionally beneficial foods
• lack of regular dental care.

Skin, hair, and nails

Age-related subcutaneous fat loss, dermal thinning, and decreasing collagen lead to the development of facial lines (crow's feet) around the eyes, mouth, and nose. Women's skin, which is thinner and drier than men's, shows signs of aging about 10 years earlier.

Also, the supraclavicular and axillary regions, knuckles, and hand tendons and vessels become more prominent, as do fat pads over bony prominences. Cell replacement decreases by 50%.

High and relatively dry

Mucous membranes become dry, and sweat gland output lessens as the number of active sweat glands decreases. Body temperature grows harder to regulate as sweat glands decrease in size, number, and function and subcutaneous fat is lost.

Pigmentary plotlines

Skin also loses elasticity with age, to the point where it may seem almost transparent. Although the production of melanocytes (skin cells that produce the pigment melanin) decreases, localized melanocyte proliferation is common. Thus, older people tend to have brown spots (senile lentigo), especially in areas regularly exposed to the sun.

Hair pigment decreases with age as the number of melanocytes declines, so the hair may turn gray or white. Hair also thins; by age 70, it may be baby fine.

Hormonal changes cause pubic hair loss. Facial hair generally increases in postmenopausal women and decreases in aging men.

News about nails

With age, nail growth slows and longitudinal ridges, thickening, brittleness, and malformations may increase. Toenails may become discolored.

Tags, tumors, and keratosis

Other common skin conditions in elderly people include:
• senile keratosis—overgrowth and thickening of the horny epithelium
• acrochordon—benign skin tags
• senile angiomas—benign tumors made up of blood vessels or lymph vessels.

Also, wounds take longer to heal.

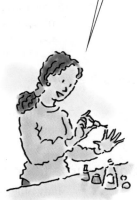

With age, nail growth slows and longitudinal ridges, thickening, brittleness, and malformations increase.

Eyes and vision

Aging brings changes to both the eye structure and visual acuity. With advancing age, the eyes sit deeper in the bony orbits and the eyelids lose their elasticity, becoming baggy and wrinkled. The conjunctiva (the membrane coating the eye's outer surface) becomes thinner and yellow, and pingueculae (yellowish spots) may develop on the bulbar conjunctiva.

No more tears?

As the lacrimal apparatus gradually loses fatty tissue, tears diminish in quantity. Tears also tend to evaporate more quickly, increasing the risk of eye infection.

The cornea loses its luster and flattens. The iris fades or develops irregular pigmentation, turning pale. Increased connective tissue may cause hardening of the eye sphincter muscles.

Let there be (more) light

The pupil shrinks, decreasing the amount of light that reaches the retina. To see objects clearly, older adults need about three times as much light as younger people.

Aging also diminishes night vision and depth perception. The sclera becomes thick and rigid, and fat deposits cause yellowing. Senile hyaline plaques may develop.

Floaters and rings

The vitreous humor (the glassy substance behind the lens) may degenerate over time, revealing opacities and floating vitreous debris on examination. Also, the vitreous may detach from the retina, appearing as an empty space. Through an ophthalmoscope, the detached vitreous looks like a dark ring in front of the optic disk.

Lens lessons

The lens enlarges and loses transparency with age. Accommodation diminishes from decreased lens elasticity. This leads to presbyopia, a vision defect in which objects very close to the eye can't be seen clearly without corrective lenses.

Color curtailment

Many older adults have impaired color vision, especially in the blue and green ranges, as the photoreceptive retinal cones deteriorate. Decreased reabsorption of intraocular fluid may predispose older adults to glaucoma.

> Don't be surprised if an older adult has poor color vision. With age, the photoreceptive retinal cones deteriorate.

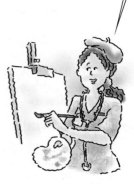

Ears and hearing

Many elderly persons lose some degree of hearing. Hearing loss sometimes results from gradual cerumen buildup in the ear. More often, though, hearing loss progresses slowly, resulting in presbycusis (sometimes called *senile deafness*). This irreversible, bilateral, sensorineural hearing loss usually starts during middle age and slowly worsens. Presbycusis affects men more than women.

A hush at high pitches

The most common form of presbycusis, called *sensory presbycusis*, results from atrophy of the organ of Corti (which contains special hearing receptors) and the auditory nerve. Hearing loss occurs mostly in the higher pitch ranges.

By age 60, most adults have difficulty hearing above 4,000 Hz. (The normal range for speech recognition is 500 to 2,000 Hz.) Many older adults have trouble distinguishing higher-pitched consonants, such as s, sh, f, ph, ch, z, t, and g.

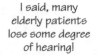

I said, many elderly patients lose some degree of hearing!

No dearth of deafness

Aging results in degenerative structural changes in the entire auditory system. In fact, hearing loss in elderly people may be more common than statistics indicate. Some people may not be immediately aware of the onset or progression of a hearing defect. Others may recognize the problem but view it as a natural part of aging—and thus not seek medical help.

Respiratory system

Age-related anatomic changes in the upper airways include nose enlargement from continued cartilage growth, tonsil atrophy, and tracheal deviations caused by changes in the aging spine.

In the thorax, anteroposterior chest diameter may increase from altered calcium metabolism and costal cartilage calcification. This, in turn, reduces chest wall mobility. Kyphosis (curvature of the thoracic spine) advances with age from such factors as osteoporosis and vertebral collapse. Respiratory muscle degeneration or atrophy may also occur, reducing pulmonary function.

Lung changes

Ventilatory capacity diminishes as the lungs' diffusing capacity declines. Also, decreased inspiratory and expiratory muscle strength diminish vital capacity. Lung tissue degeneration reduces the lungs' elastic recoil, causing higher residual volume. (In fact, aging alone can cause emphysema.)

Out of oxygen

Furthermore, closing of some airways impairs ventilation of the basal areas, decreasing both the surface area available for gas exchange and the partial pressure of arterial oxygen (Pao_2).

Thus, maximum breathing capacity, forced vital capacity, vital capacity, and inspiratory reserve volume all diminish, reducing the tolerance for oxygen debt.

Aging and alveoli

With age, the lungs become more rigid and the number and size of alveoli decline. A 30% reduction in respiratory fluids and a decrease in ciliary action and macrophages increase the risk of respiratory tract infection and mucus plugs.

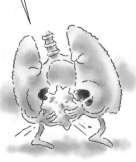

A 30% reduction in respiratory fluids—cough!—and a decrease in ciliary action and macrophages—gasp!—increases the risk of respiratory track infection and mucus plugs. Not good news!

Cardiovascular system

The heart usually becomes slightly smaller with age (except in people with hypertension or heart disease). By age 70, many people experience a 35% decrease in cardiac output at rest.

Stiffer valves, thicker walls

The heart muscle becomes less efficient and loses contractile strength, fibrotic and sclerotic changes thicken the heart valves and reduce their flexibility. The valves may become rigid and unable to close completely, leading to systolic murmurs. Also, the left ventricular wall grows 25% thicker between ages 30 and 80.

The heart's ability to respond to physical and emotional stress may diminish markedly with age; for instance, the heart rate takes longer to return to normal after exercise. Also, elderly adults may develop obstructive coronary disease and fibrosis of the cardiac skeleton.

Vessels in distress

Aging commonly contributes to arterial and venous insufficiency, as blood vessels lose strength and elasticity. These factors contribute to a higher incidence of cardiovascular disease, especially coronary artery disease.

As myocardial irritability increases with age, extra systoles may occur, along with sinus arrhythmias and sinus bradycardias. Increased fibrous tissue infiltrates the sinoatrial node and internodal atrial tracts, possibly causing atrial fibrillation and flutter.

Pressure surge

Coronary artery blood flow decreases 35% between ages 20 and 60. The aorta grows more rigid, causing systolic blood pressure to rise proportionately more than diastolic blood pressure (resulting in a widened pulse pressure).

The veins also dilate with age, and blood tends to pool in the extremities.

Electrocardiographic changes may include increased PR and QT intervals, decreased QRS complexes, and a leftward shift of the QRS axis.

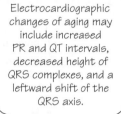

Electrocardiographic changes of aging may include increased PR and QT intervals, decreased height of QRS complexes, and a leftward shift of the QRS axis.

GI system

When assessing the elderly patient's GI system, pay special attention to the physiologic changes that accompany aging. Normal changes include diminished mucosal elasticity and reduced GI secretions, which in turn may alter digestion and absorption.

Dawdling digestion

GI tract motility, lower esophageal sphincter tone, bowel wall and anal sphincter tone, and abdominal muscle strength may decrease with age. These changes may cause signs and symptoms ranging from appetite loss to esophageal reflux to constipation.

Losses of the liver

In the liver, normal age-related changes include decreased liver weight, reduced regenerative capacity, and diminished blood flow.

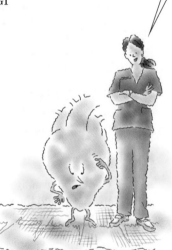

Urologic system

After age 40, renal function may diminish; by age 90, it may decrease by up to 50%. Age-related changes in renal vasculature that disturb glomerular hemodynamics reduce the glomerular filtration rate.

Renal blood flow decreases 53% from reduced cardiac output and age-related atherosclerotic changes. Tubular reabsorption and renal concentrating ability also decline as the size and number of functioning nephrons decrease.

Also, the bladder muscles weaken, possibly causing incomplete bladder emptying and chronic urine retention—conditions that set the stage for bladder infection. Residual urine, urinary frequency, and nocturia also grow more common.

Renal reductions

Other age-related changes affecting renal function include diminished kidney size, impaired renal clearance of drugs, reduced bladder size and capacity, and decreased renal ability to respond to variations in sodium intake. Blood urea nitrogen levels rise about 20% by age 70.

Female reproductive system

Declining estrogen and progesterone levels cause various physical changes in aging women. As estrogen levels decrease and menopause approaches (usually at about age 50), a host of physiologic changes occur.

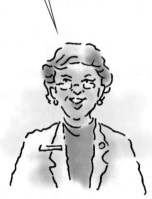

As menopause approaches, estrogen and progesterone levels decrease and various physical changes occur.

Breasts

The breast's glandular, supporting, and fatty tissues atrophy with age. As Cooper's ligaments lose their elasticity, the breasts become pendulous. The nipples become smaller, flatter, and nonerect. Inframammary ridges grow more pronounced.

Disappearing disease

Any fibrocystic breast disease present before menopause usually diminishes and disappears.

Ovaries

Ovulation usually stops 1 to 2 years before menopause. As the ovaries reach the end of their productive cycle, they become unresponsive to gonadotropic stimulation.

Pelvic support structures

Pelvic support structures typically relax after menopause. Such relaxation may first occur with labor and delivery—but clinical effects may go unnoticed until menopause, when relaxation is accelerated by estrogen depletion and loss of connective tissue elasticity and tone.

Signs and symptoms include pressure and pulling in the area above the inguinal ligaments, low backache, a feeling of pelvic heaviness, and difficulty rising from a chair. Urinary stress incontinence may become a problem if urethrovesical ligaments weaken.

Uterus

After menopause, the uterus atrophies rapidly to one-half its premenstrual weight. Uterine regression continues until the organ reaches about one-fourth of its premenstrual size. The cervix shrinks and no longer produces mucus for lubrication, and the endometrium and myometrium become thinner.

Vagina

Atrophy causes the vagina to shorten and the mucous lining to become thin, dry, pale, and less elastic. In this state, the vaginal mucosa is highly susceptible to abrasion. Also, the pH of vaginal secretions rises.

Vulva

The vulva atrophies with age. Pubic hair loss occurs, and the labia majora flatten. Vulval tissue shrinks, exposing the sensitive area around the urethra and vagina to abrasions and irritation (for instance, from undergarments). With age, the introitus (vaginal opening) constricts, vaginal tissues lose their elasticity, and the epidermis thins from 20 layers to about 5.

Despite such body changes, older women can continue to remain sexual throughout their lives.

Male reproductive system

In elderly men, reduced testosterone production may cause a decline in libido, atrophy and softening of the testes, and decreased sperm production.

Normally, the prostate gland enlarges with age, while its secretions diminish. Seminal fluid decreases in volume and viscosity.

Still sexual

During intercourse, elderly men experience slower and weaker physiologic reactions. However, these changes don't necessarily weaken the sex drive or reduce sexual satisfaction. (See *Characteristics of the male climacteric*.)

Musculoskeletal system

Decreasing height is the most apparent age-related musculoskeletal change. This decrease results from exaggerated spinal curvatures and narrowing intervertebral spaces, which shorten the trunk and make the arms appear relatively long.

Other musculoskeletal changes include:
- decreased bone mass
- reduced muscle mass, which may lead to muscle weakness
- diminished collagen formation, which causes loss of resilience and elasticity in joints and supporting structures
- greater viscosity of synovial fluid
- increased fibrosis of synovial membranes.

Characteristics of the male climacteric

Here's a list of the physiologic changes that characterize the male climacteric:
- Erections require more time and stimulation to achieve.
- Erections aren't as full or as hard as they were before.
- Testosterone production declines.
- The prostate gland enlarges and its secretions diminish.
- Seminal fluid decreases.
- Ejaculatory force diminishes.
- Contractions in the prostate gland and penile urethra during orgasm vary in length and quality.
- The refractory period following ejaculation may lengthen from minutes to days.
- Pleasure sensations become less genitally localized and more generalized.

Walking woes

An older adult may have difficulty performing tandem walking (walking heel-to-toe in a straight line). Also, he may take shorter steps and use a wider leg stance to achieve better balance and a more stable weight distribution.

Nervous system

Aging affects the nervous system in many ways. Neurons in the central and peripheral nervous systems undergo degenerative changes. Nerve transmission slows, causing the elderly adult to react more sluggishly to external stimuli.

Brain cell drain

After about age 50, the brain loses cells at a rate of about 1% per year. However, clinical effects usually aren't noticeable until aging is more advanced.

Other neurologic changes

Here are other effects of age on the nervous system:
• The hypothalamus becomes less effective at regulating body temperature.
• The corneal reflex becomes slower, so the lids close more slowly in reaction to corneal irritation.
• The pain threshold increases.
• Certain sleep stages (including rapid-eye-movement sleep) shorten.

System overlap

When testing an elderly patient's nervous system, keep in mind that neurologic changes stemming from alterations in other body systems may affect assessment findings. For instance, sensory receptor changes may lead to hearing and vision loss, cerebrovascular dysfunction, and mental status changes induced by medications.

Other factors that can influence an elderly patient's test results include fatigue, lack of sleep, depression, hyperactivity, fear, and anxiety. The patient may seem disinterested or preoccupied or he may be slow to respond.

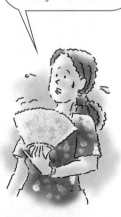

As aging occurs, the hypothalamus becomes less effective at regulating body temperature. Is it hot in here, or is it just me?

Endocrine system

A common—and important—endocrine change in elderly adults is a decreased ability to tolerate stress. The most serious sign of a diminished stress response is altered glucose metabolism.

Stress and sugar spikes

Normally, fasting blood glucose levels don't differ significantly in young and older adults. However, in an older adult, stress stimulates a rise in blood glucose that lasts longer than it does in a younger adult. In part, this stems from decreased insulin secretion and reduced responsiveness of insulin receptors. Approximately 25% of older people develop diabetes.

Thyroid slowdown

The thyroid hormones triiodothyronine and thyroxine decrease by 25% in older adults. Ordinarily, the remaining secretion of thyroid hormones is adequate for homeostasis. However, the basal metabolic rate and oxygen consumption slow.

Menstrual finale

During menopause, ovarian senescence causes permanent cessation of menstrual activity. Although changes in endocrine function during menopause vary from one woman to the next, estrogen and progesterone levels normally diminish and follicle-stimulating hormone production increases.

Estrogen deficiency in elderly women is linked to coronary artery disease and osteoporosis. In both men and women, other normal variations in endocrine function include a 50% decline in serum aldosterone levels and a 25% decrease in cortisol secretion rate.

Hematologic and immune systems

Total and differential white blood cell (WBC) counts don't change significantly with age. However, after age 65, some people have a slight decrease in the range of normal WBC counts. When this happens, B cell and total lymphocyte counts decrease and T cells decrease in number and become less effective.

Me, myself, and nonself

Immune function starts to decline at sexual maturity and continues to diminish with age. The incidence of autoimmune disease rises as the immune system starts to lose the ability to differentiate between self and nonself.

The cancer incidence increases, too, as the immune system grows less proficient at recognizing and destroying mutant cells. Decreased antibody response in elderly adults

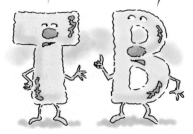

After age 65, I hear B-cell and total lymphocyte counts may decrease.

Well, I hear T cells may decrease in number and become less effective.

heightens susceptibility to infection. Tonsillar atrophy and lymph-adenopathy are common.

Assessment

Comprehensive health assessment of the older adult focuses on medical history and current health status, including a review of body systems and an evaluation of the patient's dietary regimen and ability to function. Besides establishing the patient's health status, the information you obtain during assessment helps you evaluate improvements or declines in his condition over time and helps determine whether he needs support services.

Health history

The information you elicit during the health history and interview alerts you to key areas to focus on during the physical examination. To begin the history, establish the patient's well-being as your primary concern. Talking with him about health concerns promotes his health awareness, helps identify knowledge deficits, and allows you to launch your patient teaching.

Move along methodically

Because the patient may overlook some important health information, be sure to interview him methodically. When necessary, gather additional or corroborating information from his family or friends.

Current health status

Begin with the patient's current health status. Ask him to describe his health, and record his responses using his own words.

Next, record the reason he's seeking treatment (chief complaint). Ask him about current medication use and treatments, his diet, and any devices he uses (such as a cane, walker, or hearing aid).

If he seems confused or shows signs or symptoms of dementia, consider asking his permission to include a spouse, child, or significant other in the interview.

Ask the patient what medications and supplements he's taking, and find out if he uses a cane, hearing aid, or other medical device.

Medical history

During the medical history, obtain an overview of the patient's general health status, a history of his adult illnesses, a record of past hospitalizations, frequency of practitioner visits, and previous use of drugs and other treatments and their purpose.

Review of body systems

When reviewing an older adult's body systems, consider the physiologic changes normally associated with aging. Also, keep in mind that older adults commonly have atypical disease presentations. For example, subtle changes in appetite and mental status may be the only signs and symptoms of certain disorders.

Organized assessment

Assess specific body areas and systems using either the head-to-toe approach or the major body system approach. Both methods provide a systematic and organized framework, so choose the one that works best for you.

Physical examination

During the physical examination, use inspection, palpation, percussion, and auscultation to gather objective data that help validate the subjective data obtained from the health history.

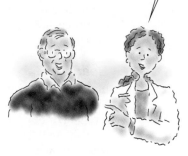

Begin your physical examination with a general head-to-toe observation.

General survey

Begin the physical examination with a general head-to-toe observation to gain an overall impression of your patient's status. Be sure to observe:
• overall appearance, including body build, skin, hygiene, and grooming
• general mobility status
• level of consciousness (LOC), affect, and mood
• overt signs of distress.
    Then take the patient's vital signs. Keep in mind that in an older adult, normal body temperature ranges from 96° to 98.6° F (35.6° to 37° C).

Skin

Inspect the skin on the patient's scalp, head, neck, trunk, and limbs. Be sure to note its color, temperature, texture, tone, turgor, thickness, and moisture. Remember that areas such as the knees and elbows may look a bit darker because of sun exposure and that calloused areas may look yellow.

Turgor testing

When assessing skin turgor, keep in mind that turgor may not reliably reflect hydration in older people, who have less subcutaneous tissue. For more accurate results, check turgor by gently pinching the subcutaneous tissue of the forehead or over the xiphoid process, and then watching for a quick return to baseline.

Skin scrutiny

Inspect the skin for tears, lacerations, scars, lesions, and ulcerations. Look for early signs of pressure ulcers such as local redness over pressure sites.

Stay alert for common benign skin lesions found in older adults; these must be differentiated from precancerous or malignant lesions. Note lesion size, distribution pattern, shape, color, consistency, and borders. Also, ask about the lesion's onset. Any suspicious lesion warrants further evaluation.

Hair and nails

Inspect and palpate the patient's hair, noting its color, quantity, distribution, and texture (fine, silky, or coarse). Know that hair thinning and sparseness are common around the axillae and symphysis pubis.

Nail ailments worth noting

Inspect fingernails and toenails, noting their color, shape, thickness, and capillary refill as well as the presence of any lesions. Some distortion of the normally flat or slightly curved nail surface is normal with aging, but other changes in color, shape, or angle may indicate a pathologic condition.

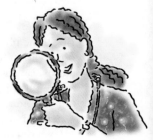

Inspect the patient's face and neck for skin color and proportion. Skin color should be evenly distributed.

Head and face

Inspect the patient's head, noting its size, contour, and symmetry. Skull size and shape don't normally change with age. Soft-tissue swelling or cranial bulging may indicate recent head trauma.

Palpate the skull, noting tenderness, masses, or lesions. Localized cranial enlargement requires further evaluation.

Reading faces

Inspect the face and neck for skin color and proportion. Skin color should be evenly distributed. Facial features should be proportionate to head size. Also observe the patient's facial expression and movements.

Nose and mouth

Examine the external portion of the patient's nose, noting any asymmetry or abnormality such as a structural deformity. Inspect the internal mucosa, noting its color and any discharge, swelling, bleeding, or lesions. The area should be pink and moist, with clear mucus and no crusting or lesions. Palpate the frontal and maxillary sinuses for tenderness, which should be absent.

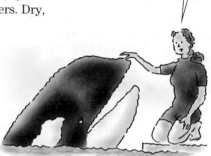

Your oral mucosa look nicely hydrated for someone of your advanced years!

Oral observations

Inspect the mouth, starting with the lips. Note their color, symmetry, and hydration status as well as any lesions or ulcers. Dry, parched lips indicate dehydration.

Note whether the patient wears a dental appliance. Inspect his mouth with the appliance in place, noting its fit and observing for sores or abscesses resulting from friction.

Then inspect the oral mucosa, noting color, texture, hydration status, and any exudate. The mucosa and gums should be pink, smooth, and moist— although in a dark-skinned person, the mucosa normally may be slightly bluish.

Palpate the oral mucosa for lesions and nodules, noting tenderness, pain, or bleeding. Inspect the gums for color, inflammation, lesions, and bleeding. They should be pink and moist. If your patient has his natural teeth, note their number and condition.

Tales of the tongue

Next, observe tongue color, size, texture, and coating. The tongue is normally pink to red, smooth, and free from involuntary movement. Assess tongue position; deviation to one side suggests a neurologic disorder.

Observe the pharynx for signs of inflammation, discoloration, exudate, and lesions. It should be pink to pale pink, without discharge or lesions.

Eyes

When examining an older adult's eyes, keep in mind that ocular signs of aging can affect the appearance of the entire eye. Also, know that age-induced fatty tissue loss may cause the eyes to sit deeper in the bony orbits.

Lids and lacrimation

Compare eyelid color to facial skin color; the lid should be free from redness and other color changes. Check for lesions and edema, and note the direction of the eyelashes. Determine whether the upper eyelid partially or completely covers the pupil—which indicates ptosis, an abnormal finding.

Inspect the lacrimal apparatus, noting discharge, redness, edema, excessive tearing, or tenderness. Examine the sclera and conjunctiva; the sclera should appear creamy white.

Pointers on pupils

Next, inspect the pupils, noting their size, shape, and reaction to light. Observe the iris, noting any margin aberrations. You may see bilateral irregular iris pigmentation, with the normal pigment replaced by a pale brown color.

Acuity analysis

Test the patient's visual acuity with and without corrective lenses, and note differences. Perform an ophthalmoscopic examination to inspect internal eye structures.

Ears

Inspect the auricle of the ears, noting color and temperature changes, discharge, or lesions. Palpate the auricle for tenderness.

Inspect internal ear structures with an otoscope. Examine the external canal and tympanic membrane, and observe for the light reflex. Note lesions, bulging of the tympanic membrane, cerumen (earwax) buildup, or (in a male) hair growth.

Can you hear me now?

To detect hearing loss early, perform the Weber and Rinne tuning fork tests. Also, evaluate the patient's ability to hear and understand speech, in case you need to recommend rehabilitative therapy. If the patient wears a hearing aid, inspect it closely for proper functioning.

Neck

Inspect the patient's neck, noting scars, masses, or asymmetry. Gently palpate any masses, noting their consistency, size, shape, mobility, and tenderness. Repeat this inspection for the lymph nodes.

Check the trachea for alignment. Normally, the trachea is midline at the suprasternal notch. Note any displacement or masses.

Spying on the thyroid

Inspect the thyroid gland while your patient sips water. Note any masses or bulging. Normally, the thyroid can't be seen or palpated.

Chest and respiratory system

Inspect the shape and symmetry of the patient's chest, both anteriorly and posteriorly. Note the anteroposterior-to-lateral diameter. During respirations, listen for inspiratory or expiratory wheezing, which may be audible from the oral airways.

Palpate the anterior and posterior chest for tenderness, masses, and lumps. Assess diaphragmatic excursion. Palpate the anterior and posterior chest symmetrically for tactile fremitus. Usually, fremitus is most evident near the tracheal bifurcation.

A percussion discussion

Percuss the patient's lung fields anteriorly and posteriorly from the bases to apices. Be sure to percuss in a symmetrical pattern for comparison. Normal lung fields sound resonant. Bony prominences, organs, or consolidated tissue sound dull.

Next, auscultate from the lung bases to the apices, anteriorly and posteriorly. Ask the patient to take some deep breaths, in and out, with his mouth open. You may hear diminished sounds at the lung bases if some of the airways are closed. Inspiration is significantly more audible than expiration.

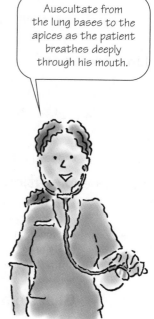

Auscultate from the lung bases to the apices as the patient breathes deeply through his mouth.

Cardiovascular system

Inspect and palpate the point of maximal impulse (PMI, or apical pulse), normally located in the fourth or fifth intercostal space just medial to the midclavicular line. In an older adult, the PMI may be displaced downward to the left.

Using the ball of your hand, palpate over the aortic, pulmonic, and mitral areas for thrills, heaves, or vibrations. You may detect a palpable thrill in a patient with valvular heart disease.

Heart sound symphony

Auscultate the heart over the aortic, pulmonic, tricuspid, and mitral areas and Erb's point, listening for the first and second heart sounds (S_1 and S_2) over each area. Also listen for extra diastolic heart sounds, or third and fourth heart sounds (S_3 and S_4).

In an older adult, S_3 heard between S_1 and S_2 (usually at the lower sternal border) isn't a reliable indicator of heart failure. Instead, it may be physiologic or occur in response to an increased diastolic flow. You may hear S_4 after S_2 and before S_1—most audibly over the heart's apex.

Vessel investigation

Next, assess blood vessels of the patient's head, neck, trunk, and extremities. Palpate the carotid arteries one at a time, pressing lightly so you don't obliterate the carotid pulse. Note the rate, rhythm, strength, and equality of both pulses. Auscultate each carotid artery for bruits—humming or high-pitched sounds that may represent narrowing of the arterial lumen.

Evaluate for jugular vein distention. Identify the level of venous pulsation and measure its height relative to the sternal angle.

A height exceeding 1¹⁄₈″ (3 cm) is considered abnormal and may indicate right-sided heart failure.

Palpate the peripheral arteries, noting the rate, rhythm, strength, and equality of pulses and checking for bruits. In an older adult, expect the arteries to be tortuous, kinked and, possibly, stiffer. However, pulses should be symmetrical in strength.

Limb look-see

When inspecting the legs, note their color and temperature and check for edema, varicosities, and trophic changes of the toes.

Using the ball of your hand, assess the temperature of the arms and legs, which should be equal bilaterally. Thrombosis is usually associated with a sensation of heat, although this response may be reduced in an older adult.

Edema exploration

Finally, check for edema, which is best assessed over bony prominences or the sacrum. Typically, edema is more pronounced in the most dependent body areas. Determine if the edema is pitting or nonpitting, and grade the degree of edema.

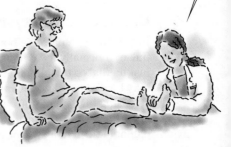

Edema may occur over bony prominences in dependent body areas such as the ankles.

GI system

When examining the GI system, be aware that older adults are more likely to have abdominal distention and less likely to have abdominal rigidity than younger adults. Inspect the abdomen, noting its shape and symmetry and any scars, masses, pulsations, distention, or striae. Describe the abdomen as obese, scaphoid, or distended.

Auscultate all four abdominal quadrants for bowel sounds. Listen over the abdominal aorta for bruits.

Next, percuss the abdomen to determine the presence of air or fluid, assess liver size, and check for bladder distention. Air in the large bowel sounds tympanic, whereas fluid sounds dull.

Palpation implications

Palpate the belly, noting masses or tenderness on light or deep palpation. Watch for peritoneal signs, such as rigidity or rebound tenderness. Masses in the lower quadrants may be impacted stool. Try to palpate the liver; normally it isn't palpable.

Genitourinary system

When you assess the patient's genitourinary system, use the same basic technique as you would in a younger patient. Note that pubic hair becomes sparse and gray with age. Normally, the testes of an older male are slightly smaller than adult size. However, they should be equal, smooth, soft, and freely movable, without nodules.

Musculoskeletal system

Assessing the musculoskeletal system helps determine the older adult's overall ability to function. Limitations in range of motion (ROM), difficulty in ambulation, and diffuse or localized joint pain can be detected easily during the physical examination.

Stay alert for signs and symptoms of motor and sensory dysfunction, such as weakness, spasticity, tremors, rigidity, and sensory disturbances.

Rating the gait

Observe the patient's walk, noting his gait and posture. Gait reflects integration of reflexes as well as motor function. Assess static balance and station by gently pushing on his shoulders while he's standing.

Then observe the patient's tandem (heel-to-toe) walking, watching for exaggerated ataxia (coordination difficulties) and observing the position of his head and neck relative to the shoulders and legs.

To evaluate posture and balance, elicit Romberg's sign by noting whether the patient sways or falls when standing with his feet close together and eyes closed. Swaying indicates a positive Romberg's sign.

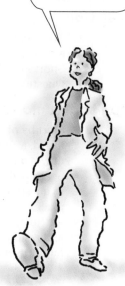

Watch for exaggerated ataxia as the patient performs tandem (heel-to-toe) walking.

Judging joints

Inspect the joints of the hands, wrists, elbows, shoulders, neck, hips, knees, and ankles. Note any joint enlargement, swelling, tenderness, crepitus, temperature changes, or deformities.

Following the feet

Assess the feet for common deformities, such as:
• hallux valgus—angulation of the great toe away from the midline or toward the other toes
• metatarsal (forefoot) prolapse
• hammer toe—bending of the second, third, or fourth toe at the middle joint.

Taking measure of muscles

Inspect each muscle group for atrophy, fasciculations, involuntary movements, and tremor. Move the joints through passive ROM exercises, and palpate the muscles for tone and strength.

Then assess for rigidity and spasticity. Rigidity is best detected in the wrist or elbow joint.

Appraising zip and grasp

Throughout the physical examination, ask the patient to show you how he buttons or zippers his clothing. This allows you to directly observe his ability to perform selected activities of daily living. Also observe him grasping items, such as a doorknob or water faucet.

Neurologic system

The neurologic examination includes assessment of LOC or awareness, affect, mood, cognition, orientation, speech, general knowledge, memory, reasoning, object recognition and higher cognitive functions, cranial nerves, motor and sensory systems, and reflexes.

Test time

To assess the older adult's cognitive status, consider using a screening tool, such as the Mini-Mental Status Examination, the Short Portable Mental Status Questionnaire, or the Mental Status Questionnaire.

Monitoring mood

Start by observing your patient's general appearance, including mood, affect, and grooming. An older adult who seems depressed may require further evaluation, as with the Geriatric Depression Scale. Note whether the patient is dressed appropriately, responds to questions appropriately, and is oriented to person, time, and place.

Next, assess the patient's speech. Evaluate his vocabulary and general knowledge level by discussing current news items or family events.

Memory, reason, and recognition

To evaluate memory, assess the patient's immediate, recent, and remote recall.
- Check *immediate* recall by naming a certain number of objects or reciting a group of numbers and having him repeat them immediately.
- To elicit *recent* memory, ask him about events that occurred during the past 24 to 48 hours.
- To assess *remote* memory, ask him to recall significant events that occurred many years ago.

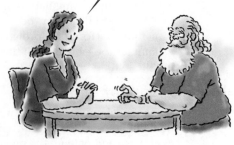

To assess remote memory, ask your patient to recall events that occurred many years ago.

Reasoning and reckoning

Next, evaluate the patient's ability to reason by asking questions that require judgment, insight, and abstraction to answer.

To assess his object recognition, point to two objects and ask him to identify each one. Grade his response as normal or agnosia (inability to name objects).

Cranial nerves

Assess each cranial nerve sequentially, beginning with cranial nerve I and progressing to cranial nerve XII.

Motor and sensory systems

Evaluate the patient's muscle and joint function. Assess for rapid, rhythmic, alternating movements, which reflect coordination. Observe whether he can repeat maneuvers, and watch for smoothness in executing them. Expect an older adult to respond more slowly than a younger person.

Probing perception

Next, check the patient's pain perception, using the sharp and dull ends of a safety pin; temperature perception, using hot and cold substances; touch perception, using a light touch of the hand; and vibration perception, using a vibrating tuning fork.

Also evaluate his two-point discrimination and position sense. His perceptions should be accurate and symmetrical.

Reflexes

Assess an older adult's reflexes as you would in any other patient. Be sure to check for the plantar and Babinski's reflexes, which may suggest upper motor neuron disease.

Special considerations

Older adults have special health needs that require skilled, knowledgeable care. For instance, people over age 65 use twice as many medications annually as people under age 65. Furthermore, age-related physiologic changes may influence drug actions, so you need to understand how drugs affect elderly patients to promote compliance and minimize adverse reactions.

You may also need to help an older adult learn to deal with such age-related concerns as managing multiple chronic illnesses and preventing falls.

Drug therapy

Four out of five older adults have chronic medical conditions. Accordingly, they buy approximately 400 million prescriptions per year—twice the number bought by people under age 65.

For elderly patients with chronic disorders, drug therapy may extend life and enhance its quality. One or more drugs may successfully manage arthritis, diabetes, heart disease, glaucoma, osteoporosis, and hypertension.

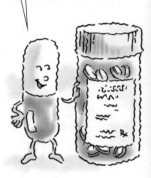

Older adults buy twice as many prescriptions annually as people under age 65.

The polypharmacy predicament

However, if your patient has multiple diseases and takes several different drugs, be sure to watch for problems stemming from polypharmacy (concomitant use of multiple medications) such as drug interactions.

Age-related changes in pharmacokinetics

Drug therapy in elderly people is complicated by age-related changes in body functions, which may influence a drug's action—how a drug is absorbed into the bloodstream, distributed throughout the body, metabolized, and eliminated. (See *How aging influences drug actions.*)

Age-related changes in pharmacodynamics

Pharmacodynamic changes can significantly alter a drug's action and effect in an older adult. Aging alters tissue sensitivity to drugs, enhancing certain drug effects. This is especially true for sleep aids, benzodiazepines such as diazepam, and alcohol.

Dearth of drug receptors

Age-related changes in the number or function of tissue and organ receptors may also alter a drug's effect. For instance, the number of beta-adrenergic receptors decreases with age, reducing beta-adrenergic receptor function and influencing the effects of drugs that stimulate or block these receptors (for example, metaproterenol and propranolol).

Similarly, changes in cholinergic and dopaminergic receptors may influence the effect of such drugs as phenothiazines, chlorpromazine (Thorazine), and other psychoactive agents. These changes may contribute to such adverse neurologic reactions as extrapyramidal effects and tardive dyskinesia. To compensate for these pharmacodynamic changes, prescribers usually reduce drug dosages for elderly patients.

How aging influences drug actions

The physiologic changes that come with aging cause changes in how the body absorbs, distributes, metabolizes, and eliminates drugs. Awareness of these changes can help you better predict the outcome of your patient's drug therapy.

Action	Pathophysiologic change
Absorption	• Increased gastric pH • Slower gastric emptying • Decreased gastric blood flow and motility
Distribution	• More fatty tissue • Less lean body mass
Metabolism	• Decreased total body water • Smaller liver • Less liver blood flow and enzymatic activity • Less air exchange • Decreased renal mass
Elimination	• Decreased nephron function • Decreased glomerular filtration rate, tubular secretion, and creatinine clearance and reabsorption

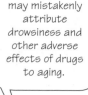

Caregivers may mistakenly attribute drowsiness and other adverse effects of drugs to aging.

Adverse drug effects

Adverse drug effects and unwanted drug interactions are common in elderly patients and result mainly from physiologic changes and multiple medication use.

One troublesome aspect of drug therapy in elderly adults is the potential for misdiagnosing or failing to detect adverse reactions, such as confusion, depression, drowsiness, and urine retention. Caregivers may mistakenly attribute these problems to aging.

Spotting adverse reactions

Careful nursing assessment can help identify adverse reactions so that the offending drug's dosage may be lowered or the drug can be replaced with a safer one. To recognize common adverse reactions, make sure you know both the intended and adverse effects of all the drugs your patient takes. (See *Recognizing common adverse drug effects in elderly patients*, page 912.)

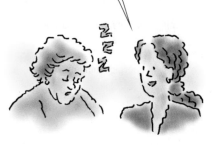

Recognizing common adverse drug effects in elderly patients

Signs and symptoms of common adverse drug effects include hives, impotence, incontinence, stomach upset, and rashes. Elderly patients are especially susceptible to adverse effects and may even experience more serious ones, such as orthostatic hypotension, altered mental status, anorexia, dehydration, blood disorders, and tardive dyskinesia.

Also, other adverse effects—such as anxiety, confusion, and forgetfulness—may mistakenly be dismissed as typical effects of aging rather than correctly identified as adverse drug reactions.

To help recognize bad reactions to drugs, be sure you know the potential adverse effects of the drugs your patient is taking.

Pharmacologic class	Potential adverse effects
Angiotensin-converting enzyme inhibitors	Dizziness, headache, fatigue, orthostatic hypotension, nasal congestion, cough
Alpha-adrenergic blockers	Dizziness, palpitation, nausea
Aminoglycosides	Ototoxicity, nephrotoxicity
Antiarrhythmics	Dizziness, tremors, blurred vision, nausea, vomiting, dry mouth
Anticholinergics, antihistamines	Drowsiness, blurred vision, fatigue, constipation, dry mouth
Anticoagulants	Bleeding
Antidiabetics	Hypoglycemia, weight gain, nausea
Antispasmodics, phenothiazines, tricyclic antidepressants	Sedation, extrapyramidal movements, anticholinergic effects
Beta-adrenergic blockers	Bradycardia, fatigue, hypotension, central nervous system (CNS) disturbances, impotence
Diuretics	Electrolyte disturbances, urinary frequency, dehydration
Histamine-2 blockers	Diarrhea, fatigue, dizziness, neutropenia
Nonsteroidal anti-inflammatory drugs	Bleeding, GI upset, renal compromise
Opioids	CNS depression, respiratory depression, dependency

Drug interactions

Many potent drugs commonly used by elderly adults can interact, resulting in hazardous consequences. For example, cimetidine

(Tagamet) interacts with aminophylline, phenytoin (Dilantin), antidepressants, propranolol (Inderal), and other drugs.

Anticholinergics, such as some antidepressants and tranquilizers, may have additive effects when used together. Digoxin (Lanoxin) may have increased toxic effects when taken with a diuretic or other drug that decreases body potassium levels.

Hindering interactions

To help prevent harmful drug interactions, make sure you know all the drugs your patient is taking. Keep in mind that he may be taking several drugs prescribed independently by several prescribers.

Adherence with drug therapy

An elderly adult may have any number of reasons for not adhering to the treatment regimen—for example, poor vision or hearing, physical disability, inability to afford drugs, cultural beliefs, or failure to understand the importance of taking a particular drug.

Augmenting adherence

Nonadherence can lead to treatment failure. If the prescriber misinterprets this failure as ineffective drug therapy, he may mistakenly increase the dosage or prescribe a second drug, compounding the problem.

Helping the patient overcome obstacles to adherence is an important nursing responsibility. To meet it, make sure your patient understands the purpose of each prescribed drug and knows how to take each one correctly.

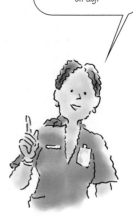

To promote adherence to drug therapy, make sure your patient understands the purpose and administration method for each drug.

Urinary incontinence

Incontinence, the uncontrollable passage of urine, is common among the elderly—but it shouldn't be considered a normal part of aging. Incontinence can result from bladder abnormalities or neurologic disorders. It may be transient or permanent and may involve large volumes of urine or scant dribbling.

Incontinence categories

Urinary incontinence occurs in four main forms.
• *Stress* incontinence refers to loss of less than 50 ml of urine triggered by increased abdominal pressure—for example, from coughing or sneezing.
• *Overflow* incontinence is an involuntary urine loss occurring at somewhat predictable intervals when a specific bladder volume is reached.

• *Urge* incontinence involves a strong, sudden need to urinate, followed immediately by a bladder contraction that leads to involuntary urine loss.
• *Total* incontinence is complete lack of urinary control, resulting from the bladder's inability to retain urine.

What causes it

Urinary incontinence may result from a wide range of conditions, including:
• benign prostatic hyperplasia
• bladder calculi (stones)
• bladder cancer
• chronic prostatitis
• diabetic neuropathy
• drugs, such as diuretics, sedatives, hypnotics, antipsychotics, anticholinergics, and alpha-adrenergic blockers
• Guillain-Barré syndrome
• multiple sclerosis
• prostate cancer
• spinal cord injury
• stroke
• urethral stricture.

    In some patients, incontinence follows a prostatectomy (prostate removal) that damaged the urethral sphincter.

What to look for

If your patient has urinary incontinence, be sure to cover these factors in your assessment:
• Ask the patient when he first noticed the problem and whether it began suddenly or gradually.
• Have him describe his typical urinary pattern: Does incontinence usually occur during the day or night? Does he have any urinary control or is he totally incontinent? If he sometimes urinates with control, what are the usual times he voids and the amounts of urine voided?
• Ask about other urinary problems, such as hesitancy, frequency, urgency, nocturia, and decreased force or interruption of the urine stream.
• Evaluate the patient's fluid intake.
• Obtain a medical history, especially noting urinary tract infection, prostate conditions, spinal injury or tumor, stroke, or surgery involving the bladder, prostate, or pelvic floor.
• Determine if the patient is taking any medications, particularly sedative-hypnotics, anticholinergics, or diuretics.

Memory jogger

The mnemonic **OUTS** can help you remember the main forms of urinary incontinence:

Overflow incontinence: urine loss occurring when a specific bladder volume is reached

Urge incontinence: urine loss from a bladder contraction that follows a strong, sudden need to urinate

Total incontinence: complete loss of urinary control, as from a nonfunctioning urethral sphincter muscle

Stress incontinence: loss of small amounts of urine (less than 50 ml) when abdominal pressure increases, such as when a person coughs, sneezes, or lifts a heavy object.

Correcting incontinence with bladder retraining

An incontinent patient typically feels frustrated and embarrassed—sometimes even hopeless. Fortunately, bladder retraining—a program that aims to establish a regular voiding pattern—may help correct the problem. Here are some guidelines for establishing such a program.

Assess elimination patterns

Before you start the program, assess the patient's fluid intake pattern, voiding pattern, and behavior (for example, restlessness or talkativeness) before each voiding episode.

Establish a voiding schedule

Encourage the patient to use the toilet 30 minutes before he's usually incontinent. If this isn't successful, readjust the schedule.

Once he can stay dry for 2 hours, increase the time between voidings by 30 minutes each day until he achieves a 3- to 4-hour voiding schedule.

Provide consistency and privacy

When the patient voids, make sure the sequence of conditioning stimuli is always the same. Also, ensure his privacy while voiding; any inhibiting stimuli should be avoided.

Record results and stay positive

Keep a record of continence and incontinence for 5 days to help reinforce the patient's efforts to remain continent.

Remember, your positive attitude—and the patient's—are crucial to successful bladder retraining.

Here are some additional tips that may help your patient succeed.
• Make sure the patient is near a bathroom or portable toilet.
• Leave a light on at night. If the patient needs help getting out of his bed or chair, promptly answer his call for help.
• Encourage him to wear his accustomed clothing, which conveys that you're confident he can remain continent. Acceptable alternatives to diapers include condoms for a male patient and incontinence pads or panties for a female patient.
• Encourage the patient to drink 2 to $2\frac{1}{2}$ qt (2 to 2.5 L) of fluid each day. A lower fluid intake doesn't prevent incontinence—but does promote infection. To help him stay continent overnight, limit his intake after 6 p.m.
• Reassure the patient that if he has an episode of incontinence, that doesn't mean the program has failed. Encourage him to maintain a persistent, positive attitude.

• After completing the history, have the patient empty his bladder. Inspect the urethral meatus for obvious inflammation or anatomic defects. Have a female patient bear down; note any urine leakage.
• Gently palpate the abdomen for bladder distention, which signals urine retention.
• Perform a complete neurologic assessment, noting motor and sensory function and muscle atrophy.

Nursing interventions

• Prepare the patient for diagnostic tests, such as cystoscopy, cystometry, and a complete neurologic workup.
• As appropriate, implement a bladder retraining program. (See *Correcting incontinence with bladder retraining.*)
• Make sure the patient receives an adequate fluid intake.

- Have him void regularly.
- If his incontinence has a neurologic basis, monitor him for urine retention, which may warrant periodic catheterizations.
- If appropriate, teach the patient how to catheterize himself.

Falls

In people age 75 and older, falls cause three times as many accidental deaths as motor vehicle accidents. Several factors can make falls ominous for elderly patients—lengthy convalescence and immobility, the risk of incomplete recovery, and inability to cope physiologically. Also, injuries caused by falls can be psychologically devastating, leading to loss of independence and self-confidence.

Accident or omen?

Falls can be accidental or result from temporary muscle paralysis, vertigo, postural hypotension, or central nervous system (CNS) lesions. Accidental falls commonly result from environmental factors, such as poorly lighted stairs, throw rugs, and highly waxed floors. Sometimes, an accidental fall stems from physiologic factors, such as decreased visual acuity, loss of muscle strength, or poor coordination.

Temporary muscle paralysis may explain falls that occur with no apparent cause. This phenomenon presumably results from compromised blood supply to the reticular formation in the brain's medulla. This, in turn, is caused by spondylosis (vertebral joint fixation or stiffness) that results from head and neck movement in the presence of cervical arthritis.

Other falling factors

Vertigo, as from a middle-ear disturbance or infection, may cause the patient to lose his balance and fall. Orthostatic hypotension may cause dizziness, which leads to a fall when the patient rises too quickly from a lying or sitting position. CNS lesions, as from a stroke, may affect nerve impulses and set the stage for falls.

What to look for

If your patient is found on the floor or reports falling, don't move him until he has been evaluated. Relieve his anxiety as you rapidly assess his vital signs, mental status, and functional capacity.

Note such signs and symptoms as confusion, tremors, weakness, pain, dizziness, or shortening of one leg. Take steps to control any bleeding, and assess whether the patient hit his head.

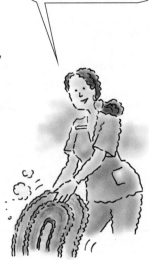

Accidental falls commonly result from environmental factors such as throw rugs. So don't clean those throw rugs—make a clean sweep and get rid of them!

Obtain an X-ray if you suspect a fracture. Observe and monitor the patient's status for the next 24 hours.

Chasing down clues

After the patient's condition is stabilized, include these factors in your assessment:
• Review events that preceded the fall to help avoid future episodes. Did the patient make an abrupt position change or other movement? If he normally wears corrective lenses, was he wearing them when he fell?
• Review his use of such medications as tranquilizers and opioids, which can cause drowsiness that leads to a fall.
• Assess for other contributing factors, such as gait disturbances, poor vision, improper use of assistive devices, and environmental hazards.

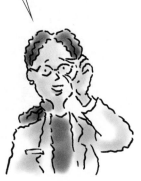

Teach your patient ways to reduce the risk of accidental falls—including wearing eyeglasses if he needs them.

What to do

• Provide measures to relieve pain and discomfort. Give an analgesic if ordered. Apply cold compresses for the first 24 hours and warm compresses thereafter to reduce the pain and swelling of bruises.
• If the patient is bedridden, encourage him to stay as active as possible to avoid becoming bedbound and immobile.
• Provide appropriate care for the patient who has sustained a fracture.
• If indicated, arrange for visiting nurse services for the recovery period after the patient's release.

Fashion tips for safety

• Teach the patient how to reduce the risk of accidental falls by wearing well-fitting shoes with nonskid soles, avoiding long robes, and wearing eyeglasses if he needs them.
• Advise him to sit on the edge of the bed for a few minutes before rising and to use a walking stick, cane, or walker if he feels even slightly unsteady on his feet.
• Suggest ways he can adapt his home to guard against accidental falls—for instance, applying nonskid treads to stairs and installing handrails to walls around the bathtub, shower, and toilet.
• Teach the patient how to fall safely by protecting his hands and face. If he uses a walker or wheelchair, make sure he knows how to cope with a fall, should one occur. Teach him to survey the room for a low, sturdy piece of furniture (for example, a coffee table) he can use for support. Then teach him the proper procedure for lifting himself off the floor and either standing up with the walker or getting into the wheelchair.

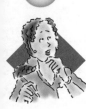

Quick quiz

1.   Which change isn't normally related to aging?
    A.   Difficulty regulating body temperature
    B.   Blurred vision caused by corneal flattening and loss of corneal luster
    C.   Enlargement of the heart
    D.   Decreased pulmonary function

Answer: C. As a person ages, the heart usually becomes slightly smaller, not larger.

2.   Which statement about urinary incontinence is *not* true?
    A.   It's a normal result of aging.
    B.   It may be associated with certain medications.
    C.   It may be transient or permanent.
    D.   It may result from conditions such as prostate cancer.

Answer: A. Urinary incontinence is not a normal result of aging.

3.   Which cardiovascular change in the older adult isn't normal?
    A.   Loss of efficiency and strength of the heart muscle
    B.   Hypotension
    C.   Decreased cardiac output at rest
    D.   Displacement of the PMI and heart sounds

Answer: B. Aging causes the arterial walls to thicken and lose elasticity, leading to higher-than-normal blood pressure, not hypotension.

4.   Which instruction may increase a patient's risk for falling?
    A.   "Use a cane or walker if you feel even slightly unsteady."
    B.   "Wear well-fitting shoes with nonskid soles."
    C.   "Rise quickly when getting out of bed."
    D.   "Install handrails around your bathtub, shower, and toilet."

Answer: C. Rather than suggesting the patient rise quickly out of bed, you should advise him to sit on the bed's edge for a few minutes before rising to avoid orthostatic hypotension and consequent dizziness.

Scoring

✩✩✩   If you answered all four questions correctly, glorious! You show wisdom beyond your years when it comes to gerontologic care.

✩✩   If you answered three questions correctly, good job! Your elder-care expertise is maturing quite nicely.

✩   If you answered fewer than three questions correctly, don't go gray with worry! If you read this chapter again, your understanding of aging is sure to ripen.

End-of-life care

Just the facts

In this chapter, you'll learn:

♦ the purpose of hospice care

♦ commonly performed end-of-life nursing care

♦ ethical and legal issues associated with end-of-life care.

A look at end-of-life care

Health care researchers and practitioners continue to improve medical technology and seek cures for practically every health condition known to humankind. However, terminal illnesses have no cure. Decades ago, patients with these illnesses had few options and commonly dealt with large amounts of pain. Today, hospice and palliative care programs are available to care for patients as they near the end of their lives. Nurses can provide certain interventions during this time to maximize the quality of life for these patients and to prepare them for death.

> End-of-life care focuses on maximizing the quality of the patient's remaining life.

Hospice care

Hospice is an organized program for delivering palliative care. Hospice focuses on support and care for people in the last phase of an incurable disease so that they may live as fully and comfortably as possible. In addition to providing personal support to these patients, hospice care includes support for the patient's family while the patient is dying as well as support to the family during their bereavement.

Palliative provisions

Palliative care strives to relieve suffering and to support the best possible quality of life for patients with advanced chronic and life-threatening illnesses.

Broadened horizons

During the early days of the hospice movement in the United States, most of the care was provided to patients diagnosed with cancer. Today, hospice and palliative care services are available to patients with any serious illness, such as cardiovascular and pulmonary diseases, neurodegenerative disorders, stroke, cancer, human immunodeficiency virus (HIV) or acquired immunodeficiency syndrome (AIDS), and renal failure. Hospice and palliative care focus on treating pain, alleviating illness symptoms and stressors, providing support to the patient and his family for daily living, assisting the patient and his family with difficult medical decisions, and ensuring that the patient's and family's wishes for care are followed. (See *Standards of hospice and palliative nursing care.*)

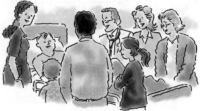

> Hospice care is about supporting not only the patient but also the patient's family.

Care settings

Today, hospice programs serve patients in hospitals, residential facilities, prisons, and long-term care facilities as well as maintain the tradition of caring for patients in their homes. The services of the hospice team supplement the care at a time when facility staff, family members, and the patient are facing the increased and urgent needs associated with the dying process.

Location, location

Hospice programs are offered by hospital systems and home health agencies. Palliative care programs are located in acute care hospitals and ambulatory outpatient settings. However, there's a growing trend for hospice organizations to provide palliative care services earlier in the patient's course of illness.

End-of-life nursing care

The nursing care given to end-of-life patients focuses on evaluation and management of symptoms and their causes. This includes providing assessments, responsive treatment modalities, and communications about therapy to your patient and his family.

Weighing the evidence

Standards of hospice and palliative nursing care

Listed here are the standards of care for hospice and palliative nursing as outlined by the American Nurses Association and the Hospice and Palliative Nurses Association.

Standard	Action
Assessment	Collect basic patient and family data.
Diagnosis	Analyze the assessment data and determine diagnoses using an accepted framework that supports hospice and palliative nursing knowledge.
Outcome identification	Identify expected outcomes relevant to the patient and his family, in partnership with the interdisciplinary team.
Planning	Develop a care plan—negotiated with the patient, his family, and the interdisciplinary team—that includes interventions and treatments to attain expected outcomes.
Implementation	Implement the interventions identified in the care plan.
Evaluation	Evaluate the patient's and his family's progress in attaining expected outcomes.

Source: Scope and standards of hospice and palliative nursing practice (2002). Hospice and Palliative Nurses Association and American Nurses Association.

Shifting nursing goals

With end-of-life care, nursing goals for the patient shift from a curative intent to comfort and supportive management. For example, you might provide written instructions for all medications, encourage deep-breathing and relaxation techniques to decrease your patient's and his family's anxiety, and discuss with your patient who should provide the hands-on care.

Changing medical priorities

Patients who are at the end of their life typically face different medical priorities than patients who are focused on returning to health. Some commonly encountered problems that take center stage include anorexia, anxiety, constipation, depression, and pain.

A patient's shift to an end-of-life focus requires you to take a time-out and switch your nursing goals—from a curative intent to one of comfort and support.

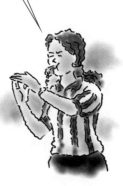

Anorexia

The loss of appetite resulting in the inability to eat, anorexia is due to the underlying disease and treatment modalities. Cachexia, or wasting syndrome, is commonly seen in cancer, HIV, and AIDS patients and may lead to anorexia in certain diseases.

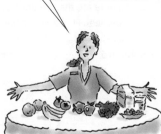

Expect patients to have difficulty taking even two bites of their favorite foods once anorexia sets in.

Be on the lookout for...

Assess your patient by asking about his eating patterns, mouth sores, taste changes, bowel patterns, pain level, sleep patterns, fatigue, anxiety, and ability to cook and feed himself. During your physical assessment, compare your patient's current weight and body mass index to baseline levels and assess his oral cavity and throat for sores or lesions.

Digesting treatment options

Common treatments include parenteral nutrition, appetite stimulants, and nutritional supplements. Effective appetite stimulants include dronabinol (Marinol), cyproheptadine, and megestrol acetate (Megace). Complementary therapies you may use to stimulate your patient's appetite include omega-3 fatty acids, ginger, and fennel. Additionally, encourage your patient to engage in such safe exercises as walking, passive range of motion, yoga, and stretching to help increase his appetite.

Quality, not quantity

Remember, the nutritional goal for your patient is quality as opposed to quantity. If your patient enjoys two bites of food, then you have been successful.

Reassurance helps

As a patient's thirst and hunger decrease in response to the slowing of his body's physiologic demands, family members commonly become particularly emotional and need reassurance. The chaplain and social worker may also lend support in dealing with the family's emotions at this time.

Anxiety

The cause of anxiety may be disease-specific (as in cardiac, endocrine, pulmonary, neurologic, and hematologic illnesses) or due to nutritional deficits and drug side effects. Anger, guilt, and spiritual distress also are common causes of anxiety in end-of-life situations.

Talking treatment

Ask your patient about past experiences with anxiety as well as his usual coping mechanisms, medication use, and support systems. Encouraging him to discuss his fears can help alleviate anxiety.

Relaxing the mind and body

Your patient may benefit from taking an antianxiety medication, such as an anxiolytic, neuroleptic, non-benzodiazepine, or antihistamine. Or he may find listening to music, reading a book, or receiving a massage to be equally helpful.

Constipation

Constipation can be uncomfortable for your end-of-life patient and can lead to fecal impaction. The leading causes of constipation are dehydration, medications, depression, and ascites.

Ask about it

Question your patient about:
- nutrition and hydration status
- bowel frequency
- stool characteristics and amount
- abdominal discomfort
- flatulence
- nausea
- rectal fullness
- incomplete evacuation.

Use your senses

Listen for bowel sounds in all four quadrants noting bowel characteristics, palpate the abdomen for tenderness or masses, and perform a digital rectal examination if your patient complains of incomplete evacuation or if you suspect he's too weak to evacuate completely.

Manager in charge

You can manage your patient's constipation by increasing fluid intake and dietary fiber and encouraging physical activity to promote intestinal motility. Most palliative care programs employ a stepped bowel regimen. Generally, you should start out with a stimulant and, if this is ineffective, progress to a saline enema, then to an oral saline agent, and then to an osmotic laxative.

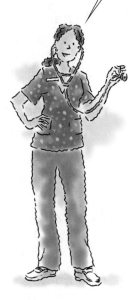

When the patient experiences constipation, listen for bowel sounds in all four quadrants noting bowel characteristics.

A stimulating conversation

Bowel stimulants may cause uncomfortable cramping in patients with neuropathies or in those who are extremely weak. For these patients, recommend stool softeners and daily or every-other-day enemas.

Pan the bedpan

Encourage your patient to use a toilet or bedside commode; these measures are much more effective than a bedpan.

Cough

Coughing is common in end-of-life patients with lung cancer, chronic obstructive pulmonary disease, and heart failure. It's a protective mechanism that clears mucus, fluids, and inhaled foreign bodies from the trachea and bronchi.

Up and out

Assess your patient's cough for:
- frequency
- duration
- aggravating factors
- alleviating factors
- sputum (color, amount, consistency).

Cancel that cough

Antitussives are useful in managing coughing when the underlying cause of cough can't be treated. Drugs such as benzonatate (Tessalon) and dextromethorphan/guaifenesin (Robitussin-DM) are particularly effective.

Don't be so naïve

You may choose to give small doses of morphine every 3 to 4 hours to your opioid-naïve patients. For patients already taking morphine, increase the dose by 25%. If this regimen isn't effective, try increasing the dose another 25%. Codeine and hydrocodone are other opioid choices.

Little bit o' Lasix

Furosemide (Lasix) decreases coughing in patients with heart failure or those who have excess fluid with pitting edema.

Other remedies and advice

Try a warm elixir of honey and lemon, ventilation from an opened window, cool cloths to your patient's face, and water to help loosen sputum. Your patient may need to be taught and reminded to cough effectively to prevent pooling of secretions in his lungs. Instruct family members not to smoke, cook, or allow overcrowding in your patient's room.

Delirium and terminal agitation

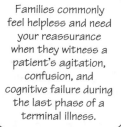

Family members commonly feel helpless as their loved one displays agitation, confusion, and cognitive failure—symptoms of delirium and terminal agitation. This helplessness stems from the inability to communicate and comfort the patient. Reassure the patient's family that this behavior isn't uncommon.

Assess and intervene

Assess your patient's psychiatric history, medications, bowel habits, infection status, respiratory patterns, and urinary habits. Useful pharmacologic interventions for delirium and terminal agitation include haloperidol (Haldol) and chlorpromazine hydrochloride. Other supportive interventions include:
• exploring your patient's concerns regarding death, unfinished tasks, and spirituality
• monitoring patient safety
• keeping your patient in a familiar environment
• discussing your patient's transition to approaching death with his family.

> Families commonly feel helpless and need your reassurance when they witness a patient's agitation, confusion, and cognitive failure during the last phase of a terminal illness.

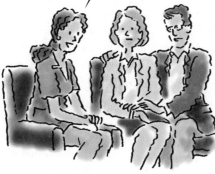

Depression

Many symptoms associated with terminal illnesses overlap the symptoms of depression. To assess your patient's depression, ask him about changes in mood, sleep patterns, diet, and fatigue. To ascertain if your patient is at risk for suicide, inquire about feelings of hopelessness, worthlessness, and helplessness.

Diminishing depression

The medications used to treat depression include tricyclics, selective serotonin reuptake inhibitors (SSRIs), serotonin/norepinephrine reuptake inhibitors, norepinephrine/dopamine reuptake inhibitors, and other antidepressants. SSRIs have less sedative side effects than other antidepressants. For those who are severely depressed, psychostimulants such as methylphenidate (Ritalin) can enhance mood, increase appetite, and reduce fatigue. Psychostimulants administered with an antidepressant relieve depression more quickly. If anxiety is a part of your patient's depressive disorder, the prescriber may also order a benzodiazepine.

Nonpharmacologic methods

The following therapies may alleviate some of the symptoms associated with depression:
- aromatherapy
- cognitive-behavioral therapy
- color therapy
- guided imagery
- music therapy
- pet therapy.

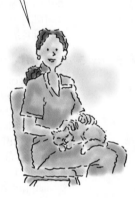

Don't underestimate the effect pets can have on a patient. They can be especially comforting to depressed patients dealing with end-of-life illnesses.

Dyspnea

Dyspnea is a subjective experience that includes difficulty breathing, an uncomfortable awareness of breathing, and shortness of breath. If your patient finds it difficult to speak or if answering questions exacerbates his problem, you may need to intervene first and ask questions later.

Assess and ask

Physical assessment includes auscultating the lungs, monitoring oxygen saturation, and assessing your patient's skin for oxygenation clues. Because anxiety almost always accompanies dyspnea, ask about the presence of anxiety before, during, and after dyspneic episodes.

Treat and take precautions

Benzodiazepines, such as lorazepam (Ativan), are very effective in treating dyspnea. Dyspneic patients should be monitored frequently and should have a mechanism to call for help.

Fatigue

Fatigue, another subjective complaint, is caused by chronic illnesses at the end of life.

Fatigue factors

Many factors contribute to fatigue, including:
- medications
- chemotherapy and radiation therapy
- stress
- depression
- infection
- inadequate nutrition and hydration.

Ask your patient about feelings of depression, causative factors, aggravating and alleviating factors, and fatigue patterns.

Fatigue busters

Effective pharmacologic interventions include psychostimulants, corticosteroids, antidepressants, and blood products. Other helpful measures include balancing activity and rest, prioritizing activities, exercising on a regular basis (if able), and participating in attention-restoring activities such as playing cards. Your patient and his family should be informed that fatigue levels increase with disease progression and impending death.

Nausea and vomiting

Between 40% and 70% of patients with advanced cancer have reported nausea and vomiting. The symptoms occur more often in women, those younger than age 65, and patients with either breast or stomach cancer.

Here comes that sinking feeling

Assessment of your patient includes:
• asking her to identify aggravating and alleviating factors
• noting the volume, color, consistency, and contents of the vomit
• noting the status of bowel movements
• identifying any treatments used
• reviewing medications for potential emetogenic agents.

Emesis nemesis

Although antiemetics and other types of drugs are the mainstay of therapy, nausea and vomiting can sometimes be controlled with nondrug therapies. Nonpharmacologic interventions include distraction, relaxation, acupuncture, dietary changes, and a celiac plexus block. Offering smaller meals consisting of foods your patient enjoys and sips of water, juice, tea, and ginger drinks may help as well.

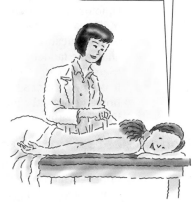

Although drugs are the mainstay in controlling nausea and vomiting, nonpharmacologic interventions, such as relaxation and acupuncture, can help, too.

Pain

Pain is a phenomenon with physical, affective, cognitive, behavioral, sociocultural, spiritual, and environmental components. It's important to remember that pain exists when the patient says it exists.

Assessment arsenal

One of the most common ways to assess pain is by asking your patient to rate his pain intensity on a scale from 0 to 10, with "0" being no pain and "10" being the worst pain possible. Besides rating the pain, include the following descriptions of the pain in your assessment:

- location
- quality
- severity
- duration
- aggravating and alleviating factors
- impact on function and quality of life
- response to current and past treatment
- goals and expectations.

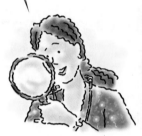

Assessment for pain includes asking the patient directly about pain and looking for nonverbal clues that indicate he's in pain. Oh, and don't forget the physical examination...that can be revealing, too.

Clued to cues

In addition to verbal communication, look for nonverbal messages communicated through gestures, posture, body movements, and facial expressions. During your physical examination, assess the patient's respiratory rate, blood pressure, pulse, and skin color and condition.

Pain-free palliation

Opioids and nonopioids alike are commonly administered to end-of-life patients for pain management. Ask your patient about his pain medication preferences and past experiences, and use the analgesic ladder as a protocol for administering pain medication. (See *The analgesic ladder*.) Long-acting opioids or extended-release medications may be supplemented with short-acting medications for breakthrough pain. Nonopioid medications may be useful in neuropathic pain.

Don't sidestep side effects

When administering morphine, be sure to address the issue of side effects, which include (among others) constipation, respiratory depression, itching, and urinary retention. Teach the patient and his family about all pain medications, including their administration and potential side effects, and provide information about alternative pain control measures, such as massage, heat or cold applications, and distraction.

The analgesic ladder

The World Health Organization uses an analgesic ladder to guide the treatment of pain. If the patient's pain persists or increases, move up the ladder. If it abates, you may be able to move down the ladder.

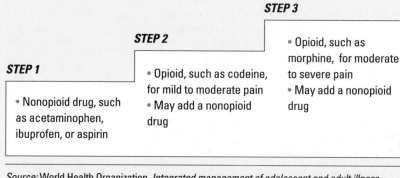

STEP 3
- Opioid, such as morphine, for moderate to severe pain
- May add a nonopioid drug

STEP 2
- Opioid, such as codeine, for mild to moderate pain
- May add a nonopioid drug

STEP 1
- Nonopioid drug, such as acetaminophen, ibuprofen, or aspirin

Source: World Health Organization. *Integrated management of adolescent and adult illness.* Palliative Care, p. 12.

Sleep disturbances

Sleep disturbances in the end-of-life patient may be due to medication side effects, diet, depression, infection, or anxiety. Evaluate these possibilities, and discuss the problem with your patient.

Catching some zzzz's

Pharmacologic options include benzodiazepine hypnotics, non-benzodiazepine hypnotics, antidepressants, and pineal gland hormones. The choice of medication depends on the type of sleep problem your patient experiences. Home remedies include reducing noise, reducing caffeine intake late in the evening, drinking herbal tea or warm milk, and exploring your patient's fears and anxieties that may be contributing to insomnia.

Spiritual distress

Many patients experience spiritual distress as death approaches. This distress may be due to regret of unfulfilled dreams, guilt over a misdeed, or fear of the dying process and death. Other feelings associated with spiritual distress include:
- abandonment
- anger

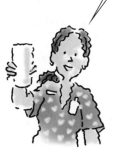

Sleep disturbances in end-of-life patients can stem from several causes. Home remedies include drinking a glass of warm milk.

- betrayal
- despair
- sorrow
- remorse
- depression.

Feel out the family

Family members may also experience spiritual distress during this time. Care of the patient and his family includes listening with empathy, understanding reactions of anger, discussing fears, and connecting with a chaplain or spiritual counselor. For some patients, it's better to talk about meaning in their life, rather than speaking directly about spirituality or religion.

Patient teaching

During the final phase of a terminal illness, you'll need to prepare the patient and his family for what to expect. This includes preparing them not only for the physical aspects of the patient's deteriorating condition but also for the act of dying itself.

> Knowing the correct way to transfer a weak patient is critical for both the patient and your back.

Physical needs

It's important to teach the patient and his family about:
- oral care
- pressure ulcer prevention
- bathing
- contracture prevention.

Active and injury-free

Show the patient and his family how to perform range-of-motion exercises and the correct method of transferring a weak person from a bed to a chair or commode.

Impending death

The patient's family may become anxious as the patient's death approaches. It's especially important to teach family members about the signs and symptoms of impending death and to reassure them that you are making the patient as comfortable as possible. (See *Signs and symptoms of approaching death.*)

Signs and symptoms of approaching death

Teaching your patient's family about the signs and symptoms of impending death can help relieve their anxiety about what to expect. Common signs and symptoms are listed here.

Body system	Signs and symptoms
Respiratory	• Shortness of breath • Cough • Mucus production • Inability to clear secretions
Gastrointestinal	• Nausea and vomiting • Sore mouth • Poor appetite and weight loss • Constipation and diarrhea
Musculoskeletal	• Obvious deterioration • Weakness • Sluggishness, lethargy, lack of energy • Muscle twitching, especially in limbs
Skin	• Irritation or dryness • Pressure areas that appear quickly • Pressure ulcers (possible) • Jaundiced, pale, or gray color • Loose skin from weight loss • Aversion to touch, including blankets
Genitourinary	• Urinary tract infections • Foul smelling, cloudy, or concentrated urine • Bladder spasms • Urine retention • Decreased or no urine production
Cardiac	• Edema of the limbs and sacral area (possible) • Abdominal swelling (possible)
Neuropsychological	• Less engagement in family activities • Less concern with talking or hearing about family news • More focus on personal needs and comfort • Less ability to empathize with others' needs or feelings • Agitation with unclear cause, including picking at covers or clothes (possible)

Permission to leave

It's crucial to explain to the family that hearing is the last sense to leave a dying person. Patients can still hear what's occurring in their surroundings even if they can't communicate. Family members should be encouraged to speak to and touch their loved one during this time. Encourage them to reassure the patient by saying something like "It's okay for you to go...We'll take care of each other when you're gone." A statement like this may allow the patient to release his emotional anxieties and die a more peaceful death.

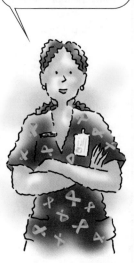

Everyone in the family is affected by the patient's illness and impending death. Be supportive, and make every attempt to address their varied and collective needs.

Social needs

The social needs of a patient and his family can be wide-ranging and warrant a detailed assessment. Focus on supporting the family as a unit as well as on individual members in their varied family roles. When possible, work with a social worker or chaplain to address the family's needs.

Lengthy laundry list

Areas to concentrate on when conducting a social assessment include:
- medical equipment
- nutritional needs
- medications
- finances
- relationships
- other social networks.

Ethical and legal issues

If your patient can make decisions, the decisions he makes should guide his care and the family's level of involvement in his care. If he can no longer make decisions and communicate them, you'll need to rely on advance directives; the patient's previously expressed wishes, values, and preferences; and appropriate surrogate decision makers.

Take the bull by the horns

When possible, urge the patient and his family to finalize their advance directives, wills, guardianship agreements, and other legal documents before the patient becomes unable to express his wishes. (See *Advantages of advance directives*.)

Ethical to the end

If ethical concerns arise, handle them according to the principles of beneficence, self-determination, confidentiality, and informed consent. Keep patient and family care consistent with the nurse's professional code of ethics. Include the hospice or palliative care team in such ethical issues as withholding nutrition and hydration, adopting "do not resuscitate" orders, and giving sedatives.

Bereavement counseling

Grieving over the loss of a loved one, in many cases, begins well before the actual death of the patient. And it isn't limited to family members only. The patient also grieves over his impending death.

Getting a grip on grief

Bereavement counseling for the patient entails:
• maintaining open communication
• assisting the patient in accepting his death
• asking the patient how he wishes to die
• ensuring that the patient's wishes are respected.

A social worker can facilitate patient and family meetings regarding financial concerns, legal issues, and care and support of family members after the patient's death.

> Make sure you remain consistent with the nurse's professional code of ethics and follow the principles of beneficence, self-determination, confidentiality, and informed consent. It never hurts to brush up on your reading.

Grief response

It's important to reassure your patient and his family that grieving is an individual process, without any time or emotional constraints. The patient and his family may experience the five stages of grief—denial, anger, bargaining, depression, and acceptance—or they may not experience these emotions at all, or at least not in the order presented.

Individuals typically manifest their grief physically, cognitively, emotionally, behaviorally, and spiritually. Remain supportive, and encourage all family members to have patience with and try to accept the emotions experienced.

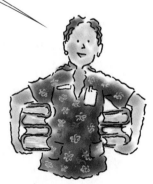

Advantages of advance directives

Advance directives offer several advantages, including:
• peace of mind for the patient that his wishes will be carried out even if he can't communicate
• clear directions for the family and significant others about the patient's wishes
• clear directions for health care providers about the patient's wishes
• prevention of family arguments and increased stress at an emotionally difficult time.

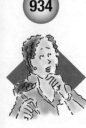

Quick quiz

1.   The focus of a hospice program is:
    A.   returning the patient to his optimal health as soon as possible.
    B.   support and care for patients in the last phase of an incurable disease.
    C.   long-term rehabilitation for patients.
    D.   keeping patients in the hospital as long as needed.

Answer: B. Hospice focuses on support and care for persons in the last phase of an incurable disease so that they may live as fully and comfortably as possible.

2.   The nutritional goal for an end-of-life patient is to:
    A.   promote quality of food over quantity of food.
    B.   eat as much as possible.
    C.   gain 1 pound a week.
    D.   eat three well-balanced meals each day.

Answer: A. The nutritional goal for an end-of-life patient is to enjoy what food he eats. It doesn't matter how much or how little the patient eats.

3.   Step three on the analgesic ladder includes:
    A.   nonopioid drug use alone.
    B.   adding a nonopioid drug to opioids for moderate pain.
    C.   giving opioids, such as morphine, for severe pain.
    D.   using anti-inflammatory drugs alone.

Answer: C. Step three on the analgesic ladder includes using opioids for severe pain. A nonopioid drug may also be added.

4.   Which is *not* a stage of grief?
    A.   Denial
    B.   Bargaining
    C.   Acceptance
    D.   Fear

Answer: D. Fear isn't one of the five stages of grief. The five stages are denial, anger, bargaining, depression, and acceptance.

Scoring

⭐⭐⭐   If you answered four questions correctly, super! You know enough to offer the support that's needed.

⭐⭐   If you answered three questions correctly, you're no slouch. You can still stand on your own.

⭐   If you answered fewer than three questions correctly, sit down, take a deep breath, reread the chapter, and take the quiz again.

Appendices and index

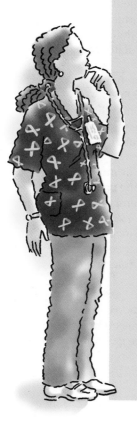

NANDA-I taxonomy II by domain

This list presents the 2009-2011 NANDA International (NANDA-I) taxonomy II according to their domains.

Domain: Health promotion
- Impaired home maintenance
- Ineffective health maintenance
- Ineffective family therapeutic regimen management
- Ineffective self-health management
- Readiness for enhanced immunization status
- Readiness for enhanced nutrition
- Readiness for enhanced self-health management
- Self-neglect

Domain: Nutrition
- Deficient fluid volume
- Excess fluid volume
- Imbalanced nutrition: Less than body requirements
- Imbalanced nutrition: More than body requirements
- Impaired swallowing
- Ineffective infant feeding pattern
- Neonatal jaundice
- Readiness for enhanced fluid balance
- Risk for deficient fluid volume
- Risk for electrolyte imbalance
- Risk for imbalanced fluid volume
- Risk for imbalanced nutrition: More than body requirements
- Risk for impaired liver function
- Risk for unstable blood glucose level

Domain: Elimination and exchange
- Bowel incontinence
- Constipation
- Diarrhea
- Dysfunctional gastrointestinal motility
- Functional urinary incontinence
- Impaired gas exchange
- Impaired urinary elimination
- Overflow urinary incontinence
- Perceived constipation
- Readiness for enhanced urinary elimination
- Reflex urinary incontinence
- Risk for constipation
- Risk for dysfunctional gastrointestinal motility
- Risk for urge urinary incontinence
- Stress urinary incontinence
- Urge urinary incontinence
- Urinary retention

Domain: Activity/Rest
- Activity intolerance
- Bathing self-care deficit
- Decreased cardiac output
- Deficient diversional activity
- Delayed surgical recovery
- Disturbed energy field
- Disturbed sleep pattern
- Dressing self-care deficit
- Dysfunctional ventilatory weaning response
- Fatigue
- Feeding self-care deficit
- Impaired bed mobility
- Impaired physical mobility
- Impaired spontaneous ventilation
- Impaired transfer ability
- Impaired walking
- Impaired wheelchair mobility
- Ineffective breathing pattern
- Ineffective peripheral tissue perfusion
- Insomnia
- Readiness for enhanced self-care
- Readiness for enhanced sleep
- Risk for activity intolerance
- Risk for bleeding
- Risk for decreased cardiac tissue perfusion
- Risk for disuse syndrome
- Risk for ineffective cerebral tissue perfusion
- Risk for ineffective gastrointestinal perfusion
- Risk for ineffective renal perfusion
- Risk for shock

- Sedentary lifestyle
- Sleep deprivation
- Toileting self-care deficit

Domain: Perception/Cognition

- Acute confusion
- Chronic confusion
- Deficient knowledge
- Disturbed sensory perception (specify: visual, auditory, kinesthetic, gustatory, tactile, olfactory)
- Impaired environmental interpretation syndrome
- Impaired memory
- Impaired verbal communication
- Ineffective activity planning
- Readiness for enhanced communication
- Readiness for enhanced decision making
- Readiness for enhanced knowledge
- Risk for acute confusion
- Unilateral neglect
- Wandering

Domain: Self-perception

- Chronic low self-esteem
- Disturbed body image
- Disturbed personal identity
- Hopelessness
- Powerlessness
- Readiness for enhanced power
- Readiness for enhanced self-concept
- Risk for compromised human dignity
- Risk for loneliness
- Risk for powerlessness
- Risk for situational low self-esteem
- Situational low self-esteem

Domain: Role relationships

- Caregiver role strain
- Dysfunctional family processes
- Effective breast feeding
- Impaired parenting
- Impaired social interaction
- Ineffective breast-feeding
- Ineffective role performance
- Interrupted breast-feeding
- Interrupted family processes
- Parental role conflict

- Readiness for enhanced family processes
- Readiness for enhanced parenting
- Readiness for enhanced relationship
- Risk for caregiver role strain
- Risk for impaired attachment
- Risk for impaired parenting

Domain: Sexuality

- Ineffective sexuality pattern
- Readiness for enhanced childbearing process
- Risk for disturbed maternal/fetal dyad
- Sexual dysfunction

Domain: Coping/Stress tolerance

- Anxiety
- Autonomic dysreflexia
- Chronic sorrow
- Complicated grieving
- Compromised family coping
- Death anxiety
- Decreased intracranial adaptive capacity
- Defensive coping
- Disabled family coping
- Disorganized infant behavior
- Fear
- Grieving
- Impaired individual resilience
- Ineffective community coping
- Ineffective coping
- Ineffective denial
- Post-trauma syndrome
- Rape-trauma syndrome
- Readiness for enhanced community coping
- Readiness for enhanced coping
- Readiness for enhanced family coping
- Readiness for enhanced organized infant behavior
- Readiness for enhanced resilience
- Relocation stress syndrome
- Risk for autonomic dysreflexia
- Risk for complicated grieving
- Risk for compromised resilience
- Risk for disorganized infant behavior
- Risk for post-trauma syndrome
- Risk for relocation stress syndrome
- Risk-prone health behavior
- Stress overload

Domain: Life principles

- Decisional conflict
- Impaired religiosity
- Moral distress
- Noncompliance
- Readiness for enhanced hope
- Readiness for enhanced religiosity
- Readiness for enhanced spiritual well-being
- Risk for impaired religiosity
- Risk for spiritual distress
- Spiritual distress

Domain: Safety/Protection

- Contamination
- Hyperthermia
- Hypothermia
- Impaired dentition
- Impaired oral mucous membrane
- Impaired skin integrity
- Impaired tissue integrity
- Ineffective airway clearance
- Ineffective protection
- Ineffective thermoregulation
- Latex allergy response
- Risk for aspiration
- Risk for contamination
- Risk for falls
- Risk for imbalanced body temperature
- Risk for impaired skin integrity

- Risk for infection
- Risk for injury
- Risk for latex allergy response
- Risk for other-directed violence
- Risk for perioperative positioning injury
- Risk for peripheral neurovascular dysfunction
- Risk for poisoning
- Risk for self-directed violence
- Risk for self-mutilation
- Risk for sudden infant death syndrome
- Risk for suffocation
- Risk for suicide
- Risk for trauma
- Risk for vascular trauma
- Self-mutilation

Domain: Comfort

- Acute pain
- Chronic pain
- Impaired comfort
- Nausea
- Readiness for enhanced comfort
- Social isolation

Domain: Growth/Development

- Adult failure to thrive
- Delayed growth and development
- Risk for delayed development
- Risk for disproportionate growth

Glossary

anemia: reduction in the number and volume of red blood cells, the amount of hemoglobin, or the volume of packed red cells

aneurysm: an abnormal dilation of an artery, a vein, or the heart caused by a weakness in the wall

angiography: radiographic visualization of blood vessels after injection of radiopaque contrast material

anorexia: loss of appetite

aphasia: loss or impairment of the ability to communicate through speech, written language, or signs, resulting from brain disease or trauma

apraxia: complete or partial inability to perform purposeful movements in the absence of sensory or motor impairment

ascites: fluid in the peritoneal cavity

ataxia: impairment of the ability to coordinate voluntary muscle movement

aura: sensations that occur before a paroxysmal attack, such as a seizure or migraine headache

auscultation: physical assessment technique by which the examiner listens (usually with a stethoscope) for sounds coming from the heart, lungs, abdomen, or other organs

autoimmune disorder: disorder in which the body launches an immunologic response against itself

bruit: abnormal sound heard over blood vessels on auscultation that indicates turbulent blood flow

cardiac output: volume of blood ejected from the heart per minute

crepitation: a crackling or grating sound heard under the skin, around the lungs, or in the joints

decerebrate posturing: associated with a lesion of the upper brain stem or severe bilateral lesions in the cerebrum; the patient typically lies with legs extended, head retracted, arms adducted and extended, wrists pronated, and the fingers, ankles, and toes flexed

decorticate posturing: associated with a lesion of the frontal lobes, cerebral peduncles, or internal capsule; the patient lies with arms adducted and flexed, wrists and fingers flexed on the chest, legs stiffly extended and internally rotated, and feet plantar flexed

disease: pathologic condition that occurs when the body can't maintain homeostasis

distal: farthest away

dysmenorrhea: painful menstruation

dyspepsia: gastric discomfort, such as fullness, heartburn, bloating, and nausea, that occurs after eating

dysphagia: difficulty swallowing

dysphasia: impairment of speech involving failure to arrange words in their proper order, usually resulting from injury to the speech area in the cerebral cortex

dyspnea: difficult, labored breathing

ecchymosis: bruise

embolism: sudden obstruction of a blood vessel by foreign substances, a blood clot, or plaque traveling through the bloodstream

exacerbation: increase in the severity of a disease

fasciculation: involuntary twitching or contraction of the muscle

Fowler's position: patient positioning with head of bed raised, knees slightly flexed

hematuria: blood in the urine

hemoglobin: iron-containing pigment in red blood cells that carries oxygen from the lungs to the tissues

hemoptysis: expectoration of bloody sputum

hemorrhage: escape of blood from a ruptured vessel

hirsutism: excessive hair growth or unusual distribution of hair

hormone: chemical substance produced in the body that has a specific regulatory effect on the activity of specific cells or organs

hypertension: high blood pressure

hypotension: abnormally low blood pressure

hypoxia: reduction of oxygen in body tissues to below normal levels

idiopathic: disease with no known cause

inspection: critical observation of the patient during which the examiner may use sight, hearing, or smell to make informed observations

insulin: hormone secreted into the blood by the islets of Langerhans of the pancreas; promotes the storage of glucose, among other functions

ischemia: decreased blood supply to a body organ or tissue

jugular vein distention: distended neck veins that may indicate increased central venous pressure

lethargy: slowed responses, sluggish speech, and slowed mental and motor processes in a person oriented to time, place, and person

lichenification: thickening and hardening of the epidermis

lithotomy position: lying on the back with the hips and knees flexed and the thighs abducted and externally rotated

lymphadenopathy: enlargement of the lymph nodes

melena: passage of black, tarry stools

murmur: abnormal sound heard on auscultation of the heart; caused by abnormal blood flow through a valve

necrosis: tissue death

nocturia: excessive urination at night

oliguria: urine output of less than 30 ml/hour

orthopnea: respiratory distress that's relieved by sitting upright

palpation: physical assessment technique by which the examiner uses the sense of touch to feel pulsations and vibrations or to locate body structures and assess their texture, size, consistency, mobility, and tenderness

pathogen: disease-producing agent or microorganism

percussion: physical assessment technique by which the examiner taps on the skin surface with his fingers to assess the size, border, and consistency of internal organs and to detect and evaluate fluid in a body cavity

peristalsis: intestinal contractions, or waves, that propel food toward the stomach and into and through the intestine

petechiae: multiple, small, hemorrhagic areas on the skin

plasma: liquid part of the blood that carries antibodies and nutrients to tissues and carries wastes away from tissues

platelet: disk-shaped structure in blood that plays a crucial role in blood coagulation

polydipsia: excessive thirst

polyphagia: consuming abnormally large amounts of food

polyuria: excessive production of urine

pruritus: severe itching

ptosis: drooping of the eyelid

renal colic: flank pain that radiates to the groin

reverse Trendelenburg's position: lying flat with the head higher than the body or legs

subluxation: partial dislocation of a joint

supine position: lying flat on the back

thrombosis: the development of a thrombus (blood clot)

tophi: clusters of urate crystals surrounded by inflamed tissue; occur in gout

Trendelenburg's position: lying flat with the head lower than the body or legs

vasopressor: drug that stimulates contraction of the muscular tissue of the capillaries and arteries

virus: microscopic, infectious parasite that contains genetic material and needs a host cell to replicate

Selected references

American Cancer Society. (2010). Retrieved November 16, 2010 from http://www.cancer.org/

American Pain Society. (2008). *Principles of analgesic use in the treatment of acute pain and cancer pain* (6th ed.). Glenview, IL: Author.

Bickley, L. (2008). *Bates' guide to physical examination and history taking* (11th ed.). Philadelphia, PA: Lippincott Williams & Wilkins.

Global Initiative for Asthma. (2009). GINA Report, Global strategy for asthma management and prevention. Retrieved November 14, 2010 from http://www.ginasthma.org/Guidelineitem. asp??l1=2&l2=1&intId=1561

Global Initiative for Chronic Obstructive Lung Disease. (2009). Executive summary: Global strategy for the diagnosis, management, and prevention of COPD. Retrieved November 14, 2010 from http://www.goldcopd.com/Guidelineitem. asp?l1=2&l2=1&intId=2180

Ignatavicius, D., & Workman, M. (2009). *Medical-surgical nursing: Patient-centered collaborative care* (6th ed.). St. Louis, MO: Elsevier Saunders.

Kuebler, K., et al. (2006). *Palliative and end-of-life care: Clinical practice guidelines* (2nd ed.). St. Louis, MO: Elsevier Mosby.

Lippincott's nursing procedures (5th ed.). (2008). Philadelphia, PA: Lippincott Williams & Wilkins.

Marquis, B., & Huston, C. (2009). *Leadership roles and management functions in nursing* (6th ed.). Philadelphia, PA: Lippincott Williams & Wilkins.

Melnyk, B., & Fineout-Overholt, E. (2011). *Evidence-based practice in nursing & healthcare: A guide to best practice* (2nd ed.). Philadelphia, PA: Lippincott Williams & Wilkins.

NANDA International (2009). *Nursing diagnoses 2009-2011: Definitions and classification*. West Sussex, United Kingdom: Wiley-Blackwell.

Nettina, S. (2009). *Lippincott manual of nursing practice* (9th ed.). Philadelphia, PA: Lippincott Williams & Wilkins.

Nursing2011 Drug Handbook. (2010). Philadelphia, PA: Lippincott Williams & Wilkins.

Polit, D., & Beck, C. (2007). *Nursing research: Generating and assessing evidence for nursing practice* (8th ed.). Philadelphia, PA: Lippincott Williams & Wilkins.

Porth, C. (2011). *Essentials of pathophysiology: Concepts of altered health states* (3rd ed.). Philadelphia, PA: Lippincott Williams & Wilkins.

Smeltzer, S., et al. (2010). *Brunner & Suddarth's textbook of medical-surgical nursing* (12th ed.). Philadelphia, PA: Lippincott Williams & Wilkins.

Taylor, C., et al. (2010). *Fundamentals of nursing: The art and science of nursing care* (7th ed.). Philadelphia, PA: Lippincott Williams & Wilkins.

Touhy, T., & Jett, K. (2009). *Ebersole and Hess' gerontological nursing & healthy aging* (3rd ed.). St. Louis, MO: Elsevier Mosby.

Woods, S., et al. (2009). *Cardiac nursing* (6th ed.). Philadelphia, PA: Lippincott Williams & Wilkins.

Yarbro, C., et al. (2010). *Cancer nursing: Principles and practice* (7th ed.). Sudbury, MA: Jones & Bartlett.

Index

i refers to an illustration; t refers to a table.

i refers to an illustration; t refers to a table.

i refers to an illustration; t refers to a table.

i refers to an illustration; t refers to a table.

i refers to an illustration; t refers to a table.

i refers to an illustration; t refers to a table.

i refers to an illustration; t refers to a table.

i refers to an illustration; t refers to a table.

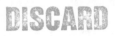

CCS0114